Exercise Therapy
Principles and Practice

Request for Your
Suggestions, Criticism and Ideas

This book is an attempt to bring basic, applied and related knowledge for exercise therapy.

We have done the best we can, given or limitations. We know the book is not perfect and that it has weaknesses and perhaps some mistakes.

We would appreciate any **S**uggestions, **C**riticism and **I**deas you may have for ways that this book might bc improved to serve the patients.

Mail at:

roshan7leo@yahoo.com

Exercise Therapy
Principles and Practice

Roshan L Meena
BPT, MPT (Ortho)
Senior Physiotherapist and Faculty Member
Pt. Deen Dayal Upadhyaya
Institute for the Physically Handicapped
(University of Delhi)
New Delhi, India

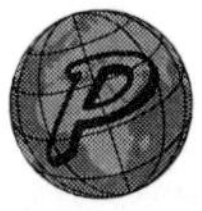

PEEPEE
PUBLISHERS AND DISTRIBUTORS (P) LTD.

Exercise Therapy
Principles and Practice

Published by
Pawaninder P. Vij and Anupam Vij
© Publishing rights with:
Peepee Publishers and Distributors (P) Ltd.
Head Office: 160, Shakti Vihar, Pitam Pura
Delhi-110034 (India)

Correspondence Address: 7/31, First Floor, Ansari Road
Daryaganj, New Delhi-110002 (India)
Ph: 65195868, 23246245, 9811156083
e-mail: peepee160@yahoo.co.in
e-mail: peepee160@rediffmail.com
e-mail: peepee160@gmail.com
www.peepeepub.com

© 2014 by Roshan Lal Meena

This book has been published in good faith that the material provided by authors/ contributors is original. Every effort is made to ensure accuracy of material, but publisher and printer will not be held responsible for any inadvertent errors. In case of any dispute, all legal matters to be settled under Delhi jurisdiction only.

First Edition: **2006**

Second Edition : 2014

ISBN: 978-81-8445-127-6

Printed by : Balaji Offset Printers,

Dedicated to
My parents
my wife and son
for
their appreciation and
encouragement

Foreword

The twin disciplines of physical therapy and occupational therapy are two of the most upcoming health related professions in our country. Exercise therapy is an integral part of treatment in majority of the disabling conditions that physiotherapists and occupational therapists are dealing with in their day-to-day practice.

The present textbook titled *"Exercise Therapy: Principles and Practice"* covers the entire subject of exercise therapy in a very lucid manner. The contents of book succinctly describe the systematic meaning of exercise therapy and its importance in the rehabilitation of person with impairments. Its illustration provides visual image and help in understanding of various methods and concepts of exercise therapy.

This will definitely prove to be one of the most comprehensive presentation of a subject which has so far failed to receive the attention of practising physical therapists and occupational therapists in India.

I have no hesitation in stating that this book will act as a guide book for physical therapists and occupational therapists. They can easily look up to the contents of this book which will help them in selecting the appropriate regimen when faced with different problems requiring exercise therapy.

Dharmendra Kumar
MS (Orthopaedic)
DNB (Physical Medicine and Rehabilitation)

Director, Pt. DUIPH, New Delhi-2
Former Dy. Director (Technical) and Officiating Director
NIRTAR, Cuttack, Orissa

Preface

"Exercise Therapy: Principles and Practice" is divided into Two Parts. Part-I consists two sections. First Section covers the principles and basic concepts of the therapeutic exercises. Second Section covers advanced therapeutic approaches. Part-II covers pathomechanics, assessments, differential diagnosis and therapeutic interventions of different conditions, commonly administered by the therapists in their day-to-day practice.

This book includes all the aspects of exercise therapy which are used by Physical therapists and Occupational therapists in the management of patients with musculoskeletal disorders, neurological disorders, pediatric and geriatric ailments, sports injuries and cardiovascular diseases.

It has been observed that the importance of exercises in the rehabilitation field is decreasing day by day and therapists are relying more on electrotherapy. This book empowers professionals and students by giving them knowledge about various exercises as well as all other related aspects without which comprehensive management through exercise therapy is not possible.

This book is useful for Physical therapists, Occupational therapists, Orthopaedic surgeons, Physiatrists and all other health care professionals concerned with the rehabilitation of persons with physical disability. As this book is written in simple and clear form it is also useful for the students of aforesaid professionals.

Roshan Lal Meena

Acknowledgements

We profusely thank the following individuals who have contributed in so many ways to the production of this book:

- Illustrations — **Gyan Bharti**
  e-mail: *ergomedicine@yahoo.co.uk*
- Photographs — **Kamal N Arya.**
- Models/Subjects — **Patients** of Pt Deen Dayal Upadhaya Institute for the Physically Handicapped, New Delhi.
  Students of Pt DDUIPH, New Delhi.
  Imran, Birendra, Kumar Gulshan, Devesh, Amit Kachap, Vinay, Paritosh, Dharam Raj, Bhaur Singh.
  Others—Mohan Lal, Rajbir, Pradeep, Roshan L Meena.
- Proof Readers — **Rajni Kalra**—Superintendent Physiotherapist Pt DDUIPH, New Delhi.
  Prachi Raj Meena—Sr. Physiotherapist, Pt Deen Dayal Upadhaya Institute for the Physically Handicapped, New Delhi.
  AMR Suresh Kumar—Sr. Physiotherapist Pt Deen Dayal Upadhaya Institute for the Physically Handicapped, New Delhi.
  Gyan Bharti—Sr. Occupational Therapist and Director, Institute for Rehabilitation and Community Health, New Delhi.
  Ruchi Nagar—Lecturer (Occupational therapy), Jamia Hamdard, New Delhi.
  Shikha Lohia—Visiting Lecturer (Occupational therapy), Jamia Hamdard, New Delhi.
  Suchi Zindal—Physiotherapist, Akshay Pratisthan, New Delhi.
- Other support — **Gunjan**—Occupational Therapist St. Stephen's Hospital, Delhi.
- Publication — **M/s Peepee Publishers and Distributors (P) Ltd.**
  Pawaninder P Vij and Anupam Vij—Directors.
  S.K. Sharma—Editor.
  Rajesh Negi—DTP Operator.
  Pawan Sharma—Graphics Designer.

We would like to extend our sincere thanks to Director, Pt Deen Dayal Upadhaya Institute for the Physically Handicapped, New Delhi for allowing us to write this book.

Contents

PART - I

Section-I
Basic Concepts

1. Introduction to Exercise Therapy ----- 5

2. Simple and Applied Biomechanics ----- 11

3. Active and Passive Movements ----- 16

4. Basic and Derived Positions for Exercise Therapy ----- 38

5. Posture, Human Locomotion and Walking Aids ----- 47

6. Manual Muscle Strength Testing (MMST) and Goniometry ----- 93

Section-II
Therapeutic Approaches

7. Mobilization of Peripheral Joint ----- 105

8. Breathing Exercises ----- 131

9. Therapeutic Massage (Soft Tissue Manipulation) ----- 135

10. Suspension Therapy ----- 157

11. Hydrotherapy ----- 164

12. Relaxation ----- 172

13. Stretching Techniques of Soft Tissue Structures ----- 178

14. Proprioceptive Neuromuscular Facilitation (PNF) ----- 198

15. Mat Activities ----- 214

16. Group Exercises -- 219

17. Balance and Coordination Exercise ----------------------------------- 221

18. Disability, Function and Activities of Daily Living (ADL) ------------ 245

19. Therapeutic Approaches in Neurological Conditions ------------------- 254

20. Therapeutic Approaches in Orthopaedic Conditions -------------------- 271

21. Yoga and Asanas -- 283

PART - II

22. Orthopedic Assessment -- 293

23. Soft Tissue Injuries --- 304

24. Arthritis -- 328

25. Shoulder Injuries -- 366

26. Cervical Spine --- 412

27. Low Back Pain -- 462

28. Sacroiliac Joint Pain -- 518

PART - ONE

Basic Concepts

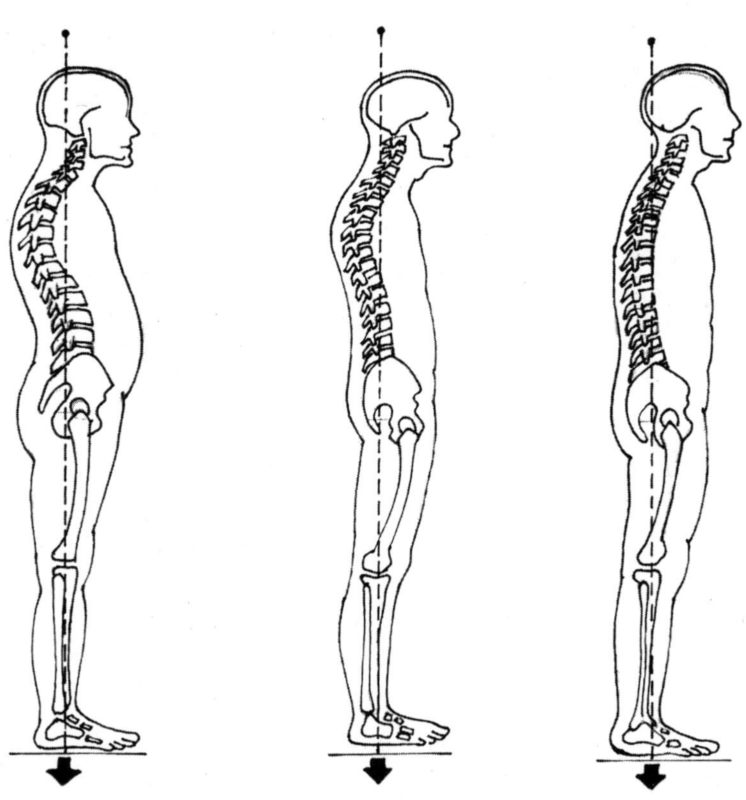

CHAPTER-1

Introduction to Exercise Therapy

INTRODUCTION

Before discussing the field of exercise therapy, the concept of exercise must first be defined and explained. When we contract skeletal muscles to cause movement, or maintain a given posture, it is generally explained that we are being active. This is in contrast to being inactive, where we are not voluntarily contracting our skeletal muscles.

The Webster's dictionary provides three important definitions of exercise:

i. "Regular or repeated use of a faculty or body organ."
ii. Bodily exertion for the sake of developing and maintaining physical fitness.
iii. Something performed or practised in order to develop, improve, or display a specific power or skill.

The term exercise therefore can be used to denote activity that is performed for the purpose of improving, or expressing a particular type of physical fitness.

The organised and purposeful implication of exercise that separates it from activity is a complication, when going to market to get vegetables, we are being active, simply we are performing this act for a task rather than for physical fitness means that it does not suit the previous definition of exercise. Similarly, when workers lift object or force to exert themselves with repeated periods of muscular contraction (e.g., Labourers, farmers, construction workers, hawkers), they are active yet once again are not exercising. This definitional inadequacy of exercise has caused the term physical activity to be more widely used. Physical activity pertains to the activity performed by the body for purpose other than the specific development of physical fitness. Research has shown that physical fitness is improved from regular physical activity, just as it is from exercise. Thus individuals who are physically active in general lifestyle and vocation can be physically fit without (necessarily completing what we know to be exercised) exercise.

Exercise–Activity that is performed for the purpose of improving maintaining or expressing a particular type of physical fitness.

Physical activity–The activity performed by the body for purpose other than the specific development of physical fitness.

Physical fitness–A state of bodily function that is characterized by the ability to tolerate exercise stress. Exercise training the repeated use of exercise to improve physical fitness.

Exercise therapy–Is the systematic and planned performance of bodily movement postures or physical activities intended to provide a patient or client with means to:
- Remediate or prevent impairment.
- Improve, restore or enhance physical function.
- Prevent or reduce health-related risk factors.
- Optimise overall health status fitness or sense of well-being.

Therapeutic exercise programs designed by therapist are individualized to the unique needs of each patient or client. A patient is an individual with impairment and functional limitations diagnosed by a therapist, receiving therapeutic care to improve functions and prevent disability.

A client is an individual without diagnosed dysfunction who is engaged in therapeutic services to promote health and wellness to prevent dysfunction.

EFFECTS OF THERAPEUTIC EXERCISES

Every normal muscular contraction affects not only the musculoskeletal system but also neuromuscular and cardiopulmonary system of human body. These systems respond according to the force and stress created by such contractions. An external and constant force i.e. gravity also affects these systems. These forces and stresses altogether are essential for normalcy of the body and its system. When these forces and stresses decrease or increase than the normal requirement, bodily dysfunction occur in the form of osteoporosis, muscle atrophy, deformity, pain and poor cardiopulmonary fitness etc.

Therapeutic exercises are not only controlled, progressive and planned but are also as per the capability of the patient resulting into the improvement of their functional ability.

Therapeutic exercise affects the development, improvement and maintenance of normalcy.

The goals of exercise therapy:

To improve or maintain the following:

- Muscular strength.
- Muscular power.
- Muscular endurance.
- Cardio-respiratory endurance.
- Joint mobility.
- Joint flexibility.
- Agility.
- Body and mental relaxation
- Coordination.
- Motor control.
- Balance.

TYPES OF MUSCULAR CONTRACTION/ACTION

Traditionally the word contraction has been used to describe different muscle actions, i.e. isometric, isotonic, concentric and eccentric contraction.

Recently a suggestion has been made to replace the word contraction with the term action. The proposed change in terminology was made on the base that the term "contraction" (which means drawing together) does not adequately or accurately reflect what happens to the entire muscle during activity and is contradictory when used to describe eccentric muscle activity, that is lengthening contraction.

Isotonic (iso = equal, tonic = muscle tone, the tone of muscle remains same throughout the contraction of muscle).

This is the contraction in which the intramuscular tension or tone remains same/constant as the muscle shortens or lengthens. The intramuscular tension is accompanied by a change in the length of the muscle.

The use of the term isotonic "contraction" is not used by some authors, because it refers to equal or constant tension which is unphysiological. The tension generated in a muscle cannot be controlled or kept constant.

Isometric (iso = equal, metric = length, the length of muscle remains same throughout the contraction of muscle)

When both the distal and proximal attachments of a muscle are fixed and the torque produced by a muscle is equal to the torque of the resistance the visible muscle length will remain unchanged, although shortening occurs at the myofibrils level. When there is no noticeable change in the length of muscle that is developing tension the muscular action is called an isometric contraction. No mechanical work is performed in an isometric contraction because work is equivalent to the product of $F \times d$ (F = force, d = distance). There is no distance involved in an isometric contraction because both bony components are fixed and do not move during the contraction. However energy is being expended to produce cross-bridge cycling.

Static

The muscle remains in partial or complete contraction without changing its length. These are two different conditions under which this type of contraction is likely to occur:

1. Muscles which are antagonistic to each other contract with equal strength, thus balancing or counteracting each other (co-contraction of the agonist and the antagonist). The part affected is held tensly in place without moving. Tensing the Biceps to show off its bulge is an example of this. The contraction of the triceps prevents the elbow from further flexing.

2. A muscle is held in either partial or maximal contraction against another force such as the pull of gravity or an external mechanical or muscular force. Example of this are holding a book at stretched hand, a tug of war between two equally matched opponents and attempting to move an object which is too heavy to move.

Concentric-Toward the Centre

The muscles contract isotonically in shortening to produce movement.

The attachments of the muscles are drawn closer together and movement is in the direction of the muscle pull (Fig. 1.1).

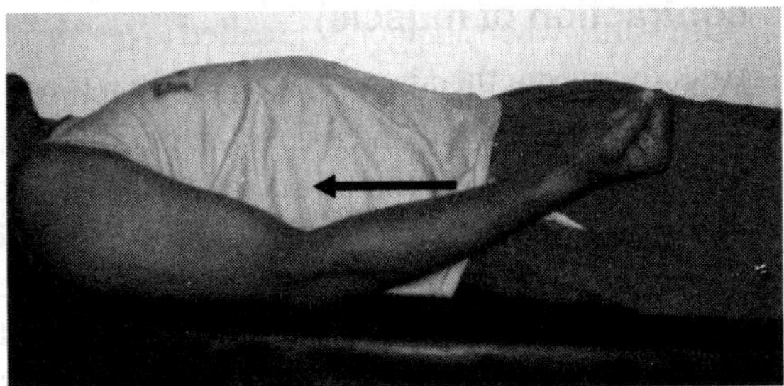

Fig. 1.1: Concentric contraction of elbow flexors

Usually during functional activities, one attachment of a bone is stabilized and the other attachment is free to move. If the proximal attachment is fixed and the distal attachment is free (as in an open kinematic chain) the muscle action will pull the distal bony component toward the proximal component. If the distal component is fixed and proximal bony component is free (in a closed kinematic chain), reverse action will occur and the proximal bony component will be pulled toward the distal bony component.

Positive muscular work is done during concentric exercise because when a concentric contraction occurs the muscular moment acts in the same direction as the angular velocity of the joint and by convention both are considered to be positive.

Eccentric-Away from the Centre

When a force that a muscle generates is insufficient to offset an opposing force on a lever, the muscle will undergo a lengthening or eccentric contraction. In this type of contraction the muscle acts as a brake and controls the movement of a bony component (Fig. 1.2).

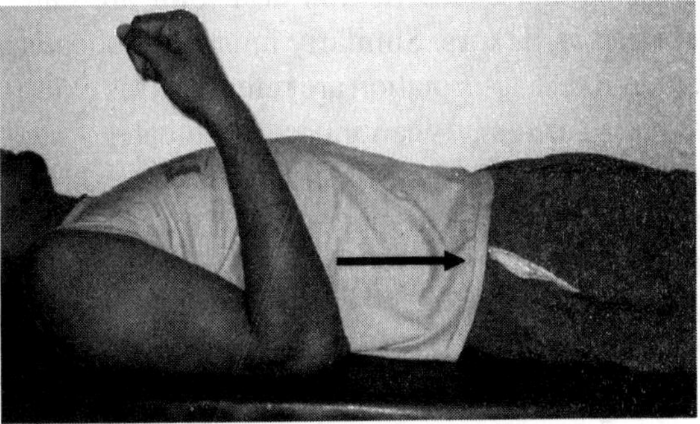

Fig. 1.2: Eccentric contraction of elbow flexors

When the hand holding a glass moves from the face to the table the flexor muscle of the elbow undergo a lengthening or eccentric contraction as they control the gravity-produced descent of the hand. In this activity the two ends of the muscle moves apart or away from each other. The muscle acts as the resistance to the gravitational effect and a second class lever is formed. Eccentric muscle action like concentric muscle action can occur as motion of either the distal or proximal bony lever or normal and reverse actions, respectively. The mechanical work that is done by a muscle during an eccentric contraction is called negative work because work is done on the muscle rather than by the muscle. The energy cost of an eccentric contraction is considerably less than that of a concentric contraction when equal loads are used.

The Group Muscle Action

Under normal circumstances a smooth purposeful desired movement cannot be produced by a single muscle action. To produce such type of efficient movement, and maintain the stability of the joint during movement integrated activity of many/ several muscles is required. This is known as group muscle action.

Group of muscles are categorized on the basis of either the action they perform or the particular role they serve during specific action. When muscles are categorized on the basis of action, muscles that cause flexion at a joint are categorized as flexors. Similarly muscles that cause either extension/rotation are referred to as extensors or rotators. When muscles are categorized according to role individual muscles or group of muscles are described in terms of that demonstrate the specific role that the muscle plays during action.

Functionally muscles work together in groups, although each muscle may have some specific part to play in relation to the action of the whole group.

For example determining the precise direction of the movement or by maintaining its progress in a particular part of the range.

Movers

Mover is a muscle which is directly responsible for producing a movement. In the majority of movements there are several movers some of them have greater importance than others.

Principal Movers

When a movement is performed by several muscles, some of them have greater importance than other. These are known as prime or principal movers.

For example Dorsiflexors of ankle joint are– tibialis-anterior, extensor hallucis longus, extensor digitorum longus. But principal mover is tibialis anterior.

Assistant Movers

The muscles which help to perform the movement but which seem to be less important, or which contract only under certain circumstances are assistant movers.

Emergency Muscles

Muscles which help only when an extra amount of force is needed, as when a movement is performed against resistance are sometimes called emergency muscles.

Agonist and Antagonists

Agonist is used to designate a muscle that is responsible for producing a desired motion at a joint. If flexion is the desired action, the flexor muscles are the agonists and extensors that are working directly opposite to the desired motion are called the *antagonists*. The desired motion may not be opposed by antagonists but these muscles have the potential to oppose the action.

Ordinarily when antagonist is called to perform a desired motion, the agonist is inhibited (reciprocal inhibition) if however, the agonist and potential antagonist contract simultaneously, then *co-contraction* occurs. Co-contraction of muscles around a joint can help to provide stability for the joint and represents a joint synergy that may be necessary in certain situations. Co-contraction of muscles with opposing function can be undesirable when a desired motion is prevented by involuntary co-contraction such as occurs in disorders affecting the control of muscle function.

Synergists

Muscles that help the agonist to perform desired action are called *synergists*.

For example, if flexion of the wrist is the desired movement/action, the flexor carpi radialis and flexor carpi ulnaris would be referred to as the "agonists" or "prime movers" because these muscles produce flexion. The wrist extensors would be the potential antagonists. The synergists that might directly help the wrist flexors would be the finger flexors.

Synergists may assist the agonist directly by helping to produce the desired movement such as in the wrist flexion, or indirectly either by stabilizing a part or by preventing an undesired action.

True synergists act, *for example* when using the long finger flexors as agonists to grip an object in the hand. The unwanted action of these muscles in flexing the wrist nccds to be controlled or opposed. This is done by the simultaneous contraction of the wrist extensors acting as true synergists.

Helping synergists act simultaneously. Flexor carpi radialis and extensor carpi radials longus are usually antagonistic to each other in producing wrist flexion and extension, respectively. However, they can act simultaneously as helping synergists to produce radial deviation at the wrist.

Neutralizer is a muscle which acts to prevent an undesired action of one of the movers. Thus if a muscle both flexes and abducts, but only flexion is desired in the movement, an adductor contracts to neutralize the abductor actions of the mover.

Mutual Neutralizers: Occasionally two of the movers have one action in common but can also perform second action which are antagonistic to each other. For instance one muscle may upward rotate and adduct while the other may downward rotate and adduct. When they contract together to cause adduction, their rotatory function counter act each other. Muscles which behave this way in a movement are mutual stabilizers as well as movers.

Stabilizers or fixators are muscles which contract to control the position of a bone so that it may act as a steady base from which the agonist can act. They thus provide a fixed attachment for another muscle.

For example, during elbow flexion the shoulder girdle muscles act as fixators to control the position of the arm.

RANGE OF MUSCLE WORK

The range of muscle work is the extent of the muscular contraction which result in joint movement.

The excursion of muscle, i.e. the amount of shortening or lengthening possible during contraction, is estimated to be about 50% of the muscles maximum extended length. The maximum excursion possible is called the full range of muscle work and any excursion which falls short of this is called inner, outer or middle range to specify the particular part of the range in which movement takes place (Fig. 1.3).

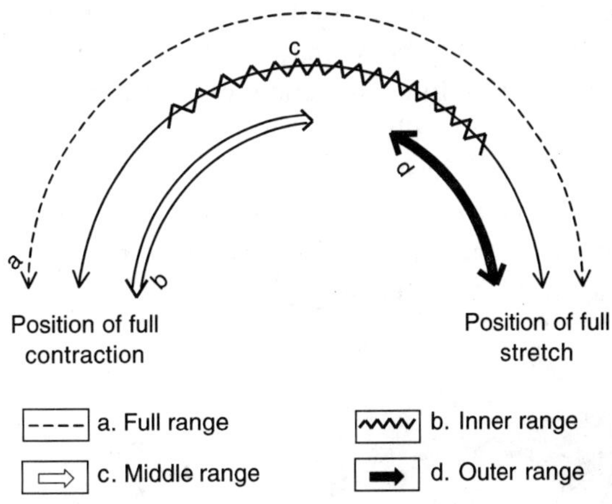

Fig. 1.3: Range of muscle work

Full Range

The joint is moved as the muscles work concentrically from the position in which they are fully stretched to the fully contracted, or concentrically, or from the position of the fully contracted to the fully stretched (Fig. 1.4).

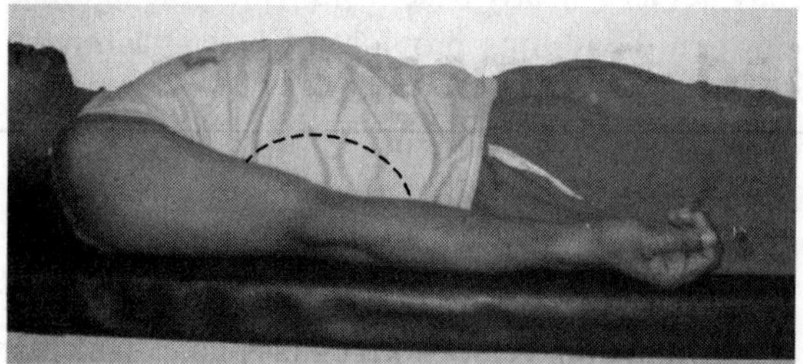

Fig. 1.4: Range of muscle work (full range) of elbow flexors

Under ordinary circumstances muscles are rarely required to work in full range, but in emergencies they may have to do so. Active full range of exercises are used for patients as they maintain its mobility, increase the circulation and ensure that the emergency reserve of powers and mobility is preserved.

Inner Range

The muscle works either concentrically from a position in which it is partially contracted (approximately half-way between the limit of full range) to position of full contraction, or vice versa if it works eccentrically (Fig. 1.5).

Exercises in inner range is used to gain or maintain movement of a joint in the direction of the muscle pull, and to train some extensor muscles responsible for stabilising joints.

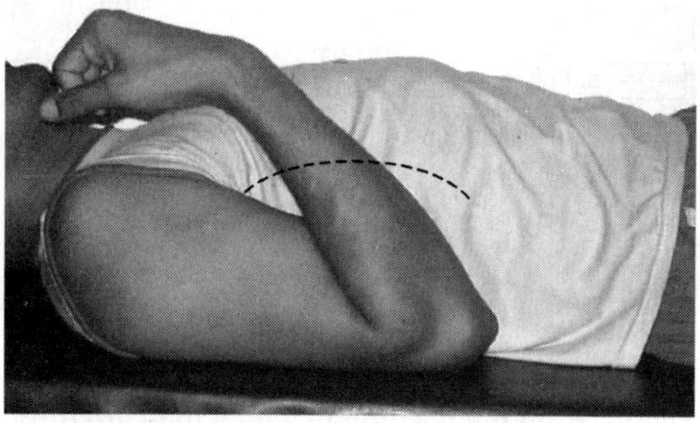

Fig. 1.5: Inner range of elbow flexors

Middle Range

The muscles are usually neither fully stretched nor fully contracted, this is the range in which muscles are most often used in everyday life. Generally speaking, they are most efficient in this range (Fig. 1.6).

Exercises in this range maintain muscle tone and muscle power.

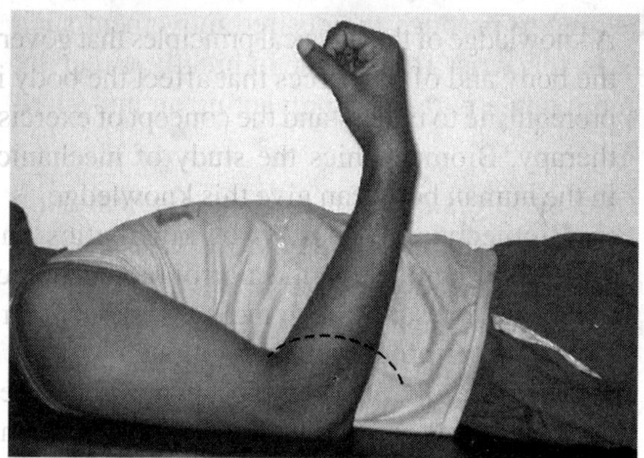

Fig. 1.6: Middle range of elbow flexors

Outer Range

The muscles work concentrically from the position in which they are fully stretched to a position in which they are partially (held) contracted, or vice versa if working eccentrically.

The outer range work is used extensively in muscle re-adduction as a contraction is initiated more easily from stretched position in most muscles (Fig. 1.7).

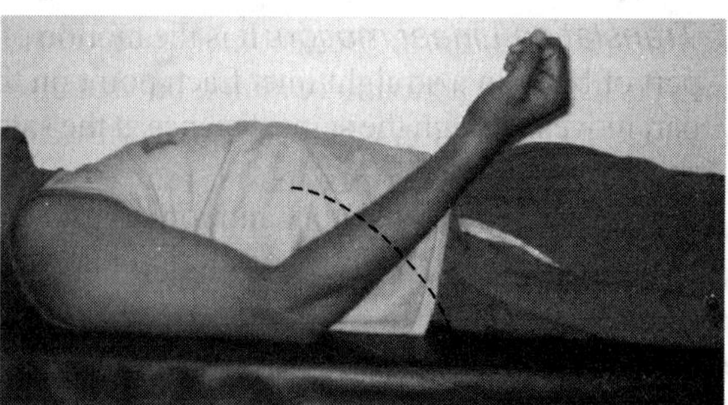

Fig. 1.7: Outer range of elbow flexors

CHAPTER-2

Simple and Applied Biomechanics

INTRODUCTION

A knowledge of the physical principles that govern the body and of the forces that affect the body is prerequisite to understand the concept of exercise therapy. Biomechanics the study of mechanics in the human body can give this knowledge.

Biomechanics consists of kinematics and kinetics. Kinematics is the area of biomechanics that include description of motion without regard for the forces producing the motion.

Kinetics is the area of biomechanics concerned with the forces producing motion or maintaining equilibrium.

Kinematics consists of:
- Type of motion.
- Location of motion
- Direction and magnitude.

Type of Motion

Angular or rotatory motion: It is the movement of a part of body around a fixed axis in a curved path. Each point on the part moves through the same angle at the same time at a constant distance from the axis of rotation.

Translation/Linear motion: It is the motion of a part of body in a straight line. Each point on the part moves through the same distance at the same time in parallel paths.

Angular and translatory motion combine to produce the third path way of motion known as *curvilinear motion.*

Location of Motion

Consists of various planes and axis.

The universal x-coordinate corresponds to the cardinal transverse (horizontal) plane. This plane divides the body into upper and lower halves. Movement in this plane occur parallel to the ground. For e.g. Neck rotation. Rotating movement occur around a vertical or longitudinal axis of motion. The term longitudinal axis is used when the axis of motion passes through the length of a long bone. (The axis of movement is always found prependicular to its corresponding plane).

The Y–coordinate corresponds to the frontal (coronal) plane. The frontal plane divides the body into front and back halves, for example neck lateral flexion in this movements occurs around an anterior posterior or AP axis.

The Z–coordinate corresponds to the sagittal plane and divides the body into right and left halves. For e.g. forward flexion and backward extension of neck. In this plane movement occur around coronal or mediolateral axis.

Direction and Magnitude

Direction is basically the movement in terms Flexion/Extension, Abduction/Adduction and rotations (Internal/External).

While magnitude is the measure of movement in degrees or radians.

Kinetics

It is the study of forces which can make body or its part to move or at rest.

External forces—Come from outside the body, gravity is one of the important external force which greatly influence human body position and motion.

Internal forces—Come from within the body. Muscles are the structures which provide such forces.

Centre of gravity—While gravity acts at all points or segment of an object, its point of application is given as the gravity (COG).

It is a hypothetical point at which all mass would appear to be concentrated and is the point at which the force of gravity would appear to act.

The action line and direction of the force of gravity on an object are always vertical downward toward the center of the earth regardless of the orientation in space of the object.

The gravity vector is commonly referred to as the line of gravity (LOG).

COG of the Human Body

When all the segments of the body are combined and the body is taken as a single solid object in anatomic position, the COG of the body lies approximately anterior to the second sacral vertebrae.

Also each segment in the body is acted on by the force of gravity and has its own COG.

Stability and COG

For an object to be stable the COG must fall with in the base support, when the COG falls outside the base of support, the object will tend to fall.

Other factors which affect stability:

i. The larger the base of support of an object, the greater the stability of that object.

ii. The closer the COG is to the base of support, the more stable is the object.

For e.g.: In cricket wicket keeper widely opens his legs (larger base of support) and flexes his knees (COG closer to base of support).

Newton's Laws of Motion

These laws are also applicable to human motion and therefore their concept should be reviewed to understand exercise therapy.

First Law—States that an object will remain at rest or in uniform motion unless acted upon by an unbalanced force.

Inertia is the property of an object that makes the object resist both initiation of motion and a change in motion.

Second Law—States that the acceleration of an object is proportional to the unbalanced forces acting on it and inversely proportional to the mass of that object

$$a = F/m$$

(a-acceleration, F-force, m-mass)

i.e. the greater the force more will be acceleration and on contrary greater the mass lesser will be accleration.

Third Law—States that for every action there is an equal and opposite reaction.

Pulleys

Pulleys are frequently used in exercise and traction equipment to change the direction of a force or to increase or decrease the magnitude of a force.

Anatomic Pulley–Muscles or muscle tendons are found to be wrapped or deflected by bony prominences or sesamoid bone like patella.

When the direction of pull of a muscle is altered the bone or bony prominences causing the deflection form an anatomical pulley. Pulley changes the direction.

Example: The tendon of the quadriceps not only changes its direction of pull as a result of the interposed patella but its leverage also improves.

They are commonly used in two forms.

1. Single fixed pulley
2. Movable pulley

Single Fixed Pulley–The line of action of force may be changed by means of a pulley such pulley does not provide any mechanical advantage to the force, but only changes its direction (Fig. 2.1).

Example–cervical traction.

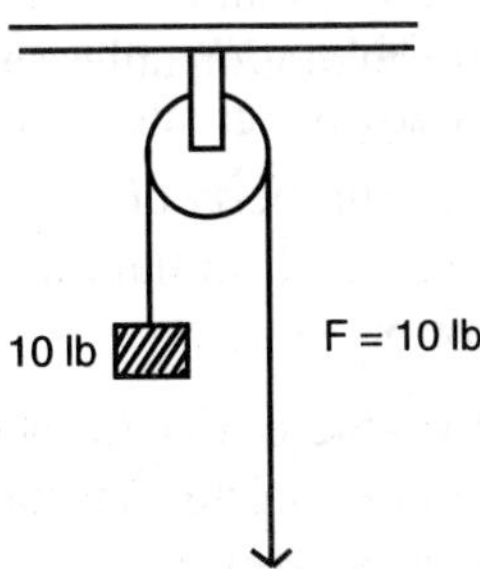

Fig. 2.1: Fixed pulley (example-cervical traction)

Movable Pulley—If a weight is attached to a movable pulley, half of the weight is supported by the rope attached to stationary hook and half by the rope on the other side of the pulley. Therefore the mechanical advantage of the force F is 2. The rope however, must be moved twice the distance that the weight is raised, and what is gained in force is lost in distance (Fig. 2.2).

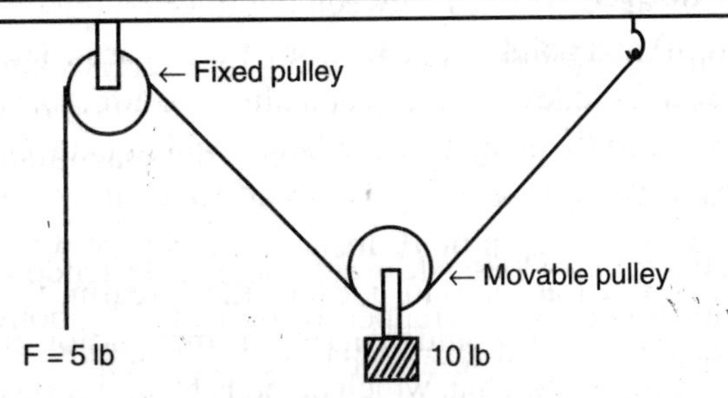

Fig. 2.2: Movable pulley (example–Leg traction, russal traction)

LEVERS

A lever is a simple machine that magnifies force and speed of the movement, and commonly defined as rigid bar that rotates about a fixed point, the fulcrum. In biomechanics the principles of the lever are used to visualise the more complex system of forces that produce rotatory motion in the body. In the human body levers are primarily the bones and axis (fulcrum) are the joints where bones meet.

Elements of lever—There are three elements of the lever (Fig. 2.3):

a. The fulcrum (F)—It is represented by the joint or is a point on the axis about which the rigid mass rotates.

b. The effort arm (EA)—Effort (E) is the point where contracting muscle is attached to the moving bone. EA includes all parts of the rigid mass between the fulcrum and the point at which energy is applied to the rigid bar.

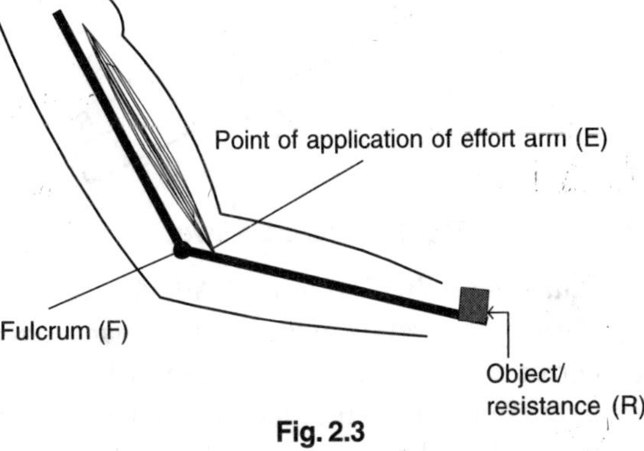

Fig. 2.3

c. The resistance arm (RA)—Resistance (R) is the point where object is held . RA includes all parts of the rigid mass between the fulcrum and the point at which energy is applied to the object to be moved by the lever .

These three elements may be found in any arrangement and any one of the three may be between the other two.

Classification of levers—Basically three types of levers are found in the body and are classified on the basis of arrangement of the three elements i.e. Fulcrum (F), point of application of effort (E) and point of application of resistance (R).

• If the fulcrum is in the between point of application of effort (E) and point of application of resistance (R) or EFR it is termed as first class lever.

- If the point of application of effort is between fulcrum and point of application of resistance or FER it is termed as second class lever.
- If the point of application of resistance is between fulcrum and point of application of effort or FRE it is termed as third class lever.

First Class Lever

As the figure 2.4 shows that the fulcrum lies between two resultant forces one applied on either side. In description of body levers the EFR will not be exactly located.

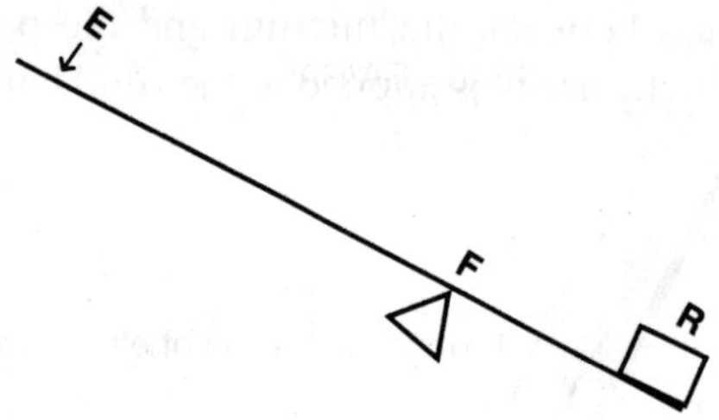

Fig. 2.4: First class lever

Examples of Ist class lever— Atlanto occipital joint where the weight of the head is balanced by posterior neck muscle force. Similarly at the intervertebral joints where the weight of the trunk is balanced by the erector spinal muscle forces. The first class lever is also seen during extension of elbow (Fig. 2.5).

The first class lever are used for maintaining postures and balance.

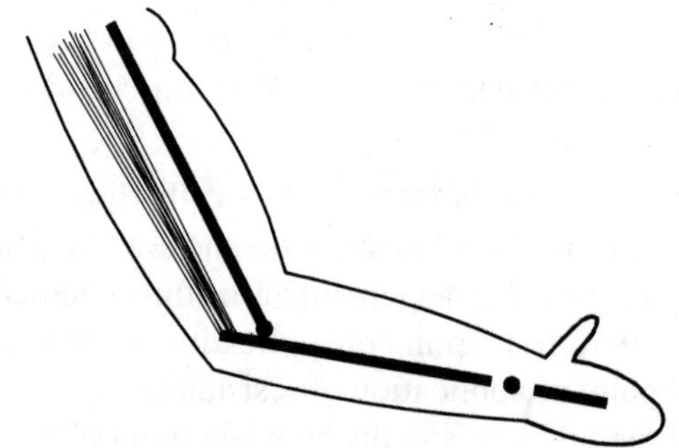

Fig. 2.5: Example of first class lever. The fulcrum (F) lies between the point of application of resistance (R) and effort (Triceps), or EFR

Second Class Lever

In the second class the resistance arm lies between the fulcrum and effort arm (FRE) or whenever two parallel forces are applied at some distance from the fulcrum or axis (F) with the resistance arm closer to the fulcrum. In a second class lever effort arm is always greater than the resistance arm.

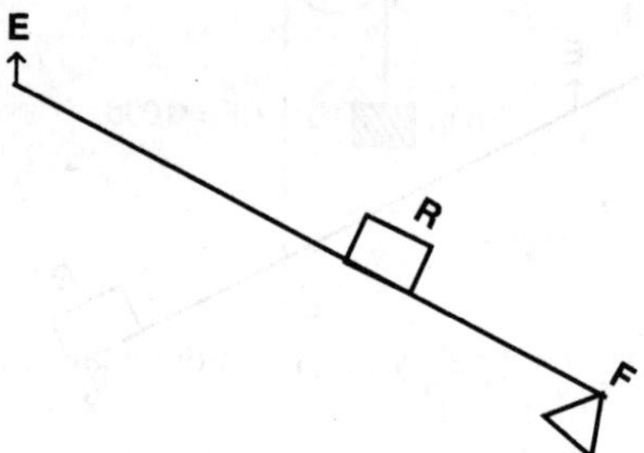

Fig. 2.6: Second class lever

In the human body there are limited examples of the second class lever. It commonly occurs when gravity is the effort force and muscles are the resistance. The only muscle example is the pull of the brachioradialis and wrist extensors to maintain the position of elbow joint, therefore the resistance arm lies between the fulcrum (elbow joint) and point of application of effort arm. The lever includes the radius and ulna; the effort arm includes the length of the bones which extends from the axis to the point of attachment of the muscle, a length of 10 inches. If a weight were suspended at the mid point of the forearm, the resistance arm would then include that portion of the radius and ulna, which extends from the axis to the weight a distance of 5 inches. However this system changes to a third class lever if any heavy object is held in the hand. This example of lever is because in case of paralysis of the biceps brachii and brachialis, patient can use the brachio-radialis and wrist extensors to hold the elbow in a flexion position. Normally however, brachio-radialis and wrist extensors do not act in this isolated manner.

There are no apparent examples of second class lever in the body.

Third Class Lever

It is the most common lever formed in the body. The effort arm lies between the fulcrum and resistance (Fig. 2.7).

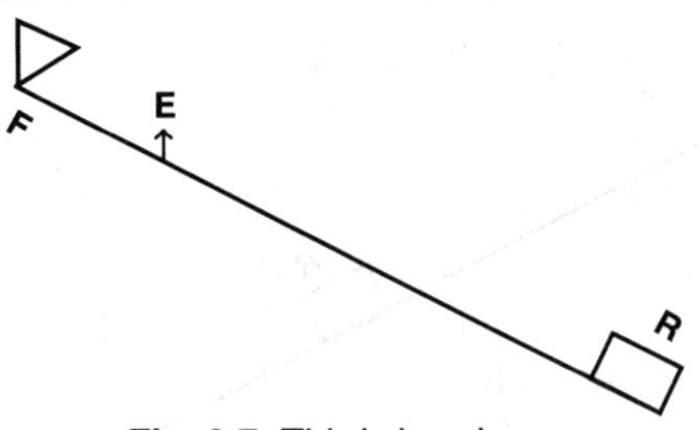

Fig. 2.7: Third class lever

The point of application of effort is always closer to the fulcrum therefore effort arm is smaller and resistance arm is larger and mechanical advantage may be 0.1 or even low. This arrangement is designed for producing speed of the distal segment or for moving a small weight a long distance (Fig. 2.8).

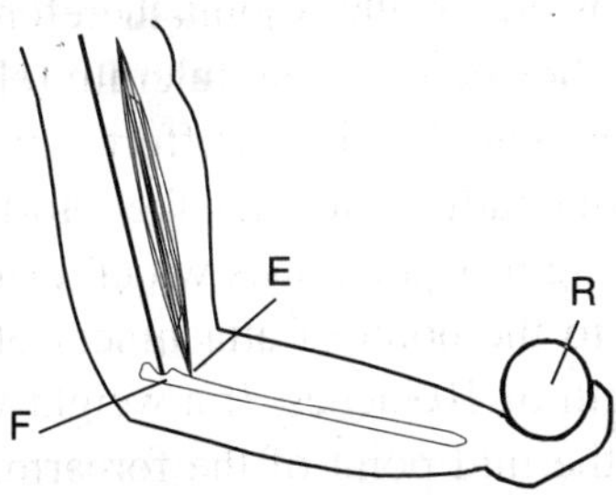

Fig. 2.8: Example of third class lever, the point of application of effort (E) is located between fulerum (F) and resistance (R), (or FER) therefore it forms the third class lever

Example—Forces on the forearm. The fulcrum will be a point on the axis and in the joint. The point of application of effort is at point where the brachialis attaches to the bone and the effort arm is between the fulcrum and point where the brachialis attaches to the bone which may be approximately 1 inch in length.

The resistance is the object held in the hand and the resistance arm extends from fulcrum (F) to the object or the resistance arm includes the total length of the radius and ulna, the wrist and metacarpal and the portion of the proximal phalanges, approximately 16 inches in length.

Mostly third class lever is common in open chain motions of the activities.

Mechanical Advantage of Lever

Is a measure of the efficiency of the lever. It is the ratio of the effort arm to the resistance arm or

$$MAd = EA/RA$$

MAd : Mechanical Advantage
EA : Effort Arm
RA : Resistance Arm

Whenever mechanical advantage is greater than one, the magnitude of the effort force can be smaller than the magnitude of resistance. That is, a small effort can create more torque and overcome a large resistance.

– In all second class lever, the mechanical advantages of the lever will always be greater than one as effort arm is larger than resistance arm (EA > RA)
– In all third class lever mech. advantage will always be less then one. Hence more effort force is required to overcome resistance force. (as RA > EA)
– Ist class lever follows no rules relative to mech advantage. EA can be greater than, less than, or equal to RA.

Use of Levers in Exercise Therapy

By learning the concepts of various types of lever these principles can be applied in almost all aspects of therapy.

To make exercises more resistive long lever arm can be selected. Contrary in the beginning short lever arm is preferred.

These concepts are also be used in gait training with crutches, canes etc.

CHAPTER-3

Active and Passive Movements

ACTIVE MOVEMENTS/EXERCISES

INTRODUCTION

Movement which is performed by the patient on his own efforts with little or without external support.

Classification of Active Movements/ Exercises

- Active free movement/exercise.
- Active assisted movement/exercise.
- Active assisted and resisted movement/ exercise.
- Active resisted movement/exercise.

Free Exercises

Free exercises are those exercises which are performed by the patient's voluntary muscular effort in the absence of any assistance or resistance of external force except gravity.

Effects of Free Exercises

- Relaxation
- Maintenance of muscle tone
- Improving strength and power (depends upon speed, leverage and duration of the exercise).
- Improving co-ordination maintaining flexibility and mobility.

Advantage: after learning the concept of the exercise patient can perform and practice it of his own.

Disadvantage:

- Neurologically affected patients who have poor voluntary control cannot perform it.
- Weak muscles can be strengthened upto certain extent only.

Classification of Free Exercises

Free exercise can be classified on the basis of the extent of the area involved into localized and generalized forms.

Localized free exercises: are those which are to mobilize a particular joint or to strengthen a particular muscle/muscle group. e.g. Active movements of shoulder joint; pendular movement of shoulder.

Generalized free exercises: are those which involve the use of many joints and muscles all over the body and the effect is generalized as in running, jogging, cycling etc.

Free exercise can also be classified on the basis of character of a particular exercise. They may be subjective or objective free exercises.

Subjective free exercises: are usually formal and consist of more or less anatomical movements performed in full range, the emphasis is on form and pattern of the exercise.

Objective free exercises: are those in which patient's aim is to achieve a particular goal during performance. e.g. to reach a point marked on the wall, here goal is a stimulating factor for the performance. But care should be taken to maintain the accuracy of movement, it should not be compromised in an effort to reach for the goal.

Indications and Uses of Free Exercises

The indication and use of any particular free exercise depend on the nature of exercise, its extent and intensity and duration of its performance.

1. *Relaxation:* Rhythmical swinging and pendulum movements are used for relaxation of muscles in the region of the joint moved. The alternating and reciprocal contraction and relaxation of the opposing muscle group cause state of relaxation which is prerequisite for contraction.

   Relaxation exercises are used for relieving wasteful tension in the muscles which limits joint mobility and reduces the efficiency of neuromuscular coordination.

2. *Joint mobility and flexibility* are maintained and improved by free exercises (Figs 3.1a to c).

3. *Muscle strength power and endurance* are maintained or increased in response to the tension created in the muscles (Figs 3.2a to d).

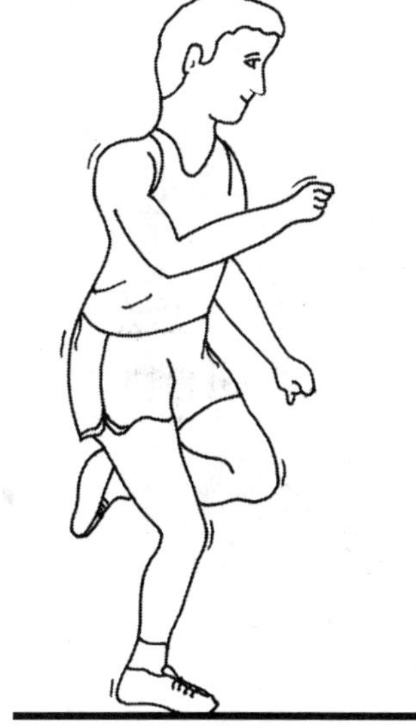

Fig. 3.1b: Running

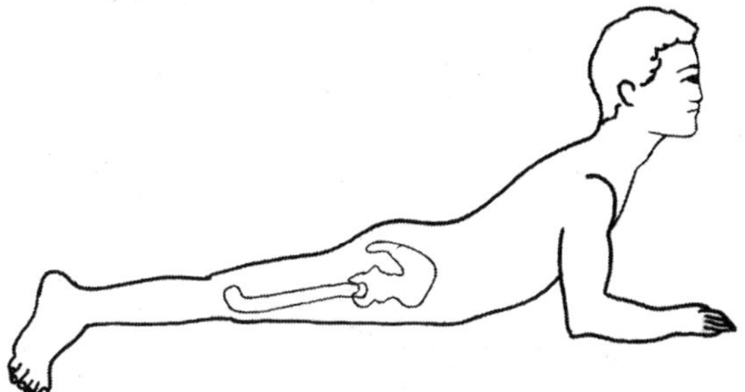

Fig. 3.1c: Prone on elbows

Free exercises which are performed against resistance of body weight or gravity and/or with long leverage, mainly improve strength and power. While those which are performed for longer duration with slow speeds tends to improve endurance.

4. *Tone:* Muscles are toned up; when free exercises performed. On contrary it also reduces the tone in hypertonic muscle groups.

5. *Neuromuscular coordination* improves by practice and repetition. As the pattern of movement is established it is simplified and becomes more efficient, and the conduction of the necessary impulses along the neuromuscular pathways is facilitated. With

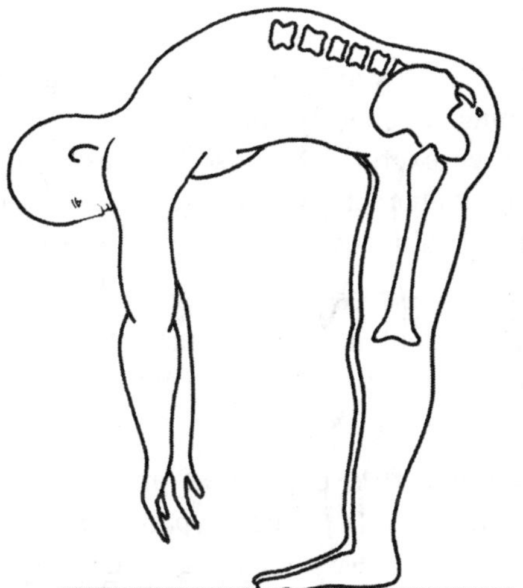

Fig. 3.1a: Forward bending

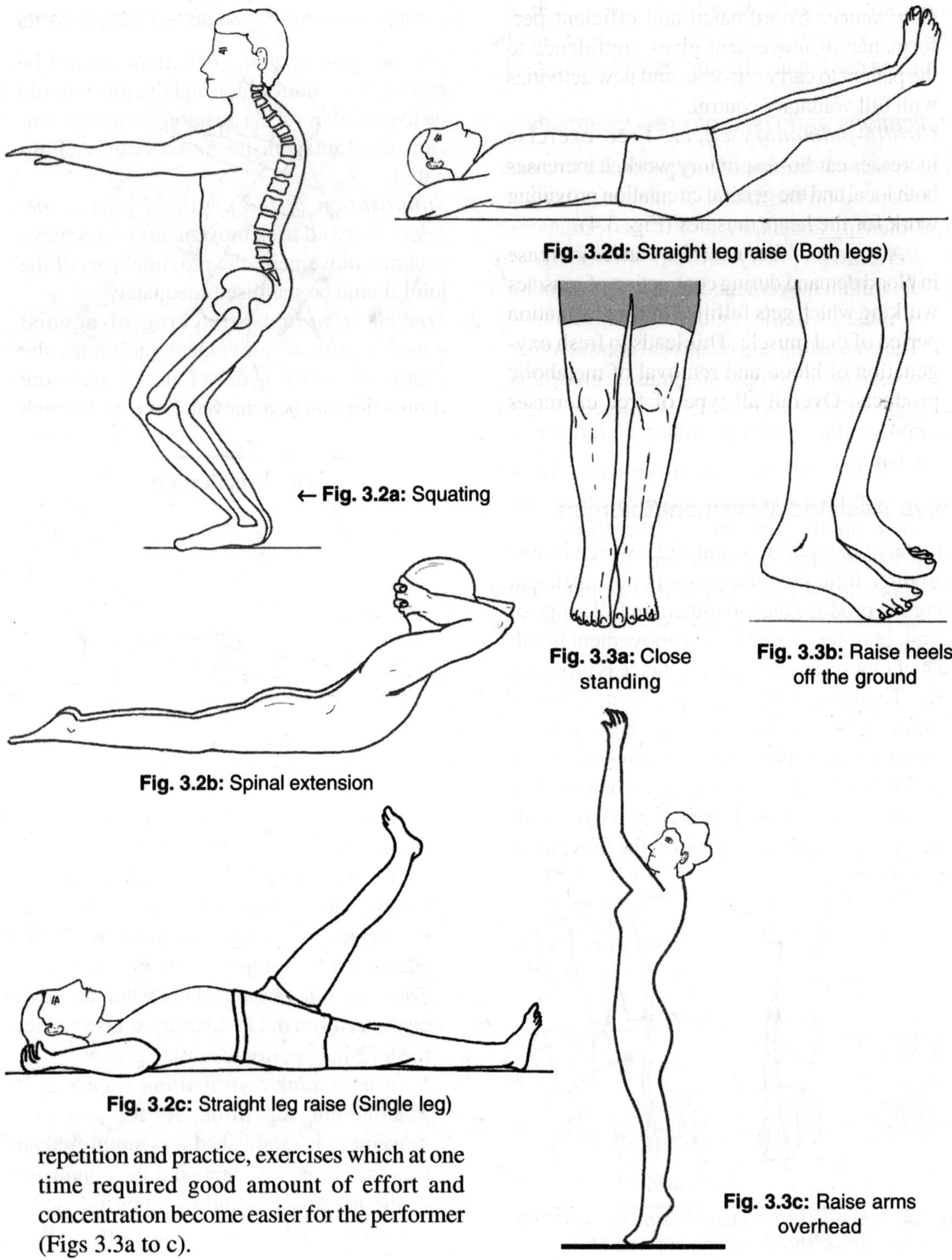

Fig. 3.2a: Squating

Fig. 3.2b: Spinal extension

Fig. 3.2c: Straight leg raise (Single leg)

Fig. 3.2d: Straight leg raise (Both legs)

Fig. 3.3a: Close standing

Fig. 3.3b: Raise heels off the ground

Fig. 3.3c: Raise arms overhead

repetition and practice, exercises which at one time required good amount of effort and concentration become easier for the performer (Figs 3.3a to c).

6. *Confidence:* Coordinated and efficient performance of movement gives confidence to the patient to carry out other and new activities with full voluntary control.
7. *Cardio-pulmonary effect:* Free exercise increases cardio-respiratory work, it increases both local and the general circulation providing work for the heart muscles (Fig. 3.4).

Any type of free exercise causes increase in blood demand during contraction of muscles working which gets fulfilled during relaxation period of that muscle. This leads to fresh oxygenation of blood and removal of metabolic products. Overall all type of free exercises improves the cardiopulmonary endurance of the patient.

Active Assisted Movement/Exercise

Voluntary contraction of a muscle, which is able to produce little movement but is not sufficient enough to produce the movement in full range of motion. In order to produce the movement in full range of motion an external assistance is provided by the Therapist, with voluntary contraction of the muscle. In some individuals where muscles are severely weak/paralysed, movement can not be performed but contraction can be palpated. In such patients or individuals assistance by the hands of therapist is required to perform the movement (Fig. 3.4).

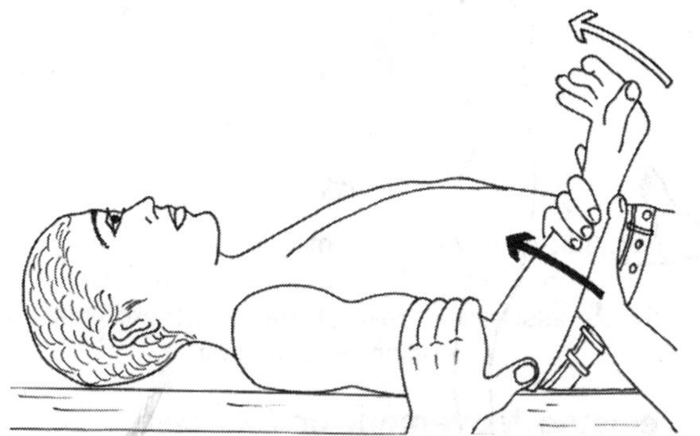

Fig. 3.4: Active-assistive elbow flexion (initial ROM) white arrow shows movement and black assistance toward the movement

Techniques of Active Assisted Movements

1. *The position of patient:* Patient should be relaxed and comfortable and the joint should be to placed in such a position so that the tension of the antagonistic muscles can be eliminated.
2. *Stabilisation of the proximal part of the joint:* To avoid trick movements and achieve accurate movement, the proximal part of the joint should be stabilised adequately.
3. *Stretch stimulus:* Stretching of agonist muscles prior to movement facilitates the contraction of the agonist muscles and more contraction can be achieved. For e.g., a stretch stimulus is given to the agonist (dorsiflexors) before the active assisted exercise.
4. *Direction of movement:* Patient may have difficulty to perform the movement in desired direction. Therefore, it is important to explain the direction of movement and it can be taught by active movement of the contralateral limb or passive movement of the same joint.
5. *Suspension* (discussed in Ch-10).
6. *Assisting force:* Therapist's hand(s) provide assistance to the agonist muscles to perform the movement in full range of motion. An assistance force should not be higher than the contraction of the agonist muscles as it is given to augment the contraction of muscle.

An assistance is given in the direction of movement and patient is given command to contract the muscle as maximum as possible. A muscle is formed by number of muscle fibres and different muscle fibres work in different range of the movement. Generally more assistance is required in initial and end ROM because the middle ROM is completed by more muscle fibres than the initial and end range.
7. *The nature of the movement:* The movement is performed in smooth manner in the anatomical range. When an assistance is given to strengthen the muscles in gravity eliminated position, great support is required to perform the movement.

Assistance is always given to facilitate the contraction of muscle fibres, therefore therapist must keep observing the patient whether he/she is contracting the muscle or not. There will not be any use of assisting the movement if patient does not contract the muscle while performing the movement.

8. *Repetitions* of active assisted movement depends on the condition of patient and age. Inorder to strengthen the muscles PRE techniques may be followed, which includes 10 repetition (one set) with minimal assistance followed by brief restart the interval of 3 sets per session.

Indications of Active Assisted Exercises/Movements

1. *Strengthening of the weak muscles:* Prolonged immobilisation of joint can cause disuse atrophy of muscles and patient finds difficulty to perform the movement in available ROM against gravity or in gravity eliminated positions. An external assistance by the hands of therapist or suspension therapy unit is given to complete the ROM. To strengthen the muscles an assistance is given to support the movement and during this period patient is asked to contract the muscle as maximum as possible. After 1-2 weeks an external assistance may be eliminated as patient starts moving the joint without any assistance against the gravity or in gravity eliminated position.
Example: Post fracture disuse atrophy, post tendon transfer muscle weakness.

2. *Co-ordination of movement:* It has been observed that prolonged immobilisation of joint can cause loss of memory of brain to the movement and patient finds difficulty to initiate the movement. Passive or Active movement of the same joint of contralateral limb is performed to stimulate motor pathway. The patient may re-learn the movement as the conduction of impulses is facilitated in the neuro-muscular pathway. As patient re-learns the movement an external assistance is given to perform the movement in available range of movement.

Active Assisted Resisted Movement

A muscle is formed by number of muscle fibers, different muscle fibres work in different ranges (outer range, middle range and inner range). Some muscle fibres initiate the range, while others are engaged to perform the movement in middle and end range.

Trauma or pathology in the muscle can hamper the movement in different ranges. Patient finds difficulty to initiate the movement, but has strong contraction of the muscle in the middle range.

Active assisted-resisted is a combination of both assisted and resisted movement in which an assistance is given to initiate the movement and resistance is given in the middle range where patient has strong contraction of muscle (Figs 3.5 and 3.6).

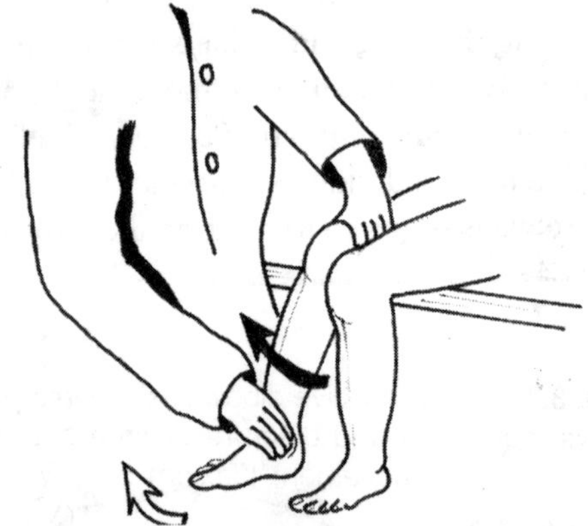

Fig. 3.5: Active assistive movement, white arrow shows movement (extension) and black arrow shows assistance toward the movement (initial extension of knee joint

Resisted Movement or Exercise

A movement or exercise is carried out against the resistance in available range of motion. The

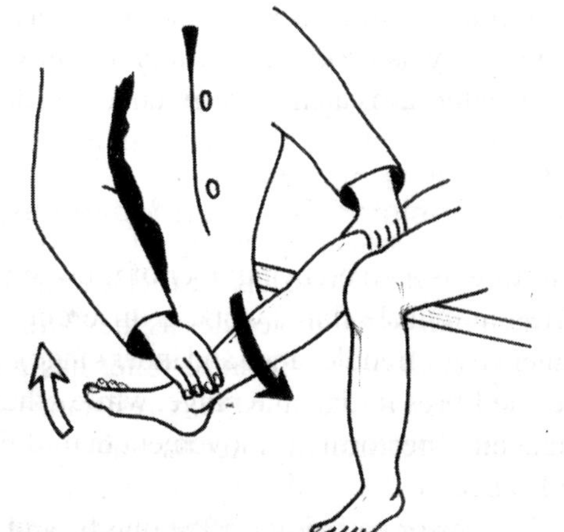

Fig. 3.6: Ascitve assistive movement, white arrow shows movement and black resistance against movement terminal extension of the knee joint

intramuscular tension is increased as the resistance is applied against isometric or isotonic contraction of muscle (Fig. 3.7).

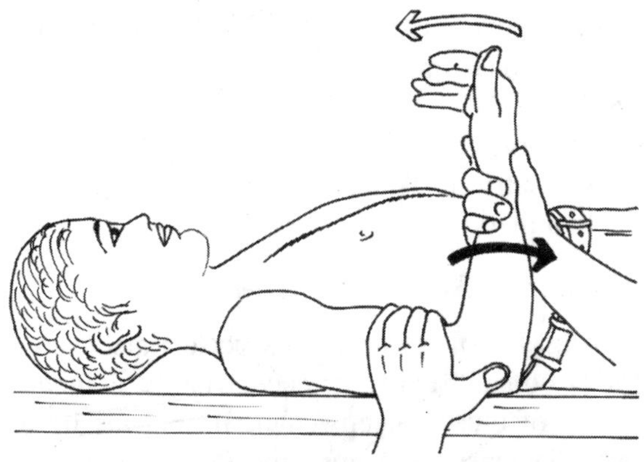

Fig. 3.7: Active-resistive elbow flexion white arrow shows movement and black resistance against the movement (flexion)

Methods/Apparatus Used to Provide Resistance Include

1. Multygymnasium apparatus-weights, pulley, dumbells
2. Highly sophisticated computer driven-isokinetic
3. Suspension therapy unit
4. Hydrotherapy
5. Therabands
6. Sponge balls and medicinal ball.
   Resistance can also be applied by:
   - Therapist (Manual resistance)
   - Patient (auto resistance)
   - Springs.

1. Resistance by the Therapist

a. *The position of patient:* should be comfortable
b. *Stabilisation:* The proximal part of the joint should be stabilised by straps or therapist's hand, or body weight
c. *Pattern of movement:* Explain the direction of movement to the patient to perform the smooth and coordinated movement in anatomical range. This can be taught by passive or active movement of same limb.
d. *Resisting force:* Therapist stabilizes the proximal part of joint by one hand while other hand is used to apply resistance.

2. Resistance by the Patient

The patient can apply resistance by his/her contralateral limb.

3. Resistance by Weight

The apparatus which are used to apply weight are sandbags, dumbell, metal weights, medicinal ball etc. In U/E while stabilising the proximal part of the joint patient is asked to hold the weight and lift it in full ROM (isotonic resisted exercise). In L/E straps can be used to attach the weight to a shoe or quadriceps table can also be used. This technique is also known as Heavy Resistance Training.

4. Resistance by Springs

The springs and therabands in sports physiotherapy clinic is widely used to provide resistance.
• *Advantage:* Can be arranged easily.

- *Disadvantage:* Resistance which is applied by spring does not remain same, increases gradually and becomes very high in the end range of movement. The resistance which is calculated for the particular muscle cannot be achieved by the springs as the resistance does not remain same throughout the range of motion.

5. Resistance by Therabands

The resistance is also applied by therabands. Therabands are elastic straps which are specially designed to strengthen a particular group of muscles.

Example: Theraband kit for-tennis elbow, this type of theraband kit contains therabands which are used to strengthen the extensors of the wrist to prevent tennis elbow. Different sizes of *theraband exercise balls* are inflatable balls used for strengthening and *balance training*. Each ball comes with two plugs and an inflation adapter alongwith poster illustrating 24 exercise. *Five sizes* are available which are *prescribed according* to the *height* of *patient*. Theraband exercise balls also have specific role on cerebral palsy patient to strengthen *spinal extension* and *abdominals against gravity* and to improve balance.

6. Resistance by Weighted Medicinal Ball

Medicinal weighted ball is another means of giving resistance during the management of weak muscle groups. These are available in different sizes and weight, prescribed according to the strength of particular group of muscles and mainly given for upper extremity and spinal muscles.

Muscles are strengthened by giving the weighted medicinal ball in various forms of movement and activities.

Example: Hold the weighted medicinal ball in both hands, with extended elbow and raise it over the shoulder (strengthening exercise for shoulder flexors).

Further it can also be used to develop coordination and balance in standing and sitting position by throwing and catching activities.

7. Resistance by Water

Water possesses the property of viscosity-the resistance of fluid flow. It is the friction that occurs between individual molecules as they attempt to move by each other. Because water has greater viscosity than air, there is more resistance when one is moving through water than air.

As a body moves through the water the pressure is increased infront of the body and decreased behind it. Water runs to the area of decreased pressure causing turbulence that tend to drag the body backward. The faster the movement the greater the turbulence and the longer the drag force or resistance to movement. This property of water may be used along with streamlined or blunt object for less or more resistance respectively.

Types of Resisted Exercises

1. Isotonic resistance exercise
2. Isometric resistance exercise
3. Isokinetic resistance exercise.

1. Isotonic Resistance Exercise

During isotonic resistance exercise, muscle contracts concentrically or eccentrically it means length of muscle keeps changing but the intramuscular tension remains same. Positive muscular work is done during concentric exercise because when concentric contraction occurs the muscular moment acts in the same direction as the angular velocity of the joint and by convention both are considered to be positive. The mechanical work that is done by a muscle during an eccentric contraction is called negative work because work is done on the muscle rather than by the muscle. The energy cost of an eccentric contraction is considerably less than that of a concentric contraction when equal loads are used.

Uses of isotonic resistance exercise—Isotonic resisted exercise is designed to increase:

- Muscle power
- Muscle strength
- Muscle endurance
- Cardio-pulmonary endurane.

2. Isometric Resistance Exercise

Iso means equal and metric means length—it is the types of resistance exercise in which the length of muscle remains same or constant but an intramuscular tension changes.

Types of isometric resistance exercise: An isometric resistance exercise is devised on the basis of its amount of resistance, duration of exercise, degree of movement and contraction. The following isometric exercises are being in current use.

- Muscle setting exercises
- Stabilization exercises
- Multiple angle isometric exercise.

Muscle setting exercises: It is a type of isometric exercise in which little or no resistance is applied. Exercise is generally indicated after an injury at the acute stage (although the application of this exercise depends on the severity of injury), to promote muscle relaxation (By decreasing muscle spasm) and blood circulation and decrease pain. The purpose of exercise is to increase or restore the vital functions of the muscle and increase the healing process. It is a low intensity exercise carried out against no or little resistance, thus exercise does not improve the muscle strength although some weak muscles may show improvement in muscle strength but not much markable.

Stabilization exercise: It is a type of isometric exercise which is carried out against submaximal resistance, generally at the mid range to enhance postural stability. The muscles contract isometrically against the gravitational resistance (force) or resistance applied by the hands of therapist.

Multiple-angle isometric exercise: This exercise is indicated to improve the strength of muscle when the isotonic resistance exercise is not recommended because of pain or instability. Isometric contraction of muscle is carried out against resistance applied by the hands of therapist or mechanical devices at different angles in the available range of motion. This exercise is carried out against maximal resistance for at least 6 seconds or count of 10. An alternate method of multiple-angle-isometric exercise is isokinetic machine, where desired angles, resistance, duration of resistance during single angle and duration of whole treatment session are set, and exercise is carried out smoothly. This machine also provides accurate improvement in the muscle strength which is measured after fortnight or at therapist's convenience.

3. Isokinetic Resisted Exercise

Its a type of isotonic resisted exercise in which resistance is applied by mechanical device so that the speed of movement remains same throughout the range of motion. The speed of movement can not be maintained same through the range of motion against the resistance applied by the hands of therapist, therefore this type of exercise is performed by highly sophisticated machine which is known as isokinetic machine (Such as *Kincom, Biodex* etc.).

Progressive Resisted Exercises (PRE)

PRE was developed by De Lorme in 1946, which is *based on 10 RM* (RM = Repetition maximum). He calculated 10 RM and executed on soldiers suffering from muscle weakness following trauma in second world war. A set of exercise was repeated from 7 to 10 times during treatment session. Exercises prescribed 5 days a week and in the last day of week (Friday) 10 RM was to be calculated and new exercise programme used to introduce for the next week. De Lorme called this method "Heavy Resistance Exercises".

The muscles strengthened by him were not disused but they had lost muscle strength from disuse. Later De Lorme implemented same exercises on Poliomyelitis patients.

In 1948 De Lorme revised his original method and adopted the name *PRE* because he believed the original name bore false implications since even muscles which could not contract against the force of gravity could be strengthen by this method. PRE has been explained in Chapter 20.

Active movements of upper and lower extremities (Figs 3.8a to z).

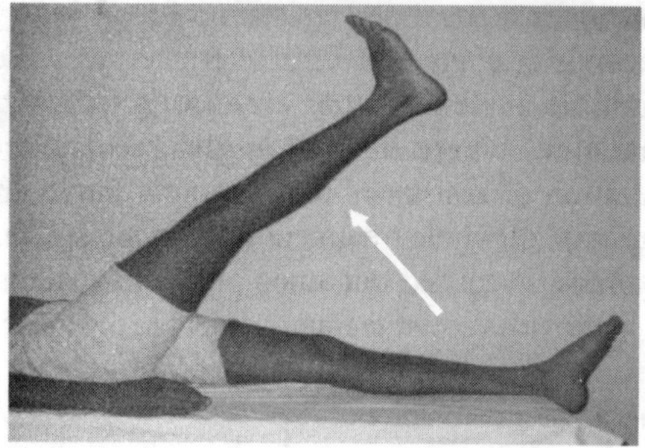

Fig. 3.8a: Hip flexion with knee extended

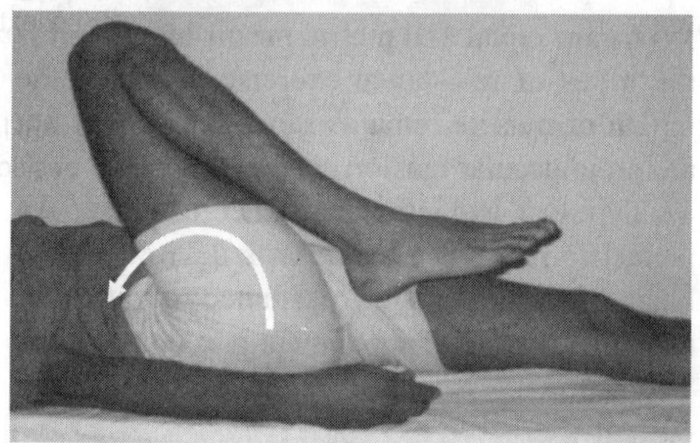

Fig. 3.8b: Hip flexion with knee flexion

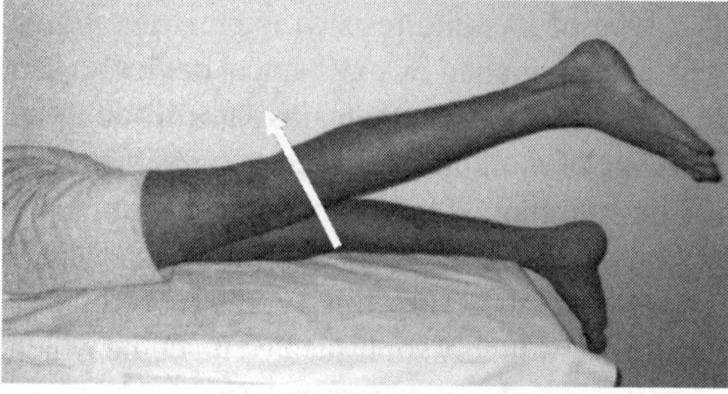

Fig. 3.8c: Hip extension

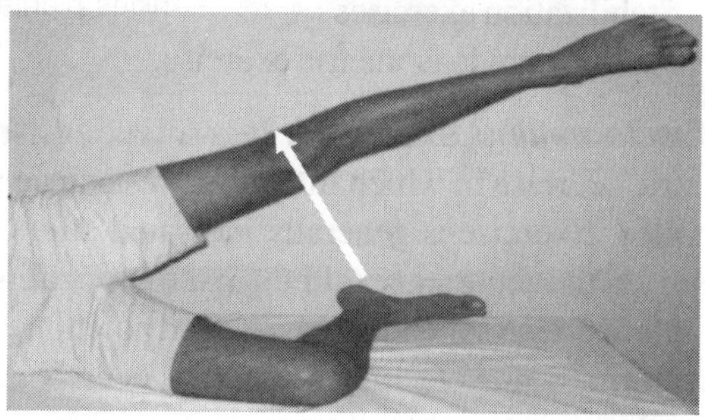

Fig. 3.8d: Hip abduction

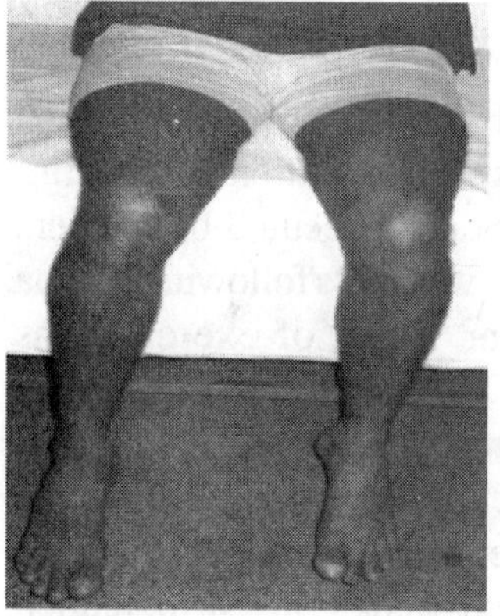

Fig. 3.8e: Hip at neutral position

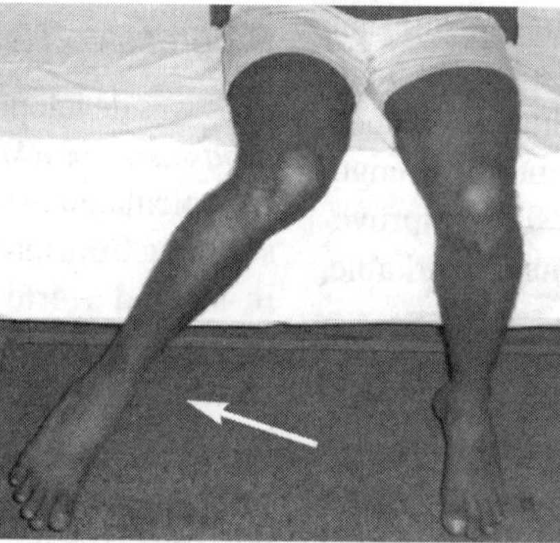

Fig. 3.8f: Hip internal rotation

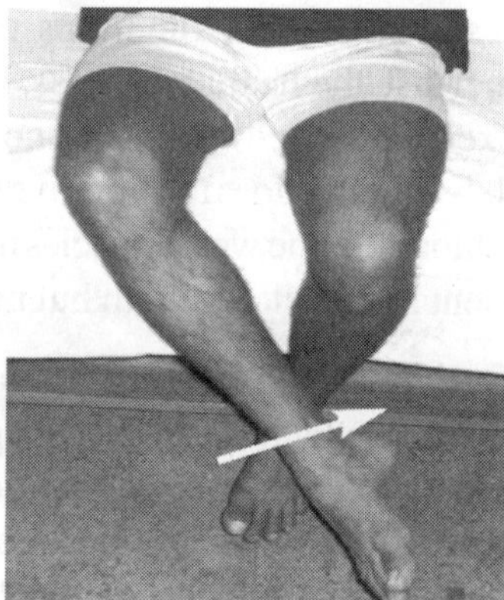

Fig. 3.8g: Hip external rotation

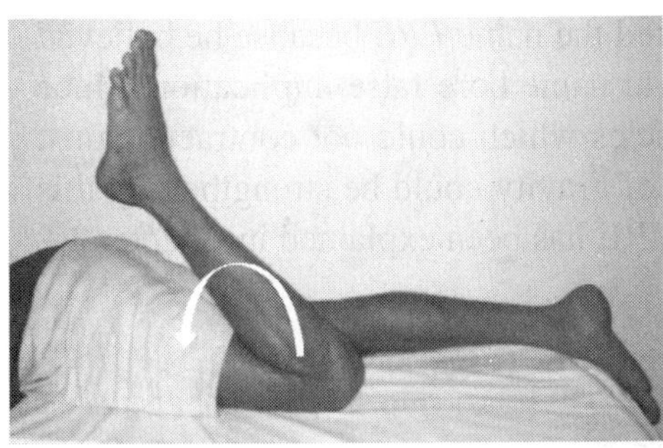

← **Fig. 3.8h:** Knee flexion

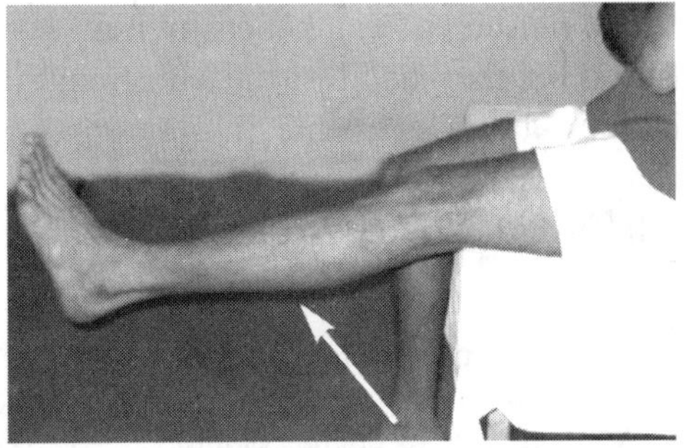

Fig. 3.8i: → Knee extension

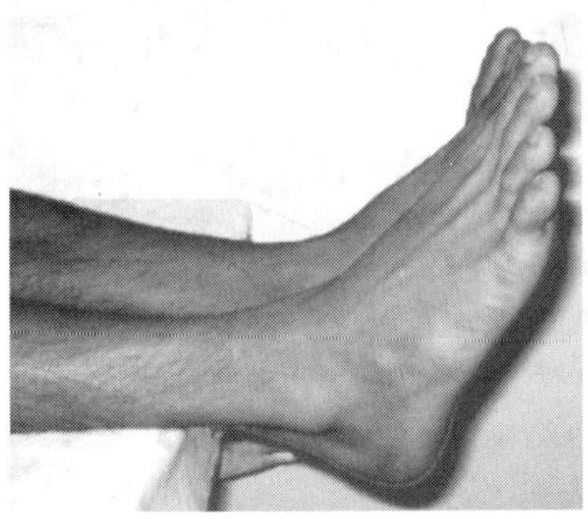

← **Fig. 3.8j:** Ankles at neutral position

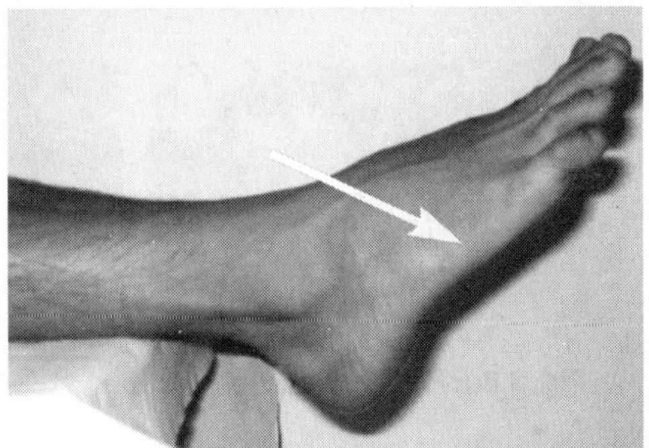

Fig. 3.8k: → Ankles plantar flexion

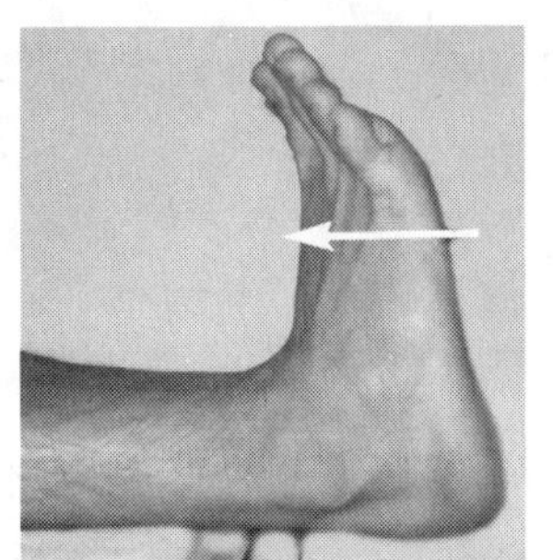

Fig. 3.8l: Ankles dorsi flexion

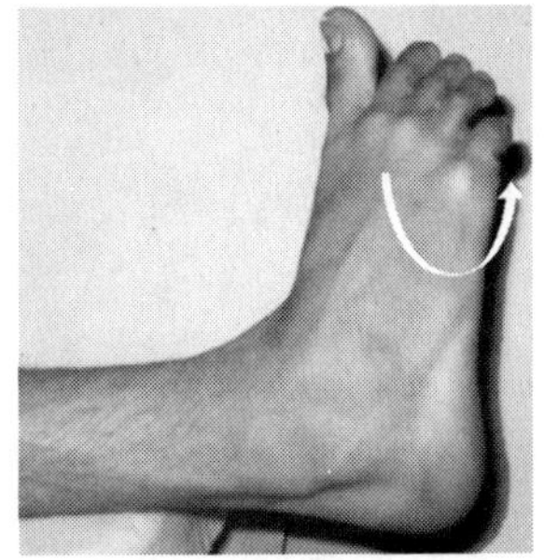

Fig. 3.8m: Ankle inversion

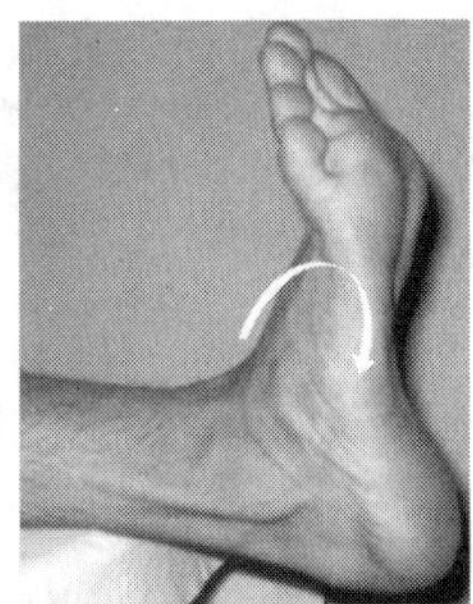

Fig. 3.8n: Ankle eversion

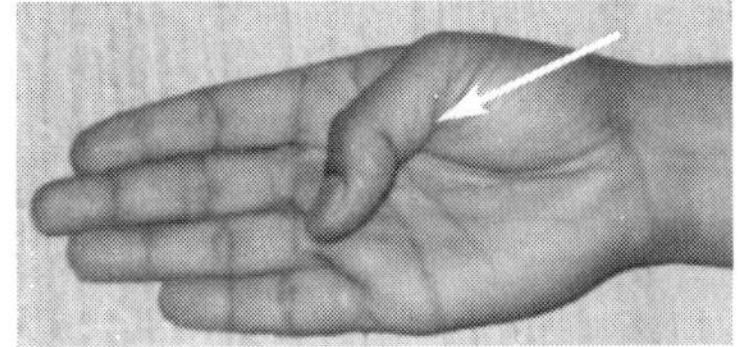

Fig. 3.8o: Thumb flexion

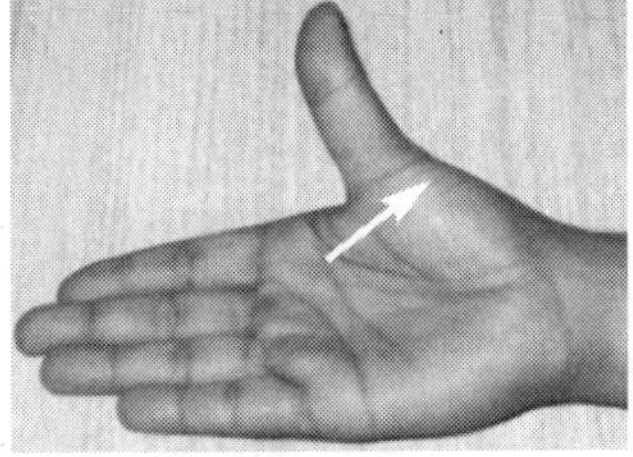

Fig. 3.8p: Thumb extension

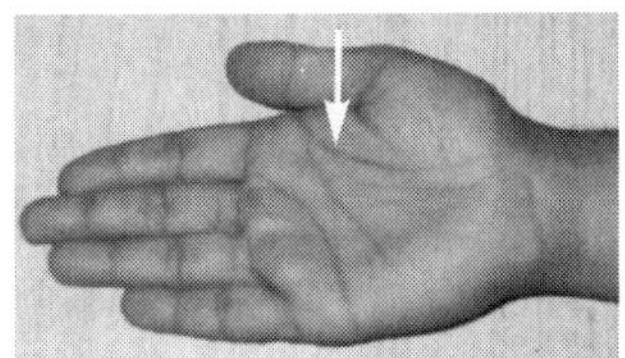

Fig. 3.8q: Thumb adduction

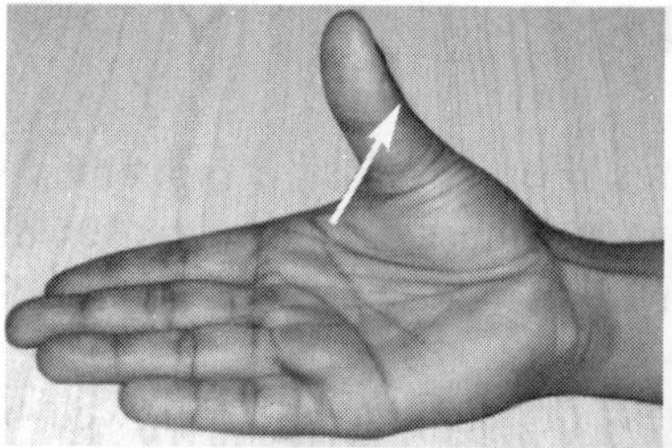

Fig. 3.8r: Thumb abduction
(Perpendicular to palmar plane)

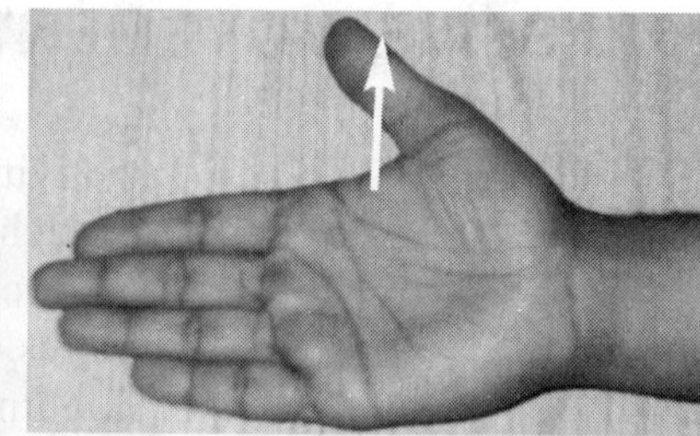

Fig. 3.8s: Thumb abduction
(Parallel to palmar plane)

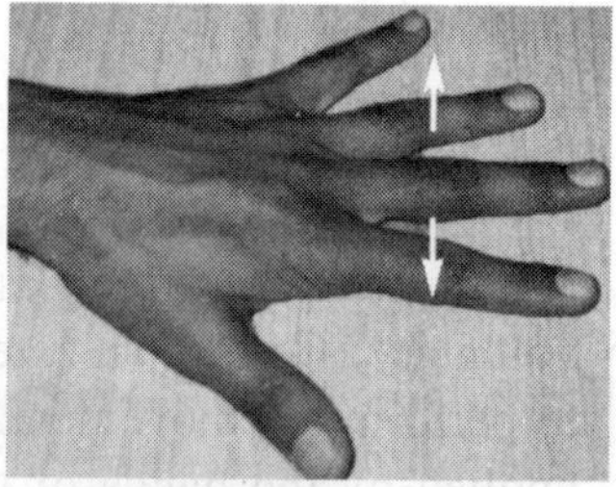

Fig. 3.8t: Finger abduction

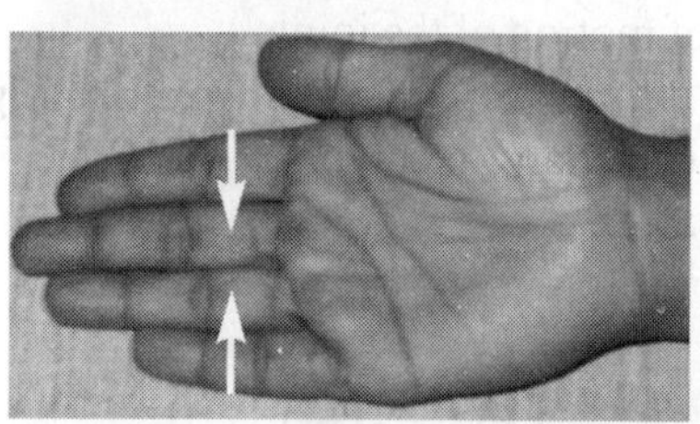

Fig. 3.8u: Finger adduction

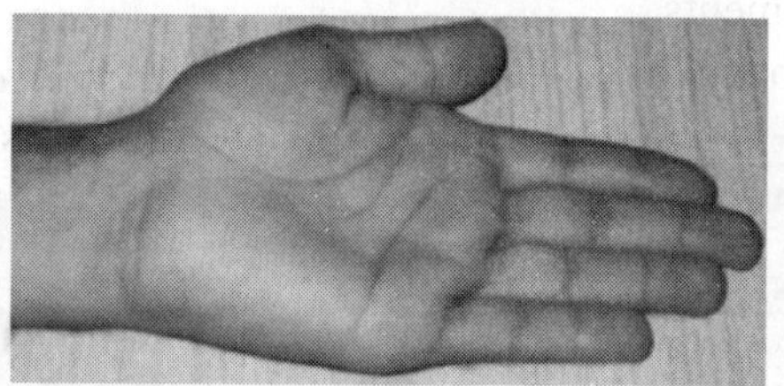

Fig. 3.8v: Wrist (Neutral)

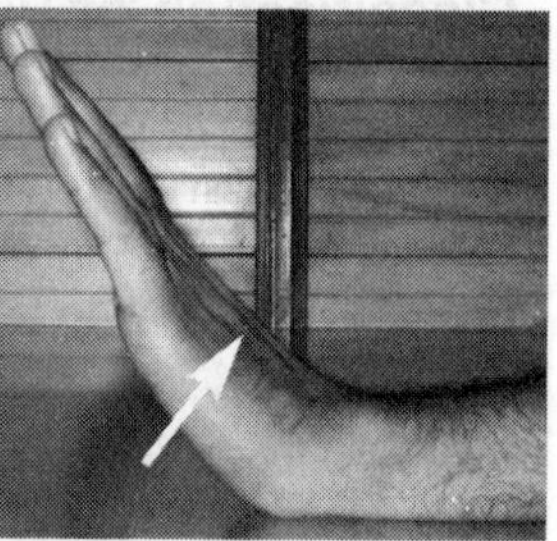

Fig. 3.8w: Wrist extension

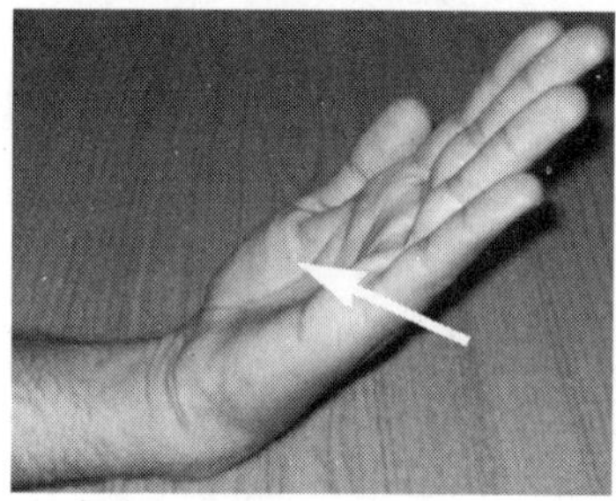

Fig. 3.8x: Wrist flexion

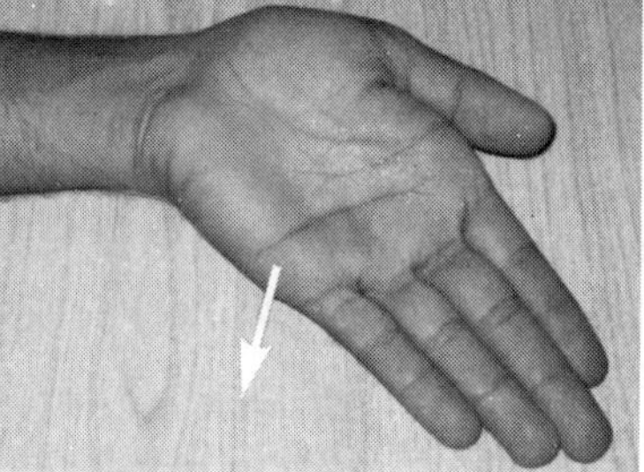

Fig. 3.8y: Wrist ulnar deviation

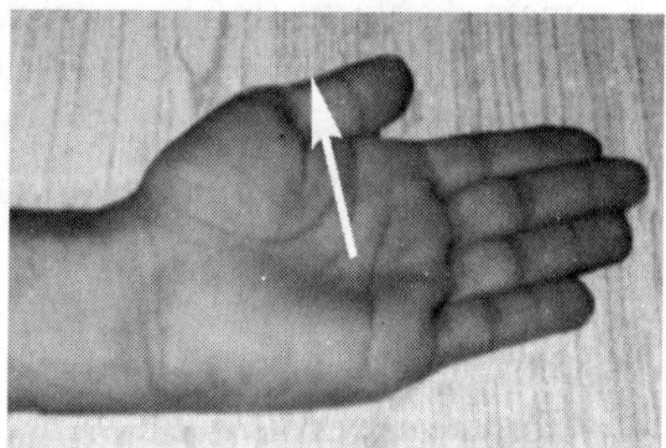

Fig. 3.8z: Wrist radial deviation

PASSIVE MOVEMENTS

INTRODUCTION

The movement which is not produced by a voluntary effort, so an external force is required to perform the movement. An external force is applied by the hands of therapist, mechanical device and or patient itself.

Classification of Passive Movements

- Relaxed passive movements.
- Forced passive movements.
- Passive manipulation.
- Passive accessory movements.

Uses, Goals and Indications of Passive Movements

1. *Maintain range of motion of the joint:* In some inflammatory conditions such as rheumatoid arthritis (RA) and ankylosing spondylitis (AS)—during the exacerbation phase, erythrocyte sedimentation rate increases (increased inflammation) which causes severe pain when patient attempts to move the joint voluntarily (actively). If joint is not allowed to move for prolonged period of time it can cause fibrous ankylosis of the joint (more common in RA and AS) and decreases range of motion as well as joint space. Gentle relaxed passive movements are given to maintain the joint range of motion. Movements should be performed in available range of motion. Forced passive movements in this stage may increase the inflammation and pain. Ice can be applied for 15-20 minutes prior to relaxed passive movements to avoid pain.

2. *Increase joint range of motion:*
   a. Tightness of the muscles followed by trauma or immobilization restricts the articular surfaces to move in full range of motion actively and prevents functional activities. Forced passive movements, stretches the muscles and increases the plasticity and extensibility of the muscle fibres.
   b. Tightness of joint capsule followed by immobilization of the joint restricts the range of motion. Passive accessory movements (glides) of the articular surfaces stretch the joint capsule thus increase range of motion of the joint.

3. *Decrease pain:* Activates pain inhibiting receptors (mechano receptors).

4. *Relaxation:* Relaxed passive movements decreases the muscle spasm and fatiguability. These movements give soothing effects to the joint if performed with soft tissue manipulation (massage) techniques.

5. *Decrease spasticity:* In upper motor neurone lesion spasticity is the most dominant clinical feature, where patient can not move the joint voluntarily which causes tightness and contracture of the spastic muscles and lengthening of antagonistic muscles. Relaxed passive movements decrease the spasticity temporarily and helps in the rehabilitation programmes. To decrease the spasticity, movement should be fairly slow, controlled and rhythmical. If the movement is preformed with high speed this can increase further spasticity by stimulating the spastic muscle fibres.

Relaxed Passive Movements

These are slow, rhythmical movements performed in the available range of motion of the joint by the hands of therapist.

Relaxed passive movements are generally given to:
- Maintain joint range of motion and connective tissue mobility.
- Prevent adhesion in the joint space.

- Enhance synovial movements for articular cartilage nutrition.
- Minimize the tightness of myofibrils.
- Decrease the spasticity temporarily.
- Increase blood circulation.
- Decrease pain.

Techniques of relaxed passive movements:

- *Position of the patient:* Position of the patient must be comfortable and appropriate instructions are given to patient to relax the antagonistic muscles. Contraction of antagonistic muscles can change the accuracy, speed, force and rhythm of the movement, therefore patient is asked to relax the antagonistic muscles to allow smooth and controlled movement.
- *Position of the Therapist:* Position of the patient also should be comfortable and as close as possible to the part which is being treated. Therapist grasps the distal end of the joint with one hand while other hand may be placed over the proximal part of the joint to stabilize it.
- *Stabilization:* The proximal part of the joint is stabilized with the straps, weight of the body, or by the hand of the therapist. Straps should not be too tight to allow the contraction of muscles.
- *Traction:* Little traction may be given to draw the articular surfaces apart, which is always given in the longitudinal axis of the joint. The traction is maintained through the range of motion and does not release unless the distal part of the joint comes to the original or starting position.
- *Repetitions:* The number of time the movement is performed depends upon the goal for which it is applied.
- *Speed of movement:* The speed of movement must be slow, uniform, controlled and rhythmical.

Forced passive movement: It is a movement which is performed by the therapist with force at the end range of motion, which can be resisted or controlled by the patient. The movement is directed at the joint without any high velocity and within the range of motion. These type of movements are commonly used to stretch the joint capsule and periarticular structures to increase range of motion and decrease pain. The forced passive movements are described in Chapter 13.

Passive accessory movement: These are the movements which take place between the joint surfaces and can not be performed voluntarily by the patient. The accessory movements which are performed by the therapist or an external force is known as passive accessory movements. The metatarsal movements can not be performed by the patient voluntarily but these movements can be performed passively by the therapist. These movements are commonly used to stretch the joint capsule and subsequently to increase range of motion and decrease pain (Passive accessory movements are described in Chapter 7).

Passive manipulation: is a very rapid, passive movement performed at the end rang of a joint. It is far more forceful than mobilization and can not be controlled by the patient.

Relaxed Passive Movements of Upper Extremity

Shoulder Joint

Flexion and extension: The patient is in supine position and therapist stands close to the shoulder joint. One hand of therapist grasps the arm at the elbow joint while other hand stabilizes the shoulder joint.

- Movement—the extremity is lifted with the one hand and is moved slowly and rhythmically through the available flexion of the shoulder then returns to the starting position. Several repetitions may be performed as per the condition (Fig. 3.9a).

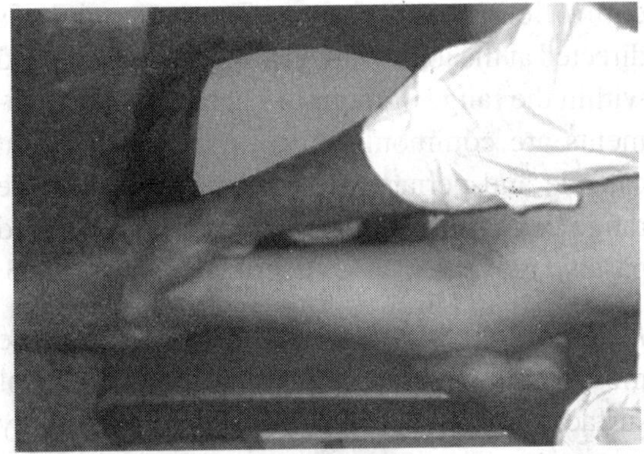

Fig. 3.9a: Flexion

Hyperextension: The patient lies on unaffected side, therapist stands behind the patient, faces the posterior aspect of the joint. The shoulder joint remains at the neutral position, elbow is flexed 45° to 60° for the convenient of therapist.

- *Placement of hands*—the upper hand is placed over the shoulder joint while lower hand grasps elbow and forearm of patient rests on therapists forearm.
- *Movement*—joint is moved from neutral position to the hyperextension (toward the therapist's body) in available range (Fig. 3.9b).

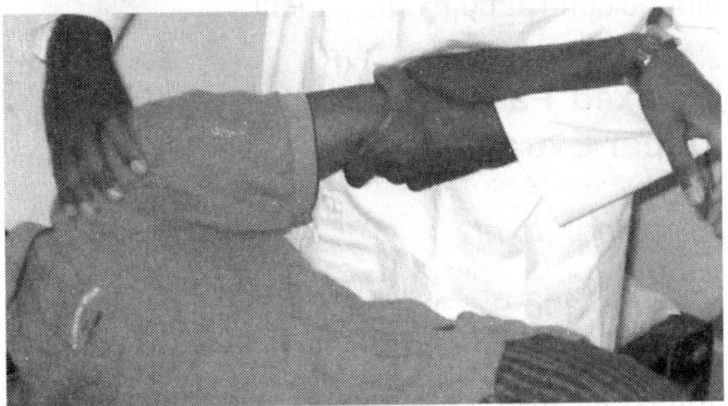

Fig. 3.9b: Shoulder hyperextension

Abduction and adduction: The patient lies in supine position, and therapist stands at the side of shoulder joint with wide base of support.

- *Placement of hands*—like flexion and extension movement one hand grasps extremity at the shoulder joint while other hand grasps at the elbow joint.
- *Movement*—the extremity is moved with little traction through the available abduction range then return to the starting position.
- **Note**—during abduction the extremity is rotated externally after 90° to avoid impingement between head of humerus and acromion process of scapula. Traction is maintained throughout abduction and adduction range till it comes to the starting position (Fig. 3.10).

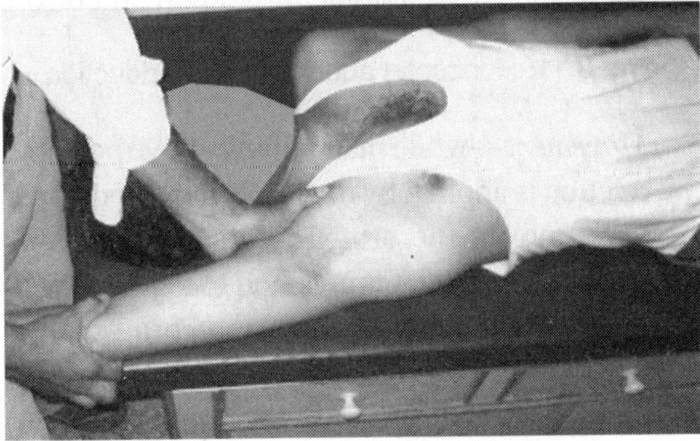

Fig. 3.10: Abduction and Adduction

Horizontal adduction and abduction: The patient lies in supine position and therapist stands close the body and faces the patient's face, starting position of shoulder is 90° of abduction.

- *Placement of hands*—remains same as shoulder flexion-extension.
- *Movement*—extremity is moved by one hand horizontally across the body through available range (Fig. 3.11).

Internal (medial) and external (lateral) rotation: The patient is in supine or in sitting position and therapist at side of patient, the shoulder joint is abducted at 90° and elbow flexed at 90°.

- *Placement of hands*—one hand grasps the extremity at wrist while other hand grasps the flexed elbow joint.

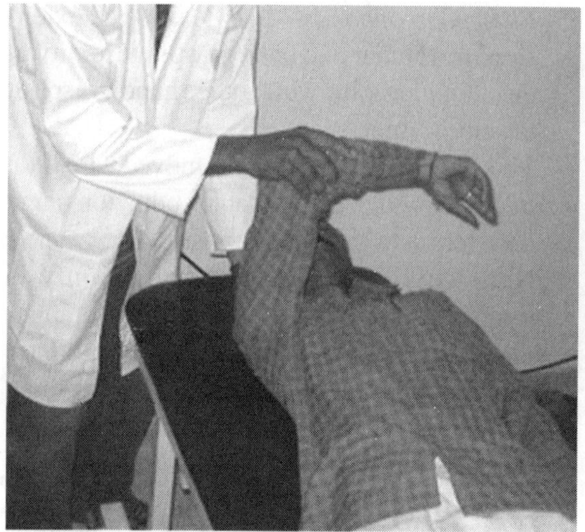

Fig. 3.11: Horizontal abduction and adduction

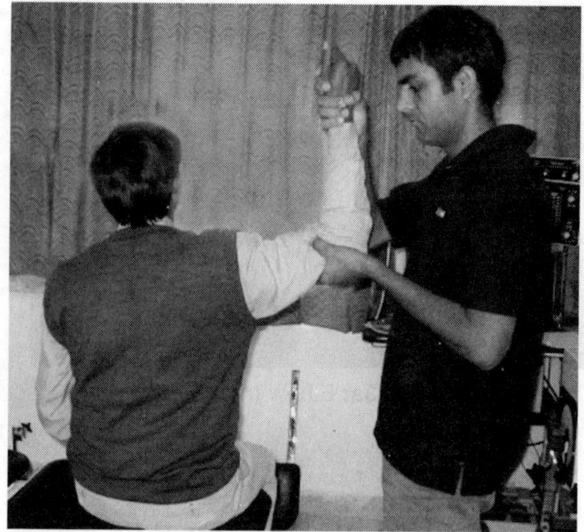

Fig. 3.12b

- *Movement*—while maintaining above position, traction is applied by the lower hand and upper hand moves the arm through the available external rotation (taking hand to the head with maintaining elbow flexion) then brings to the neutral position and traction is released. Now hand is moved towards the hip joints with traction through the available internal rotation, then returns to the neutral position (Figs 3.12a to c).

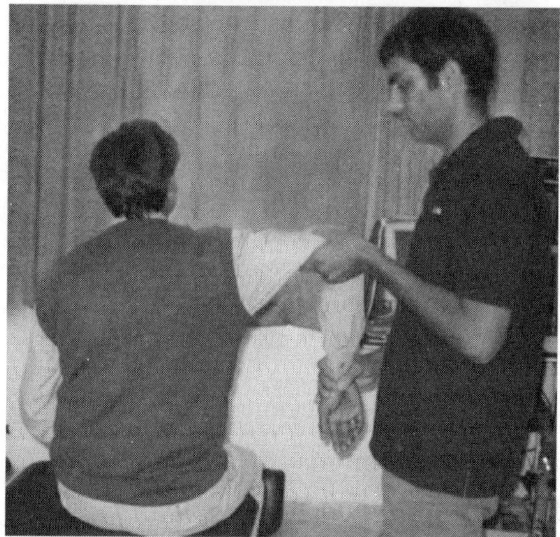

Figs 3.12a to c: Internal and external rotation

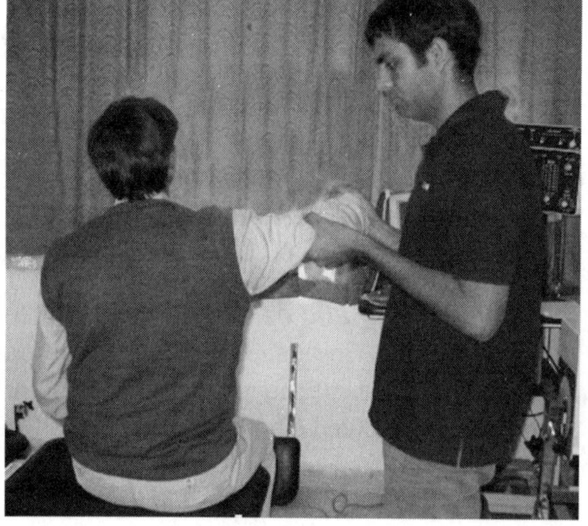

Fig. 3.12a

Elbow Joint

Flexion and extension: Patient lies in supine position, and therapist stands at the side of patient. The proximal part of the elbow may be stabilized by the hand of therapist, the hand grasps the wrist joint and moves the elbow through available range of flexion then returns to the neutral position i.e. extension (Figs 3.13a to d).

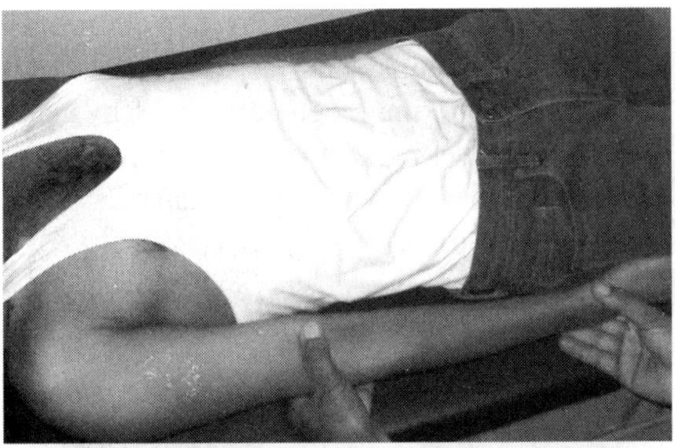

Fig. 3.13a: Elbow (neutral)

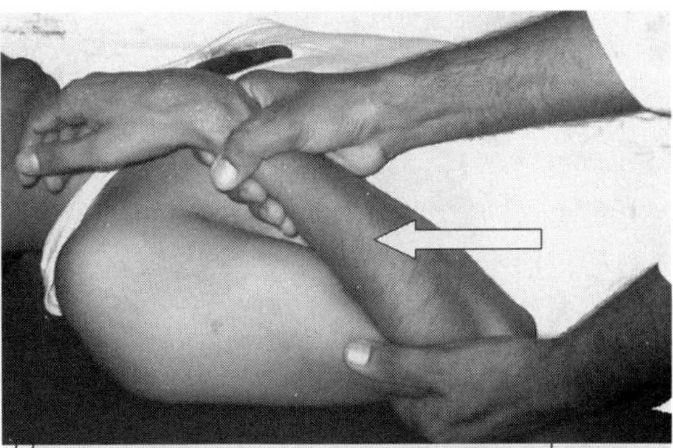

Fig. 3.13c: Elbow flexion (end range)

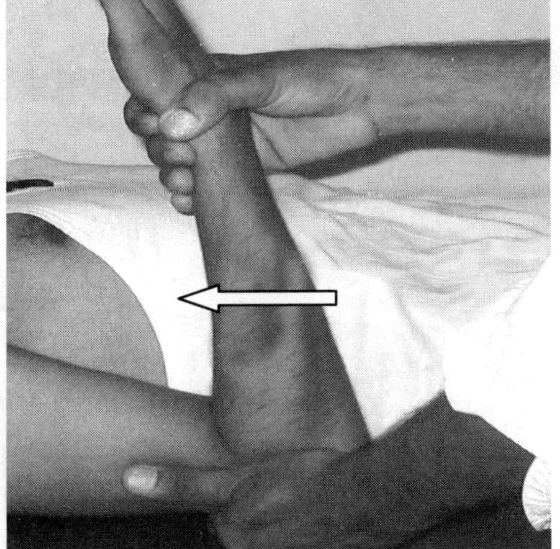

Fig. 3.13b: Elbow flexion (mid range)

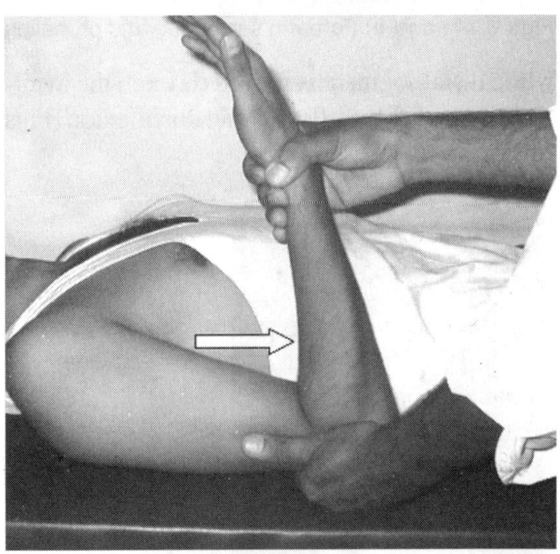

Fig. 3.13d: Elbow extension

Radio-ulnar Joint

Forearm pronation and supination: The position of patient and therapist remains same as elbow flexion and extension. Therapist holds the distal forearm and rotates it alternatively into supination and pronation, the upper hand stabilizes the elbow joint (Figs 3.14a and b).

Wrist Joint

Palmar flexion and dorsiflexion: Patient lies supine or sitting, and therapist stands at the side close to the wrist joint, the proximal part of the wrist is stabilized by the therapist's upper hand

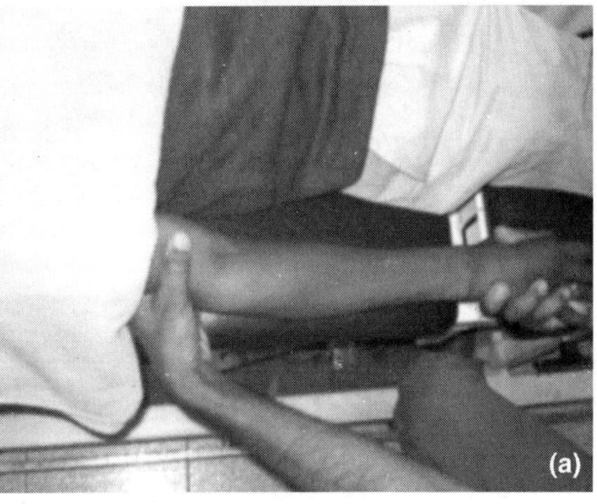

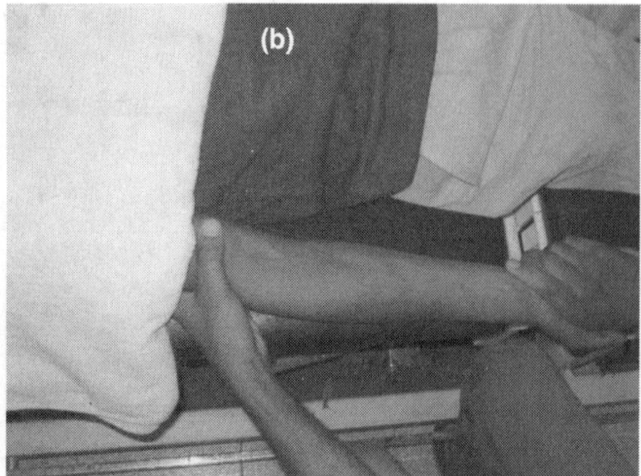

Figs 3.14a and b: Forearm supination and pronalion

while distal segment is moved through the available range of palmar flexion and dorsiflexion (Figs 3.15a and b).

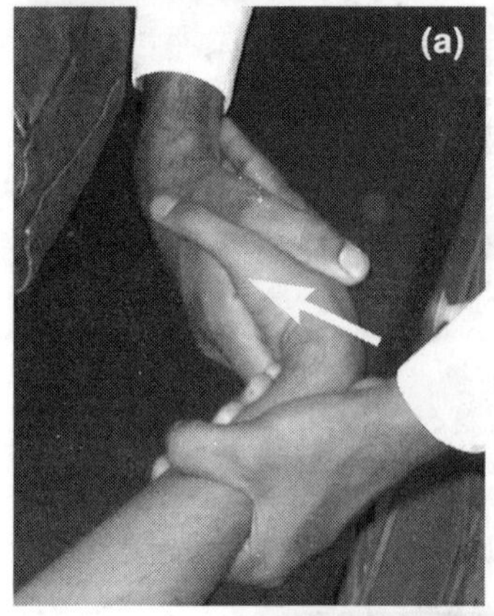

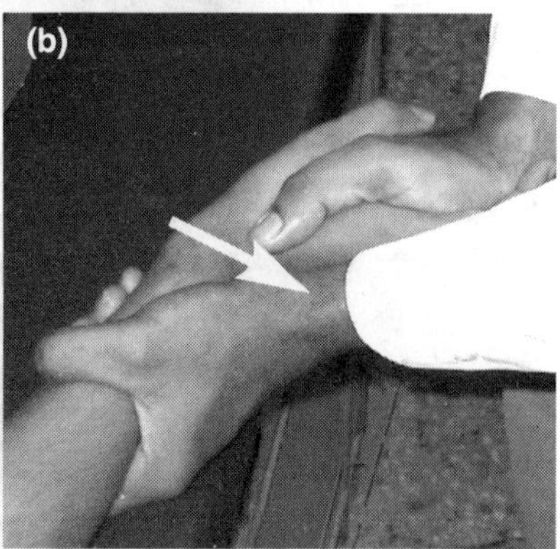

Figs 3.15a and b: (a) Wrist flexion (palmer flexion), and (b) Wrist extension (dorsi flexion)

Radial and ulnar deviation: Position of therapist and patient remains same as above, therapist stabilizes the proximal segment of wrist by upper hand while lower hand grasps the patient's hand and moves into radial deviation and ulnar deviation (Figs 3.16a to c).

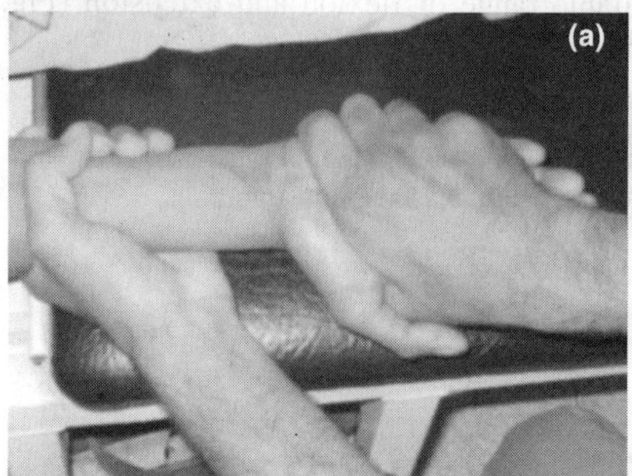

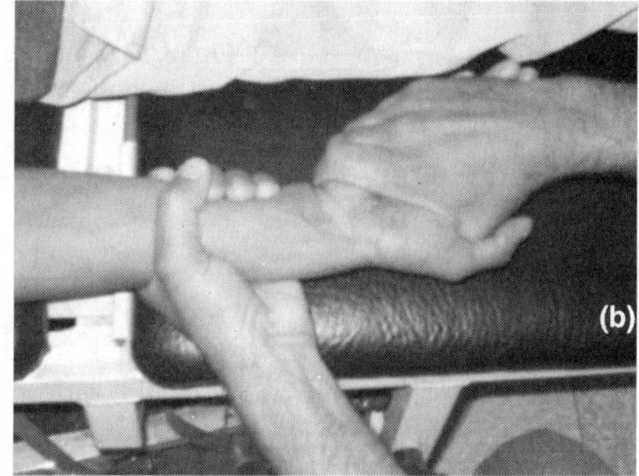

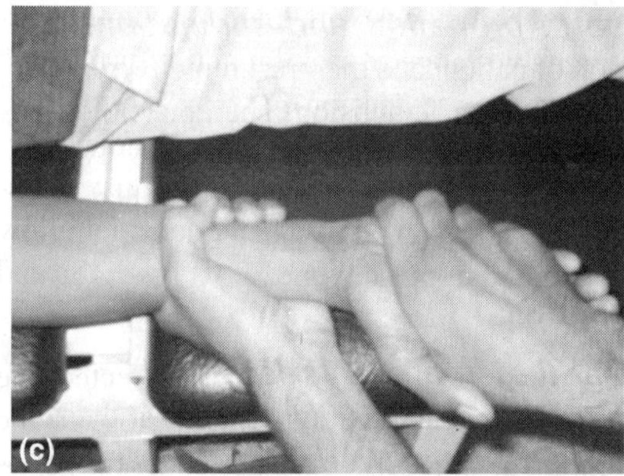

Figs 3.16a to c: Wrist Radial/ulnar deviation

Metacarpo-phalangeal and interphalangeal joint: The position of patient and therapist remain same as wrist flexion and extension. Procedure also remains same as proximal part of joint is stabilized by one hand while other hand grasps the distal part of the joint and moves through available range of flexion and extension (Fig. 3.17).

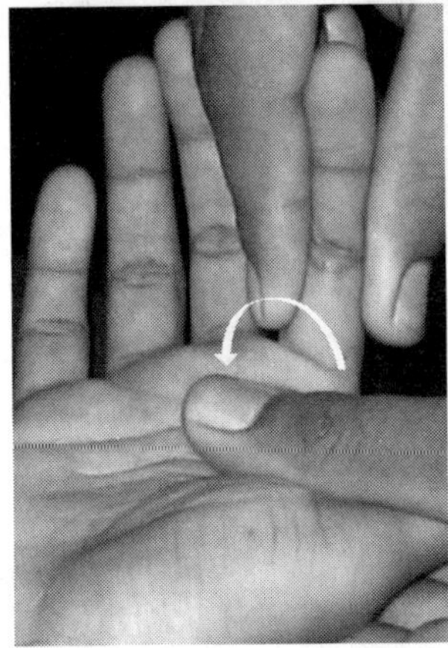

Fig. 3.17: Metacarpal joint flexion-extension

Relaxed Passive Movements of Lower Extremity

Hip Joint

Flexion and extension: Patient lies in supine position, the therapist stands at the side of hip joint, upper hand grasps extremity at the knee joint while lower hand holds the heel. The joint is moved by both hands with knee flexion through the available range of flexion and return to the neutral position (extension).

- **Note**—full flexion of hip joint can not be performed with the knee extended, because hamstring muscles get tighten and does not allow the joint to move beyond 80° (Figs 3.18a and b).

Hyper-extension: Patient lies on unaffected side therapist stands behind the patient close to the hip joint. The upper hand is placed over the pelvis to stabilize it, while lower hand grasps the knee,

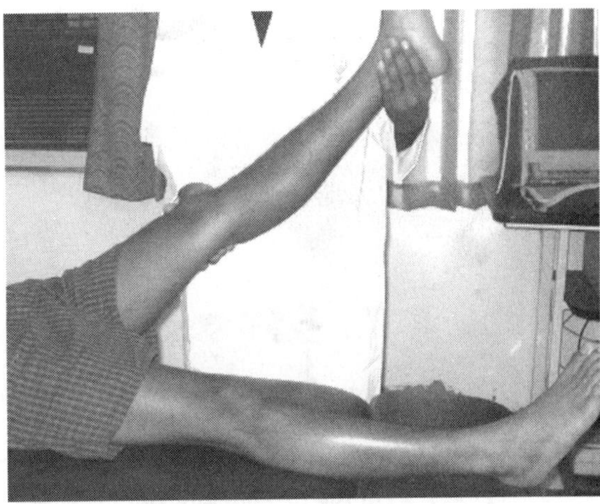

Fig. 3.18a: Hip flexion with knee extension

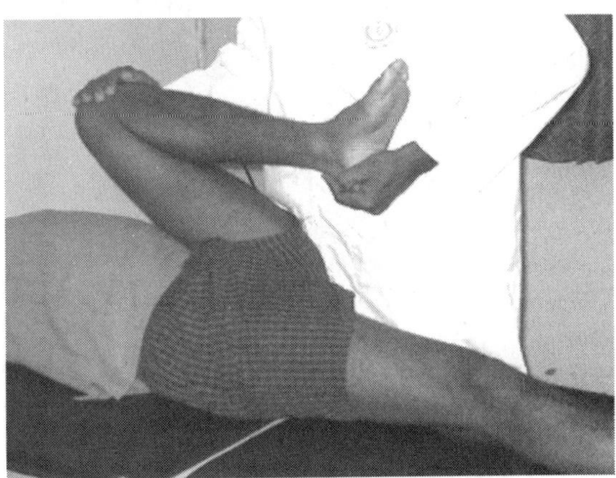

Fig. 3.18b: Hip flexion with knee flexion

the patient's leg rests on the forearm of therapist (knee flexes at 90°). While maintaining above position therapist hyperextends the hip joint by bringing the leg toward his or her body, through the available range of motion (Fig. 3.19).

- **Note**—knee joint should not be flexed beyond 80° as rectus femoris gets tighten and prevents the hyperextension.

Abduction and adduction: Patient lies in supine position, therapist stands at the side of patient. The upper hand of therapist grasps the extremity at knee joint while other grasps at the ankle joint (Fig. 3.20).

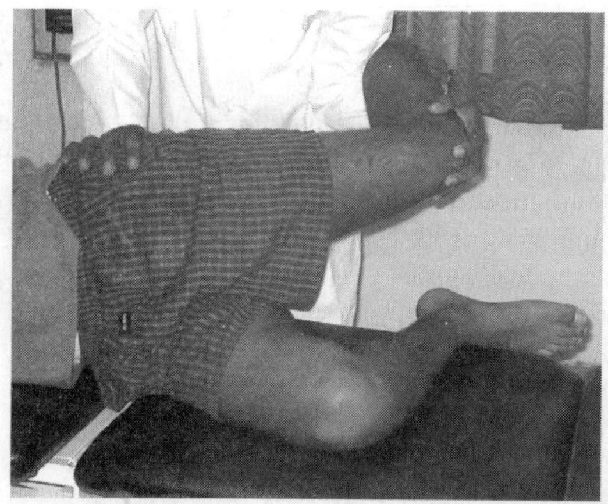

Fig. 3.19: Hip hyperextension

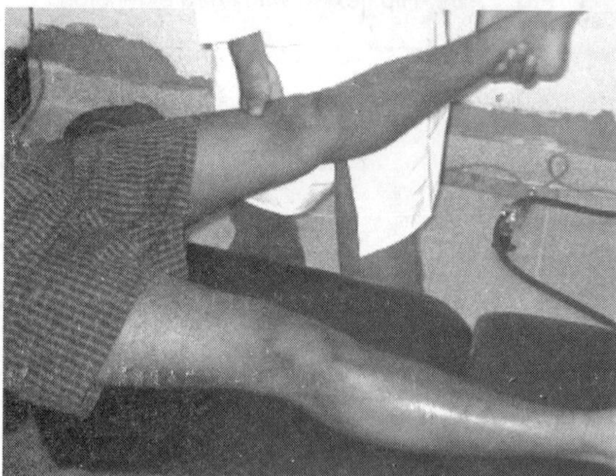

Fig. 3.20: Hip abduction-adduction

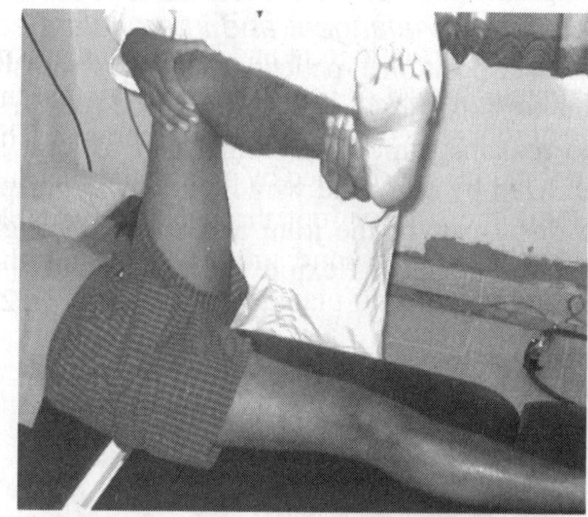

Fig. 3.21a: Hip external rotation

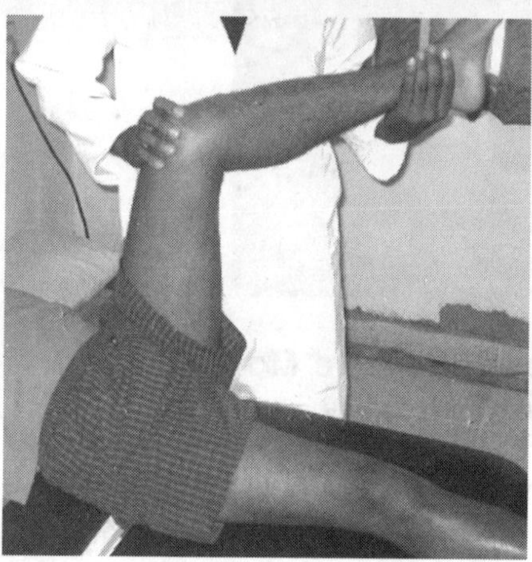

Fig. 3.21b: Hip internal rotation

- *Movement*—therapist move the limbs by taking toward his or her body through the available range of abduction then brings back to the neutral position (adduction).

Internal and external rotation: The patient lies in supine position and therapist stands at the side of patient. The knee and hip is flexed at 90°, therapist grasps the knee joint and ankle joint (Figs 3.21a and b).

- *Movement*—while maintaining above position the leg is rotated inward (external rotation) and outward (internal rotation).
- **Note**—during inward and outward rotation hip and knee should remain at 90° of flexion.

This movement may also be done in high sitting position.

Knee Joint

Flexion and extension: The procedure remains same as flexion and extension of the hip joint.

Flexion and extension of knee joint may also be performed in prone position.

Ankle Joint

Dorsiflexion and plantarflexion: The patient lies in supine position and therapist stands at the side of ankle joint. The upper hand is placed over the dorsum of the ankle joint and lower hand grasps the plantar aspect of heel in such a way that the sole of foot rests on the forearm of therapist. The dorsiflexion is performed by pulling the heel and pushing the sole of foot through the available range then upper hand gradually pushes the dorsum of foot into plantar flexion (Figs 3.22a and b).

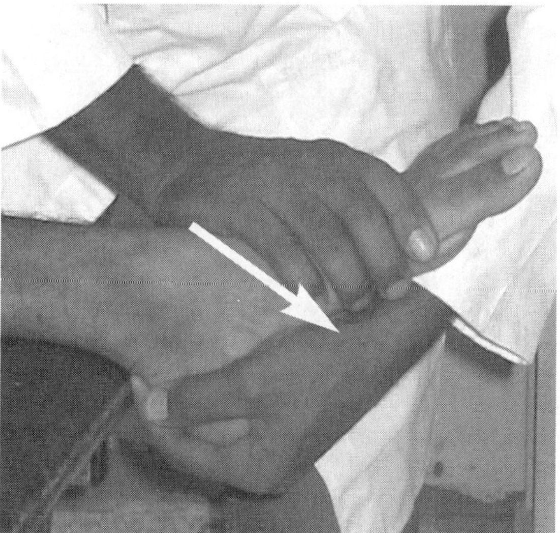

Fig. 3.22a: Ankle plantar flexion

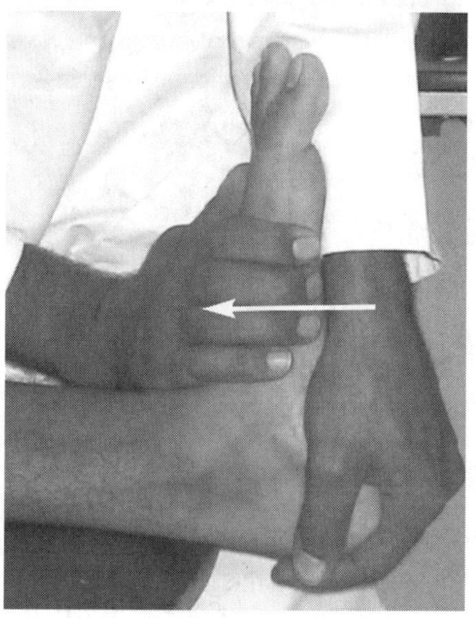

Fig. 3.22b: Ankle dorsiflexion

Subtalar Joint

Varus and valgus: The ankle joint is placed out of the table, therapist holds the heel with the both hands and moves inward (varus) and outward (valgus) (Fig. 3.23).

- *Movement*—Therapist moves the heel inward (varus) and outward (valgus).

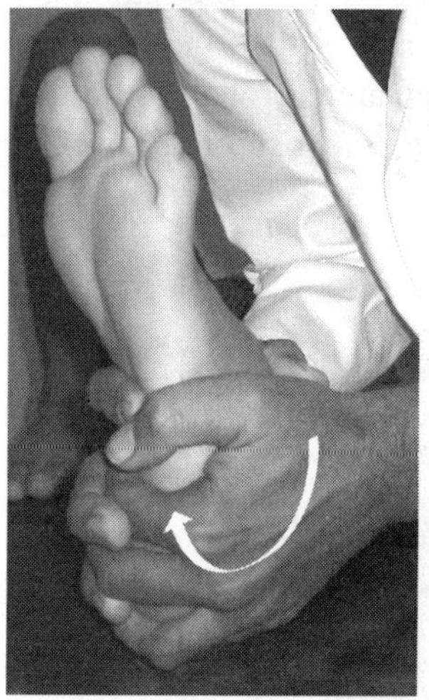

Fig. 3.23a: Varus

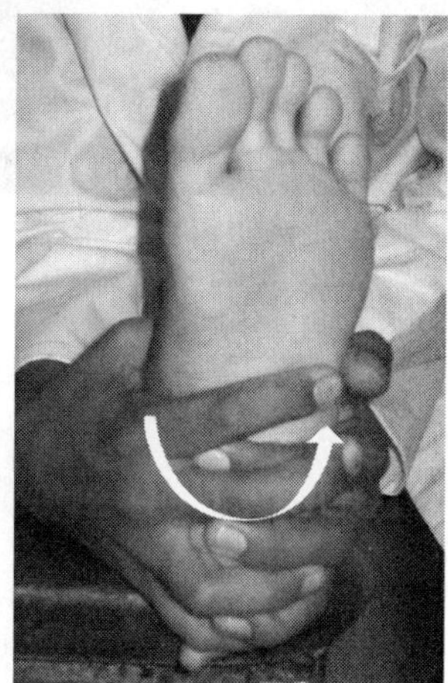

Fig. 3.23b: Valgus

Transverse Tarsal Joints

Supination and pronation: Position of patient and therapist remain same as dorsiflexion and plantarflexion of ankle joint. Therapist places both hands over the dorsum of foot in such a way that the thenar surface of one hand rests dorsum and fingers grasp the plantar surface. The thenar aspect of other hand lies on the dorsum foot and fingers grasp the plantar surface.

- *Movement*—the forefoot is taken inward by raising the middle arch (supination) and after performing available range of supination it is taken back to the normal then into outward by raising the lateral arch (pronation) of foot and back into the neutral position (Figs 3.24a and b).

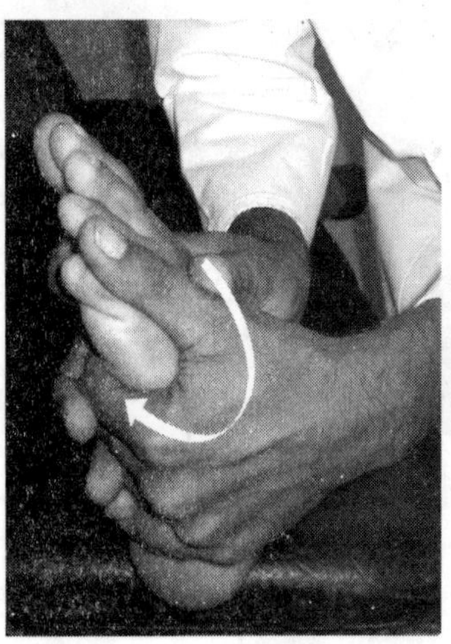

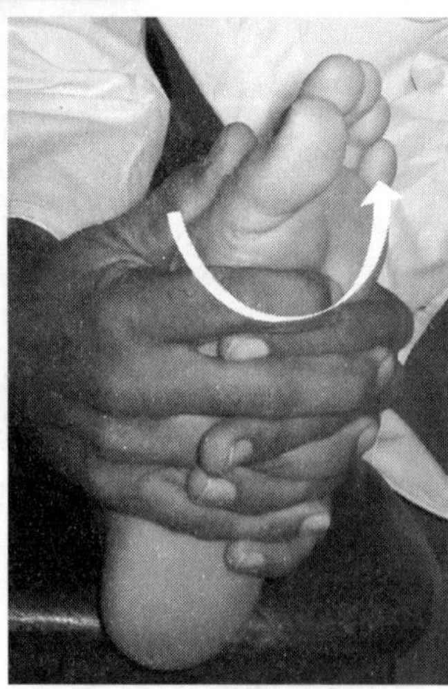

Figs 3.24a and b: (a) Ankle supination, and (b) Ankle pronation

Metatarsophalangeal and Interphalangeal Joint

Flexion and extension:

- *Metatarsophalangeal (MTP) joint:* The proximal part of the joint is stabilized by one hand and the distal part moved by the other hand into available range of flexion and extension (Figs 3.25a and b).

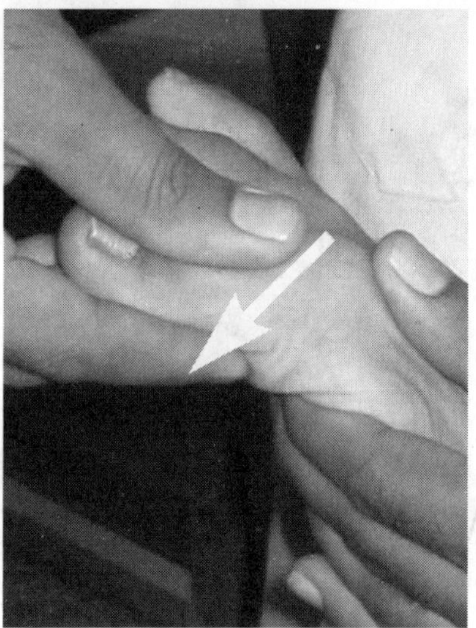

Fig. 3.25a: MTP joint flexion

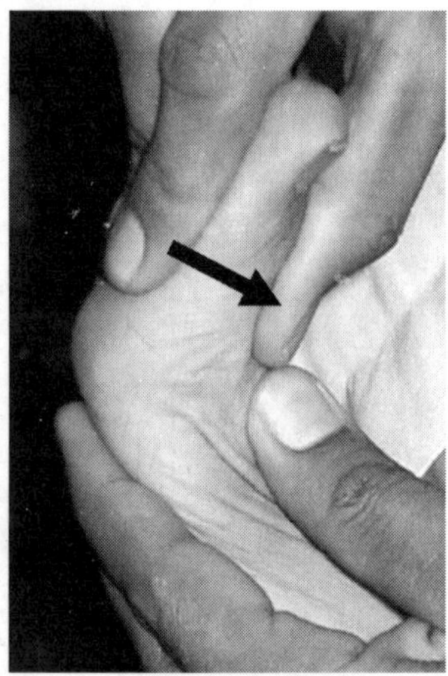

Fig. 3.25b: MTP joint extension

- *Interphalangeal (IP) joint:* Procedure remains same as MTP flexion extension (Fig. 3.26).
- *Interphalangeal (IP) joint (flexion and extension):* The patient lies in supine or sitting position, therapist stabilized the proximal phalange with one hand, while other hand grasps the distal phanges. The distal phalange is moved in flexion and extension. Each interphalangeal joint is mobilized separately.

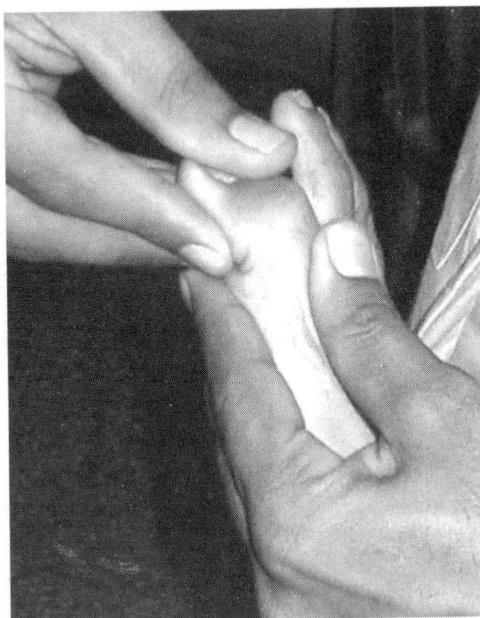

Fig. 3.26: IP flexion

CHAPTER-4

Basic and Derived Positions for Exercise Therapy

INTRODUCTION/BASIC FUNDAMENTAL POSITION

Mobility depends upon stability or success of every movement lies on its posture. Postures are fundamental to movements.

Many authors have given five basic positions (along with their derivatives) in which exercises may be given. These are lying, sitting, kneeling, standing and hanging. Out of these hanging is rarely used in clinical practice, hence first four and its derivative are discussed.

1. Lying (Supine)

The body is supine, with the arms by the sides and legs straight. The body is fully supported with a longer base of support and low centre of gravity. The muscle work is minimal and body is fully relaxed.

The derived positions are:

a. *Side lying:* Clinically this position is used for exercise therapy by bending the under arm with slight hip and knee flexion of under leg. The base of support is smaller as compared to supine lying (Fig. 4.1).

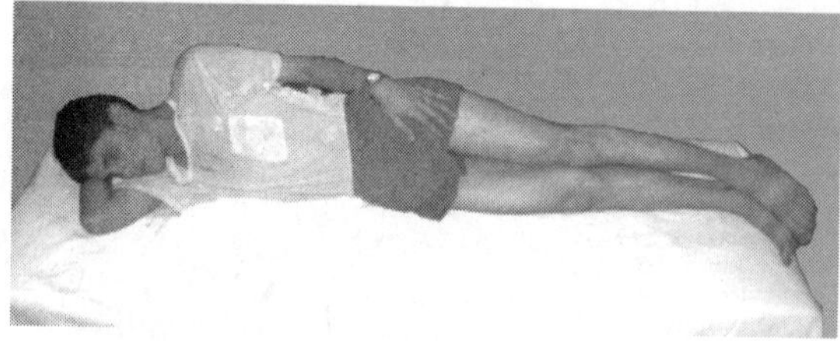

Fig. 4.1: Side lying

b. *Prone lying:* The base of support is almost same as of supine lying. Neck may be rotated to one side or pillows may be used to support forehead. This position is mainly used for spinal extensors, hip extensors and knee flexors exercises (Fig. 4.2).

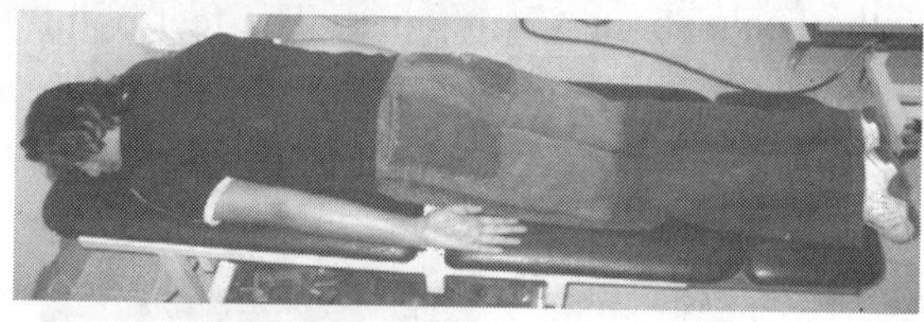

Fig. 4.2: Prone lying

c. *Across-prone lying:* It is further modified form of prone lying position in which the upper body with arms lie out side the supporting surface and the anterior superior iliac spine just off the front edge of the support. This position is usually used in pediatric group for spinal extensors exercises. The hands may be supported on stool bars or by therapist. The therapist may also hold the legs of the patient (paediatric) just above the ankle (Fig. 4.3).

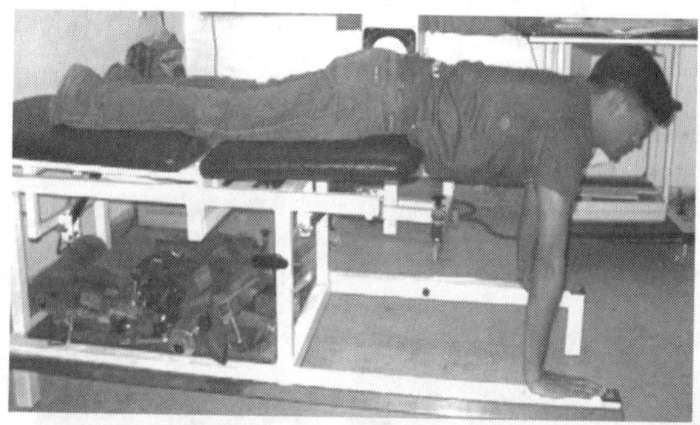

Fig. 4.3: Across prone lying

d. *Crook lying:* Lying with the soles of the feet resting on the floor. The knees are flexed to varying degrees (usually 90°) (Fig. 4.4).

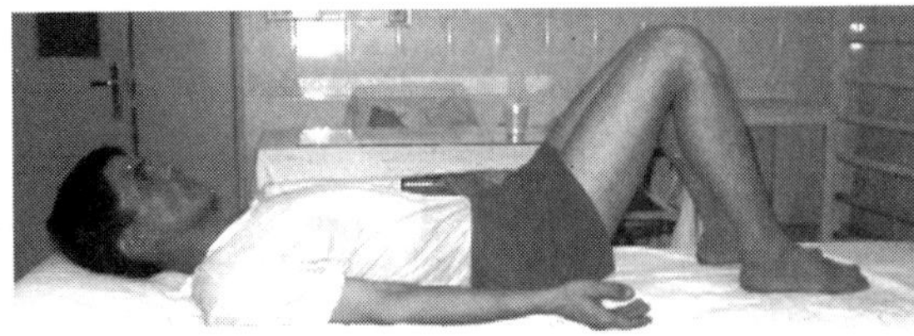

Fig. 4.4: Crook lying

e. *Stride crook lying:* As crook lying, but the legs and feet are placed astride apart, with the heels about 45 cm apart. The feet point obliquely outward in line with the legs (Fig. 4.5).

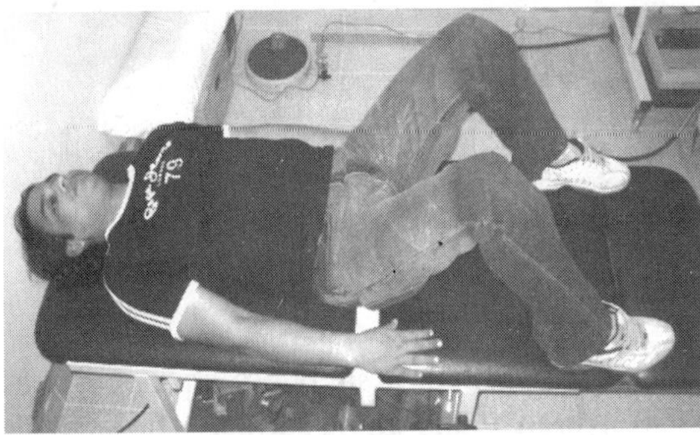

Fig. 4.5: Stride crook lying

f. *Crook lying with pelvis raised:* From crook lying position the pelvis is raised until there is a straight line between the trunk and thighs (Fig. 4.6).

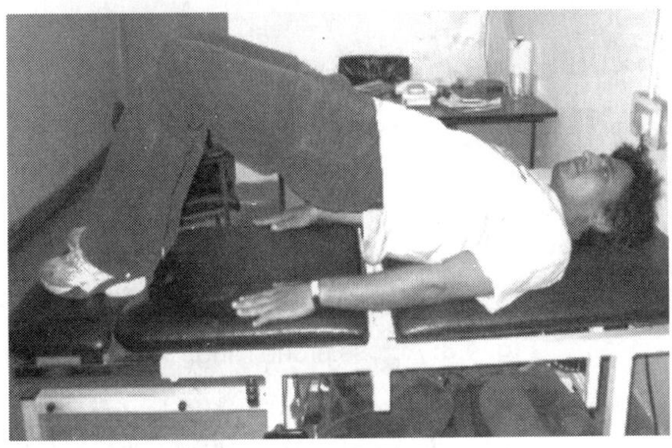

Fig. 4.6: Crook lying with pelvis raised

g. *Leg lift lying:* Lying with the legs raised (the range of movement must be indicated) (Fig. 4.7), also known as straight leg(s) raising.

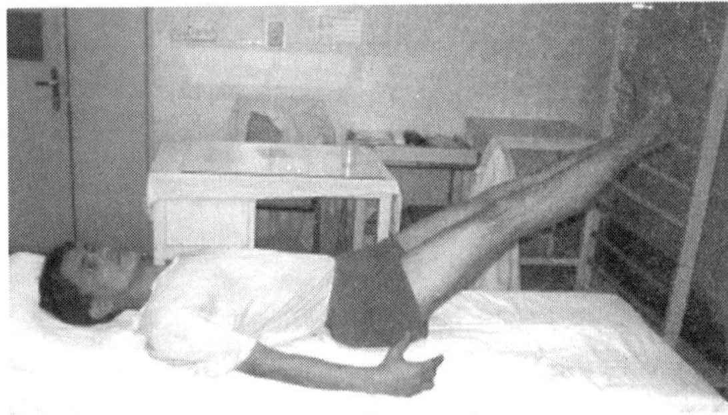

Fig. 4.7: Leg lift lying

h. *Stride lying:* Lying with feet astride apart (Fig. 4.8).

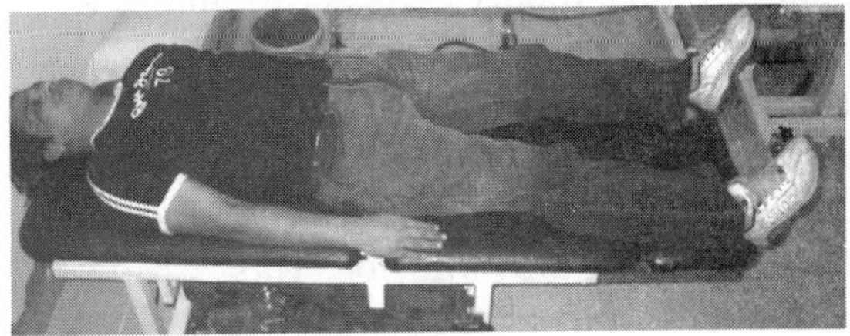

Fig. 4.8: Stride lying

i. *Half lying:* Lying on a plinth or bed with the trunk supported by a back rest or pillows in a position midway between lying and sitting upright. The legs are straight and fully supported (Fig. 4.9).

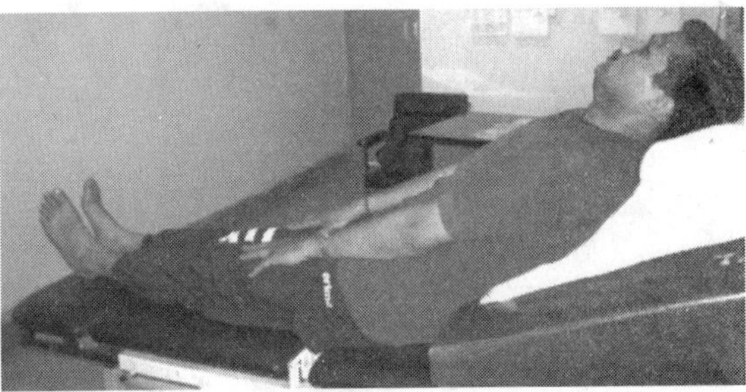

Fig. 4.9: Half lying

j. *Crook half lying:* As half lying, but the knees are flexed and the feet rest on the plinth or bed as in crook lying (Fig. 4.10).

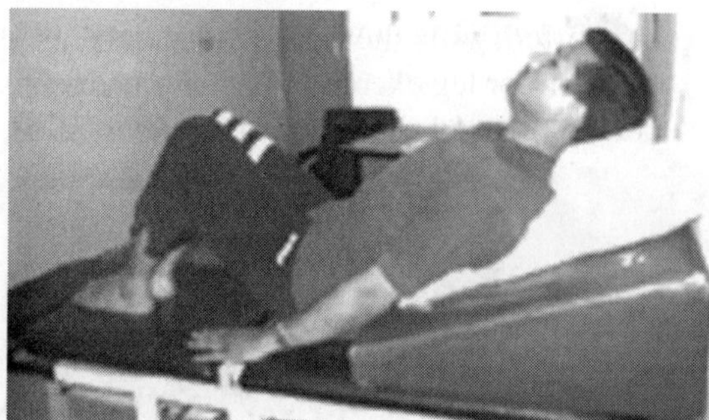

Fig. 4.10: Crook half lying

2. Sitting

Chair or stool should be used for this position. Height of chair or stool should be adjusted to keep the hip and knee 90° flexed and ankle in plantigrade position. Stools are better for movements which occurs posterior such as shoulder hyper extension. In this position muscular work of lower extremity is zero as these are fully supported on the floor. Hip flexors are in stage of static contraction to maintain hip in flexion. This is also very comfortable and stable position and most commonly used position for therapy.

The practice derived positions are:

a. *Long sitting:* Legs are straight with hips flexed at 90° and knees extended trunk is erect, commonly used for stretching purposes (Fig. 4.11).

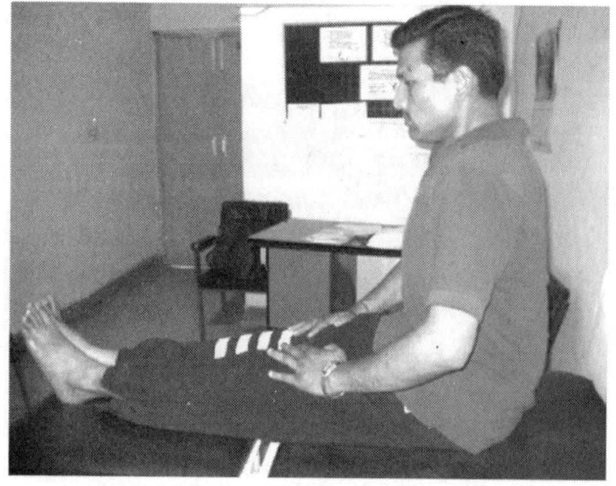

Fig. 4.11: Long sitting

b. *Sitting with legs unsupported:* The position is commonly sitting position only difference is that the legs are not supported on the floor instead they dangle in the air. The position is used mainly for knee and ankle exercises (Fig. 4.12).

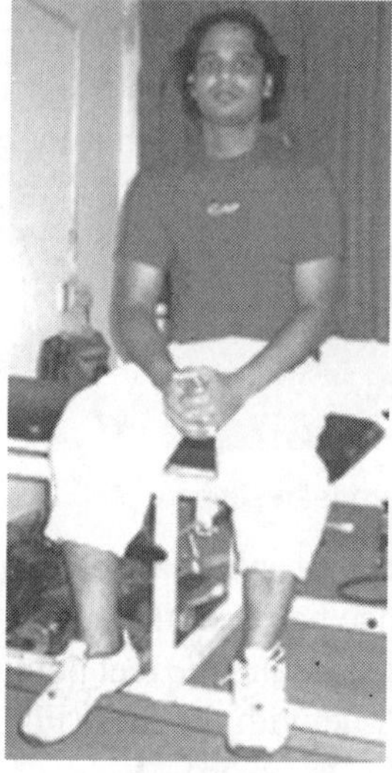

Fig. 4.12: Sitting with leg unsupported

c. *Half sitting:* Subject sits only with one buttock supported on the sitting surface. The knee of unsupported is usually flexed (Fig. 4.13).

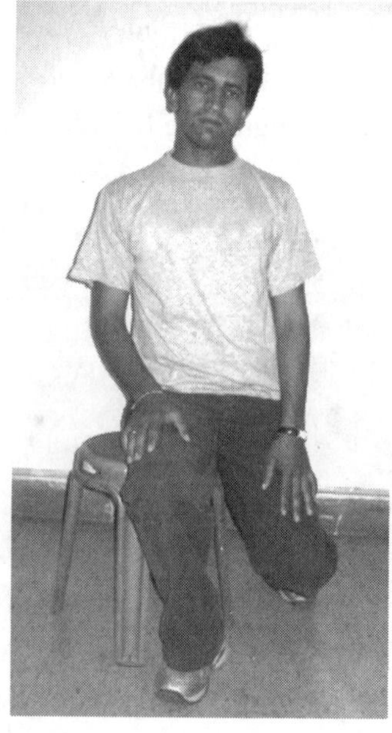

Fig. 4.13: Half sitting

d. *Forward lean sitting:* The trunk is bent forward and head supported on table with pillows (Fig. 4.14), while sitting on stool.

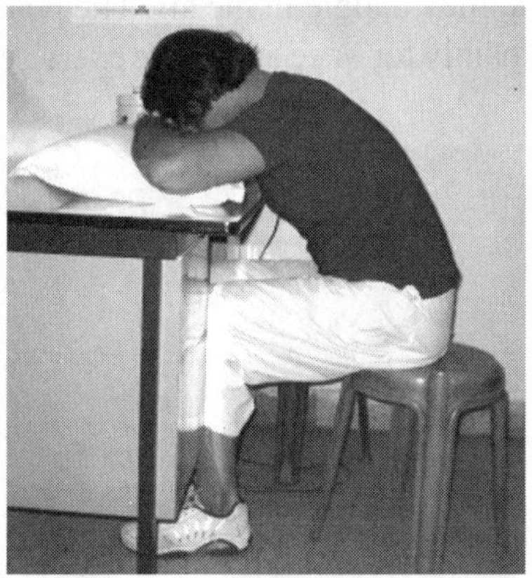

Fig. 4.14: Forward lean sitting

e. *Stride sitting:* The feet and ankles are placed apart, (one foot distance between the heels). The knees are flexed to 90° and the feet point obliquely outward in line with the legs (Fig. 4.15).

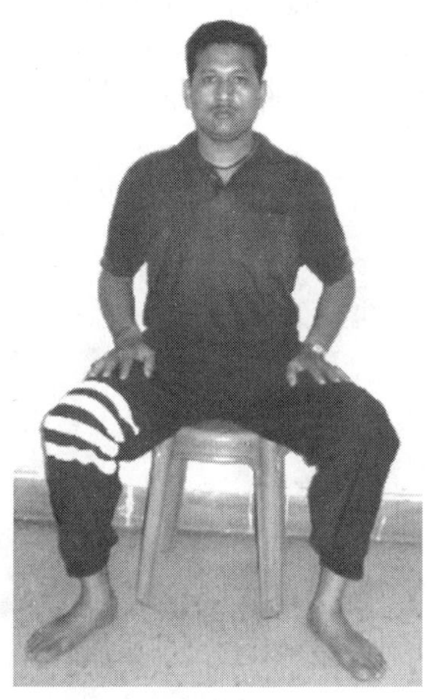

Fig. 4.15: Stride sitting

f. *Long sitting with trunk inclined backwards:* As long sitting, trunk inclined backwards

supported with the hands, a widely used position for leg exercises such as quadriceps contraction and single leg raising (Fig. 4.16).

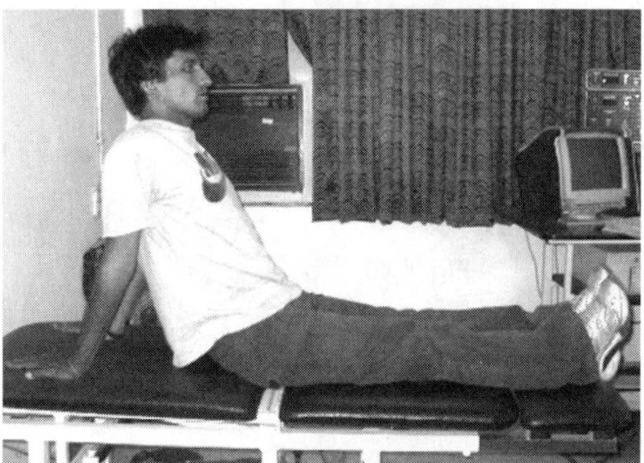

Fig. 4.16: Long Sitting with trunk inclined backward

3. Kneeling

The position is like standing the only difference is that the knees are flexed and are in contact with the surface (ground/plinth). The whole body weight comes on the knees.

The muscles below knee are in rest while others contract to maintain the posture. Extensors of the hip and flexors of the lumbar spine contract strongly to maintain the proper alignment of pelvis. This position is slightly stable than standing but uncomfortable for the subject. This is the preparatory position for the standing and used to strengthen the extensors of the hip and trunk.

The derived positions are:

a. *Kneel sitting:* It is a sitting position adopted from knee standing position with lower legs coming under the thigh (when legs are the part of body which are in contact with ground/sitting surface) (Fig. 4.17).

b. *Side sitting:* From kneel sitting position the buttocks are moved side ways so that one or both buttocks are moved sideways so that one or both buttocks rest on the ground/sitting surface (Fig. 4.18).

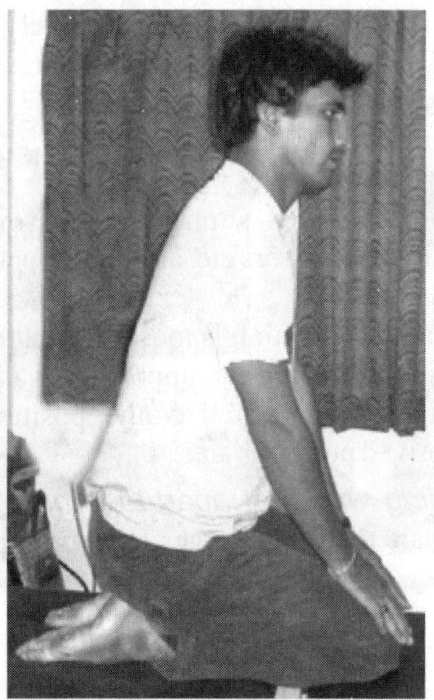

Fig. 4.17: Kneel sitting

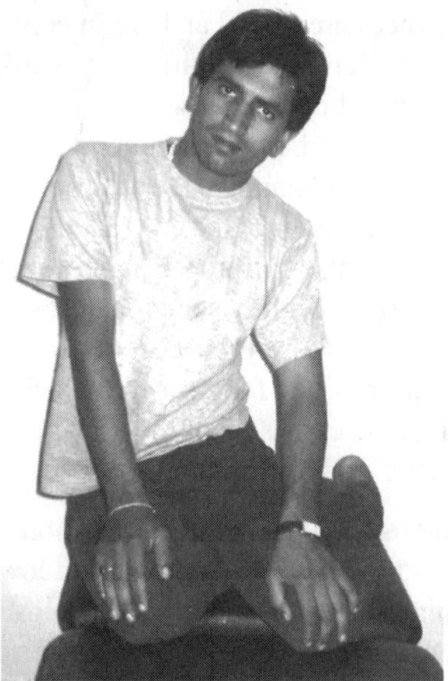

Fig. 4.18: Side sitting

c. *Half kneeling:* From kneeling position one leg is taken forward to be flexed at 90° at the hip, knee and ankle. This is a transfer stage position of standing from kneeling (4.19).

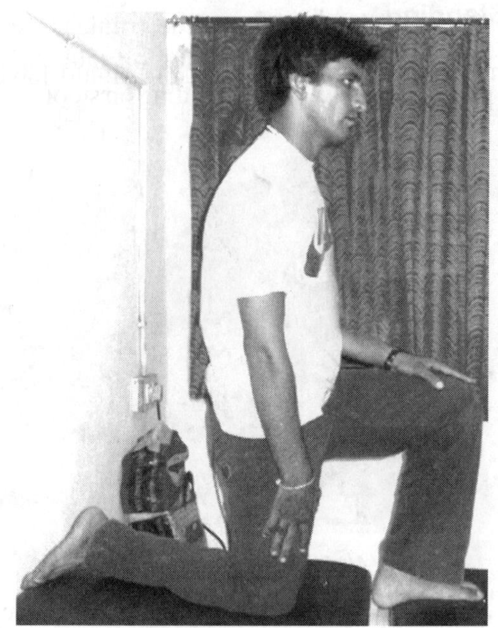

Fig. 4.19: Half kneeling

d. *Prone kneeling:* or quadruped position in which body weight is equally supported on all four limbs. Shoulder should be flexed at 90° elbow fully extended and wrist dorsiflexed with finger extended (Fig. 4.20).

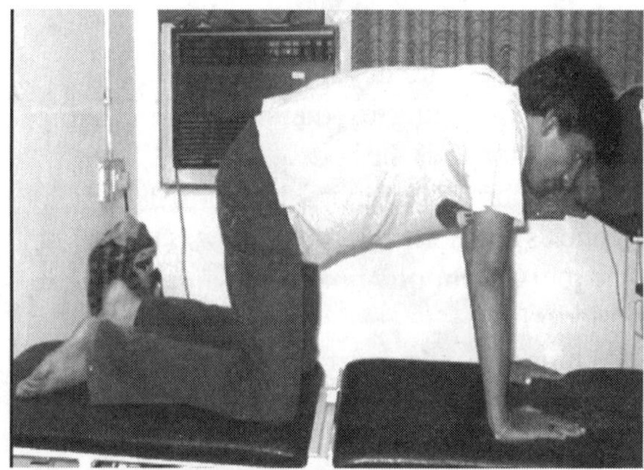

Fig. 4.20: Prone kneeling

The hip and knee should be at 90° flexion and the ankles may be plantarflexed or dorsiflexed.

4. Standing

Ideally normal standing position should have following component (Fig. 4.21):

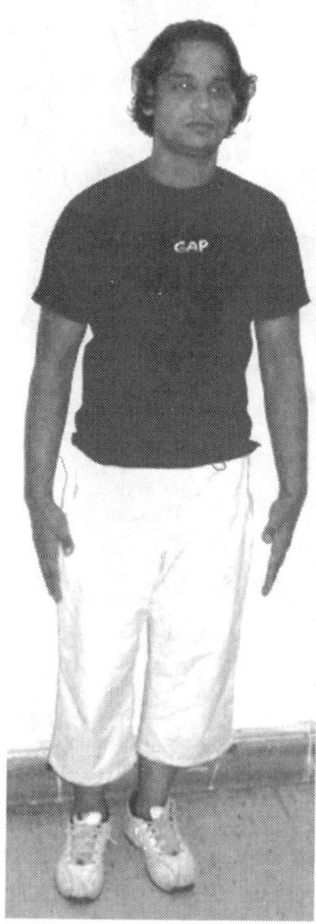

Fig. 4.21: Standing

- The head should be erect.
- The shoulders are down and back.
- The arms hanging by the sides palm facing medially towards the body.
- Spine in normal curvature (i.e. normal thoracic kyphosis and normal lumbar lordosis)
- The pelvis should not tilted anteriorly or posteriorly
- The hips are extended and slightly in external rotation
- The knees are fully extended
- The heels are together with feet apart at angle not more than 45°.

The muscles of the body part contract to maintain the normal standing posture. The main groups participating are:

1. Neck extensors
2. Spinal flexors and extensors
3. Hip extensors
4. Plantar and dorsi flexors of ankle
5. Intrinsic foot muscles.

(*Other muscles such as retractors of scapulae, knee extensors etc. also participate but in less amount).

The standing position is most difficult of all basic positions as base of support is small and COG is higher as compared to other positions.

The derived positions are:

a. *Standing with feet apart/together:* With feet apart there is a larger base of support and the subject is more stable to stand up with less muscular effort (Fig. 4.22).

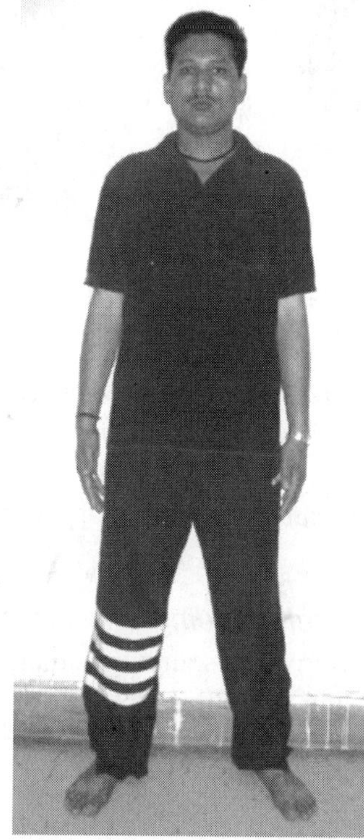

Fig. 4.22: Standing with feet apart

While with feet together base of support is narrower and the subject needs more muscular energy to maintain stability (Fig. 4.23).

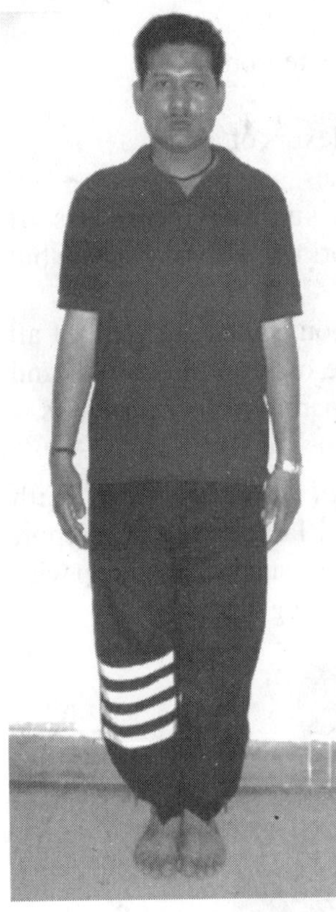

Fig. 4.23: Standing with feet together

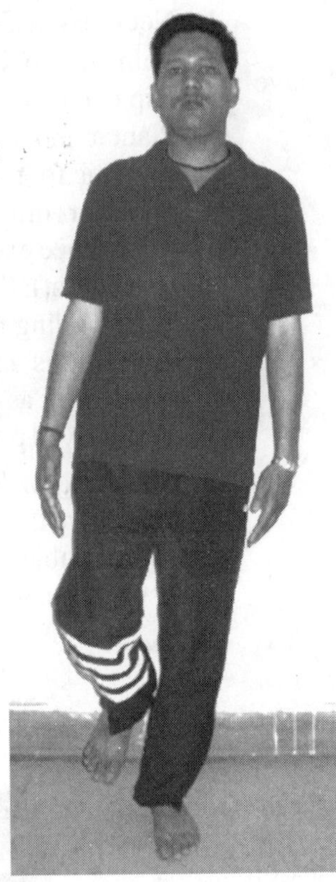

Fig. 4.24: One leg standing

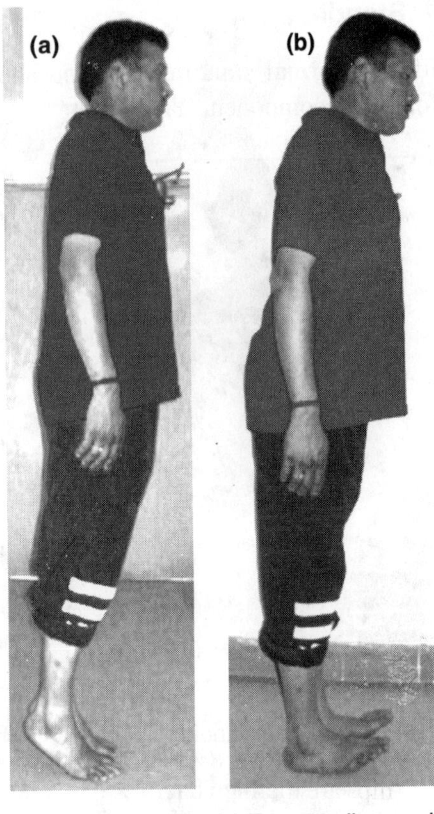

Figs 4.25a and b: (a) Toe standing, and (b) Heel standing

b. *One leg standing:* Base of support is more narrower and leg which is in contact with ground has to bear whole body weight. One of the hand can be used to support the body (Fig. 4.24).

c. *Toe and heel standing:* Smallest base of support is there. Toe standing is mainly used for increasing muscular strength of plantar flexors and also for improving balance (Figs 4.25a and b).

d. *Step standing:* Standing with one foot on a higher level than the other, as in standing on stairs with one leg on one step while other leg on other step. Foot stools or steps can also be used for this position. This position is usually used for teaching weight shift (Fig. 4.26), for stair climbing/descending.

e. *Walk forward standing:* One leg is moved/placed directly forward, so that there is a distance of 1.5 to 2 feet length between the heels (Fig. 4.27).

f. *Stoop standing:* The trunk is inclined forward from the hip joints with the spine kept straight. The movement is generally taken as far as the length of the hamstring muscles allows. The hips are inclined backwards by plantar flexion at ankle joints (Fig. 4.28).

g. *Lax stoop standing:* The spine and hip joints are flexed in a completely relaxed manner. The arms hang loosely downward, and the

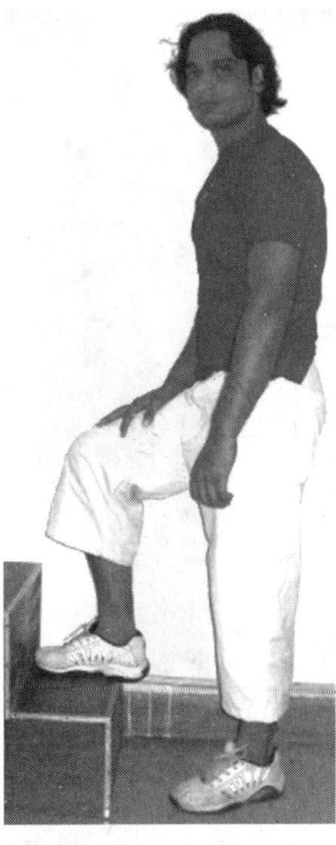

Fig. 4.26: Step standing

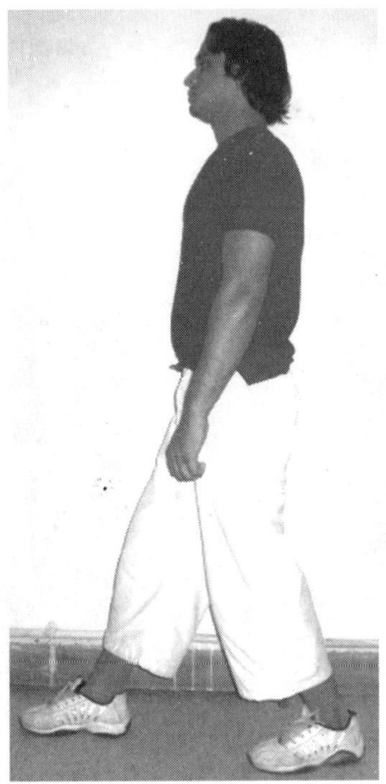

Fig. 4.27: Walk forward standing

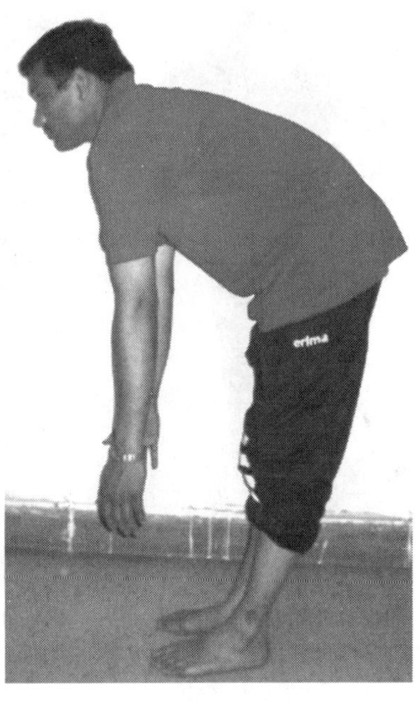

Fig. 4.28: Stoop standing

hips are inclined backward by plantar flexion at ankle joints (Fig. 4.29).

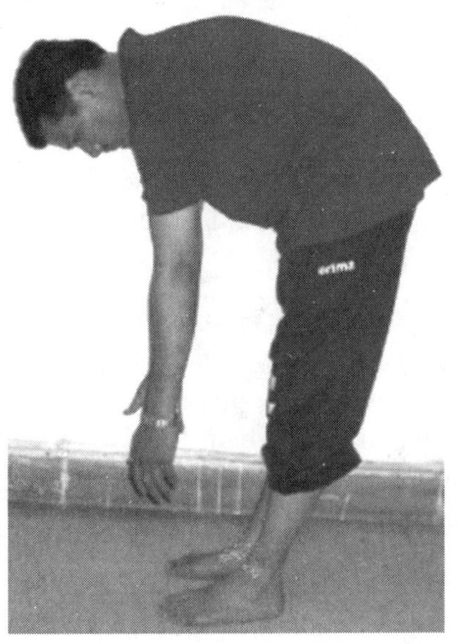

Fig. 4.29: Lax stoop standing

h. *Wing standing:* Hand rests on iliac crest, with fingers pointing forward and thumbs behind. The shoulders are dropped and the elbows kept in line with the trunk (Fig. 4.30).

i. *Neck rest standing:* Arms are held sideways in line with trunk, with shoulder joints laterally rotated and elbow joint flexed, so that fingers are placed on occiput. Palms face forward, tips of fingers touch each other, wrist and fingers are straight (Fig. 4.31).

j. *Head rest standing:* As neck rest standing but hands are placed on top of the head, with palms facing downward (Fig. 4.32).

k. *Lumbar rest standing:* As neck rest standing but shoulder joints are rotated medially and hands are placed behind lumbar spine, palm facing backward (Fig. 4.33).

l. *Reach standing: The* arms are held parallel with each other in front of the body at shoulder

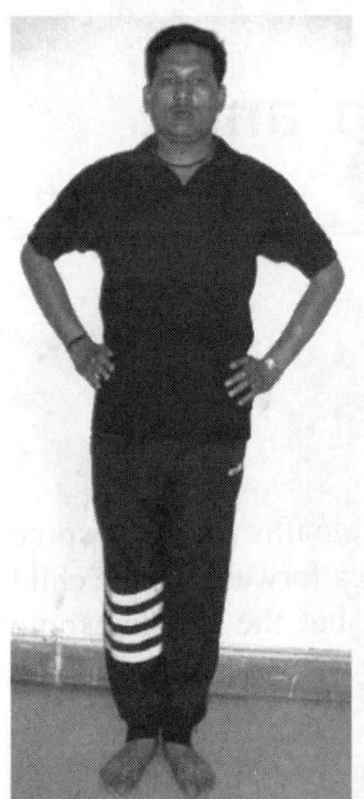

Fig. 4.30: Wing standing

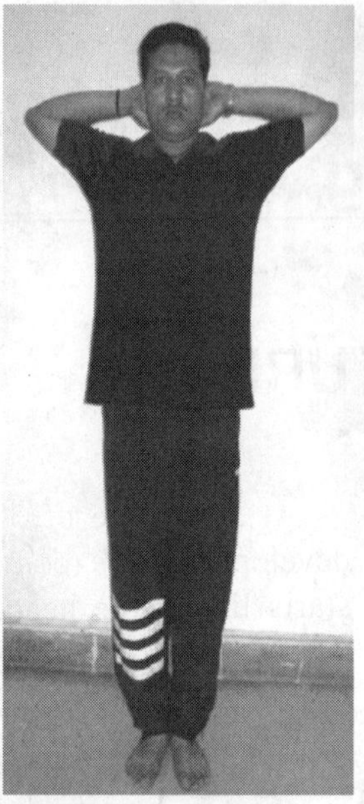

Fig. 4.31: Neck rest standing

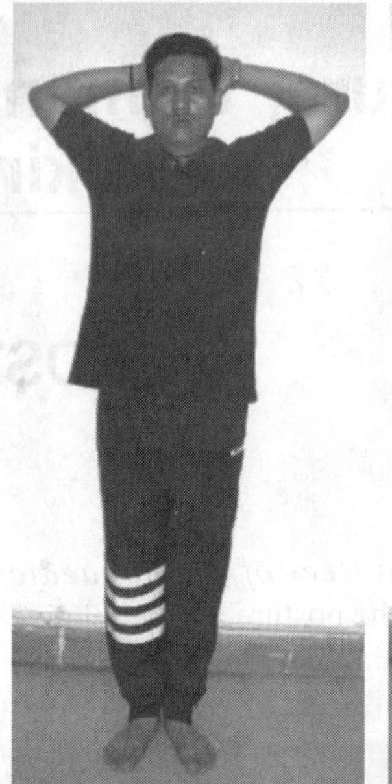

Fig. 4.32: Head rest standing

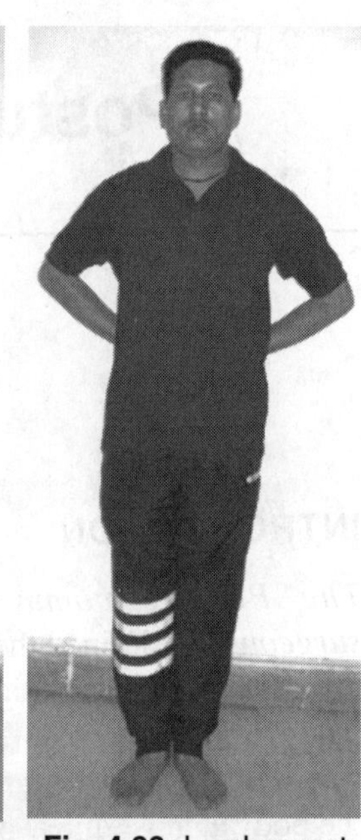

Fig. 4.33: Lumbar rest standing

level, with palm facing each other. The elbows, wrists and fingers are straight (Fig. 4.34).

Reach standing can be low or high depending upon the position of arms below or above horizontal respectively.

m. *Yard standing:* The arms are held sideways at shoulder level, with palm facing downwards (Fig. 4.35).

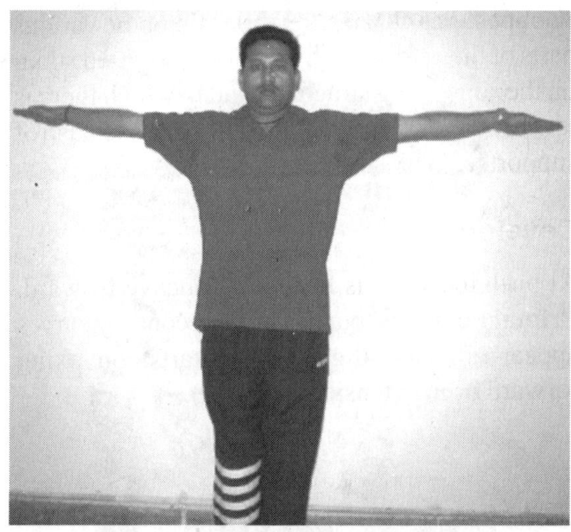

Fig. 4.35: Yard standing

Yard standing can be low or high depending upon the position of arms below or above horizontal respectively.

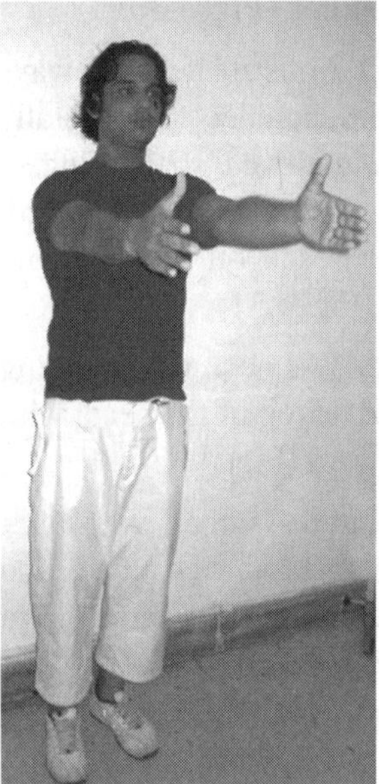

Fig. 4.34: Reach standing

CHAPTER-5

Posture, Human Locomotion and Walking Aids

POSTURE

INTRODUCTION

The Posture committee of orthopaedic surgeons has defined the posture as: the relative arrangement of the parts of the body. Good posture is the state of muscular and skeletal balance that protects the supporting structures of the body against injury or progressive deformity irrespective of the attitude (e.g. erect, lying, squatting), in which these structures are working or resting. Under such conditions, the muscles function efficiently, and the optimum positions are afforded for the thoracic and abdominal organs. Poor posture is a faulty relationship of the various parts of the body, which produces increased strain on the supporting structures and in which there is less efficient balance of the body over its base of support.

Development

At birth the spine is flexed or concave forward. **Primary curve** is found at birth, secondary curves appear as the child grows and starts convexing forward or in extension (Fig. 5.1).

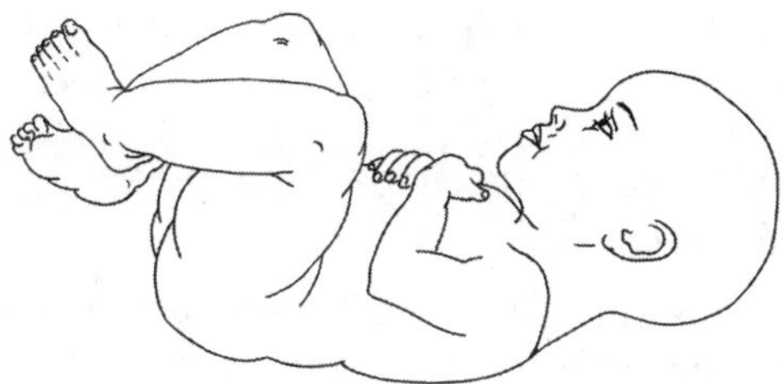

Fig. 5.1: Flexed posture in new born

At about age of 3 months cervical spine develops lordosis (convex forward) as the child starts lifting the head, but the lumbar spine develops secondary curve lumbar lordosis (convex forward) slightly later as the child begins to sit up and walk (Figs 5.2 and 5.3). The centre of gravity

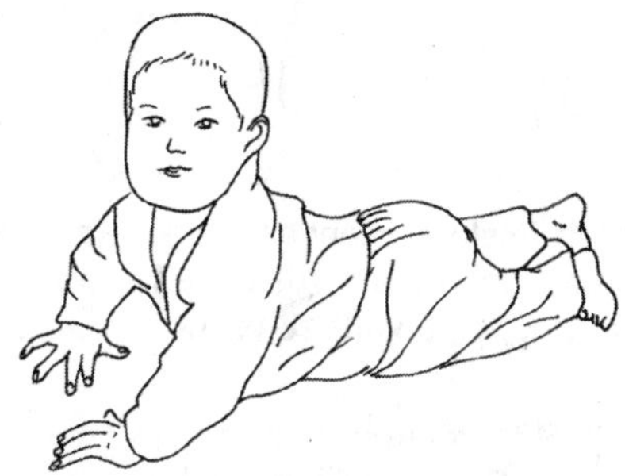

Fig. 5.2: Development of secondary curve of cervical spine

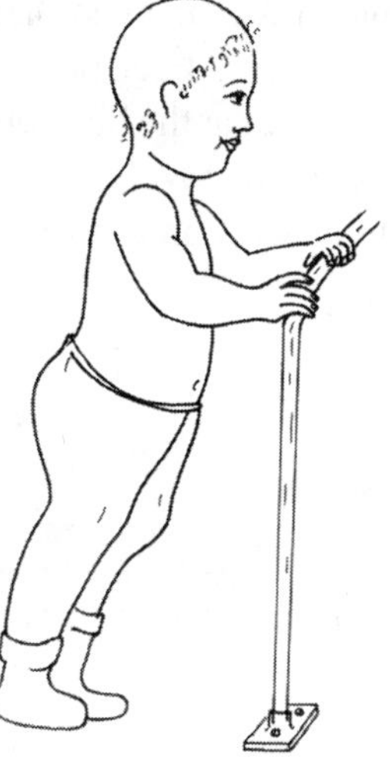

Fig. 5.3: Development of secondary curve of lumbar spine

passes through the T_{12} vertebra but as the child grows older, the centre of gravity drops, eventually reaching the level of the S2 vertebra in adult. It remains slightly higher to S2 in males. The lordosis of spine increases as the weakness of muscles of abdominal and presence of large abdominal contents, and the small pelvis characteristic of children this age (Figs 5.4a to f).

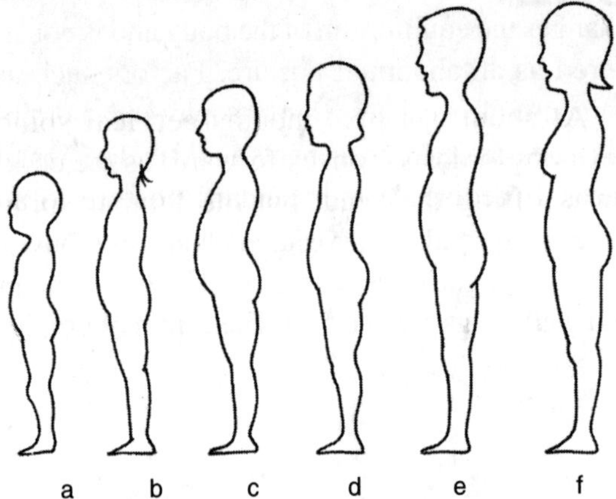

Fig. 5.4: Postural changes at age—(a) 2 years, (b) 4 years, (c) 6 years, (d) 10 years, (e) 14 years and (f) 18 years

Child starts standing at the age of 11 months with knees flexed and wide base to maintain balance. Knees remain bowed (genu varum) until about 18 months of age, then become knocked (genu valgum) until the age of 3 years, and then straighten by the age of 6 years. Feet do not develop any arch and remains flat at the birth but as the child grows medial arch develops and gradually fat pad increase in size, and muscles become strong.

Types of Posture

Static and dynamic posture

Static—lying, kneeling, sitting: The body and its segments are aligned and maintained in certain position.

Dynamic posture—walking running, jumping, thrusting and lifting—refers to postures in which the body and its segments do not remain static/constant.

Postural Control

Maintenance of Body and its Segments

Stability either in static or dynamic posture is known as postural control. Postural control requires activity of different systems of body. Mainly postural control depends on the integrity of central nervous system, visual system, vestibular and musculoskeletal system. Proprioceptors which are situated in the joints give information about the joints to central nervous system and intact central nervous system detects, predicts and receives *inputs,* and responds to all of these inputs with appropriate output to maintain the posture (equilibrium) of the body.

According to Horak the ability to maintain stability in the erect standing posture is a skill that the central nervous system learns using information from passive biomechanical elements, sensory system, and muscles. The central nervous system interprets and organizes inputs from the various structures and systems and selects responses based on past experience of the goal of the response.

Role of Muscles in Posture Control

Muscles play an important role to maintain the center of gravity of the body in its position. In erect standing the center of gravity passes through the S2 vertebra and requires minimal muscle interaction. The center of gravity passes from lumbar/vertebra through the S2 to between the feet.

Stabilization of the Spinal Column by the Muscles of Trunk

The trunk muscles including-the abdominals, erector spinae, psoas major, quadratus lumborum and the muscles of the neck such as trapezius, scalenes, and levator scapulae all serve as a stabilizing guide wire. These muscles provide dynamic control of the posture against the force of the gravity as the weight of various segments shift away from the base of support.

– When the body moves forward, the center of gravity shifts anteriorly, the extensor muscles such as the erector spinae, and posterior neck muscles such as trapezius contract eccentrically and provide the stability to the spine.

– When the body moves backward, the center of gravity shifts posteriorly, the flexor muscles such as rectus abdominals, and intercostals as well as psoas major, anterior scalenes, the capitis musculature and sternocleidomastoid (SCM) contract eccentrically and provide the stability to the spine.

– When the body moves to one side, the center of gravity shifts to the lateral side, the muscles of contralateral side such as psoas major, quadratus lumborum, erector spinae, the internal and external oblique, the sternomastoid, scalenes, and intercostal muscles provide the stability to the spine.

Standard Posture

It refers to an ideal posture rather than an average or normal posture. The standard posture is examined from two views (back and side). In the back view, a line of reference represents a plane that coincides with the midline of the body. This begins from a point in between the heels and extends upward between the lower extremities through the mid point of the pelvis, spine and skull, and divides the body into right and left halves. Both right and left of the skeletal structures are essentially symmetrical. The two halves of the body are assumed in equilibrium.

In the side view, the vertical line of reference begins at the calcaneocuboid joint and extends to a point slightly anterior to the center of the knee joint, slightly posterior to the center of the hip joint,

through the sacral promontory, through the bodies of the lumbar vertebrae, through the dens, through the external auditory meatus and slightly posterior to the apex of the coronal sutures. This vertical line of reference divides the body in to anterior and posterior parts. Around this line of reference, the body is hypothetically in a position of equilibrium.

Any deviation from the standard posture, changes the equilibrium of the body and is considered as an abnormal posture. Factors such as pain, muscle weakness (hypertrophy and shortening), anatomical impairments and developmental factors predispose the standard posture to an abnormal posture.

FAULTY OR ABNORMAL POSTURES

1. An Excessive Lordosis (Fig. 5.5)

Lordosis is the normal curve (anterior covexity) of the cervical and lumbar spine which is found in all normal individuals. In normal lumbar lordosis the angle of pelvis is found approximately 30°. In excessive lumbar lordosis the pelvis tilts anteriorly and the angle of pelvis increases to 40°. In excessive cervical lordosis there is sagging of the shoulders, medial rotation of the arms and poking forward of the head so that it is in front of the center of gravity.

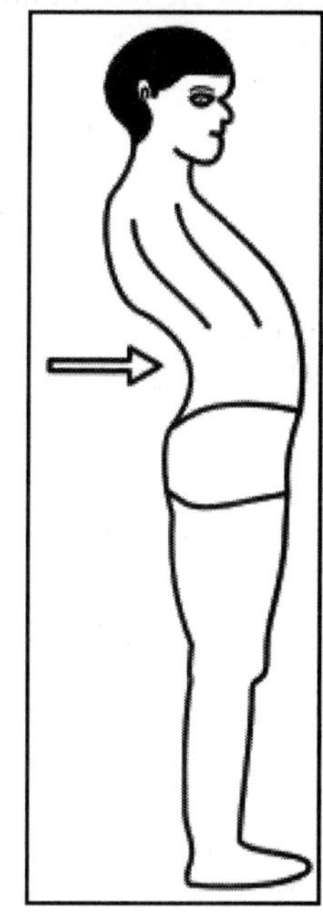

Fig. 5.5: Excessive lumbar lordosis

Common Causes of Excessive Lumbar Lordosis:

1. Weakness of muscles (Abdominals).
2. Tightness or contracture of hip flexors (Ilio psoas).

3. Congenital problems, such as bilateral congenital dislocation of the hip.
4. Pregnancy.
5. High heel shoes/foot wears.
6. Spondylolisthesis.
7. Postural deformity.
8. Anterior tilt of pelvis as result of weak extensor of hip and abdominals.
9. Tightness or shortening of cervical extensors.

2. Kyphotic Lordotic Posture

It's a faulty posture in which lumbar spine and cervical spine get hyperextended while thoracic spine gets flexed and head becomes slightly forward. The pelvis tilts anteriorly and hip joints get flexed. Slight hyperextension of knees and plantar flexion of ankle joints may also be noted (Fig. 5.6).

Causes:
1. Shortening or tightness of extensors of cervical spine and lumbar spine and flexors of hip joint.
2. Weakness of neck flexors, upper back extensors (Erector spinae) and hamstring muscles.
3. Bony anomaly.

Generally in anterior tilt of pelvis, abdominals get elongated but in this posture excessive flexion of thoracic spine offsets the effect of the anterior pelvic tilt.

3. Sway Back Posture

Sway back is a faulty posture in which head becomes slightly forward, there is extension of the cervical spine, flexion of thoracic and loss of lordosis of lumbar spine. Extension of hip and knee joint during standing are also the features of sway back posture. Ankle joints remain in neutral position (Fig. 5.7). Pelvis rotates posteriorly.

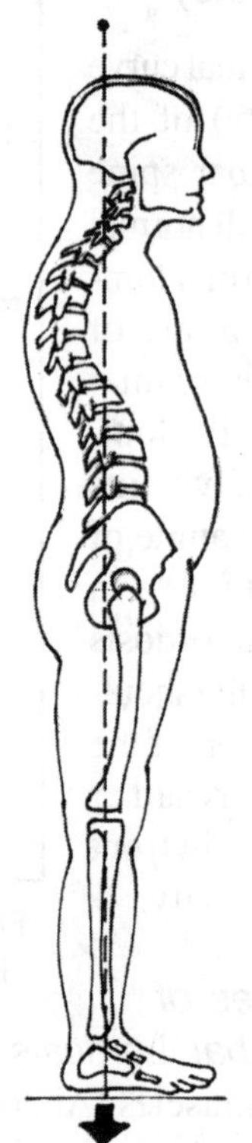

Fig. 5.6: Kyphosis-Lordosis posture

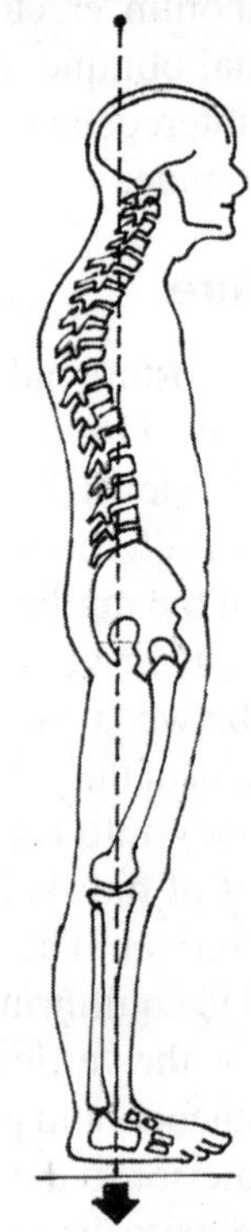

Fig. 5.7: Sway back posture

Causes of Sway Back

1. Tightness of hamstrings, and abdominal muscles.
2. Weakness of one joint iliopsoas.
3. Bony anomaly.

Mechanisms of Sway back tightness of hamstring muscles pulls the pelvis posteriorly, which causes extension at the hip and flexion at the lumbar spine. Flexion or decreased lordosis of lumbar spine causes compensatory curve in the thoracic spine in which thoracic spine flexes and gets deviated in backward direction (upper back).

4. Flat Back Posture (Fig. 5.8)

Flat back is a faulty posture in which whole lumbar and thoracic spine gets flattened. Although the causes and symptoms of both flat back and sway back are common but can be differentiated by excessive flexion and backward deviation of the upper thoracic spine in sway back posture, while in flat back posture spine becomes almost straight.

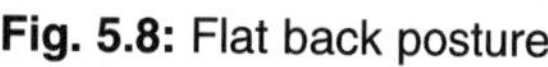

Fig. 5.8: Flat back posture

5. Forward Head Posture

It is a faulty posture which is characterized by excessive extension of the cervical spine and flexion of the lower cervical and upper thoracic spine (Fig. 5.9).

Common causes: This posture is generally caused by occupational activities which require forward head posture such as:

1. Working on computer which is slightly higher than the position of head,
2. Enthusiastically watching match on television for prolonged time also predisposes to this type of faulty posture.
3. Using of high pillow under the neck.

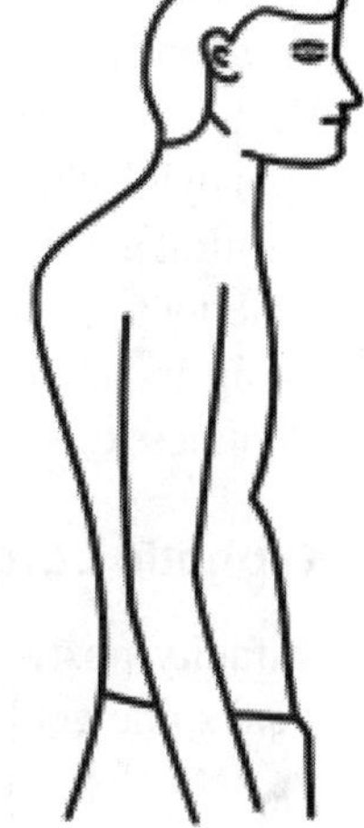

Fig. 5.9: Forward head posture

6. Flat Neck Posture

It is an abnormal posture which is characterized by any increased flexion of the occiput on atlas and decreased lordosis of the cervical spine.

Common causes: Activity which requires straightening of cervical spine predisposes to this type of posture. Such as soldiers keep their upper back straight (attention position) for prolonged period of time, using high pillow under the head, and spasm of cervical muscles.

7. Scoliosis

Bending of the vertebral column to one side, combined with rotation of the vertebral bodies toward the convexity, and the spinous processes toward the concavity. It may be single structural curve, double structural curve, S-shaped curve and gravity collapsed C curve. Scoliosis can be measured on X-rays by using cobes and rib-vertebral angle methods (Fig. 5.10).

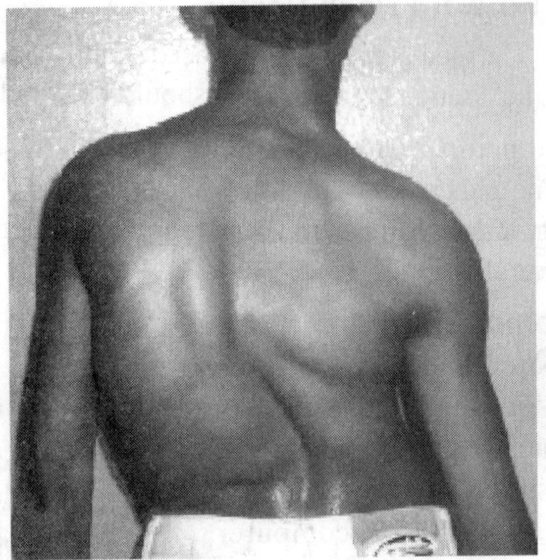

Fig. 5.10: Scoliosis

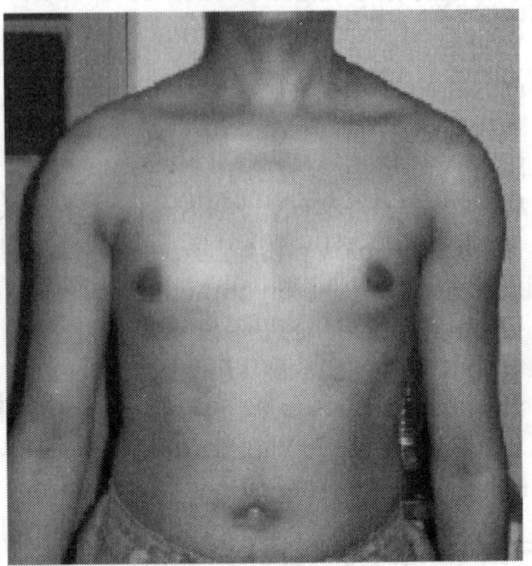

Fig. 5.12: Anterior view

ASSESSMENT OF POSTURE (ADULT)

It is always difficult to assess the posture, as patient *(usually females)* feels uncomfortable while undressing. Ideally male patient should be in shorts and female patients be in a bra and shorts, without wearing shoes. For privacy of female patient sometimes male therapist can be assisted by female therapist. On observation, therapist must observe the bony anomalies, muscle wasting/atrophy, muscle tightness, position of joints, range of motion, swelling and curve of spine (Fig. 5.11).

Assessment of Posture in Standing

The whole posture is assessed from head to toes in different views lateral view, posterior view and anterior view.

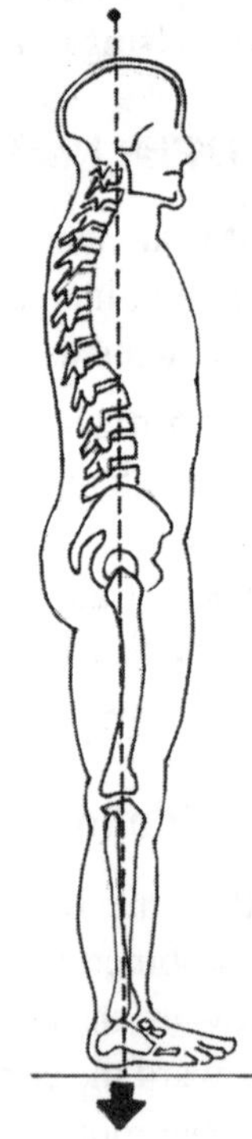

Fig. 5.11: Normal posture

Anterior View (Fig. 5.12)

Position of head: Any deviation of head should be noted. Muscle tightness or contracture (sternocleidomastoid) can cause the head to rotate to one side. This condition is known as torticollis.

In normal individual when line is drawn from tip of the nose it passes through the manubrium, sternum, xiphisternum, and umbilicus. Any deviation should be noted and considered as abnormal.

The sternoclavicular and acromio clavicular joint should be in symmetry. Any abnormality swelling, subluxation or dislocation should be noted.

Shoulders: should be in level generally dominant shoulder lies slightly lower.

Muscle atrophy of upper trapezius (bilateral) and pectoralis should be observed carefully.

Any protrusion, depression and lateral deviation of the sternum, ribs, or costocartilage should be noted.

Waist angles should be equal and the arms should be equidistance from the waist. In scoliosis waist angle is disturbed and it should be measured carefully.

- The carrying angle at each elbow should be observed carefully, normal carrying angle varies from 5° to 15°.
- The high points of the iliac crest should be at the same height on each side. In scoliosis the one iliac crest becomes higher than the other.
- In normal person when he or she is standing, both the ASIS should have same distance from umbilicus The distance changes with scoliosis and limb length discrepancy.
- Both knees should be straight and any deviation such as genu valgum and varus should be noted. In normal person while standing, when both feet are together both knees should not touch each other.

Tibial Torsion

In normal person the quadriceps angle is found 14° in males and 18° in females. In valgus the quadriceps angle is increased and is associated with lateral deviation of the tibia. The quadriceps angle is decreased in varus and is associated with internal rotation of the tibia. Examination of quadriceps angle → a line is drawn from anterior superior iliac spine to the tip of patella and another line is drawn from tip of patella to the tibial tuberosity, the goniometer's fulcrum is placed over the tip of patella, the static arm over the line above the patella and movable arm is placed over the line which is drawn from tip of patella to tibial tuberosity, then the quadriceps angle is measured.

Bilateral bow legs can be recorded by measuring the distance between the knees with the legs held in full extension and heels touching. It should be less than 6 cm.
- Bow legs in babies and knock knees in 4-year-old children are so common that they are considered to be normal stage of development.

The feet angle: It is usually measured as 10° (both tibias are normally rotated laterally at 10°) which is considered normal.

Medial arch which is present in the medial border of the foot should be equal on both feet, decreased arch is known as flat foot (Pes planus) and increased arch is known as Pes cavus.

The medial malleolus is placed slightly anterior to the lateral. Any deviation should be noted.

Posterior View

Clinician should observe the following structures carefully (Fig. 5.13):

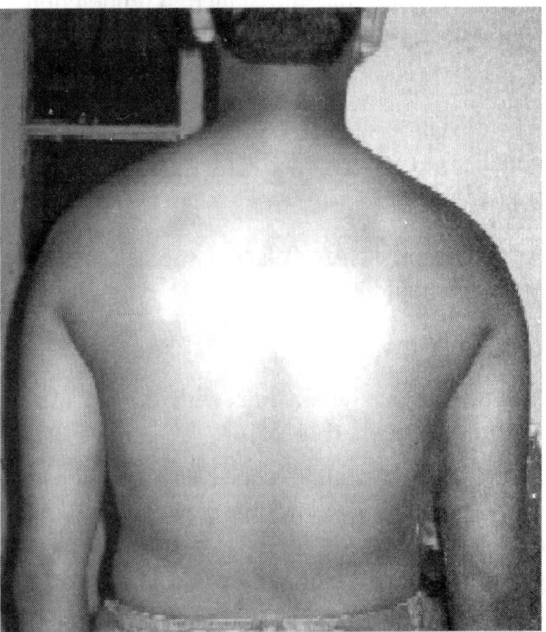

Fig. 5.13: Posterior view

Cervical spine: Lateral deviation and rotation.
Shoulder girdle:
- Subluxation and dislocation
- Level of tip of acromion process
- Muscle wasting—trapezius, rhomboides, serratus anterior etc.

Thoracic spine-level of scapula: The inferior angle of both scapula should be at the same level. In scoliosis the convexity side's scapula and the shoulder become higher than the concavity side scapula and shoulder. When the distance is measured from mid thoracic to the arms, the convexity side arm is closer than the concavity side arm.

Pelvis and Lumbar Spine

- Normal curve of the lumbar spine
- Level of both PSIS
- Level of iliac crests
- Drooping of pelvis.

Hip Joints

May be observed in single and both limb loading to see the muscular imbalance. Trendelenburg sign is observed in single limb loading.

Knees

Any deviation such as valgus or varus should be noted.

Feet

Any deviation such as pronation, supination, valgus or varus should be noted.

Lateral View

Head: The ear lies in line with the tip of the acromion process (Fig. 5.14).

Neck: The curvature of cervical spine—the cervical spine has got lordotic curve at the upper region, which is considered as a normal curve of the cervical spine. Normally when a line is drawn from ear it passes in the line of tip of acromion process. In excessive lordosis of cervical spine, line passes anterior to the tip of acromion process and posteriorly in case of straightening of cervical spine.

Shoulder girdle: Alignment of glenohumeral joint—sulcus appearance between the head of humerus and acromion process gives clues about inferior subluxation of the glenohumeral joint. To confirm it a finger is placed on the sulcus (between head of humerus and acromion process) and is pushed into the joint. The normal joint does not allow the finger to move into the joint. If finger moves slightly into the joint and allows the articular surfaces (head of humerus and glenoidfossa) to get separated, a subluxation is considered. A large sulcus between head of humerus and acromion process gives appearance of dislocation.

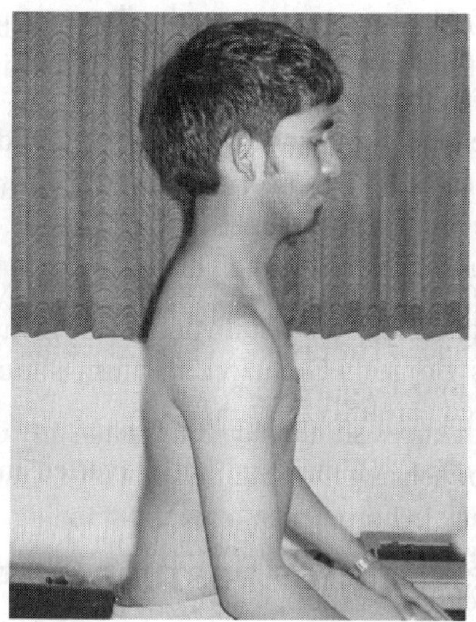

Fig. 5.14: Lateral view of posture

Thoracic spine and chest—Thoracic spine has got the normal kyphotic curve. Excessive kyphosis of the thoracic spine places head forward (decreases lumbar lordosis).

Lumbar spine and pelvis—Lumbar spine has got normal lordotic curve. Normal pelvic angle is considered as 30°. Weak abdominals and tight iliopsoas muscle causes excessive lumbar lordosis and anterior tilt of pelvis. While spasm or tightness of lower back extensors and hamstring muscles flatten the lumbar spine (posterior tilt of the pelvis).

Forward bending—During this movement 70° flexion occurs at hip joint and 40° at lumbar spine this is also known as lumbopelvicrhythm. Patients with restriction of lumbar spine movement flexes hip joint excessively and compensates the lumbar movement. Similarly restriction in the hip joint, compensates by excessive flexion of the lumbar spine. Clinician must observe the abnormal movement of lumbo-pelvic rhythm. Patient is allowed to stand up in erect standing position, or sitting (if not able to stand up). Therapist stands by the side of patient (facing lateral view of the body) and observes following structures from head to toes:

Hip joint—In erect standing hip joint lies in neutral position. Weakness of iliopsoas places the hip joint into extension. While weakness of gluteus maximus or tightness of iliopsoas cause flexion in standing position with excessive lordosis of lumbar spine.

Knee joint—Knee joint lies at 0°-5° of flexion in erect standing. Contracture of hamstring muscles causes flexion. Genu recurvatum should be observed carefully.

Ankle joint—Remains slightly everted in individuals.

ASSESSMENT OF POSTURE (INFANT)

When a baby's posture is assessed an examiner must keep the normal limits of the developmental milestones in mind. Normally baby starts standing and walking at the age of 12 months soon after the crawling. To assess the posture of baby before the age of 12 months an examiner needs to hold the baby at both the axilla. In abnormal cases where developmental milestones are delayed examiner has to hold the baby even after 12 months.

The head, trunk, upper extremities and lower extremities are observed carefully when the baby stands with or without support (0-12 months). Detection of abnormal developmental milestones helps the therapist to make an appropriate scheme of management.

If child does not poses normal posture, it may have one of three types of abnormal posture:
a. Floppy
b. Spastic
c. Athetoid.

Head

Normal Development

0-03 months: Hold the baby at the both axilla your fingers lies at the axilla while the thumb over the anterior aspect of the shoulder joint.

Response: Bobbing of head (Fig. 5.15).

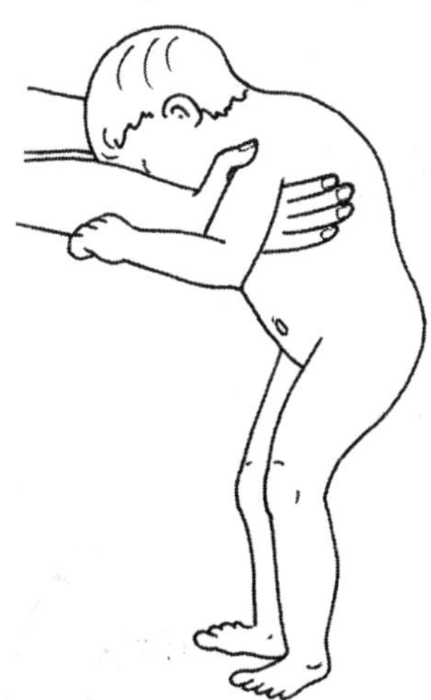

Fig. 5.15

03 months and above: The baby is held in the same position as 03 months.

Response: The baby is able to hold the head upright in mid position (Fig. 5.16).

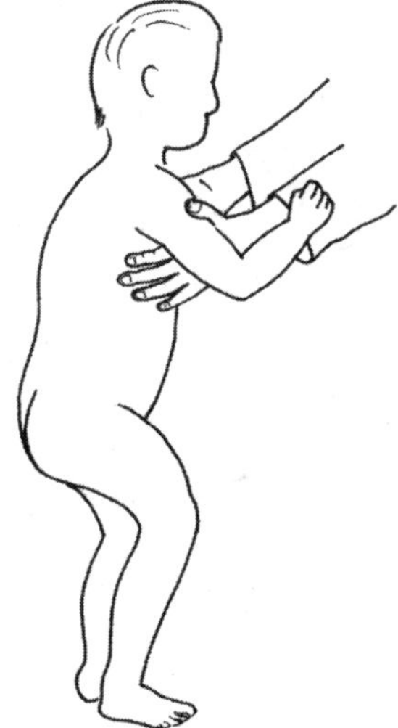

Fig. 5.16

Abnormal Development

Following abnormal responses of head may be observed by an examiner when baby is held at the axilla:

1. Flopping of head backward (Fig. 5.17).
2. Flopping of head forward (Fig. 5.18).
3. Retraction of the head to either the right or the left side (Fig. 5.19).
4. Head stiffly flexed (Fig. 5.20).

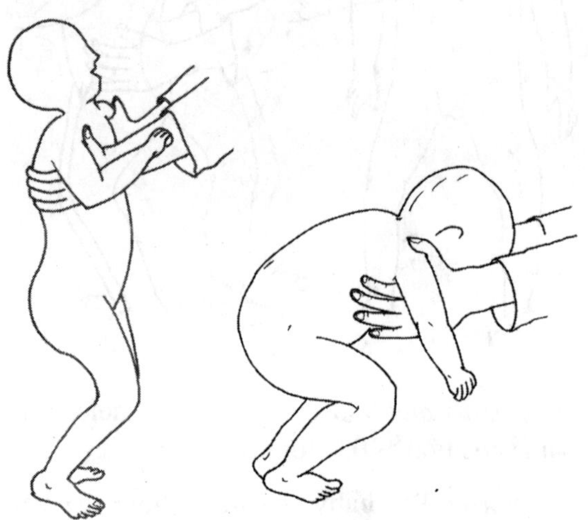

Fig. 5.17   **Fig. 5.18**

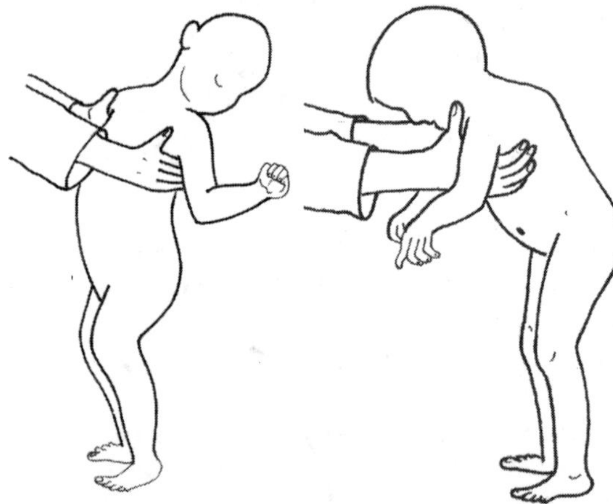

Fig. 5.19   **Fig. 5.20**

Shoulders

Normal Development

0-03 months baby is held in standing position.

Response: Elevation of both shoulders (Fig. 5.21).

0-03 months and above baby is held in standing position.

Response: Both shoulders are kept in neutral alingment with head upright position (Fig. 5.22).

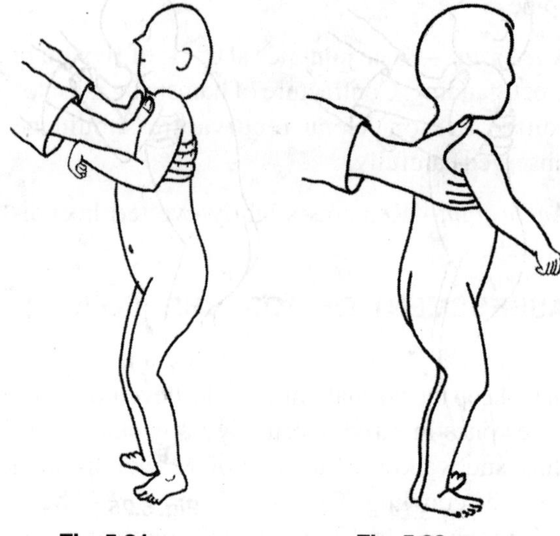

Fig. 5.21   **Fig. 5.22**

Abnormal Development

Baby is held in standing position by the examiner, the following abnormal response of shoulders may be noted:

1. Retraction of one or both shoulders (Fig. 5.23).

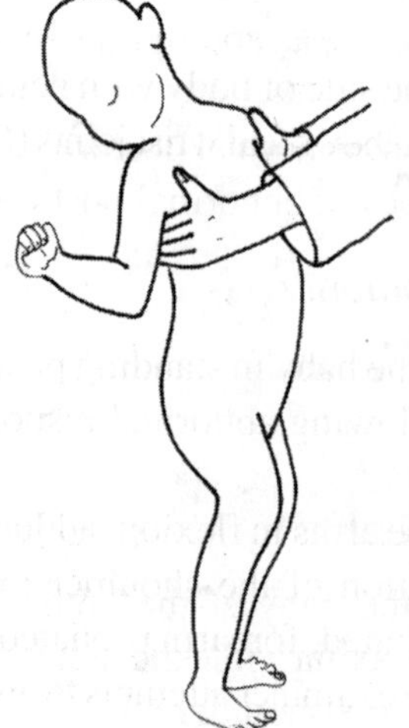

Fig. 5.23

2. Protraction of one or both shoulders (Fig. 5.24).
3. Elevation of the shoulders because of hypo-tonicity of the muscles (Fig. 5.25).

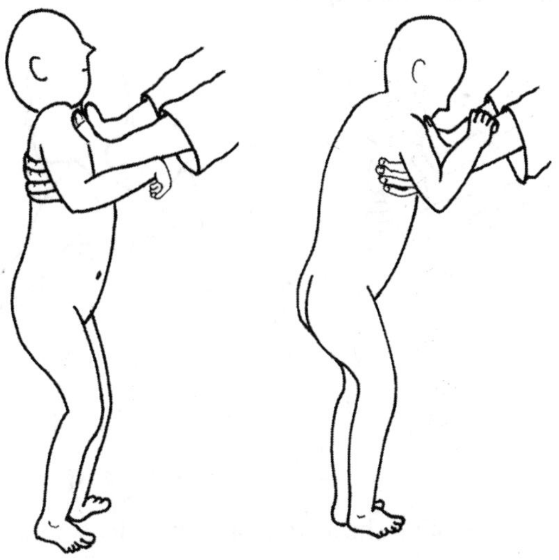

Fig. 5.24   Fig. 5.25

Arms

Normal Development

0-03 months baby is held in standing position.

Response: Arms remain at semiflexed position (at shoulders, elbows and wrist joints).

03 months and above baby is held in standing position.

Response: Arms at the side of body with neutral position at shoulders, elbows and wrist joints (Fig. 5.26).

Abnormal Development

The examiner holds the baby in standing position and observes the following abnormal responses of the arms:

1. Baby positions the arms in flexion, adduction and internal rotation of the shoulder joints, keeps elbow extended, forearm pronated and wrist flexed. If the examiner attempts to abduct

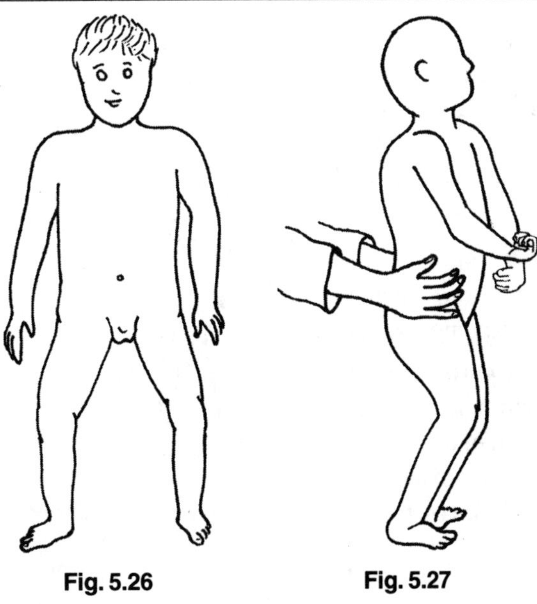

Fig. 5.26   Fig. 5.27

the shoulder joint, flex the elbow, supinate the forearm and extends the wrist joint, the baby offers resistance to all these movements (Fig. 5.27).

2. Wide abduction of the shoulder with flexion of elbows, pronation of forearm and flexion of wrist. If examiner attempts to extend the elbow joint, supinates the forearm and extends the wrist joint the baby offers resistance to all these movements (Fig. 5.28).

Trunk

Normal Development

0-03 months baby is held at the axilla in standing position.

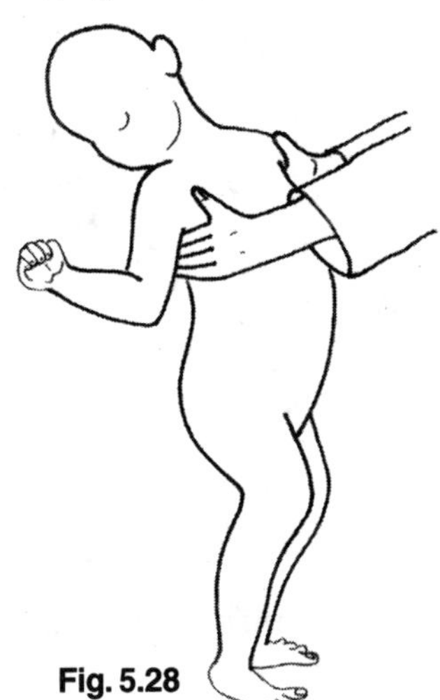

Fig. 5.28

Response: Generalized flexion of the trunk in symmetrical alignment with the head and the limbs.

0-03 months and above baby is held in standing position.

Response: Upright symmetrical alignment of the trunk in relation to the head and extremities (Fig. 5.29).

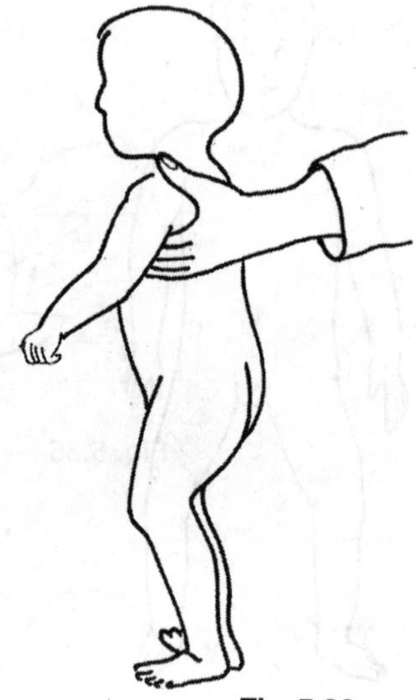

Fig. 5.29

Abnormal Development

The examiner holds the baby at the axilla in standing position and observes the following abnormal responses:

1. The infant tends to fall forward or side- ways caused by *flexor* hypertonicity. Hypotonicity of the *extensors* of the trunk are unable to hold the trunk in upright symmetrical alignment (Fig. 5.30). This posture is very uncommon.

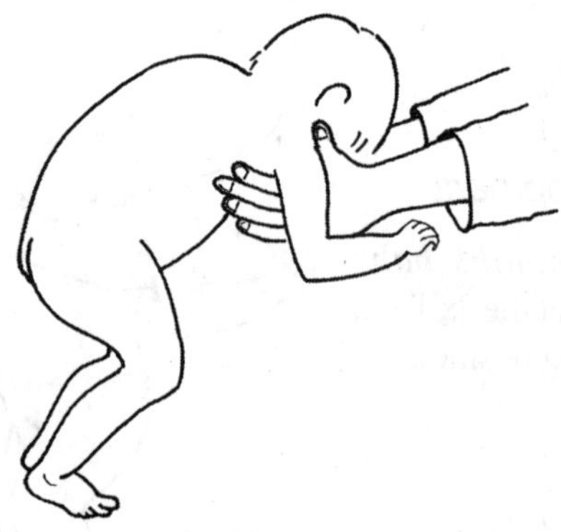

Fig. 5.30

2. The infant attempts to fall backward. *Cause*—hypertonicity (spasticity) in the extensors of back (extensor synergy-cervical,

dorsal and lumbar) causes excessive extension of the trunk (Fig. 5.31).

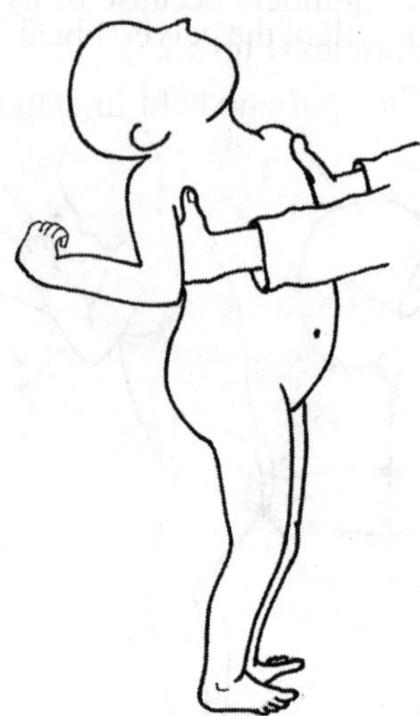

Fig. 5.31

3. The infant shows dystonic pattern by a sudden excessive extension of the trunk which is followed by trunk flexion (Figs 5.32a and b).

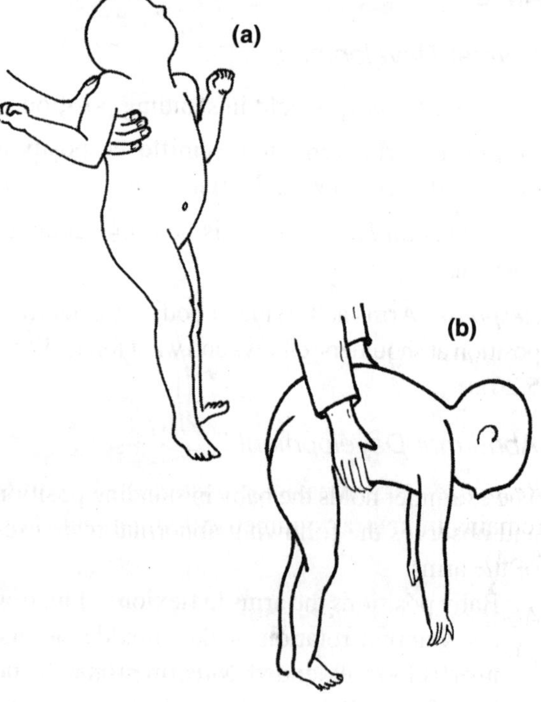

Figs 5.32a and b

Pelvis

Normal Development

0-03 months Anterior tilt of the pelvis (Fig. 5.33).

03 months and above baby is held in standing position.

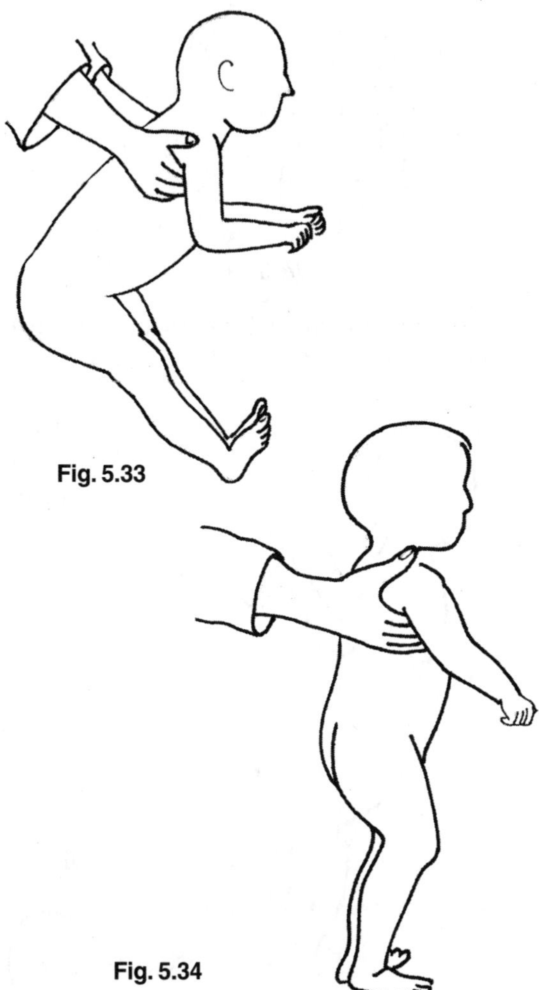

Fig. 5.33

Fig. 5.34

Response: No anterior or posterior tilt, pelvis remains in neutral symmetrical alignment (Fig. 5.34).

Abnormal Development

1. Anterior pelvic tilt caused by increased flexor spasticity.

2. Posterior pelvic tilt—(Fig. 5.35).
3. Retraction of pelvic—(Figs 5.36a and b).

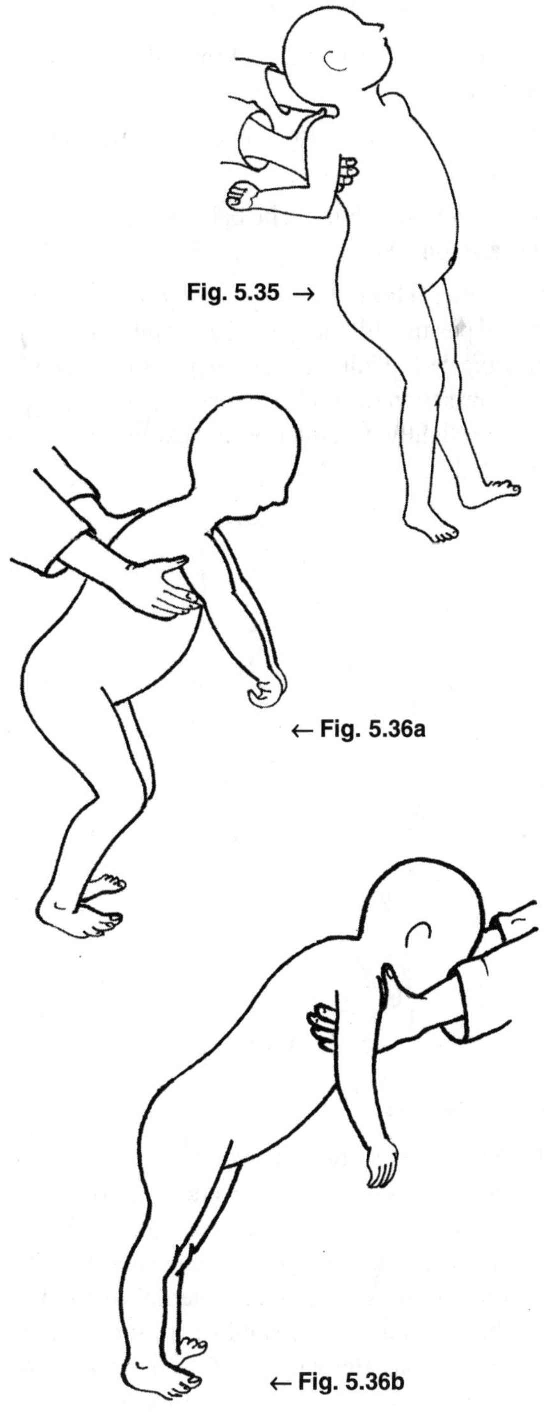

Fig. 5.35 →

← Fig. 5.36a

← Fig. 5.36b

60 Exercise Therapy

Hip Joints

Normal Development

0-03 months: The infant is held at axilla in standing posture.

Response: Flexion (45°) abduction and external rotation.

03 months and above: The baby is held in standing position.

Response: The baby keeps hip joints at semi-flexed position till the age of six months and starts keeping the hip joints in neutral position gradually by contraction of hip extensors. The baby keeps the hip slightly in abduction and external rotation (Fig. 5.37).

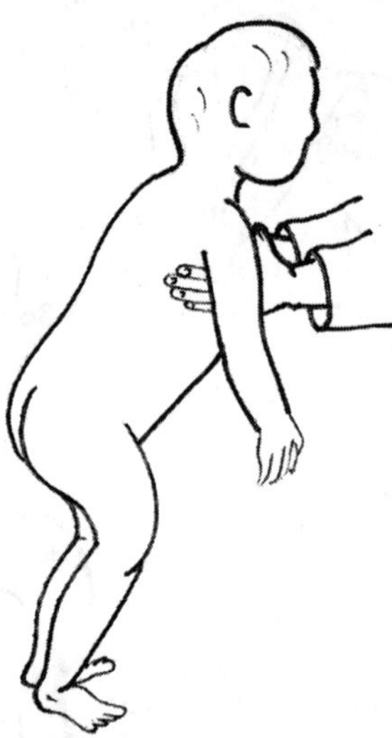

Fig. 5.37

Abnormal Development

1. Flexion, abduction and external rotation of the hip joint when examiner attempts to extend the hip joint, baby offers resistance to extension cause-flexor hypertonicity (Fig. 5.38).
2. Extension adduction and internal rotation of the hip joint. When examiner attempts to flex, abduct and externally rotate the hip joint, baby offers resistance to all these movements cause

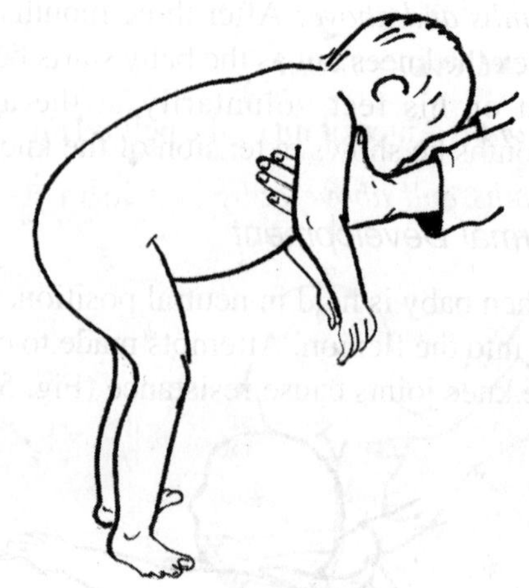

Fig. 5.38

hypertonicity of the adductors (extensor hypertonicity) (Fig. 5.39).

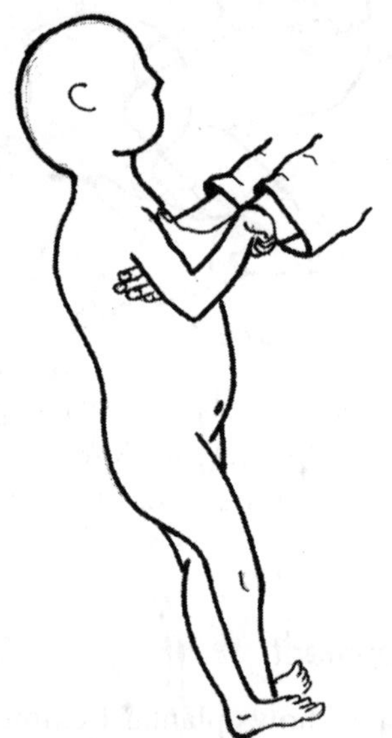

Fig. 5.39

Knees

Normal Development

0-03 months: The infant is held at axilla in standing position.

Response: Baby keeps the knees in extended position.

03 months and above: After three months baby may flex the knees but as the baby starts bearing weight on his feet voluntarily at the age of 5-6 months he shows extension of the knees.

Abnormal Development

1. When baby is held in neutral position, knees go into the flexion. Attempts made to extend the knee joints cause resistance (Fig. 5.40).

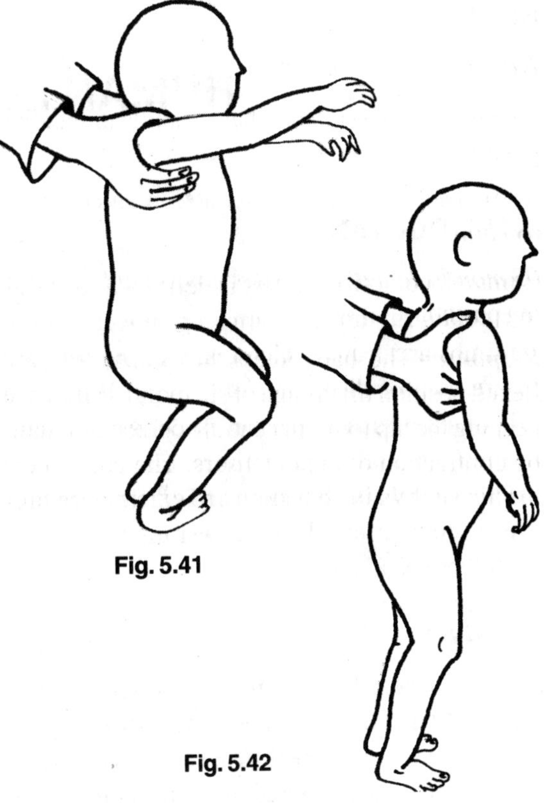

Fig. 5.41

Fig. 5.42

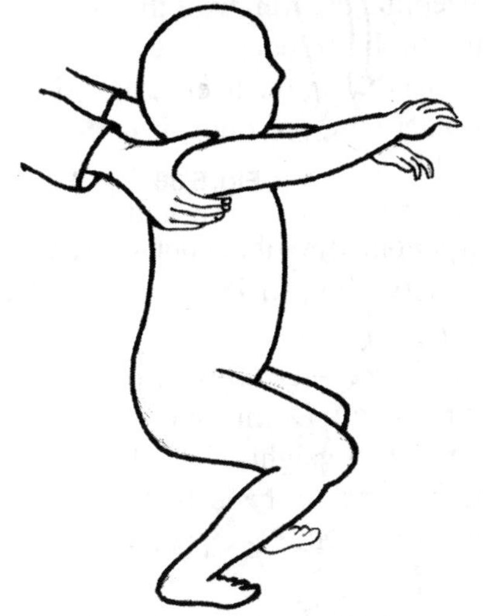

Fig. 5.40

2. When examiner holds the baby in standing position knees go into the flexion. Attempts made to extend the knee joints cause resistance.

Feet

Normal Development

0-03 months: Baby shows plantar flexion when held at axilla in standing position (Fig. 5.41).

03 months and above: At the age between 3 and 6 months the feet go into dorsiflexion and baby starts bearing weight on heels, keeps the ankle joints dorsiflexed (5-6 months) and after this the ankle joints are kept in neutral position. The infant offers no resistance against plantar-flexion/dorsiflexion (Fig. 5.42).

Abnormal Development

1. The infant bears whole weight of body on toes with eversion or inversion and offers resistance to dorsiflexion (Fig. 5.43).

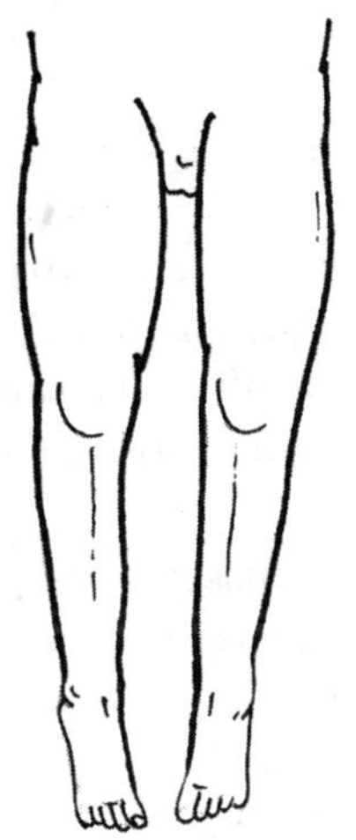

Fig. 5.43

HUMAN LOCOMOTION

INTRODUCTION

Human locomotion or gait is defined as a series of smooth, rhythmic, alternating movements of the limbs and trunk which result in the forward progression of the center of gravity. When the gait of one normal person is compared with another normal person there may be slight difference in walking patterns, this difference falls within comparatively narrow range which is considered as a normal gait.

Gait Cycle

The gait cycle is the time interval or sequence of movement that occurs between heel strike of one limb and subsequent heel strike of the same side, or between two consecutive initial contacts of the same foot. For example, time interval between one heel strike (initial contact) of the right foot to the next heel strike of the same foot consists of a gait cycle. Gait cycle is divided into two phases (i) stance and (ii) swing.

Phases of Gait

A. Stance Phase

Stance phase is the phase of gait cycle which begins with heel strike (touching of heel with the ground) and ends with toe off of the same foot. The stance phase contributes 60% of the gait cycle.

Subdivisions of stance phase:
1. Heel strike (initial contact).
2. Foot flat (load response).
3. Mid stance (single leg stance).
4. Push off (heel off and toe off).

- *Heel Strike*—The stance phase begins as soon as the heel of the limb touches the floor, or the heel touches the ground and starts accepting the weight of the body, at the same time the other foot prepares to leave the ground so that during the heel strike both feet are in contact with the floor, it is thus a period of double-leg support or double leg stance, and contributes 10% of the gait cycle (Fig. 5.44).
- *Foot Flat*—Shortly after heel strike, the whole sole (heel to toes) of the foot touches the floor (Fig. 5.45).
- *Mid Stance*—It begins with foot flat and ends with heel off. During mid stance one leg alone carries the weight of whole body, while the other leg passes beneath the body, and this is known as single leg support or single leg stance (Fig. 5.46).

  The foot flat and mid stance contributes 40% of the gait cycle.
- *Push off*—Begins with heel off and ends with toe off of the same foot. This subphase of

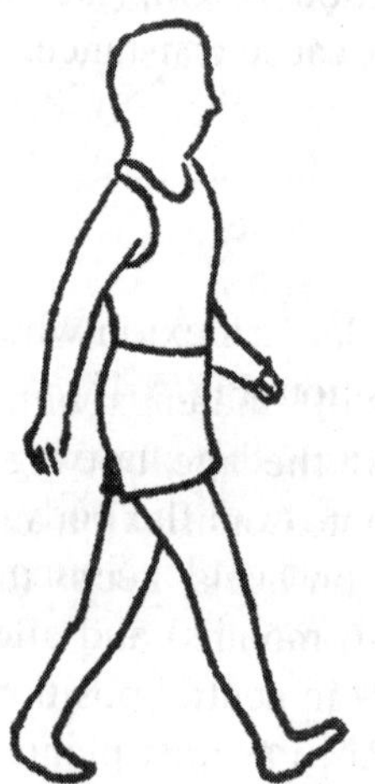
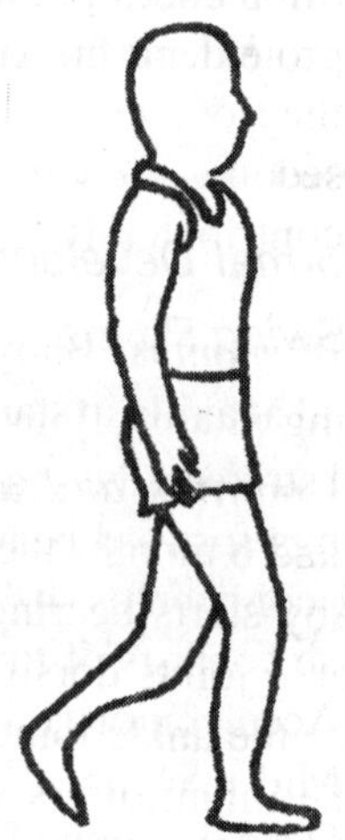

Fig. 5.44: Heel strike   **Fig. 5.45:** Foot flat

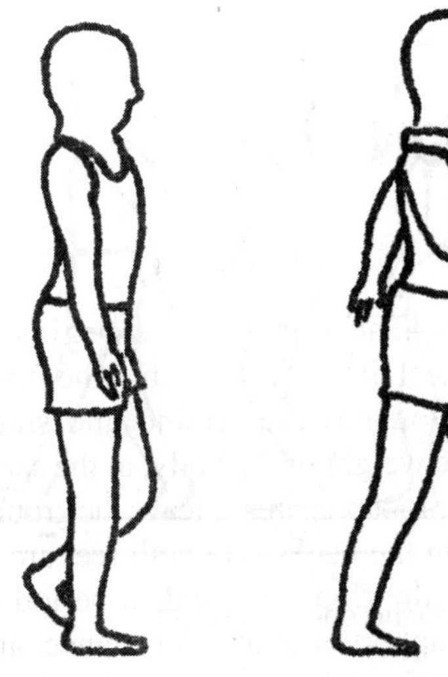

Fig. 5.46: Mid stance   **Fig. 5.47:** Push off

stance is the interval between heel off and toe off position of the same foot. This phase is known as push off because it pushes the weight of body to the another leg and prepares for swing phase (Fig. 5.47).

Heel off is the end stage of mid stance where heel leaves the ground and prepares for push off, while the weight of body is being transferred to contralateral leg.

Toe off is the end stage of push off and of course stance phase where body weight is propelled to the contralateral leg. During toe off the contralateral limb's heel strikes the ground and both feet are again in contact with the floor so that double stance occurs for the second time during gait cycle. The push off contributes 10% of the gait cycle.

B. Swing Phase

Swing phase begins with toe off and ends with heel strike of the same foot, during this phase leg swings forward bearing no weight of the body, and contributes 40% of the gait cycle. Swing phase consists of three sub phases.
1. Acceleration (Initial Swing).
2. Mid swing.
3. Decceleration (Terminal swing).

- *Acceleration (Initial Swing)*–It begins at the instant the toe leaves the ground. After leaving the ground the leg accelerates forward, with knee flexion and dorsiflexion of the same limb (Fig. 5.48).
- *Mid Swing*–This begins after initial swing. The accelerated leg (swing leg) passes directly beneath the body. During this stage rapid knee flexion and dorsiflexion occur and shorten the limb to clear the ground for mid swing (Fig. 5.49).
- *Deceleration (Terminal Swing)*—Begins after mid swing and the leg slows down in preparation for heel strike with the floor. During this phase the moving leg is controlled by extensors and flexors of the knee joint (Fig. 5.50).

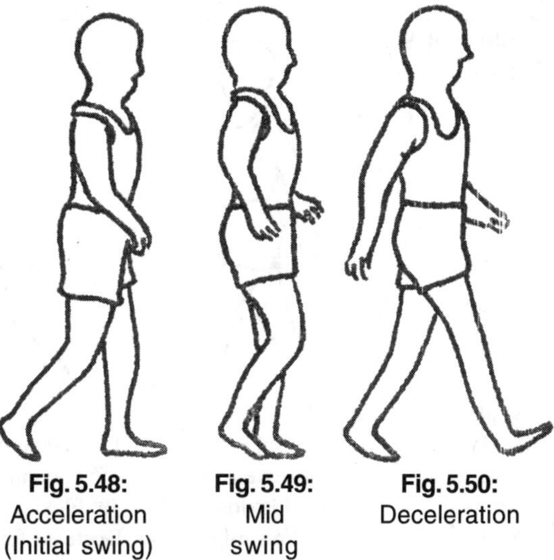

Fig. 5.48: Acceleration (Initial swing)   **Fig. 5.49:** Mid swing   **Fig. 5.50:** Deceleration

Muscular Activity During Stance Phase (Fig. 5.51) (Table 5.1)

The Ankle Joint

Heel strike–at the instant of heel strike the dorsiflexors (tibialis anterior, extensor digitorum longus and extensor hallucis longus) of the ankle joint generate great force. The EHL and EDL show the greater activity than the tibialis anterior (according to the electromyography studies).

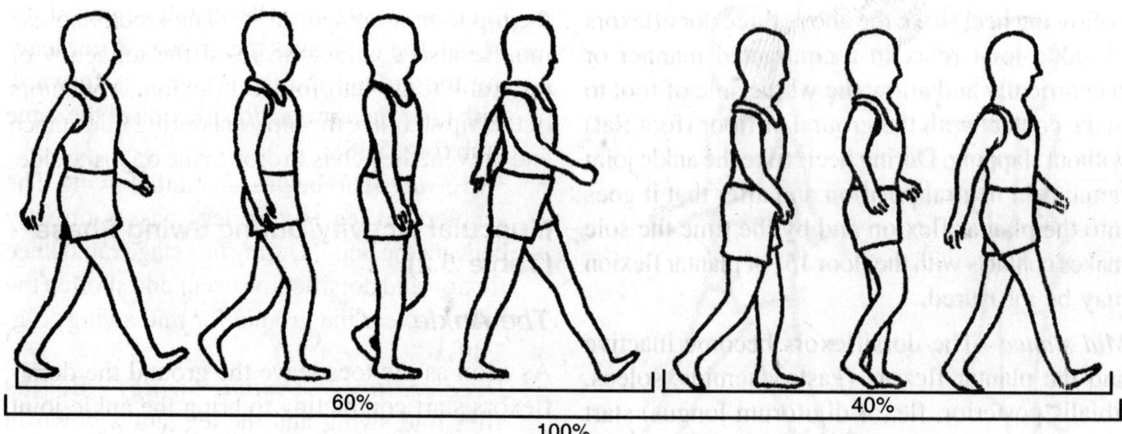

Fig. 5.51: The distribution of time in percentage spends during one Gait Cycle
(Stance = 60%) (Swing = 40%)

Table 5.1: ROM and Contraction of muscles during stance phase (right lower limb)

Sub-phase of Stance Phase	*Heel Strike*	*Foot Flat*	*Mid Stance*	*Push Off*
ROM of:				
– Ankle Joint	Neutral	15° Plantar flexion	10° Dorsiflexion	Neutral
– Knee Joint	Full extension	15° Flexion	Neutral	Full extension
– Hip joint	30° Flexion	30° Flexion	Neutral	10° extension
– Pelvis	5° Foward rotation	Decrease forward rotation	Neutral	5° Backward rotation
– Trunk	Erect neutral	Erect neutral	Erect neutral	Erect neutral
Contraction of muscles required	Dorsiflexors	Plantar flexors	Plantar flexors	Plantar flexors
	Quadriceps	Quadriceps	Quadriceps	Toe flexors
	Gluteus maximus	Gluteus maximus	Gluteus maximus	Hamstrings
	Hamstrings		Ilio-psoas	Quadriceps
	Erector spinae		Gluteus medius	Iliopsoas
			Quadratus magnus	
			Adductor longus	
			Gluteus medius	
Weakness of muscles causes	Foot drop	Excessive dorsiflexion	Excessive dorsiflexion	No sequence from heel off to toe off

Following heel strike the above three dorsiflexors of ankle joint relax in a contracted manner or eccentrically and allow the whole sole of foot to make contact with the ground or floor (foot flat) without slapping. During heel strike the ankle joint remains in neutral position and after that it goes into the plantar flexion and by the time the sole makes contacts with the floor 15° of plantar flexion may be measured.

Mid stance—The dorsiflexors become inactive and the plantar flexors (gastrocnemius, soleus, tibialis posterior, flexor digitorum longus) start contracting and the activity of plantar flexors continues beyond the point of mid stance. During end of mid-stance the ankle joint remains approximately two to three degrees in dorsiflexion.

Push off—In mid stance the plantar flexors contract eccentrically. From mid stance to heel off, plantar flexors of ankle joint contract concentrically while the flexors of toes contract eccentrically.

The Knee Joint

At heel strike the quadriceps (knee extensors) contract eccentrically in order to control the knee joint as it moves from complete extension to position of 15° to 20° of flexion.

At the point of heel strike the knee joint remains straight which is controlled by quadriceps. from heel strike to foot flat, the quadriceps contract eccentrically and allow the knee joint to flex from 0° to 15–20° of flexion. The nature of the contraction as soon as the whole foot approaches to the ground changes and quadriceps muscles contract concentrically which allows the knee joint to extend from 15°–20° to full extension.

The Hip Joint

At the heel strike the contraction of gluteus maximus and hamstrings resist the moment of force that tends to flex the hip joint following heel strike. Concentric contraction of these muscles extend the hip joint after heel strike. The erector spinae muscle also contracts to resist the tendency of the trunk to go into forward flexion. Abductors of the hip stabilize the hip joint during mid stance and prevent the pelvis to drop to the opposite side.

Muscular Activity During Swing Phase (Table 5.2)

The Ankle

As soon as the toes leave the ground the dorsiflexors start contracting to bring the ankle joint from plantar flexion to neutral position and prevent the toes from dragging on the floor. The dorsiflexors keep contracting from acceleration to the end of swing phase.

The Knee Joint

The hamstring muscles (biceps femoris–short head), gracilis and sartorius contract concentrically from acceleration to mid swing while quadriceps remain inactive and knee is flexed between 40° and 60°. After mid swing the quadriceps contract concentrically and prepare the leg for heel strike.

The Hip Joint

At the beginning of swing phase the joint remain close to the neutral position. As soon as toes leave the ground the iliacus, and psoas major muscles contract concentrically and flexes the hip joint to 25° at the time of mid-swing.

GENERAL CHARACTERISTICS OF A NORMAL GAIT

1. *Vertical displacement of the centre of gravity (Pelvic tilt)*—During normal walking pattern the vertical pelvic shift (pelvic tilt) keeps the centre of gravity (COG) moving rhythmically upwards and downwards. Total amount of pelvic displacement an adult male rarely exceeds 50 mm. The

Table 5.2: ROM and Contraction of muscles during swing phase

Sub-phase of Swing phase	*Acceleration*	*Mid Swing*	*Decceleration*
ROM of:			
– Ankle joint	10° Plantar flexion	Neutral	Neutral
– Knee joint	60° Flexion	60°–30° Flexion	Neutral
– Hip joint	20° Flexion	20°–30° Flexion	30° Flexion
– Pelvic joint	5° Backward rotation	Neutral	5° Forward rotation
– Trunk	Erect neutral	Erect neutral	Erect neutral
Contraction of muscles requires	Dorsiflexors	Dorsiflexors	Dorsiflexors
	Biceps femoris (Short head)	Hamstrings	Quadriceps
	gracilis and sortorius		Iliacus and Psoas major
Weakness of muscles causes	Dragging of foot (toes)	Dragging of foot (toes)	Draggind of foot (toes)
	unable to flex the knee joint	no forward progression	no forward progression
	unable to flex the hip joint	of leg	of leg

highest vertical displacement (50 mm) occurs during the mid stance (single limb support) and lowest point occurs at the heel strike (double leg support). In abnormal cases such as fused knee joint, vertical pelvic displacement increases more than 50 mm as the person requires more vertical pelvic displacement to clear the ground (Figs 5.52a and b).

2. *Lateral pelvic shift or Pelvic List (Lateral displacement of the centre of gravity):* During normal walking the pelvis moves side to side as it is necessary to keep the body weight over the stance leg for balance. The normal lateral pelvic shift is 2.5 to 5 cm (Figs 5.53a and b).

3. *Horizontal dip of the pelvis*—Anterior and posterior rotation of pelvis during gait is necessary to lessen the angle of the femur with the floor, result lengthening of the femur. It decreases the centre of gravity path amplitude of displacement and thus decreases the centre of gravity dip. 5° forward and 5° backward rotation is considered as a normal pelvic rotation during gait. To maintain the balance the thorax rotates in the opposite direction of the pelvis. Thus when the pelvis rotates clockwise, the thorax rotates counter clockwise and vice versa.

4. *Flexion of the knee joint during stance*— Immediately after heel strike knee begins

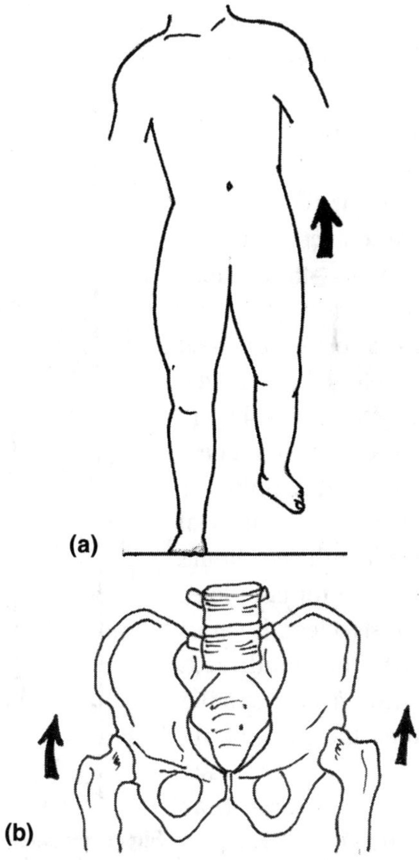

Figs 5.52a and b: Vertical shift of pelvis

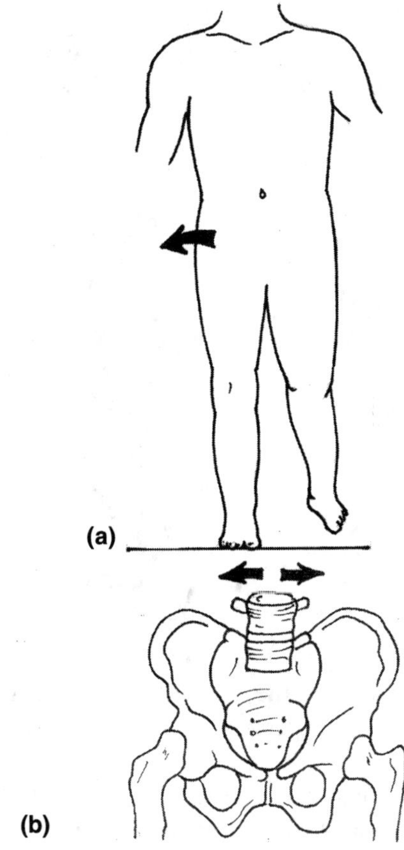

Figs 5.53a and b: Lateral shift of pelvis

flexing which is continued till it reaches to approximately 15°. This motion is coordinated with the motions at the ankle, and keeps the centre of gravity approximately at the same level for some time as it moves forward. **Knee flexion during stance phase is of special importance in minimising the vertical displacement of the centre of gravity in walking.**

5. *Cadence*—The number of steps taken per minute is known as cadence. It varies from slow walking to fast running (70 to 140 per min respectively). An average cadence for a normal adult male is considered as 90 steps per minute and he can cover four kilometer in an hour.

6. *Double support*—When both feet are simultaneously in contact with the ground it is known as double support. For example, when a stance phase commences the heel contacts (heel strike) with the ground, at the same time the toes of the contralateral limb make contact with the ground. Each gait cycle consists two double supports. Double support is a characteristic feature of normal gait when person walks. The double support decreases as the walking speed increases, and it disappears when person runs (Fig. 5.54).

7. *Single support*—It is a part of stance phase where one limb bears whole weight of the body while another limb swings forward for

preparation of stance phase without carrying weight of the body. During a gait cycle only one single support occurs (Fig. 5.55).

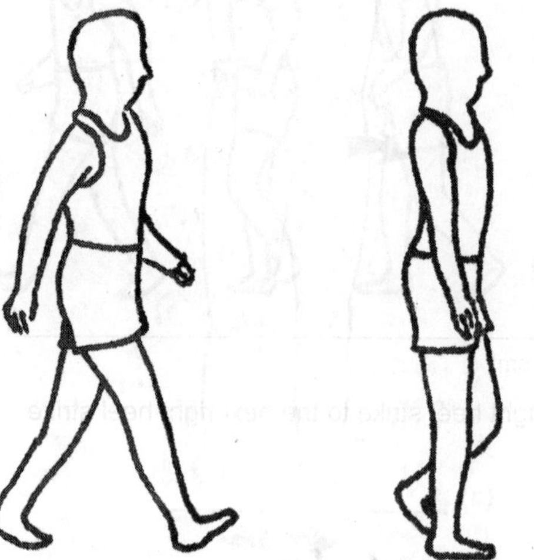

Fig. 5.54: Double support

Fig. 5.55: Single support

8. *Base width*—is the distance between the two feet when person is in erect standing posture. 5 to 10 cm distance between the feet is considered normal range of base width, more than 10 cm and below 5 cm width is considered as abnormal base width (Fig. 5.56).

9. *Step length or Gait length*—is the distance between two successive contact points. For example—the distance between right heel strike to the left heel strike is known as step length. 35 to 41 cm between two successive contact points is considered as a normal step length and should be equal for both legs. The step length varies with age and sex. Children take smaller steps than the adult, and females take smaller steps than males (Fig. 5.57).

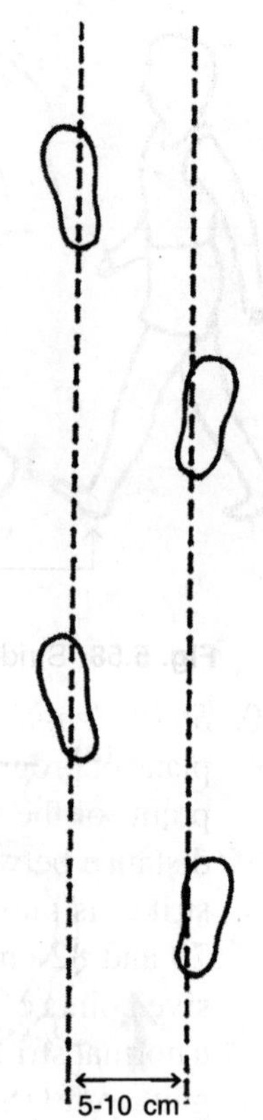

Fig. 5.56: Base width

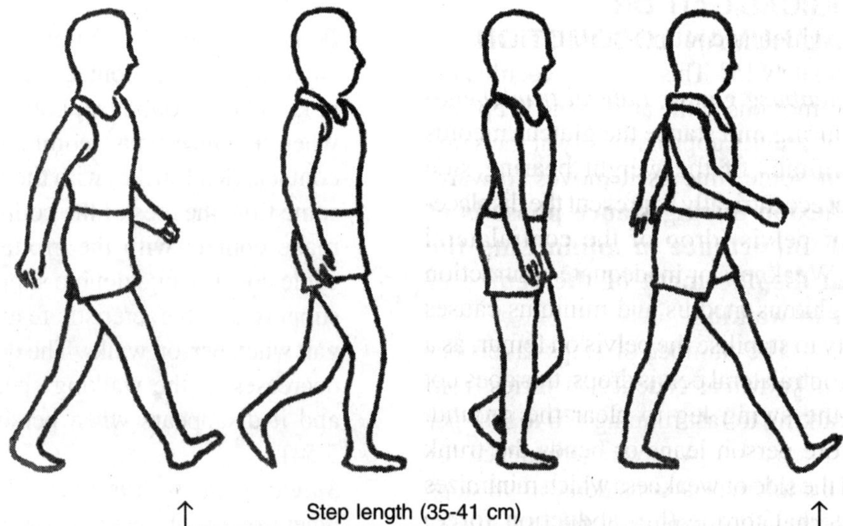

Fig. 5.57: Step length or Gait length—distance between two succesive points (right heel strike to the left heel strike)

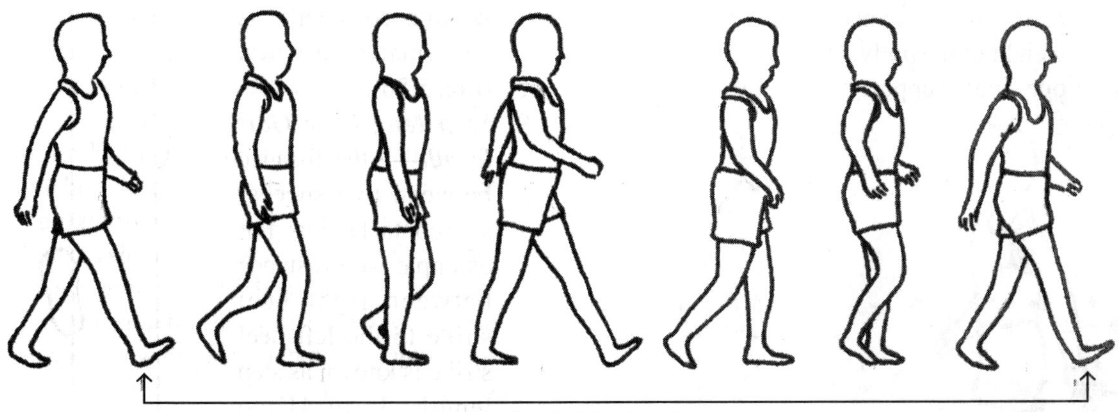

Fig. 5.58: Stride length (Gait cycle)—distance between right heel strike to the next right heel strike

10. *Stride length*—is the linear distance in the plane of progression between two successive points of the same foot. (For example—the distance between two successive right heel strikes is known as stride length). Between 70 and 82 cm length between two successive points of the same foot is considered as a normal stride length. 70-82 cm covers one gait cycle. (Stride length = one gait cycle) (Fig. 5.58).

PATHOLOGICAL GAIT OR ABNORMAL HUMAN LOCOMOTION

1. *Trendelenburg gait or Lateral trunk bending*—During mid stance the gluteus medius and minimus of the weight bearing side contract eccentrically to prevent the displacement of pelvis (drop of the contralateral pelvis. Weakness or inadequate contraction of the gluteus medius and minimus causes inability to stabilise the pelvis on femur, as a result contralateral pelvis drops, this does not allow the swing leg to clear the ground. Therefore person leans or bends the trunk toward the side of weakness which minimizes the external torque (hip abduction force) demand due to body weight on the abductor muscles of the stance leg (Figs 5.59a and b).

When an individual has one side hip abductors weakness then he or she bends the trunk only toward the involved side during stance phase. Weakness of one side hip abductors is known as Trendelenburg sign.

If both sides of hip abductors are weak then an individual leans the trunk on both sides

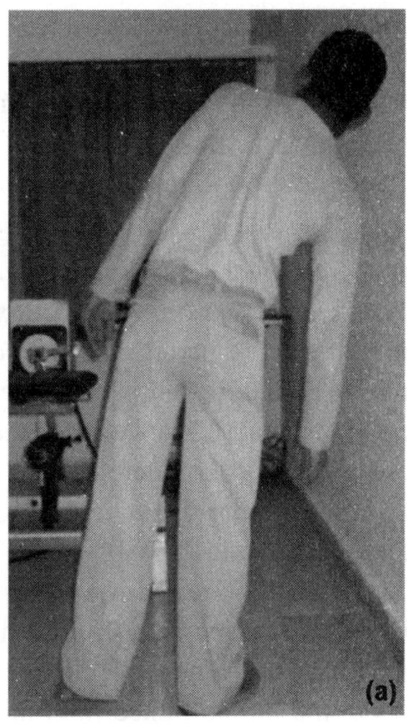

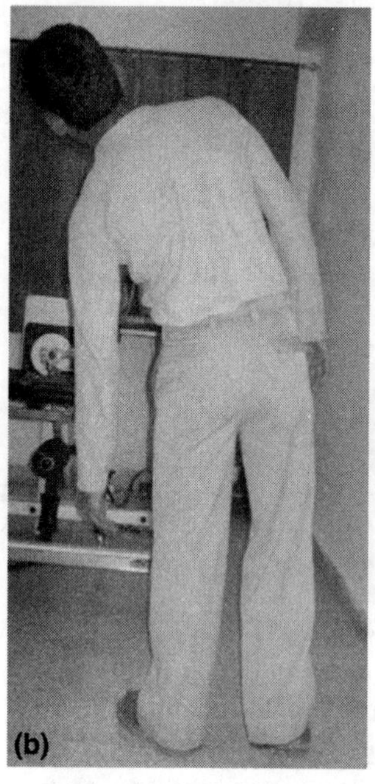

(b)

Figs 5.59a and b:
Waddling gait

alternately which is called as waddling gait (Figs 5.59a and b).

Other possible causes of lateral trunk bending

1. Hip dislocation, coxa vara and slipped capital femoral epiphysis.
2. Hip pain
3. Involved limb relatively shorter-Hip or knee flexion contracture.
4. Compensation for abducted gait.

2. *Circumductory gait*—Commonly seen in hemiplegic patients. Spasticity, decreased voluntary control, abnormal reflexes and abnormal synergy pattern are the common neurological manifestation of post cerebro-vascular accident (CVA), which predispose the patient to circumductory gait. During swing phase normal person requires 30°-60° of knee flexion and 20°-30° of hip flexion while ankle joint remains in the neutral position. These movements allow the leg to swing forward. In hemiplegia no flexion occurs at the hip and knee joint and ankle

joint remains plantar flexed which causes the limb to lengthen and patient finds difficult to swing the leg forward. To overcome this problem patient contracts the quadratus lumborum resulting in hip hiking which thrusts the limb in a circumductory manner and limb swings forward with or without dragging of the toes. Though hip hiking shortens the limb, still limb is longer and can not swing beneath the body hence the patient circumducts (pendular movement) the limb which further shortens the limb and swings it (Figs 5.60a to e).

3. *Hip hiking*—Like circumductory gait patient contracts the quadratus lumboraum of the affected side with lateral abdominals which causes hiking of the hip joint. Hiking swings the involved limb by increasing the rotation of the pelvis in the horizontal plane.

Possible causes of Hip Hiking

- The involved limb either is relatively longer or cannot be shortened/flexed during swing phase:
  - hip flexor weakness

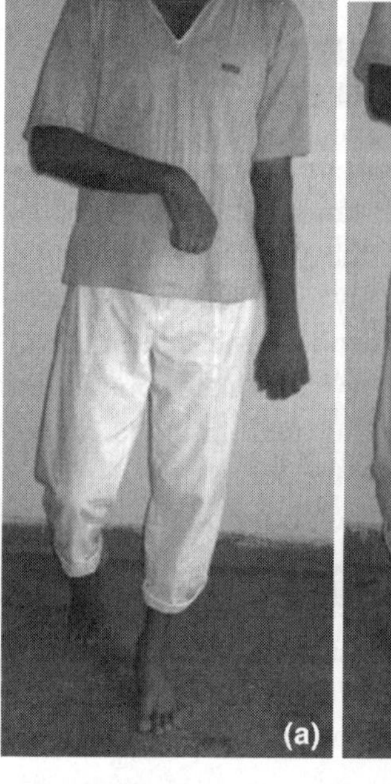
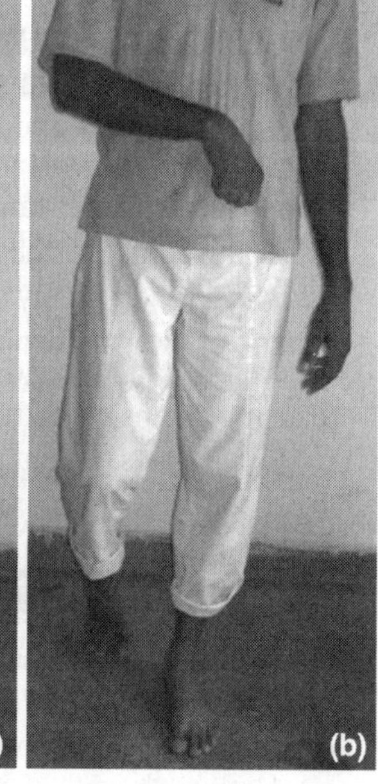

(a)

(b)

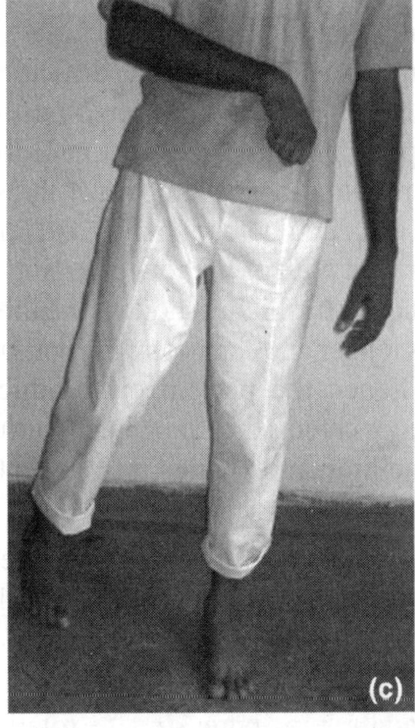 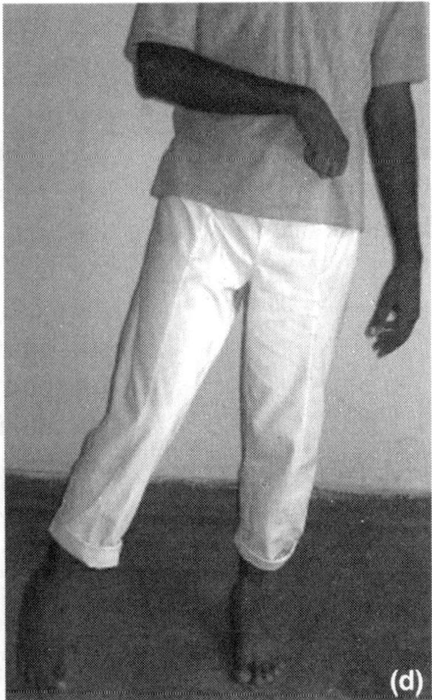 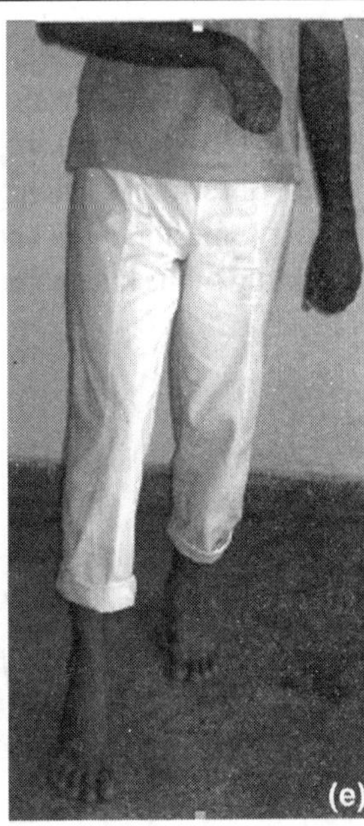

Figs 5.60a to e: circumductory gait

  - extensor spasticity
  - mechanical lock at the hip joint
  - knee ankylosis
  - weakness of dorsiflexors
- Shortening of contralateral limb (stance limb):
  - Hip or knee flexion contracture skeletal shortening:
  - Hamstrings weakness.

4. *Posterior trunk bending*—Weakness of hip extensors. Insufficient concentric contraction of gluteus maximus causes inability to extend the hip joint during stance phase. Therefore patient bends the trunk posteriorly causing extension at the hip joint (Fig. 5.61).

Some times patient places his or her hand over the gluteus maximus and pushes the buttock anteriorly which causes extension at the hip joint and trunk automatically bends posteriorly which is known as Jack knife gait.

5. *Anterior trunk bending*—Commonly seen in post polio residual paralysis (PPRP) in

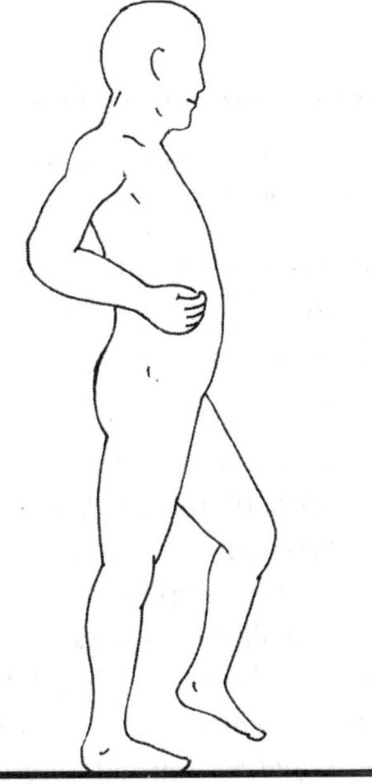

Fig. 5.61: Posterior trunk bending (Gluteus maximum gait)

which paralysis of quadriceps is combined with weakness of gluteus maximus or gastrosoleus or both. During stance phase due to weakness of these muscles knee joint buckels. To avoid buckling patient bends the trunk anteriorly which places the centre of gravity anterior to the knee joint and prevents buckling of the knee joint during stance phase (Fig. 5.62).

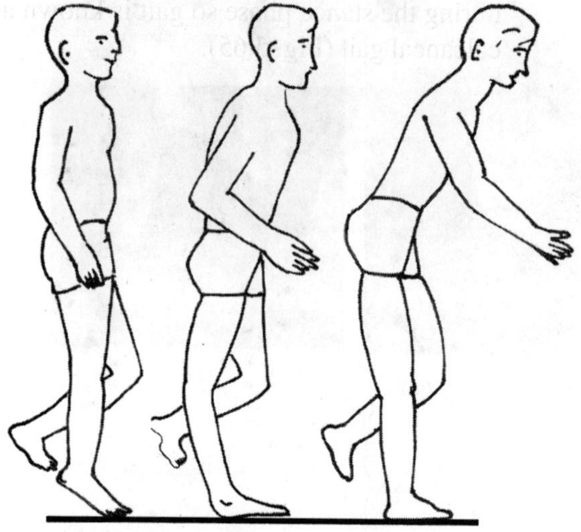

Fig. 5.62: Hyperrextended knee
(anterior trunk bending)

Some patients place their hand just above the knee joint, and walk with anterior trunk bending which is known as hand to knee gait (Fig. 5.63).

6. *Hyperextended knee*—Generally patient can not walk if his quadriceps are zero (paralysed) without stabilising the knee joint by an external support or orthosis. But patient can walk without using an external stabilisers of the knee joint if his gluteus maximus and gastrosoleus are strong. The larger proximal portion and superficial fibres of distal portion of gluteus maximus muscle inserts into iliotibial tract of fascia lata. Deep fibres of distal portion insert into gluteal tuberosity of femur. The portion of gluteus maximum muscle which inserts into iliotibial

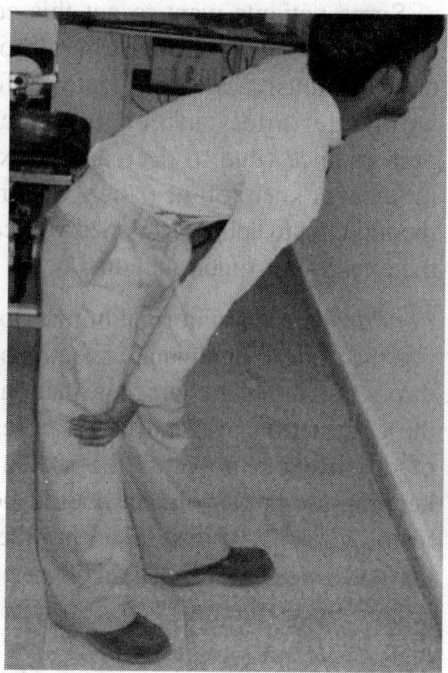

Fig. 5.63: Hand to knee gait

band contract concentrically and pulls the femur posteriorly which creates extension moment arm (knee goes behind the centre of gravity). This action of gluteus maximus prevents buckling of knee joint during the stance phase and patient can walk without hand to knee. The gastrosoleus also do the same function (pull the tibia behind the centre of gravity which causes hyperextension of the knee joint and prevent the buckling of knee joint). If patient walks frequently with this gait after some time he develops genurecurvatum (Fig. 5.62).

Some patients also prefer to walk by creating equinus at ankle. Due to which the line of gravity (LOG) shifts anteriorly to the knee joint, causing increased extensor moment at the knee joint. This extensor moment is helpful in extending knee inspite of absent or weak quadriceps. In the beginning this equinus is flexible but later on it becomes a fixed deformity.

Some patients want to get this equinus corrected surgically. But surgery should be done cautiously, as correcting the deformity would definitely affect the functional performance (due to decrease in extensor moment at knee) of the patient. It is recommended not to achieve cosmetic outcome at the expense of functional one.

7. *Foot drop gait*—In normal human locomotion the ankle joint remains at neutral position through swing phase which is maintained by the contraction of dorsiflexors. Weakness of dorsiflexors prevents the patient from keeping the ankle joint in neutral position resulting into plantarflexion and toes drag during swing phase. To get rid of this problem patient flexes the hip joint beyond 30° and then strikes the ground with the toes (Fig. 5.64). This results in toe to heel pattern instead of normal heel to toe pattern.

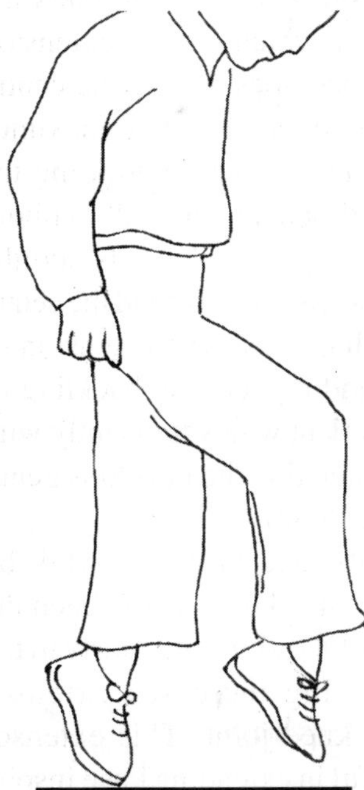

Fig. 5.64: Foot drop

8. *Calcaneal gait*—From foot flat to the end of stance phase plantar flexors (gastrosoleus,

flexor digitorum longus and brevis, and flexor hallucis longus) contract and push the ground by foot which results in heel off. Insufficient contraction of plantar flexors causes muscular imbalance and ankle joint goes into dorsiflexion, forefoot does not make contact with the ground and whole weight of body is transferred only on the heel (calcaneum) during the stance phase so gait is known as calcaneal gait (Fig. 5.65).

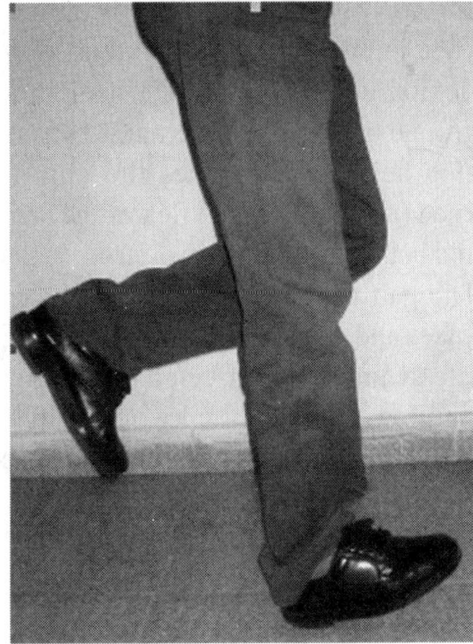

Fig. 5.65: Calcaneal

Other common causes of calcaneal gait
- Rupture of the Achilles tendon or hammer toe
- Pes calcaneus or pes varus or pes valgus
- Metatarsalgia
- Orthosis plantar stop.

9. *Vaulting*—The patient bobs up and down excessively as he walks, increasing the vertical displacement of centre of gravity by exaggerating plantar flexion of the contralateral ankle.

Possible causes:
- In all cases the involved limb is relatively longer:

- hip flexors weakness
- ankylosis of hip in extension
- extensor synergy
- mechanical lock of hip joint
- ankylosis of knee joint.
- Hamstring weakness in slow walking.

10. *Flexed knee gait*—Flexion contracture of the hamstring muscles does not allow the knee joint to extend during locomotion. Normally when heel strikes the ground, both knee joints remain fully extended. In knee flexion contracture as the heel strikes the ground the knee joint remains flexed which also deliberately forces the contralateral knee (normal knee) to flex at the same time and both knees during heel strike look flexed. The gait is characterised by flexion of the knees and excessive dorsiflexion during the late swing of the affected extremity which is followed by early stance on the uninvolved side and early heel-off during midstance (Fig. 5.66).

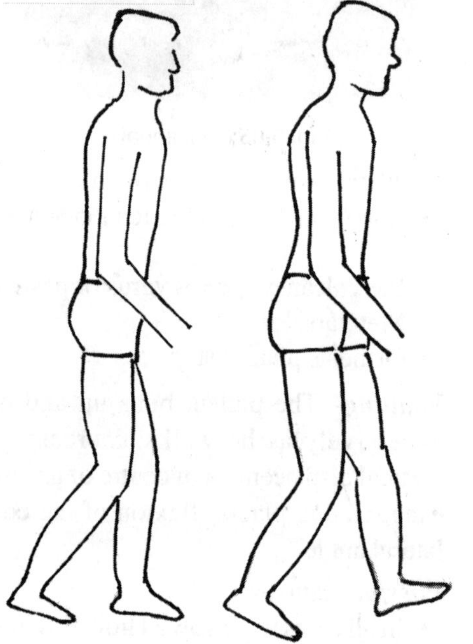

Fig. 5.66: Flexed knee gait

11. *Spastic diplegia gait*—The gait is characterised by excessive flexion at hip and knee joints during stance phase without significant heel strike child walks on forefeet.

12. *Lordotic gait*—Contracture of hip flexors can cause increase in lumbar lordotic curve during the stance phase. Normally after heel strike the hip joint goes into extension (from 30° flexion to 20° extension). The contracture does not allow hip joint to extend. Therefore, in stance phase if the hip joint remains flexed, the center of gravity moves anterior to the hip joint. The patient hyperextends his lumbar spine to retain his head over his pelvis. This lordosis also increases the posterior excursion of the limb to permit a long stride (Fig. 5.67).

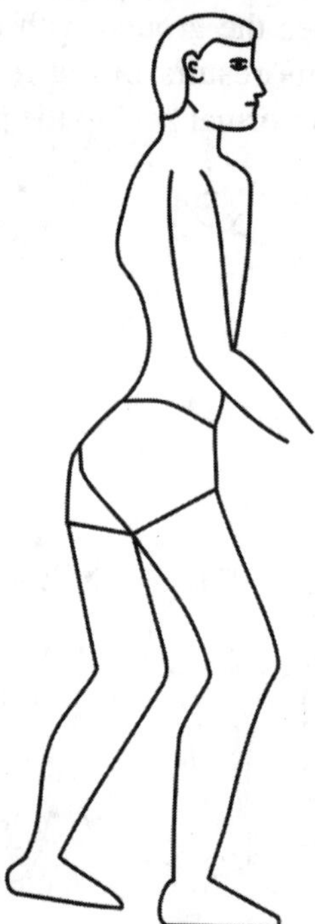

Fig. 5.67: Lordotic gait

Other possible causes
- Weak hip extensors (posterior trunk bending)
- Weak abdominal wall.

12. *Antalgic gait*—It is also known as painful gait. During stance phase, to avoid pain patient attempts to remove weight from the affected leg as quickly as possible which causes shorter stance phase. Patient may also support affected limb with the same side's hand while opposite arm acts as a counter balance and is outstretched.

    In case of painful hip patient bends the trunk toward the same side which minimises the external torque (hip abductors force) demand due to body weight on the painful side of the stance leg.

13. *Wide base gait (Ataxic gait)*—In cerebellar ataxia the patient has poor balance so he walks with broad base, and therefore he lurches, staggers, and exaggerates all movements (Fig. 5.68).

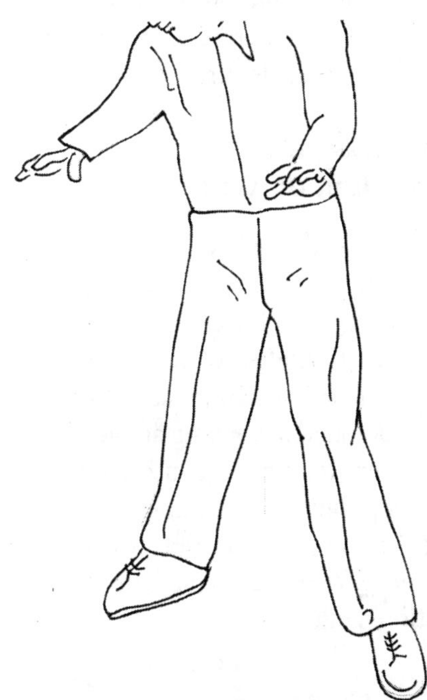

Fig. 5.68: Wide base gait (Ataxic gait)

14. *Scissors Gait*—Spasticity in the adductors of both hip joints causes great difficulty in swinging the leg forward. After push off the swing limb crosses the midline, draws the knees together and progresses forward by touching the middle thigh of the contralateral leg and both legs look like a pair of scissors (Fig. 5.69).

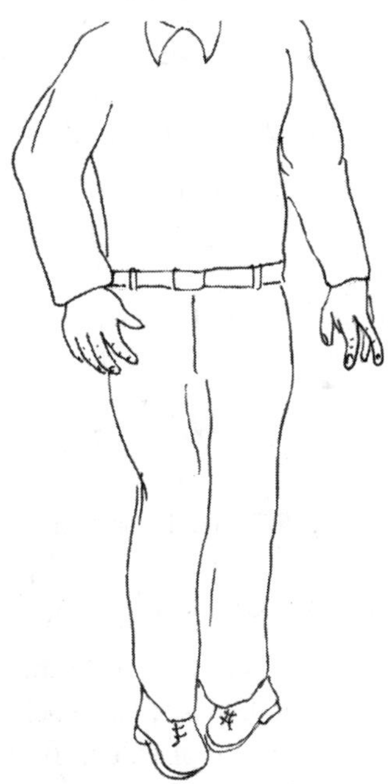

Fig. 5.69: Scissors gait

15. *Parkinsons Gait (Shuffling in Short Step, Festination Gait)*—The gait Parkinsonism is highly stereotyped and characterised by an impoverishment of movement. Decreased generalised extension of lower limb joints (hip, knee and ankle), trunk and pelvic motions. So patient walks with flexed trunk, hip, knee and ankle joints with small steps. Persistent posturing of a forward head and trunk typically displaces the patient's center of gravity forward. The patient takes multiple short steps in order to avoid falling forward and eventually breaks into a run and looks like he is running to catch the center of gravity (Fig. 5.70).

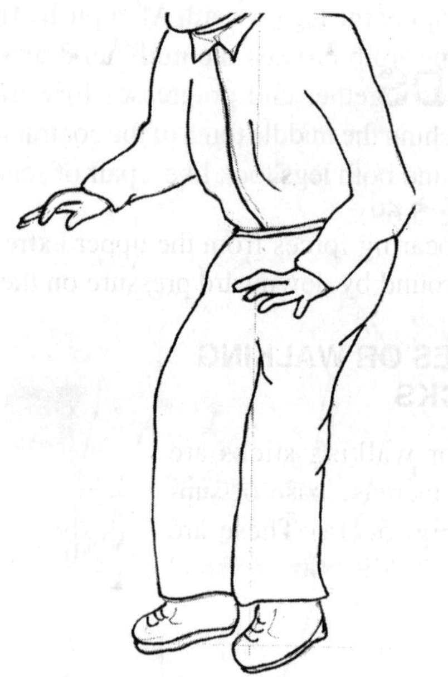

Fig. 5.70: Parkinsons gait

ASSESSMENT OF GAIT

Impairment and disability in the broad context encompass physical, mental and social functions. Walking is largely a physical function. Gait assessment may not make a diagnosis but it helps to determine physical impairment deviation from normal. It has diagnostic value when it is combined and related with results from other clinical tests and the clinical examination, such as passive and active range of motion, muscle strength, muscle spasm, pain, tenderness, and sensory and motor functions.

Following movements should be observed carefully:

Head : Movement of head to right side during midstance on the right foot.

Arm : Lateral arm swing to the left during entire stance phase on the right foot.

Trunk : Lateral movement of the trunk to the right during mid and late stance on the right foot.

Pelvis : Lateral movement of the pelvis to the right during midstance on the right foot.

Hip : Adduction of hip during midstance bilaterally. The opposite limb swings with 20° to 30° flexion during acceleration and mid swing

Knee : Extension of knee during heel strike, 15° of flexion at foot flat and remain in extension in rest of stance phase. The opposite leg swings with 60°-30° flexion during acceleration and mid swing and neutral in deceleration.

Ankle : Neutral during heel strike and 15° of plantar flexion at foot flat.

General Energetic Consideration on Gait

The important energy-saving mechanism in walking is the transformation of kinetic into potential energy and vice versa. During each stride the transformation of both energies in each other is estimated to comprise 50% to 70% of the energy demand in walking at moderate speed. Muscular work required to cause energy transformation can reduce the mechanical efficiency of walking. The negative muscle work (eccentric contraction) often reduces the kinetic translation and rotational energy.

WALKING AIDS

INTRODUCTION

Crutch walking is a highly developed art which can be improved by training and practice. All the benefits of this art is similar to that of other therapeutic exercises. This aids not only make the subject independent in walking but also act as a type of exercise for them to improve their cardiovascular, pulmonary, renal and musculoskeletal system.

In essence a crutch or a cane is an extension of the upper extremity used to provide support, balance and weight bearing normally provided by an intact functioning of lower limb. One crutch (modulate or total loss) or one cane (little loss) should be prescribed for unilateral impairment (pain, weakness etc.) but clinically one crutch is rarely used.

Walking aids are assistive devices used for supportive walking. They are broadly divided into three categories:
  i. Canes/walking sticks.
  ii. Crutches.
  iii. Walkers.

Indications

- Poor balance.
- Weakness of lower extremity muscles.
- Pain in weight bearing joints of the lower extremities.
- Joint instability.
- Fatigue.

Mechanism of Action

Walking aids eliminate weight bearing fully or partially from lower extremity. The unloading of the lower extremity is possible by transmission of weight bearing forces from the upper extremity to the ground by downward pressure on the aid.

I. CANES OR WALKING STICKS

Canes or walking sticks are used to increase base of support (Fig. 5.71a) These are used by holding in the hand opposite to affected lower extremity. The subject walks in a reciprocal gait pattern by moving the cane and affected leg together. Holding stick in contralateral upper extremity causes less later shift of centre of gravity. It reduces joint reaction force of abductor muscles at hip joint, therefore it is important to hold the cane opposite to affected lower extremity. The implication of this concept is more in hip disorders such as arthroplasty, arthritis etc.

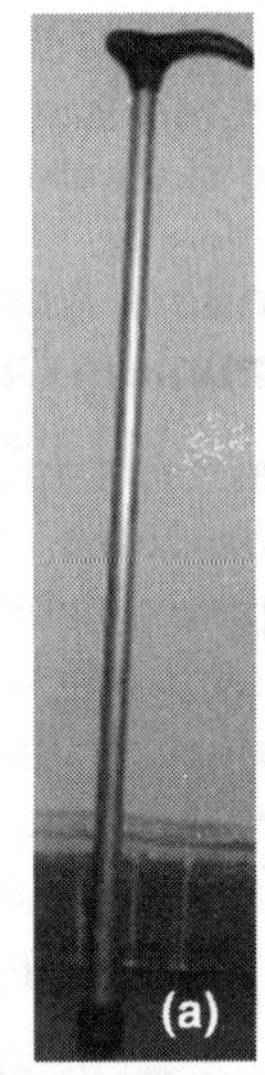

Fig. 5.71a:
Walking stick

Standard Cane/Walking Stick

Conventionally it was made of wood, but now a days mainly of aluminium and has a half circle handle. It is a single piece with a distal rubber tip of approximately 1 inch in diameter. The handle may be covered by moulded rubber or plastic coating or wood (Figs 5.71b and c). It is one of most light weighted and easy to carry assistive device for walking. The only disadvantage of this is that it is not adjustable and must be cut to fit the patient. It's point of support is anterior to hand and not directly beneath it.

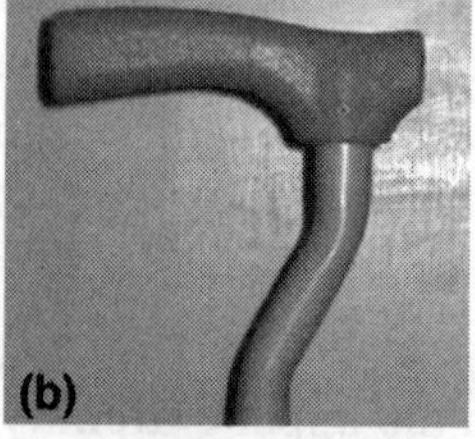

Fig. 5.71b: Hand grip with plastic coating

Fig. 5.71c: Wooden hand grip of a walking stick

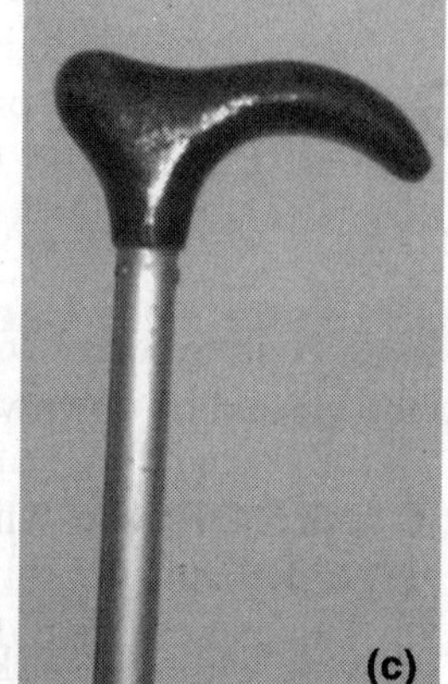

Standard Adjustable Aluminium Cane/Stick

It has the same basic design as of the regular standard cane. It can be adjusted with in the range of approximately 10 inches. It uses push button to alter height which can further be reinforced by a plastic metallic ring. Sometimes at this point the canes shows instability and make clicking sound during weight support, which does not give the feeling of adequate support to the user.

Offset Cane/Walking Stick

The proximal component of the body of the stick is offset anteriorly. This design allows weight to be born over the center of the cane for greater stability. Most of them are adjustable and more costlier than standard cane.

Quadruped Cane or Walking Stick

The characteristic feature of this cane is that they have four points (legs) floor contact which gives broad base of support (Figs 5.72a to c). All other aspects are same as in above mentioned sticks. They may also be non-adjustable, adjustable or 3-points (legs)–Tripod (Fig. 5.72d).

These canes are not practical for stair activity because of broader base which cannot be adjusted on stair steps. Further the walking speed with

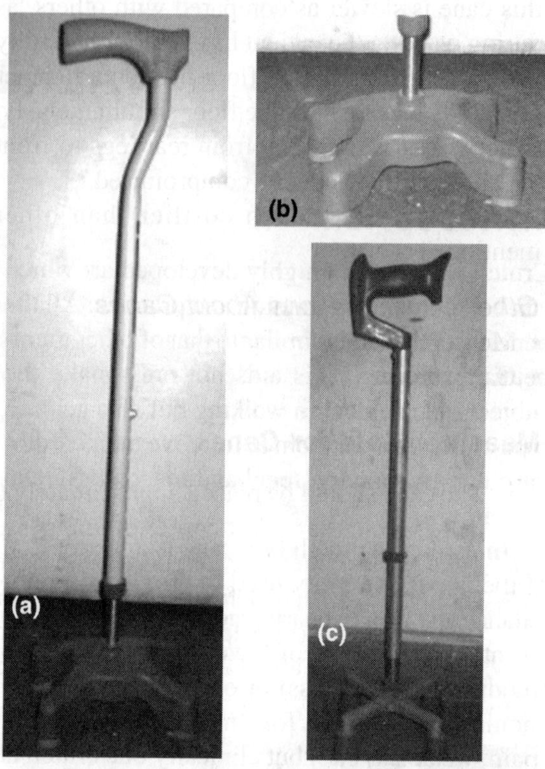

Figs 5.72a to c: (a) Quadruped, (b) Base of quadruped, and (c) A Small size quadruped

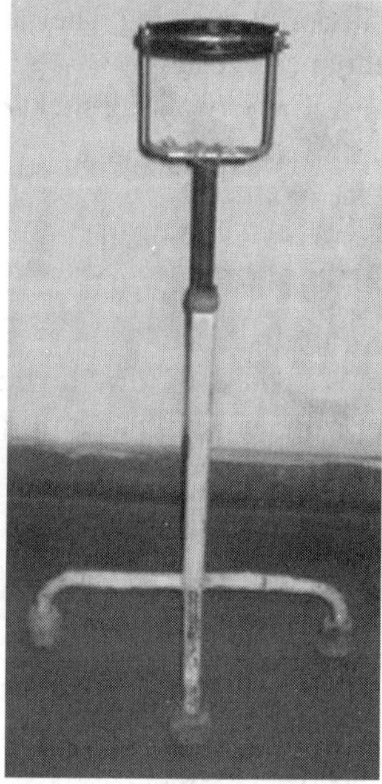

Fig. 5.72d: A Tripod

this cane is slower as compared with others, as during walking the patient has to pick stick fully and place it back on the floor in such a manner that all its legs touches the floor simultaneously. Otherwise it would rock from rear legs to front leg and stability would be compromised.

They are also much costlier than other mentioned canes.

Other Considerations About Canes

- Measurement
- Gait patterns

Measurements for Canes

i. The cane should be placed approximately 6 inches from the lateral border of the toes.

ii. Take measurement for height of cane from greater trochanter of femur to the floor or from the hand (in gripping position) with elbow flexed to about 20° to 30° degrees to the floor.

This is a more important indicator of correct cane height because of individual variation in body proportion and arm length.

iii. The cane should be assessed for client's comfort (Fig. 5.73).

Gait Pattern for Use of Canes

i. The cane should be close to the body (not to be placed ahead of the toe).

   As placing the cane far might cause threat to dynamic stability of the user.

ii. Gait pattern should be followed as shown in Figures 5.74a and b.

   - For bilateral involvement, the cane should be used on the side of comfort.
   - Or even two canes can be used in case more stability is required.

II. CRUTCHES

Crutches are commonly used to relieve weight either partially or fully on lower extremities.

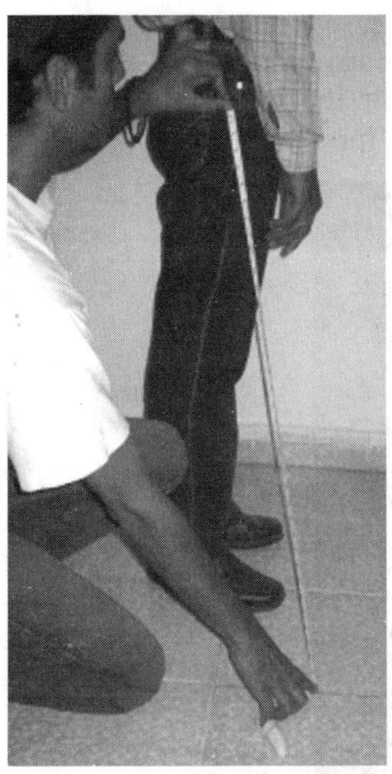

Fig. 5.73: Measurement for cane

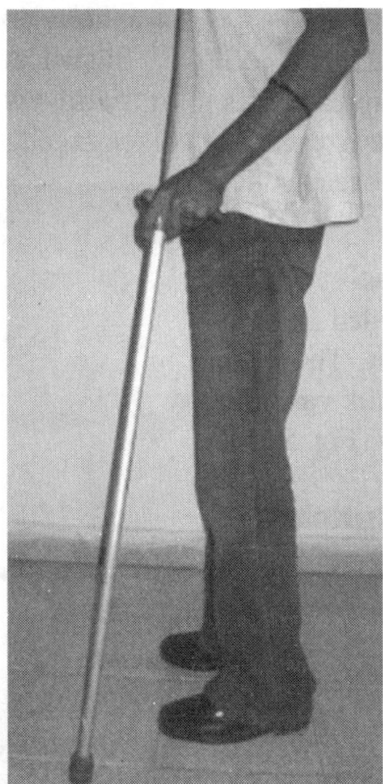
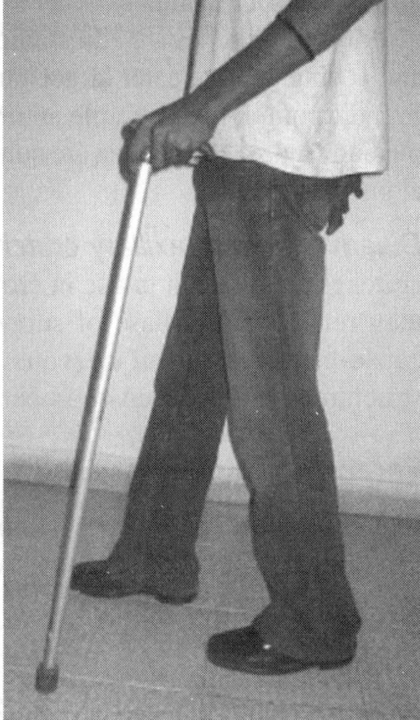

Figs 5.74a and b: Gait pattern for cane use

The common characteristics of this assistive device are:

i. Typically used bilaterally.
ii. Used to relieve weight either partially or fully on lower extremities.
iii. Used to improve balance.
iv. Increase the base of support
v. Improve lateral stability.
vi. Allow upper extremity to transfer weight to the floor.
vi. The two commonly used types are: axillary and forearm or elbow crutches.

Axillary Crutches

These are regular crutches conventionally made of wood but now aluminium is the material of choice. The components of a standard axillary crutches are:

a. An axillary bar
b. A hand piece
c. Double upright joined distally by a single leg
d. Rubber suction tip.

Most of crutches are adjustable at hand piece and at single leg to cater larger group of clients. In India commonly available in three sizes large, medium and small, wooden are quite cheaper than aluminium type.

Disadvantage of axillary crutches—Axillary crutches are difficult to use in crowded areas as they require larger base of support. They can cause compression of nervous and vascular structure in axilla if used improperly (Fig. 5.75).

Forearm Crutches or Elbow Crutches

The component of forearm crutches are (Figs 5.76a to d):

a. A single upright
b. A forearm cuff
c. A hand grip

The crutch is adjustable both proximally and distally to adjust the forearm cuff and height of crutch respectively.

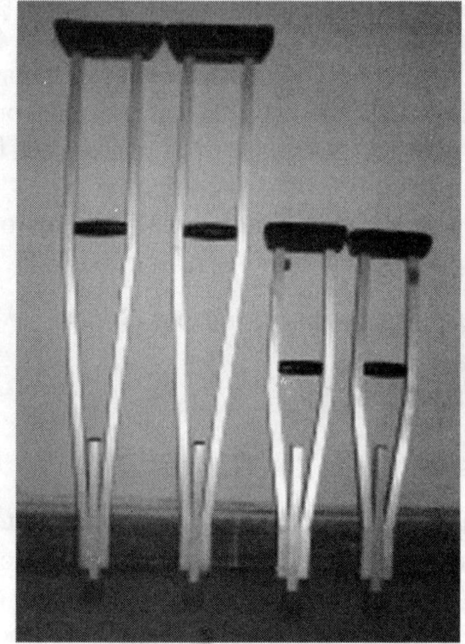

Fig. 5.75: Pair of axillary crutches (adult and small size)

They are also available in three different sizes as axillary crutch.

Significance of forearm cuff—it allows use of hands without the crutches becoming disengaged. The forearm crutches are more

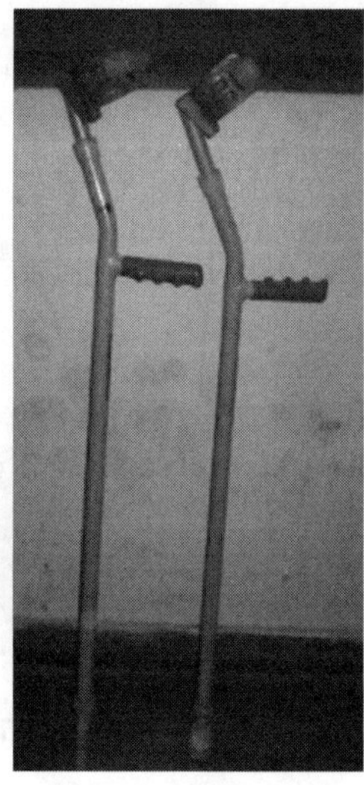

Fig. 5.76a: A pair of adult elbow crutch

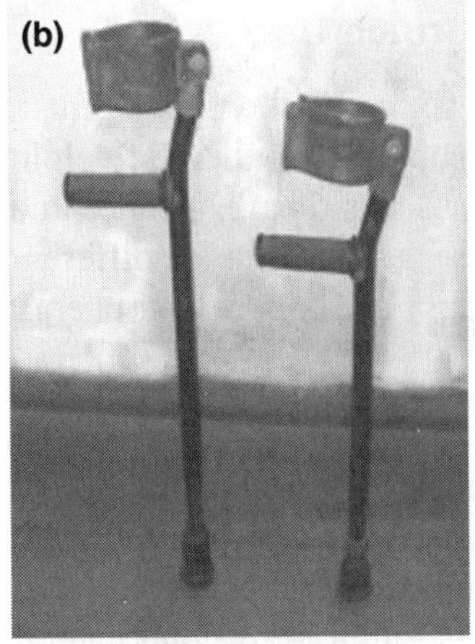

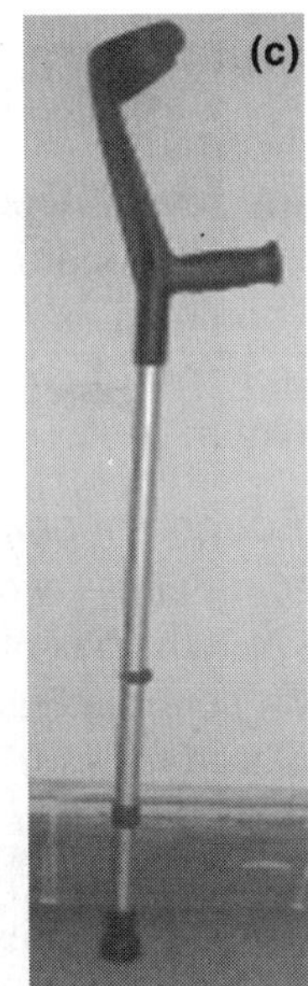

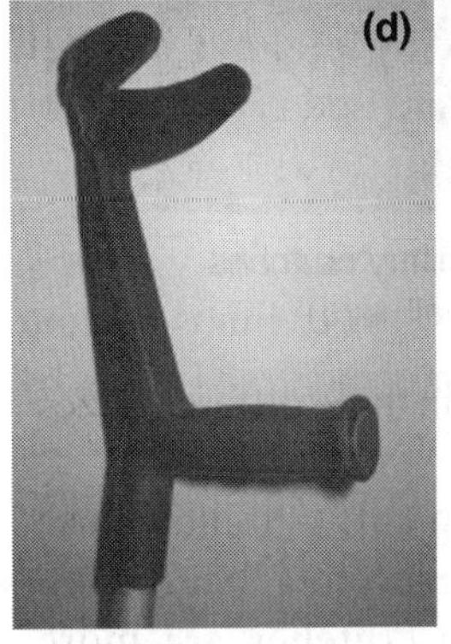

Figs 5.76b to d: (b) A pair of small elbow crutch, and (c) Elbow crutch without elbow strap (d) Forearm part of elbow crutch without elbow strap

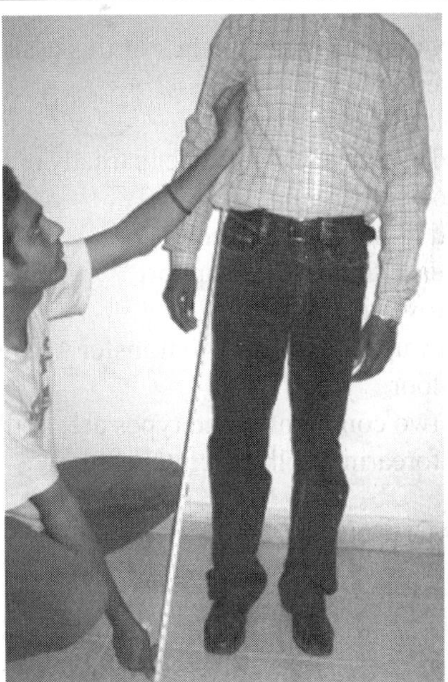

Fig. 5.77: Measurement for axillary crutch

practical to use on stairs, in buses/cars etc. Because of their smaller size client feels more comfortable with this type of crutch as compared to axillary crutch but they provide less lateral support due to absence of an axillary bar.

Other Consideration for Crutches

- Measurement
- Gait patterns.

Measurement for Axillary Crutch

Measurement for axillary crutch can be done in any of the two positions i.e. standing or supine. In standing position measurement is taken from 2 inches below the axilla to the point on floor 2 inches lateral and 6 inches anterior to the foot (Fig. 5.77).

In supine measurements are taken from axillary fold to a point on plinth 6 to 8 inches lateral to the heel.

Generally 16 inches may be substracted from body height to measure crutch height. Hand grips can be adjusted by flexing the elbow at 20 to 30° of flexion.

Measurement for Forearm Crutches

Standing position in walker or parallel bar is preferred position for taking measurement. Measurements are taken from greater trochanter to a point on the floor 2 inches lateral and 6 inches anterior to the foot. Hand grip position can further be checked by creating 20-30 degree of elbow flexion. Cuff should be positioned approximately 2 to 1.5 inches below the elbow (Fig. 5.78).

General instructions to patient for crutch use:

1. In Axillary crutches—Weight should be borne on the hands and not on the axillary bar to prevent pressure on vascular and neural structures. Axillary bars should be held near chest wall to improve lateral stability.

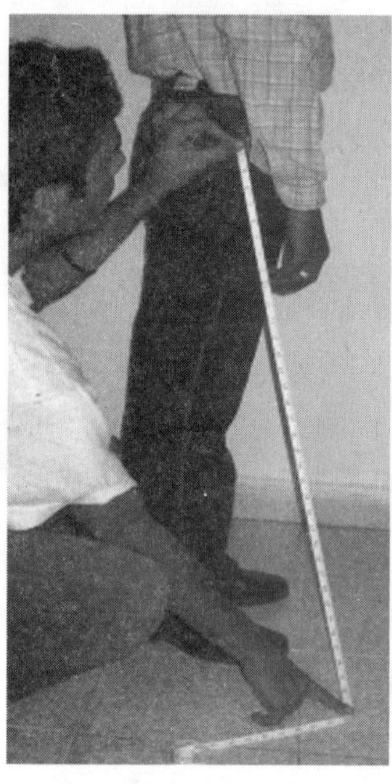

Fig. 5.78: Measurement for elbow crutch

2. The patient should use maximum possible wide base of support (BOS) by keeping crutches at least 4 inches anterior and lateral to the foot.
3. The patient should maintain good posture while using crutch.

Gait Pattern for Crutch Use

Typically there are six gait patterns for crutch use which depends upon the patient's weight bearing condition, muscle strength, balance and coordination. All these gait patterns are different in terms of speed, base of support, and energy requirement.

Four point gait—In this gait weight is borne on four points (two crutches and both extremities). One crutch is placed forward which is followed by contralateral limb, then opposite crutch is placed forward and is followed by contralateral limb. For example—right crutch is progressed forward which is followed by left limb, then left crutch is progressed forward and is followed by right limb (Figs 5.79a to e).

Two point gait—Like four point gait weight is borne on both crutches and lower limbs. In four point, progresion of cructhes and limbs is one by one, but in two point one crutch and opposite limb are progressed together For example—right crutch and left limb is progressed forward together, and weight is taken/borne on these two (right crutch and left limb) then left crutch and

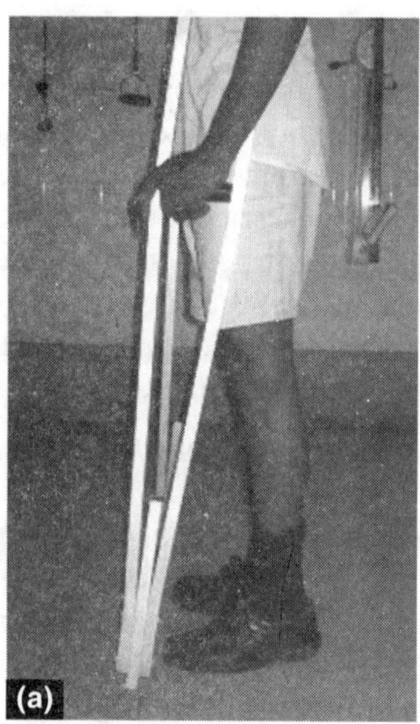

(a)

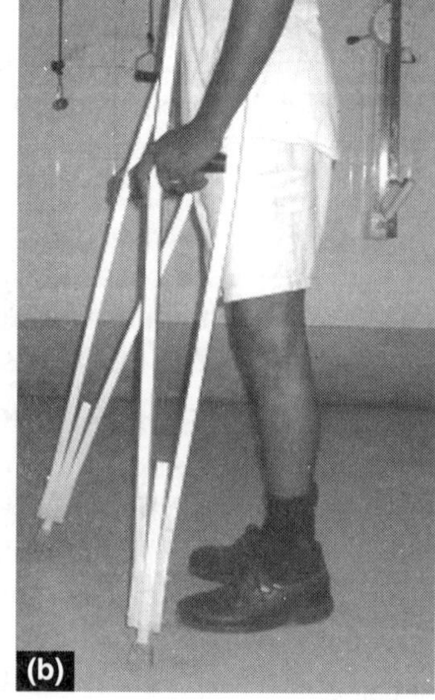

(b)

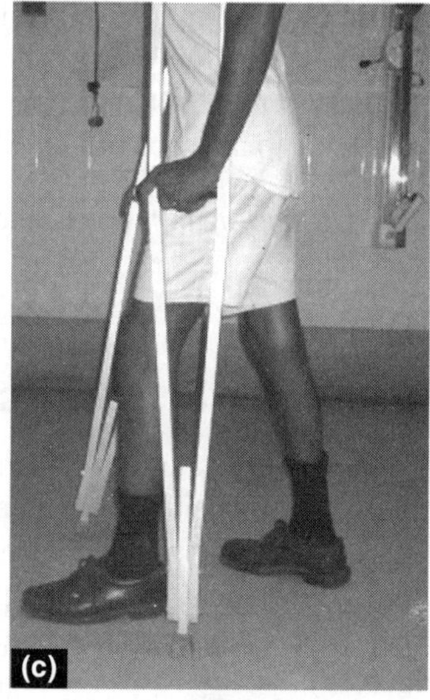

(c)

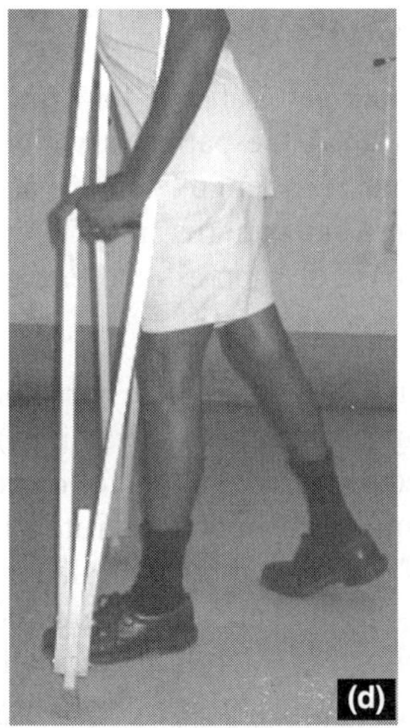
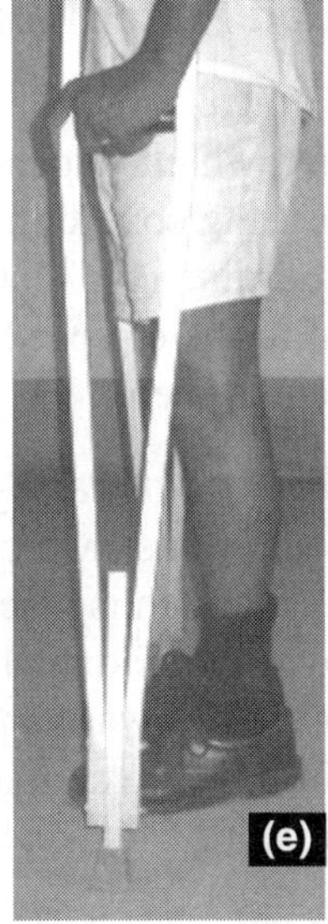

Figs 5.79a to e: Four point gait

right limb is progressed forward. Two point gait is more faster than the four point gait (Fig. 5.80).

Three point gait—In this gait both crutches are progressed forward weight is taken on these both crutches and then unaffected extremity is placed between the crutches or slightly forward. The affected extremity remain flexed at hip and knee joint and does not bear weight of the body. In the

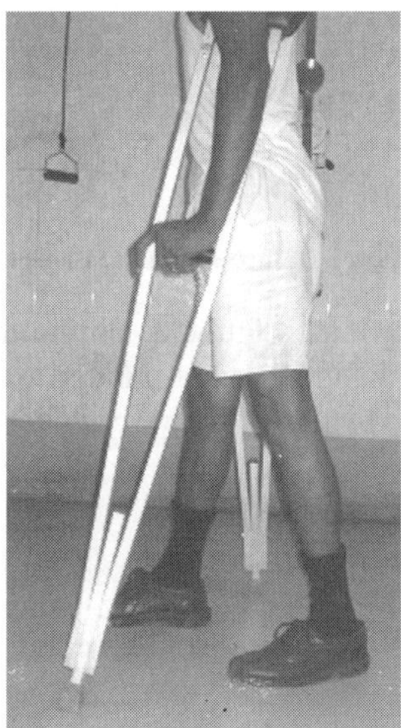

Fig. 5.80: Two point gait

next step of this gait weight is taken on the unaffected extremity and both crutches are progressed forward (Figs 5.81a and b).

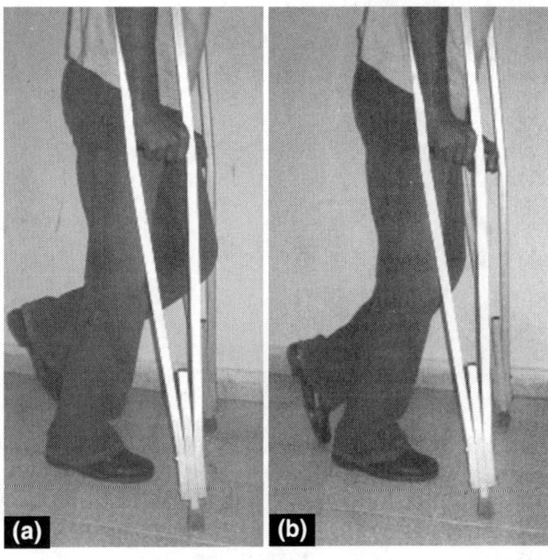

Figs 5.81a and b: Three point gait

Partial weight bearing gait—Like three point gait two axillary crutches are used. Both crutches are placed forward with proper base of support then the affected limb is placed in the same line of the crutches. After placing the affected limb between the crutches the normal leg is placed forward to the crutches, with mild to moderate weight (light weight) bearing on affected leg (Figs 5.82a and b).

Swing to and Swing Through

These gait patterns are commonly used by paraplegic patients (usually with lower extremity orthosis). In swing to both crutches are placed forward then both extremities swing with or without dragging of the feet which do not go beyond the crutches (Figs. 5.83 a to c).

In swing through, like swing to, both crutches move forward together then both extremities swing with or without draging of the feet but unlike swing to, this time extremities swing beyond the crutches (Figs 5.84a to c).

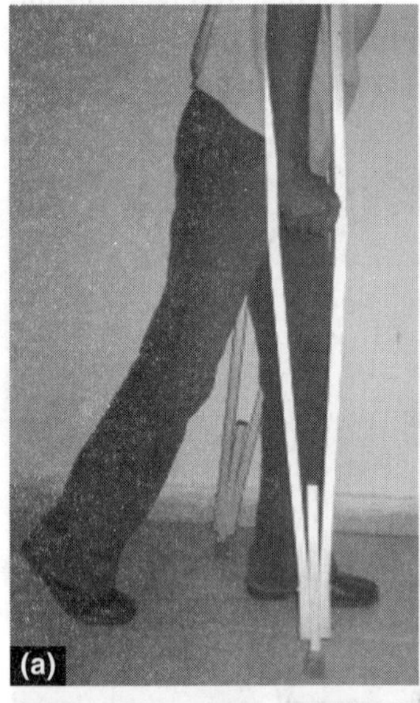
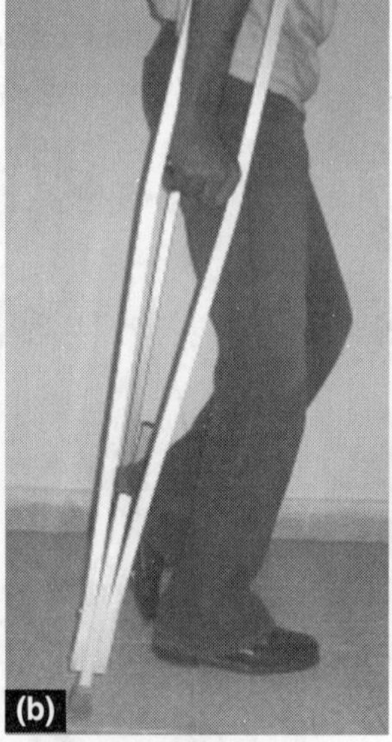

Figs 5.82a and b: Partial weight bearing gait

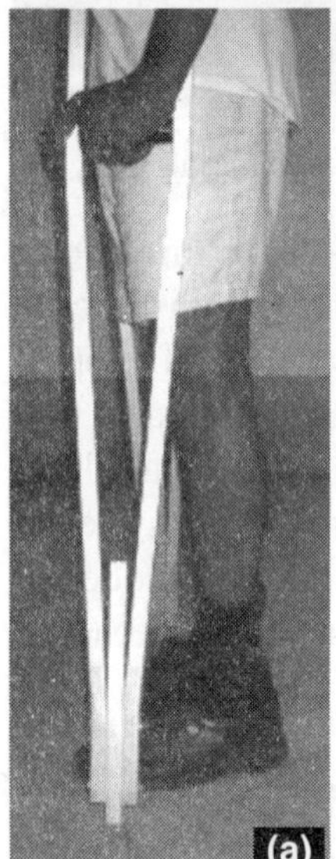
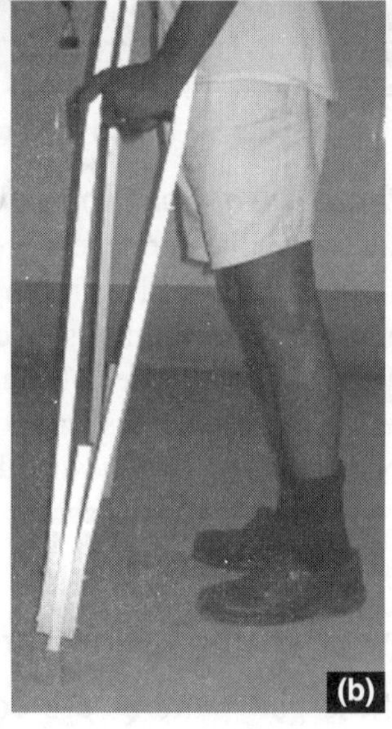
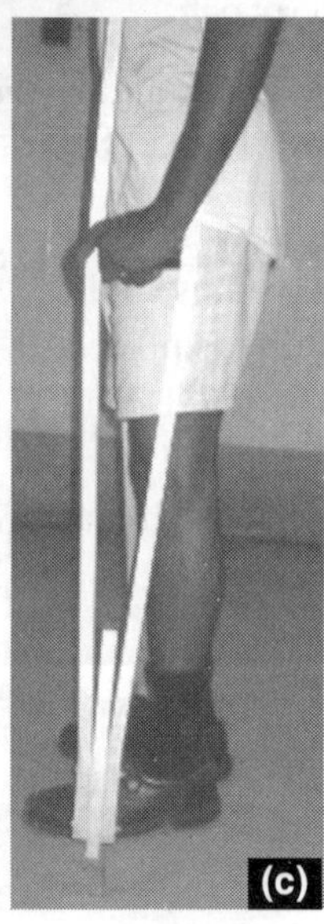

Figs 5.83a to c: Swing to gait

Both type of crutches (axillary and elbow) can be used in swing to and swing through gait.

III. WALKERS

Among all the walking aids this is the most stable aid. Walkers provide better lateral and anterior posterior stability due to wider base of support.

They are used for:

i. Relieving weight partially or fully
ii. Improve balance and stability.

They are typically made of tubular aluminium or iron frames; The hand grips are molded with rubber, foam or vinyl material. They are available in various forms such as (Figs 5.85a to g):

- Adjustable/non-adjustable
- Foldable/non foldable
- Small/medium/large size
- Rolator walker (Walker with front wheels)
- Anterior/posterior walker.

Each has some advantage over other. Like adjustable can be adjusted for taller population

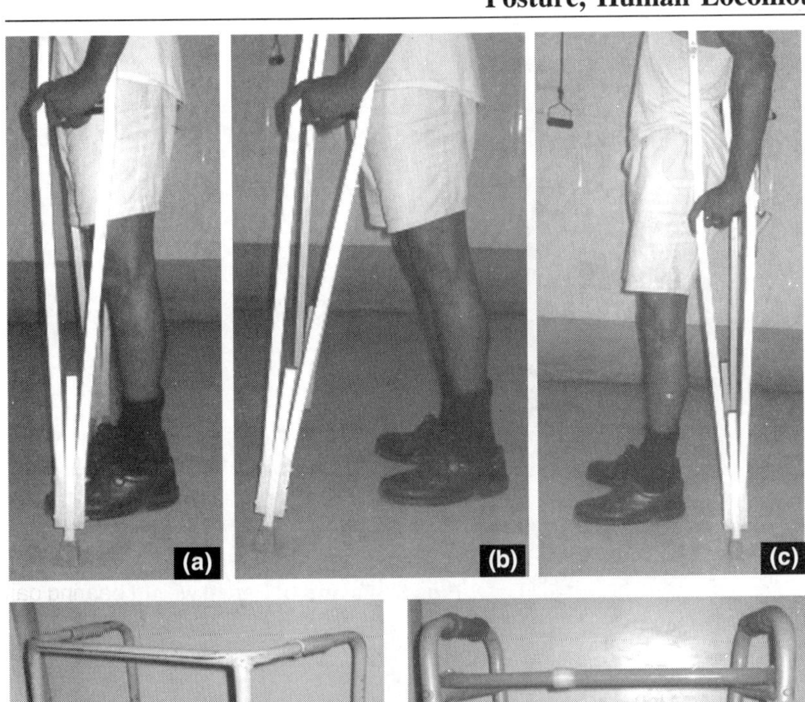

Figs 5.84a to c: Swing through gait

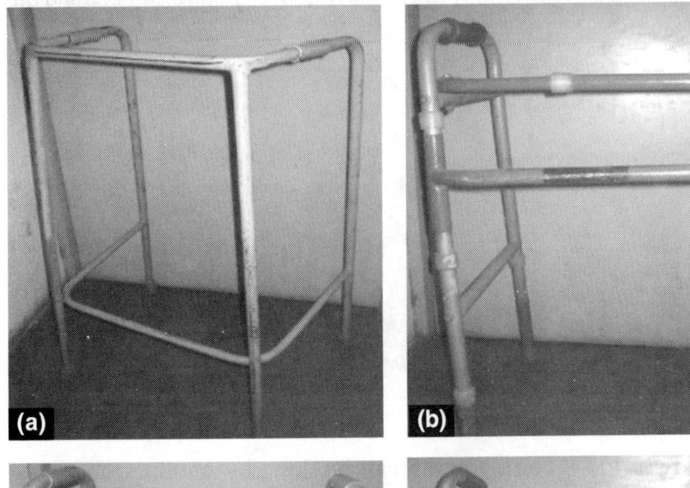

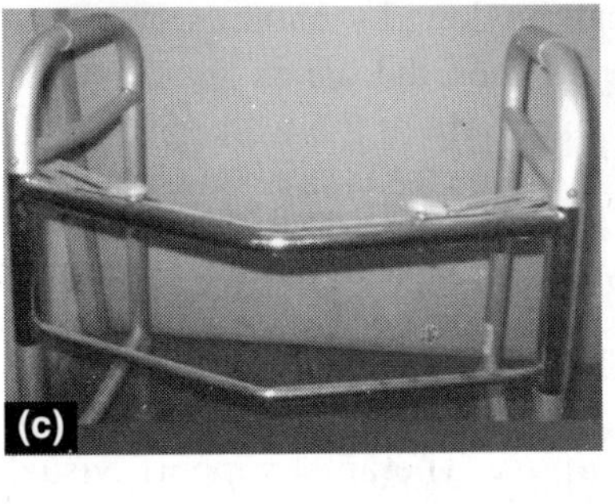

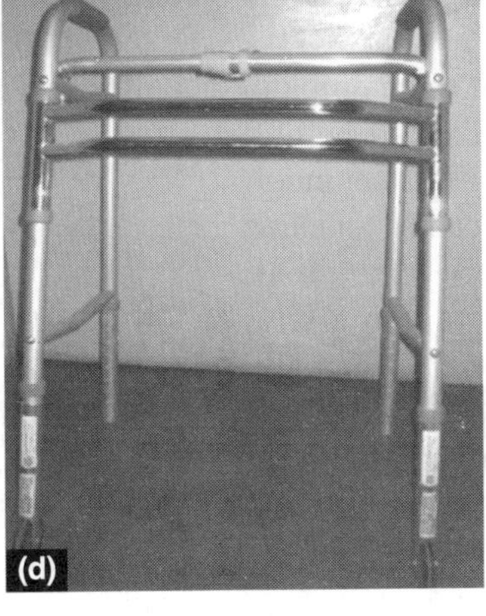

Figs 5.85a to d: (a) A non-foldable walker, (b) A foldable walker, (c) Folding mechanism of walker, and (d) Walker with front wheels

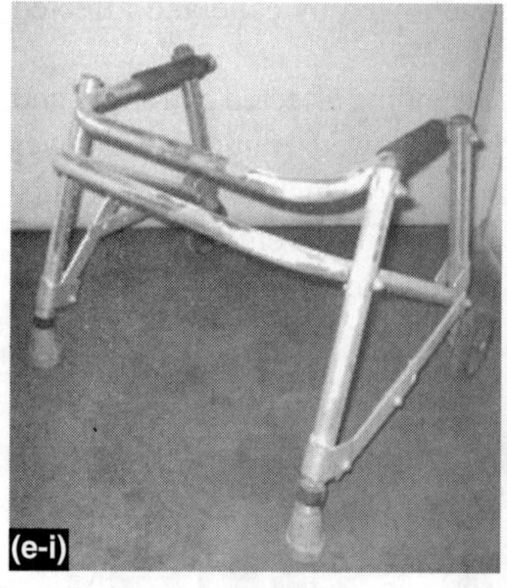

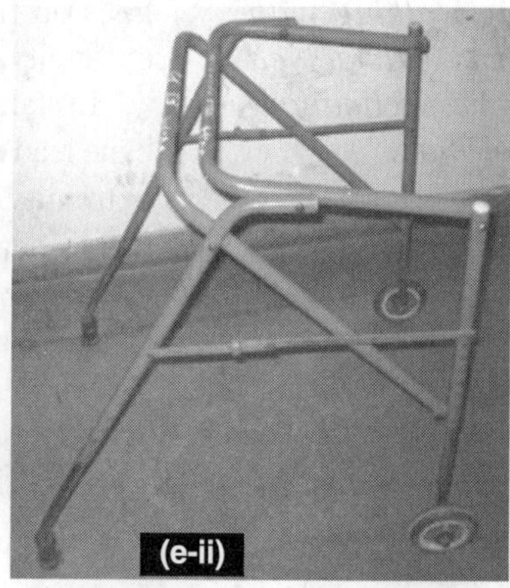

Figs 5.85e(i) and (ii): A posterior walker for children

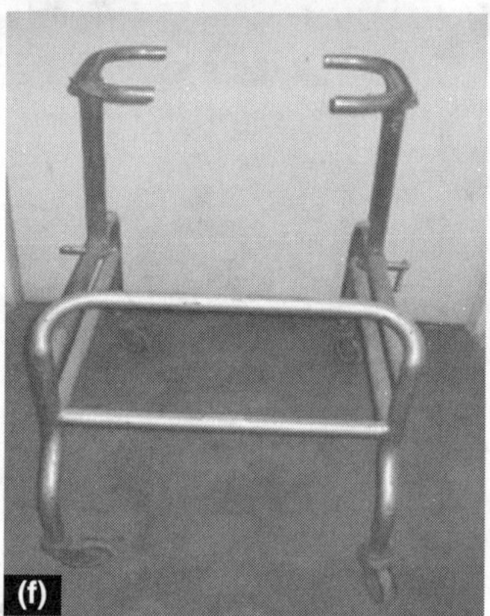

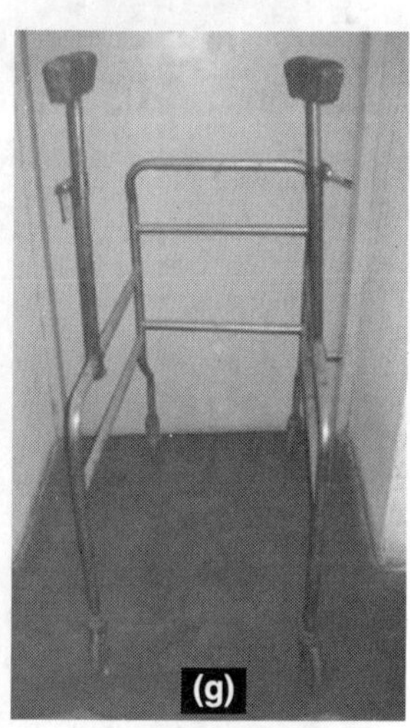

Figs 5.85f and g: (f) A para-walker for children, and (g) A para-walker for adults

but are unstable and make clicking sound at the point of adjustment.

Foldable are easy to carry but same problem of instability is there. Rolator walker are helpful for those who can't lift the usual one. Other modifications such as carry bag, seat can be attached to the walker to make it more functional. Posterior walkers are used for children with cerebral palsy who have tendency to lean forward.

Disadvantage of walker—Stair activities are not possible, difficult to carry and to use in crowded places.

Measurement—Measurement for height are taken from greater trochanter to the floor. Further confirmation can be done by making the elbow flexed at 20 to 30° and the hands should reach comfortably to hand grip of the walker.

Gait Training with Walking Aids

Gait training should be started when the patient has achieved endurance and balance for standing with or without walking aids. Parallel bar may be used for this purpose. Therapist support, visual feed back, verbral clues, ball throwing activities etc. can be used to improve balance and stability in standing. Transfer from various positions seen as sit to stand, stand to sit with or without walking should be taught to the patient.

Note: *Before actually starting walking with aids in various gait patterns (discussed earlier) patient may have some preliminary sessions of walking in parallel bars.*

STAIR ACTIVITIES

1. *Cane:* In stair ascending unaffected extremity goes up first followed by cane and affected extremity.

In stair descending affected extremity and cane lead down followed by unaffected lower extremity (as the leg which leads down later has to bear whole body weight by eccentric contraction of quadriceps) (Figs 5.86a to f).

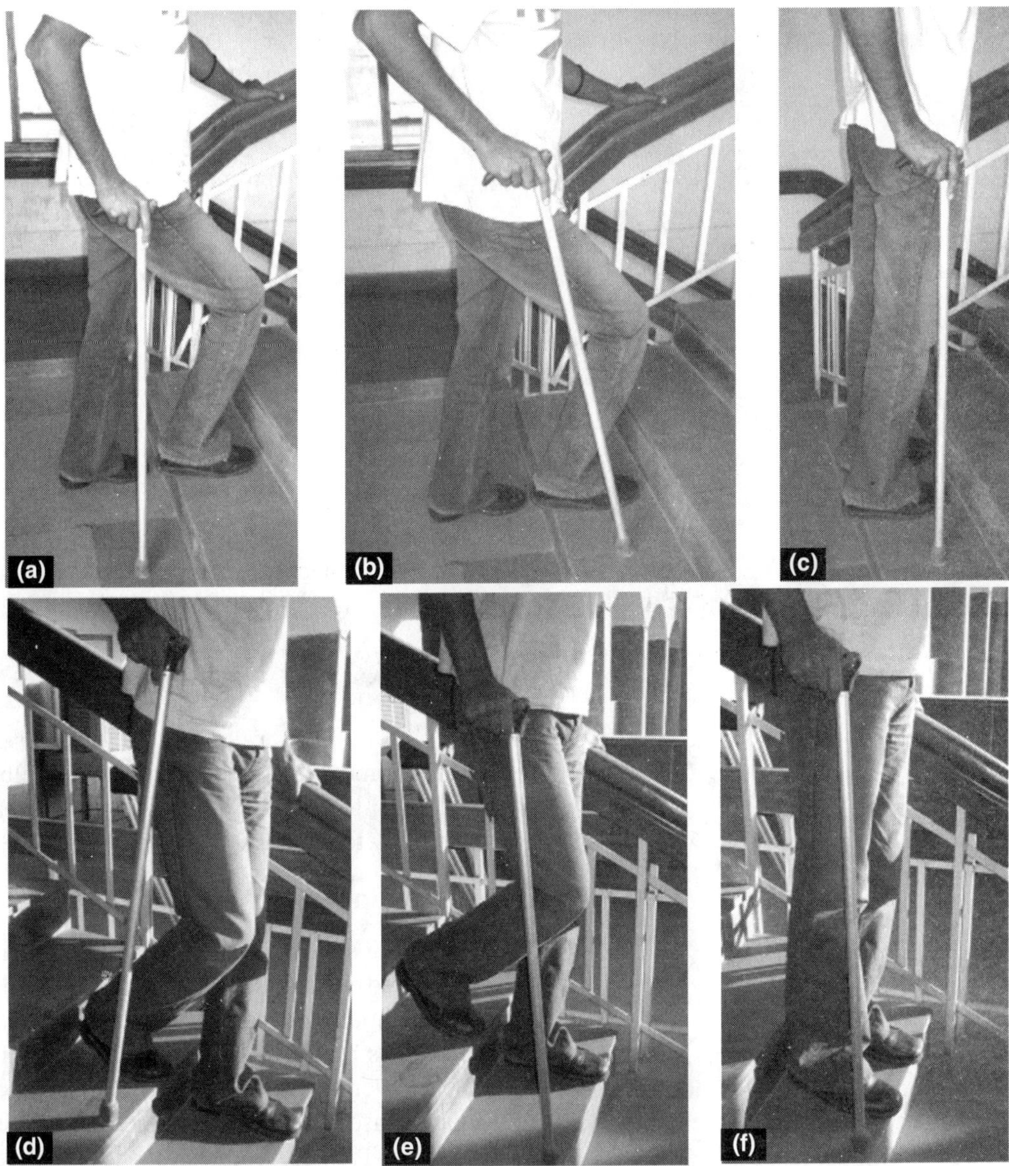

Figs 5.86a to f: (a to c) Stair ascending with cane (left extremity-affected), and (d to f) Stair descending with cane (left extremity-affected)

(Tips to remember "Sound leg takes to heaven affected leg takes to hell").

2. *Crutches:*

a. Three point gait: In stair ascending the patient stands close in front of step, giving some space for affected leg. Then he pushes down firmly on hand pieces of crutches and goes up with unaffected extremity. Which is followed by the crutches.

While descending crutches are kept on the lower step (front half) then he pushes down on the hand piece of the crutches and moves downward. Crutches follows the unaffected leg (Figs 5.87a to d).

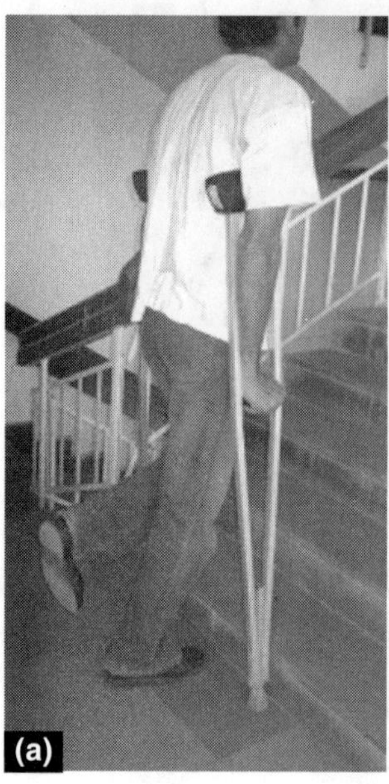

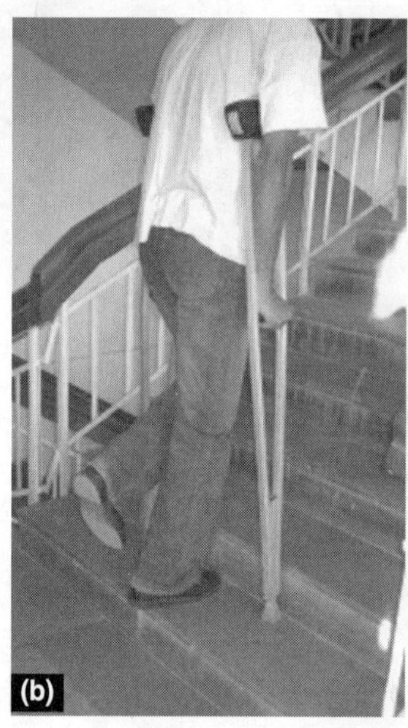

Figs 87a and b: Stair ascending with crutches–three point gait (left extremity-affected)

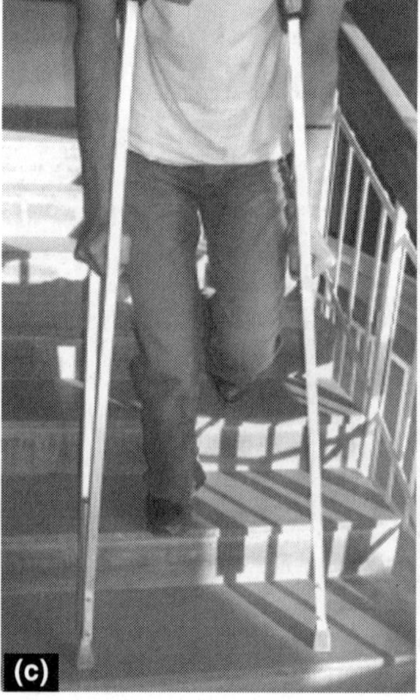

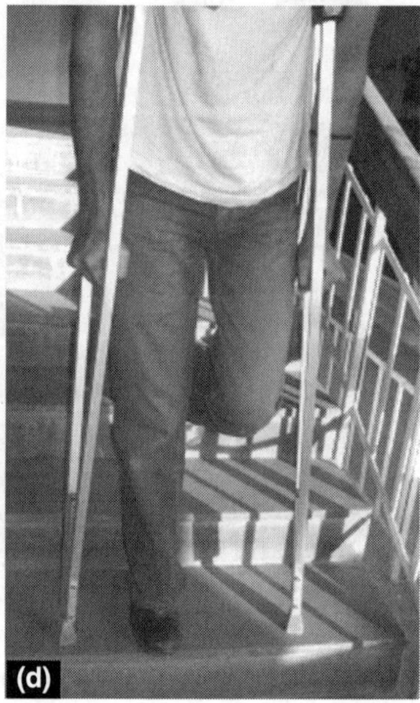

Figs 87c and d: Stair descending with crutches–three point gait (left extremity-affected)

b. Partial weight bearing gait—Pattern of ascending is same as with three point gait, except that the involved extremity also bears some weight. The involved leg and crutches follow the unaffected leg.

c. Four point and two point gait. In ascending patient moves the left lower extremity first then the right. After that crutches may either follow one by one (i.e. first right crutch then the left) or together (Figs 5.88a to j).

In descending right crutch goes down then the left (may together also).

After that right lower extremity is moved down and then the left.

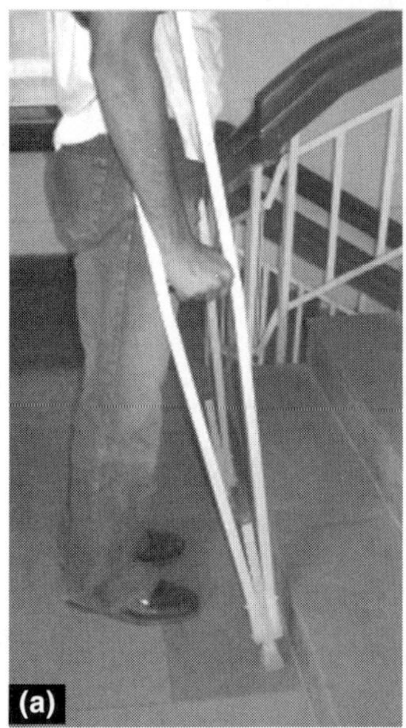

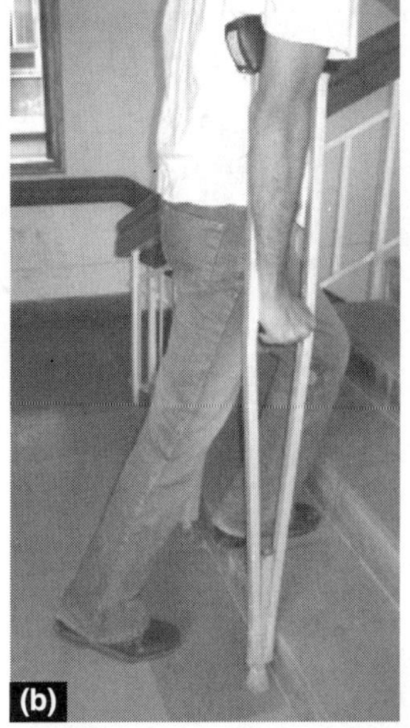

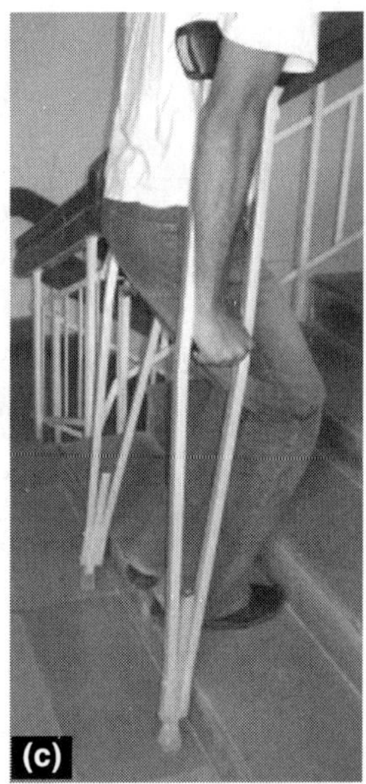

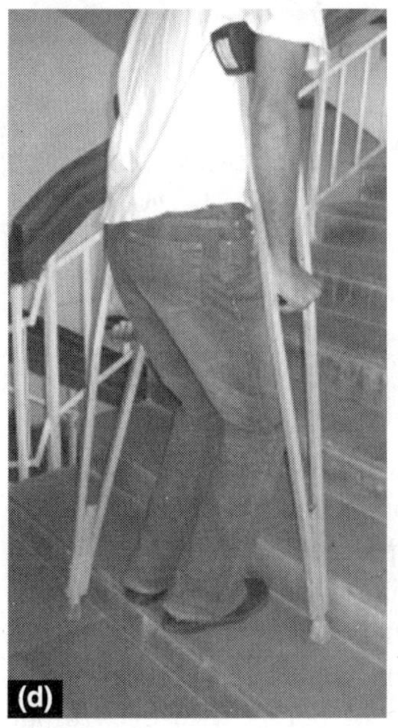

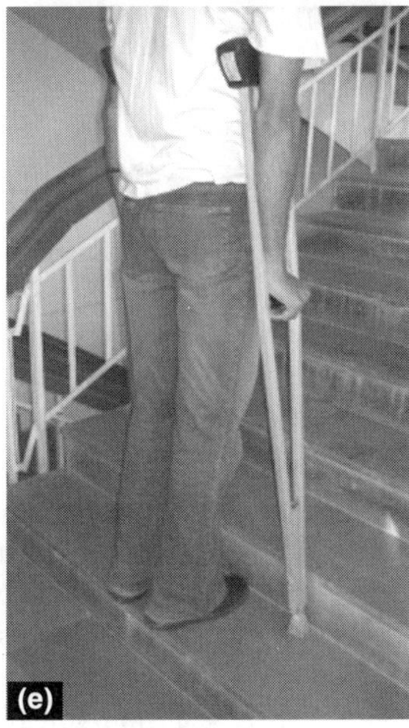

Figs. 5.88a to e: Stair ascending four point gait

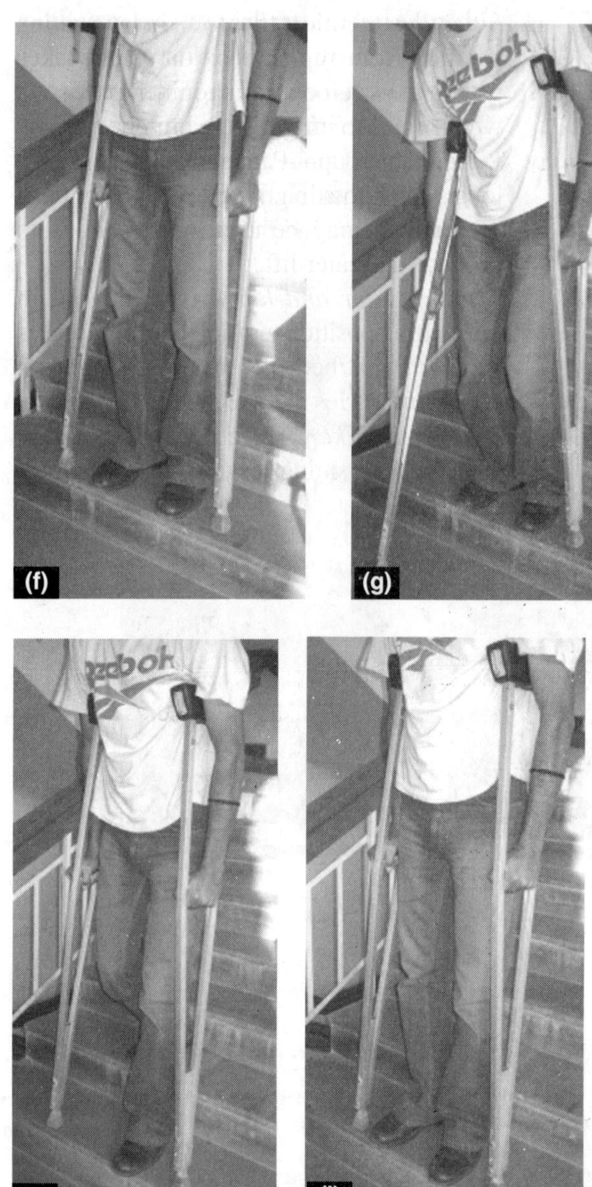

Figs 5.88f to j: Stair descending four point gait

Note: If a railing is available it should always be used. Even the aid may be placed in other hand in which it is not normally used.

CRUTCH AND CANE EXERCISES

Muscles: with their purpose required to perform crutch walking are:

i. Scapular depressors (Latissimus dorsi, lower trapezius, pectoralis minor)—To stabilise the upper limb and prevent hiking of the shoulder on weight bearing—Latissimus dorsi which is known as crutch walking muscle by virtue of its attachment with pelvis (origin point) helps in hiking of pelvis with or without quadratus lumborum to create ground clearance (Typically used by paraplegics).

ii. Shoulder adductors (pectoralis major and latissimus dorsi)—To hold the crutch close to the chest wall.

iii. Shoulder flexors, extensors and abductor especially deltoid)—For placement of the crutch forward, backward and sideward respectively.

iv. Elbow extensors (Tricpes and anconeus)—To stabilise elbow during weight bearing by preventing buckling.

v. Wrist extensors (Extensor carpi radialis and ulnaris)—To hold the wrist in proper position to bear weight on hand piece.

vi. Finger and thumb flexors (flexor digitorum superficial and profundus, flexor pollicis longus and brevis)—To adequately grip the hand piece so that the crutch can be moved to the desired position.

(The use of muscles by the patients depends on the pattern of paresis or paralysis in all the extremities and trunk).

Strengthening of the above mentioned muscles should be started as early as possible in a view to use for crutch walking. The patient whose upper extremities are normal should be taught to do weight/resistive exercises as in crutch walking these muscles have to perform more work than usual.

Preparatory Exercises for Crutch Walking

I. Mat and Bed Exercises

i. *Pelvic tilter:* Patient in supine position on bed or mat, arms at side, legs extended, tries to flatten the lumbar spine. This movement is helpful during swing gait and getting up from seated position.

ii. *Hip hiker:* Patient in supine or prone position tries to lift the hip alternately to develop coordination and skills required for gait.

iii. *Sitter upper:* Patient tries to sit in long sitting position from supine position. This makes patient to use elbow and shoulder extensors, which are also important in crutch walking.

iv. *Sitting:* Push up—Patient does push up in long sitting position. Wooden block or push up handles may be used under hands to produce a greater lift.

v. *Trunk twister and hip raiser:* Patient in long sitting position turns on one side, places hands on mat/bed then bearing weight on upper limbs tries to raise the hip.

vi. *Sitting hip hiker:* Hands on knee or hip, patient in long sitting position tries to approximate iliac crest to the lower hips on one side then the movement is repeated on other side.

vii. *Sitting swing through:* Patient in long sitting position, lifts buttocks on upper limbs by extending elbow then move buttocks backward and forward as much as possible. (These are prerequisite movements for swing through gait)

viii. *Prone push up:* Patient does push up in prone position by abducting the arm, elbow flexed and hands on the floor/mat or bed. (This exercise increases strength of almost all muscles used for crutch walking).

ix. *Tip swayer:* Patient is in quadruped position bears more weight on upper limbs, sways hip to one side then other (good for improving balance and coordination of the trunk and hips)

x. *Camel and Cat:* Patient in quadruped position, extends his neck and causes lordosis at lower trunk (camel), then flexes his neck, contracts abdominal causing rounding of back (cat).

xi. *Forward and backward reacher:* Patient in quadruped position lifts his one arm and tries to make it horizontal to the mat then repeats it with other extremity. In backward reacher exercise, everything is same except patient tries to reach back towards hips.

*(**Note:** All exercise in quadruped position should be performed exclusively on mat).*

II. Mat Exercises with Crutches and Benches

Mat exercise with crutches are done to improve balance, coordination and strength. These exercises are direct carry over of above mentioned mat and bed exercises (Mat crutches are smaller than usual crutches).

(*Crutch position:* Patient in long sitting mat crutches in the axilla, elbows flexed, wrist extended, hands grasping the hand pieces).

   i. *Crutch raiser:* Patient raises the crutch on one side while bearing more weight on other, without displacing the crutch in the axilla. Repeat the same on other side.

   ii. *Sitting crutch push up:* Patient pushes down on the hands raising the buttocks from the mat.

   iii. *Sitting crutch swing through:* After pushing up on the crutches patient moves his buttocks backward and forward as much as possible.

III. Exercises with Kneeling Mat Crutches

Patient does weight shifts, crutch raising etc to improve balance and coordination in kneeling position. This may also be preceded by kneeling balance exercises along.

IV. Wheel Chair Exercises

Patient on wheel chair can do armrest push ups to improve strength of Latissimus dorsi and triceps.

Sitting balance activities such as weight shifting, picking objects from (forward, side ward direction may also be performed.

V. Parallel Bar Exercises

Biomechanically due to bigger base of support parallel bar is the most stable among all the aids of walking. Parallel bar exercises start with standing endurance improvement. Patient stands in parallel bar, putting weight on bar through hand (level of parallel bar at the height of greater trochanter or to permit 20° to 30° of elbow flexion), with feet 4-6 inches apart. Visual feed back through mirror and verbal cues to improve posture is very important.

Patient perform following exercises in parallel bar which leads to independent and balanced walking:

- Weight shift.
- Arm raising alternately.
- Parallel bar push ups.
- Hip hiking and leg swing.
- 4-point gait (same discussed earlier with crutches. Patient shifts hands on the bar instead of crutches).
- Swing to and swing through gait (same as with crutches).
- Backward 4 point and swing gait.

The usual progression from the parallel bar is to one crutch and one bar and then to two crutches in a wide parallel bars. The final progression to 2 crutches with some passive support (wall or therapist etc.) then without any support.

CHAPTER-6

Manual Muscle Strength Testing (MMST) and Goniometry

MANUAL MUSCLE STRENGTH TESTING (MMST)

INTRODUCTION

It is a diagnostic and prognostic approach in which the therapist tests the strength of the muscle by observing the contraction or movement or applying resistance against the action of agonist (prime mover) in the anatomical available range of motion (ROM). Examination of the strength of the muscle between two time intervals provides information about the prognosis of the muscle which also helps to design the treatment.

Uses

Manual muscle strength testing is indicated in muscle weakness due to following causes:

1. *Lower motor neuron diseases*–Such as peripheral nerve injuries, spinal cord injuries, Guillain-Barre syndrome, cranial nerve dysfunctions, poliomyelitis, multiple sclerosis, amyotrophic lateral sclerosis.
2. *Primary muscle disease*–Muscular dystrophy, myasthenia gravis.
3. *Orthopaedic and other conditions*–In these conditions loss of muscle strength is caused by disuse and immobilization, rather than by a direct effect of the disease, such as–fractures, arthritis, amputation, burns.

Contraindications/Precautions

- Pain and inflammation
- Healing wound
- Subluxation and dislocation
- Fracture
- Hypermobility of a joint
- Haemophilia
- Cardiovascular conditions
- Immediate after the surgery
- Severe spasticity
- Muscle fatigue
- Osteoporosis
- Osteomyelitis
- Abdominal Hernia.

Available Range of Motion

Normally the muscle strength is examined in full range of motion but due to some circumstances/abnormal conditions full range of motion cannot be achieved. Suppose a 45 years rheumatoid arthritic patient has 15° of flexion contracture of the knee joint, it means extension is restricted at the end of 15°. So the available range of motion of the extension is 135°-15° and muscle strength should be tested in this range only (135°-15°).

Make or Break Test

The break test is the manual resistance which is used to test the strength of the muscle. At the end of available range of motion or at a point in the range where the muscle is more challenged, the patient is asked to hold the limb at that point (by contracting the muscle), at the same time the therapist applies resistance to break the hold. For example to test the biceps brachii the patient is asked to flex the elbow joint with supination of the forearm and hold the elbow at end range and therapist tries to break the hold and move the limb downward into extension. This is called break test and it is the procedure most commonly used in manual muscle testing today.

Active Resistance Test

It is an alternative of break test in which manual active resistance is applied against the action of agonist muscle throughout available range of motion. During active resistance, an amount of resistance increases gradually until it reaches the maximum level the subject can tolerate and motion ceases. This kind of manual muscle test requires considerable skill and experience to perform and is so often equivocal that its use is not recommended. An active resistance test differs from break test for resistance is against concentric contraction of the agonist muscles action while in break test resistance is applied against eccentric contraction of the agonist muscles action.

The Grading System

The manual muscle strength testing are recorded as numerical scores or qualitative scores, which represent the strength of the muscle.

Numerical Score	*Qualitative Score*
0	Zero, No muscle contraction
1	Trace or flicker muscle contraction
2	Poor—Full range of motion in gravity minimized position.
3	Fair—Full range of motion against the gravity
4	Good—Full range of motion against the gravity with moderate resistance
5	Normal—Full range of motion against the gravity with maximum resistance.

(Each grading is described with illustration of quadriceps muscles).

Grade 0

"No muscle contraction" at all on palpation or visual inspection. Muscle is completely paralysed or quiescent (Figs 6.1a and b).

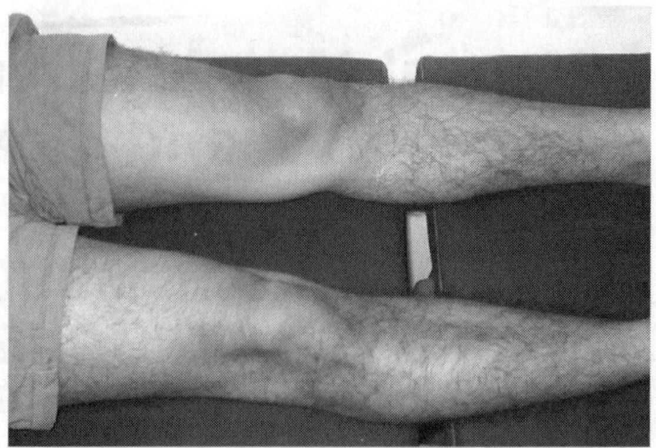

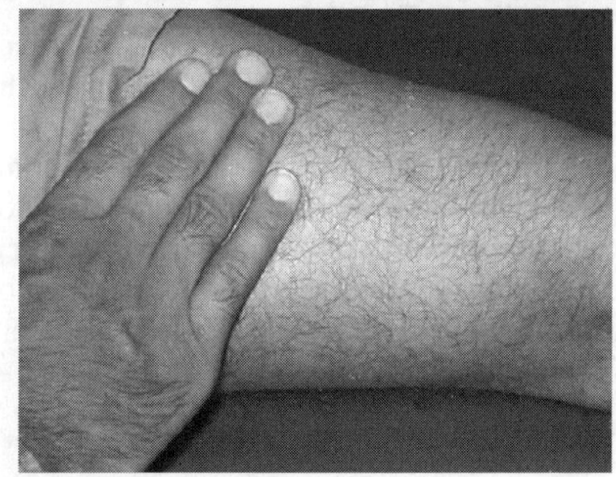

Figs 6.1a and b: Grade-0 (No contraction—Quadriceps muscles)—(a) No visible contraction, and (b) No palpable contraction

Grade 1

"Flicker muscle contraction" but no movement at all. The muscle contraction can be palpated by placing the hand over the muscle belly or therapist can also see or feel a tendon pop up or tense as the patient tries to perform the movement (Fig. 6.2).

Grade 2

"Poor" full range of motion (available range) in gravity minimized position. This position (gravity minimized) is often described as the horizontal plane of motion which minimises the force of gravity. The contraction of muscle is sufficient to perform the movement in gravity minimized position but not against the gravity (Fig. 6.3).

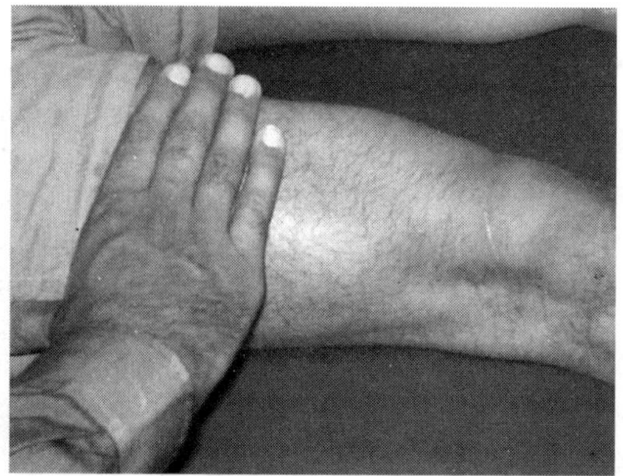

Fig. 6.2: Grade-1
(Flicker contraction—Quadriceps muscles)

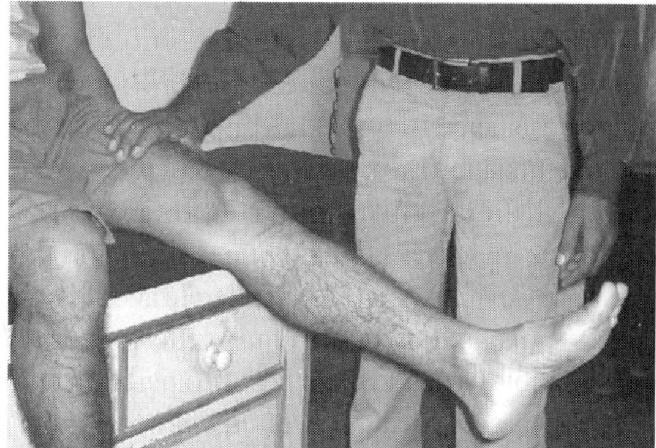

Fig. 6.4: Grade-3
(Against gravity for quadriceps muscles)

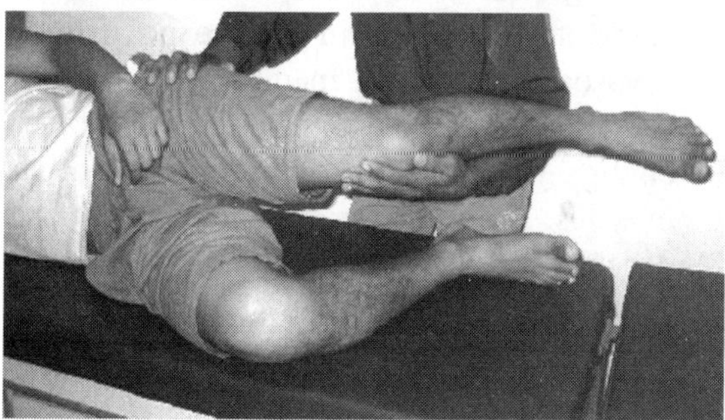

Fig. 6.3: Grade-2 (Gravity eliminated position for quadriceps muscles)

Generally the therapist applies resistance just near the distal end of the segment to which the muscle attaches. There are two common exceptions of this rule are the gluteus medius, minimus and scapular muscles which do not follow the rule (Fig. 6.5).

Grade 3

"Fair" full range of motion against the gravity.

The contraction of muscle is sufficient to perform the movement in full range of motion (available range of motion) against gravity, without an external resistance (by hand of therapist). The therapist observes the movement after stabilising the proximal part of the joint (Fig. 6.4).

Grade 4

"Good"– Full range of motion against the gravity with moderate manual resistance by the hands of therapist. The contraction of muscle is sufficient to perform the movement in available range of motion against the gravity with moderate resistance which is applied by the hands of therapist.

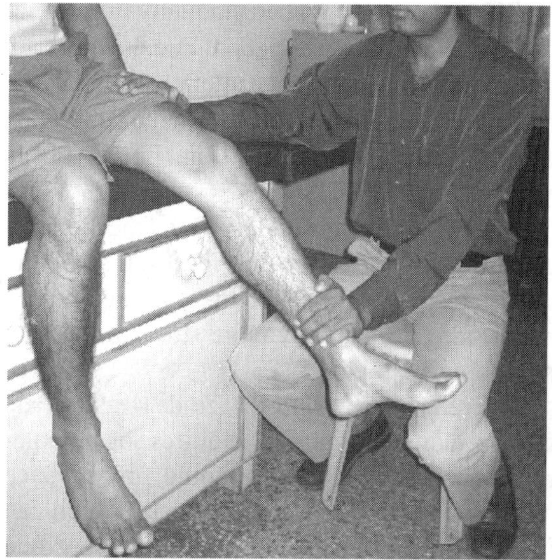

Fig. 6.5: Grade-4 (Against gravity with moderate resistance for quadriceps muscles)

Grade 5

"Normal" full range of motion, against the gravity with maximum resistance (Fig. 6.6).

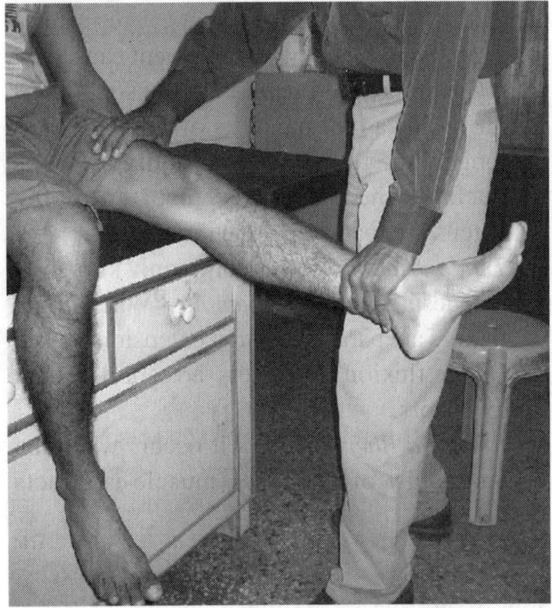

Fig. 6.6: Grade-5 (Against gravity with maximum resistance for quadriceps muscles)

The resistance is applied gradually from initial range and at end range patient is asked to hold this position while therapist attempts to break the hold. In almost every instance when the therapist cannot break the hold position the muscle is rewarded grade 5.

While testing unilateral problem, the therapist can find out the difference in strength of the muscle by testing the sound limb. Though dominated side bears slightly more strength than the non-dominated side.

Therefore, to reward the grade 4 and grade 5 to an individual muscle, requires lot of experience and skills. Students should first practice on their classmates then on patients, which can make them perfect to differentiate the grade 4 from grade 5.

General Rules of MMST

- *Patient should be relaxed:* The procedure should be explained to the patient. MMST should be done on the sound limb first.

- *Position of patient* should be comfortable. Therapist should try to test all the suspected muscles strength in the same position and should not keep changing the position again and again which irritates the patient and can cause wrong muscle testing (for example to test the muscle strength of a post polio residual paralysis, therapist selects supine position to test the lower limb muscle strength, he tests the iliopsoas and changes the position of patient to prone lying and tests gluteus maximus, after that the position of patient is changed to the supine position for gluteus medius in grade 2. To avoid this the therapist should test all the suspected muscles in supine position—iliopsoas then gluteus medius in grade 2 and adductors in grade 2 and ankle muscles then change the position of patient for other muscles. Doing this is more convenient and does not irritate the patient.

- *Position of Therapist* should be comfortable, which can be easiest to stabilise the proximal part of the joint as well as apply resistance against the agonist muscles in grade 4 and grade 5.

  To differentiate the grade 1 from grade 0 an examiner should have a knowledge of muscle anatomy (origin, insertion and muscle belly). To palpate the contraction of muscle therapist should place the hand over the muscle belly and ask the patient to contract the muscle, if therapist does not feel contraction of muscle, muscle should be rewarded grade 0, which is considered as a complete paralysis.

- *The movement should occur in anatomical range* (*For example*–When patient is asked to abduct the shoulder joint, patient lifts the shoulder between flexion and abduction that is in scapula plane and known as scaption plane which is neither flexion nor abduction) so therapist may demonstrate the movement prior to muscle strength testing.

- The proximal part of the joint which is being tested should be stabilised in three ways:
1. By using the weight of the body;
2. By one hand of the examiner; and
3. By applying straps (applying tight straps can prevent the contraction of the muscle).

Trick Movements/Substitution/ Vicarious Motions

The brain "thinks" in terms of movement and not contraction of an individual muscle. Thus a muscle or muscle group may attempt to compensate for the function of a weaker muscle to accomplish a movement. These movements are called Trick movements or substitutions or vicarious motions.

The other part of the body should also be observed during the muscle testing. Sometimes patient deliberately moves other joints, segment of the body to compensate the action of weakened muscle which is being tested. (*For example*–If abductors of shoulder joint, specially supraspinatus, is weak and as patient is asked to abduct the shoulder joint, the patient elevates the shoulder girdle of the same side and flexes the spine to the opposite side which gives thrust to arm and patient initiates the shoulder abduction. So patient is instructed prior to the test not to move other joints or segment of the body to avoid trick movements.

Classification of Trick Movements/ Substitution/Vicarious Motions

i. *Direct Substitution*: Direct substitution can be of two types. First type, which deceives the therapist. *For example*—Long extensors cause abduction of finger in a complete ulnar nerve injury.

   Second type, which successfully replace function lost by obvious paralysis. *For example*—Abduction and elevation of shoulder caused by long heads of biceps and triceps, the clavicular fibres of pectoralis major and the external rotators of the humerus in case of deltoid paralysis.

ii. *Accessory Insertion*: A very common example of this type is movement caused by abductor pollicis brevis and extensor pollicis brevis in case of paralysis of flexor pollicis longus due to radial nerve injury. This is because these muscles inserted at the extensor expansion of the thumb.

iii. *Tendon Action:* This is commonly known as tenodesis action. *For example*—When finger flexors are paralysed, wrist extension caused finger flexion as flexors are shorter than extensors.

iv. *Rebound Phenomenon*: It occurs when the antagonist of paralysed muscle contracts strongly and relaxes, it appears as if there is a contraction in the agonist. *For example*—Strong contraction of flexor hallucis longus and then relaxing it gives appearance of extension action of extensor hallucis longus.

v. *Anatomical Variation*: Almost one fifth of peripheral nerve injuries may have some anomaly of nerve supply. *For example*—Presence of action of opponens and flexor pollicis brevis in complete median nerve injury (these muscles may be supplied by ulnar nerve).

vi. *Gravity*: Action of muscles like triceps can be performed by gravity as usually patient does in triceps paralysis by depressing the shoulder and allow gravity to cause extension.

Application of Resistance

The general rule of application of resistance is to apply it just near the distal end of the segment to which muscle is attached. There are two common exceptions of this rule–the gluteus medius and minimus and the scapular muscles. To test the abductors of hip joint resistance should be applied on the distal end of femur just above the knee joint. The abductor muscles are so strong, however, that most examiners, in testing a patient with normal knee strength and joint integrity, will choose to apply resistance at the lateral aspect of the ankle joint. To test the vertebroscapular muscles (e.g. rhomboids), the preferred point of resistance is on the arm rather than on the scapula where these muscles insert.

Generally, a muscle bears most resistance at the mid range because at this point lever arm is increased (e.g. in the case of biceps brachii, when the elbow is straight, the lever arm is short; leverage increases as an elbow flexes and becomes maximal at 90° flexion, but as flexion continues beyond that point, the lever arm again decreases in length and efficiency.)

In manual muscle testing, the application of resistance at the end of the range in one joint muscles allows consistency of procedure rather than an attempt to select the estimated mid range position. In two joint muscles (e.g. medial or lateral hamstring muscles) the point of maximal resistance is generally at or near mid range.

The Plus (+) and Minus (–) Grades

Poor Minus (P⁻)   or   2⁻
Poor Plus (P⁺)   or   2⁺
Fair Minus (F⁻)   or   3⁻
Fair Plus (F⁺)   or   3⁺

Poor minus (P⁻) or grade 2⁻: the joint moves through incomplete range of motion in gravity minimized position. *For example*–The available range of motion of the elbow flexion) is 0° to 135° and when patient attempts to move the joint, he or she does not move the joint from 0°–135° in gravity minimized position, but moves from 0°–90° which is termed as grade 2⁻ or poor minus.

Poor plus or grade 2⁺: Joint moves through incomplete range of motion (less than 50%) against gravity or joint moves through complete range of motion in gravity minimized position against slight resistance.

Fair minus (F⁻) or grade 3⁻: Joint moves through incomplete range of motion (less than 100% but more than 50%) against gravity.

Fair plus (F⁺) or grade 3⁺: Joint moves through complete range of motion, against gravity and slight resistance.

The plus/minus concept with grade 4 has been discarded.

GONIOMETRY

INTRODUCTION

Goniometry is derived from two Greek words **jenio-angle, meton-measurement**.

The study of medical science in which the range of motion of the joint of human body is measured by an instrument is known a Goniometry.

Measurement Instrument

To measure the range of motion of the joint several instruments have been provided by **persons of varied professional and academic background** since early Nineteenth century.

In 1995, Salter offered a good survey of the literature but did not include references from the United States in the fields of physical therapy and occupational therapy, each of which have contributed significant studies on joint mobility.

The most widely accepted and recommended instrument is the universal goniometer called an arthrometer (Fig. 6.7a).

Many instruments are recommended to measure the range of motion of the joint but now-a-days the selection of instrument by an examiner depends on the instrument's accuracy, cost and availability.

1. Universal Goniometer

The most widely accepted and recommended instrument to measure the joint range of motion of almost all joints, designed by Moore, is known as universal goniometer. It is a type of protractor with two thin arms made of plastic or metal. The availability of the instrument is in different size

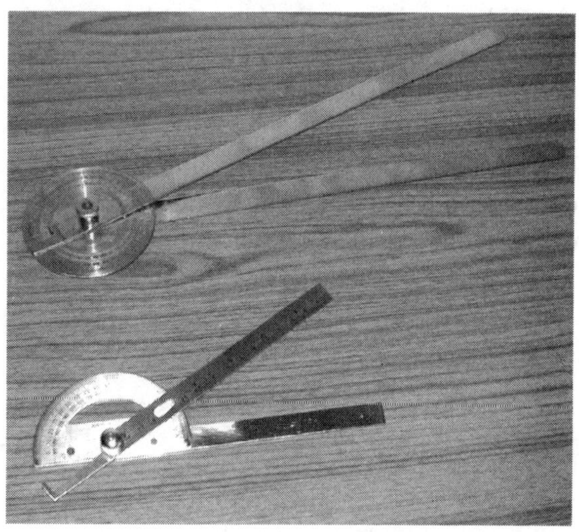

Fig. 6.7a: Half and full circle goniometer

and shape but the features (protractor and two arms) remain same in all universal goniometers.

Parts of Universal Goniometer:
1. Body or protractor .
2. Two arms.
3. Fulcrum.

Body of goniometer—it is basically a protractor on which scales are located, if the protractor is full circle then it is called as full circle goniometer in which scales are located on one or both side from 0°-360° and 360°-0° or 0°-180° and from 180°-0°.

If the protractor is half circle, then it is called as half circle goniometer and scales are located on either side from 0°-180° and 180° to 0°.

Fulcrum

It is attached to the body, or the part where moving arm attached with the body is known as fulcrum it is the type of screw which gives degree of freedom to moving arm. Fulcrum is generally placed over the joint line (Fig. 6.7b).

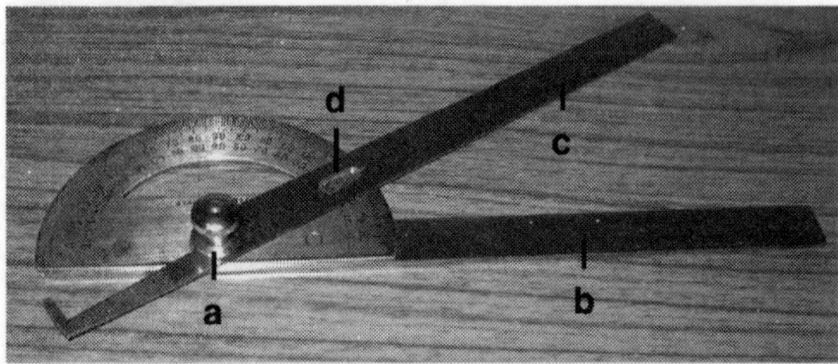

Fig. 6.7b: Parts of goniometer (a-Fulcrum; b-Stationary arm; c-Moving arm; d-keyhole)

The graduation should be large enough to be read by naked eyes. The interval on the scale may vary from 1 to 10°.

Arms

The two arms are **attached on body**, (a) stationary and (b) moving.

a. *Stationary arm:* It is fixed on body and can not be moved over it, generally stationary arm is placed over the proximal or stabilised part of the limb.

b. *Moving arm:* It is also attached on body at the centre with screw which allows it to move. Moving arm is placed on the distal part of the limb and moves along with it. Every moving arm should have one of the following character.

   i. *Keyhole indicator or cut out portion—* at the centre of moving arm over the scale a whole is made, which allows the transparency to read out the scale (degree).

   ii. A prominent line should extend from the point to the distal tip of the moving arm.

   iii. A black or white line on middle of the moving arm should extend from screw (fulcrum) to the distal tip of the moving arm.

Some Other Goniometers/Arthrometers

2. Electro Goniometers

This goniometer was designed by Kar Pavich and Karvich in 1959. It is a type of goniometer, like universal goniometer most of devices have two arms which are connected with potentio meter. The both arms of electrogoniometer placed on the proximal and distal part of the joint and a potentiometer is connected to them. Movement of the arms cause resistance in the potentiometer to vary. The resulting change in voltage can be used to indicate the amount of joint motion. Electrogoniometers are used primarily in research to obtain dynamic joint range measurement.

3. Gravity Dependent Goniometers

These are sometimes called as inclinometers (Fig. 6.8). To measure the joint range of motion the effect of gravity is used on pointers and fluid levels. These are basically of two types:

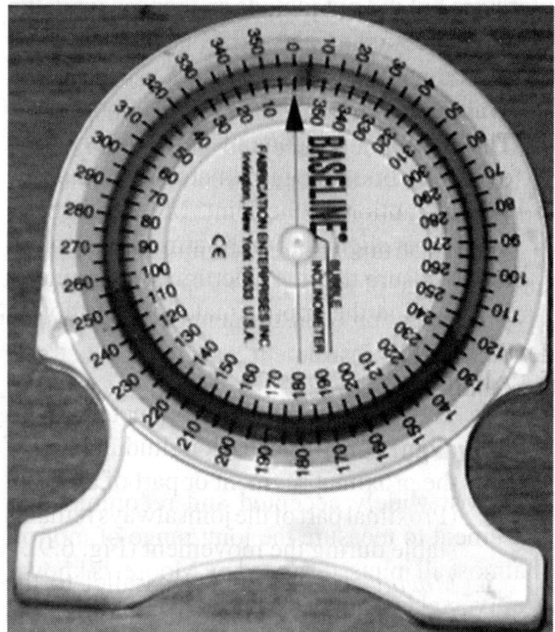

Fig. 6.8: Inclinometer (Gravity dependent goniometer)

1. *Pendulum goniometer:* It was first devised by Fox and Van Breemen in 1934. It consist a 360° protractor with a weighted pointer hanging from the center of the protractor.

2. *Fluid (Bubble) goniometer:* It was devised by Schenkar in 1956, has fluid filled circular chamber containing an air bubble.

PROCEDURES

1. To measure the ROM of the joint it is very important to select the comfortable position of patient so that he/she does not move during measurement of range of motion. The joint which is being evaluated should be adequately exposed (remove clothing), to palpate and observe the anatomical landmarks.

2. The therapist stands or sits comfortably according to his convenience and should not change the stance during measurement of ROM, it changes the alignment/position of goniometer and causes error in the measurement.

3. Selection of goniometer—Different sizes and shapes of universal goniometer are available therefore suitable size and shape of goniometer should be selected depends upon joint being evaluated.

4. The fulcrum of the goniometer which is placed over joint line or approximate location of the axis of motion of the joint. Moore suggests that proper alignment of the arms of the goniometer ensure that the fulcrum of goniometer is located at the approximate axis of motion of the joint.

5. **Alignment of arms:**
   i. The *stationary arm* of goniometer is often aligned parallel to the longitudinal axis of the proximal segment or part of the joint (Proximal part of the joint always remains stable during the movement (Fig. 6.9).
   ii. *Moving arm*–is aligned parallel to the longitudinal axis of the distal part of the joint (Fig. 6.9).
   In almost all cases the alignment of arms remain constant but in some circumstances

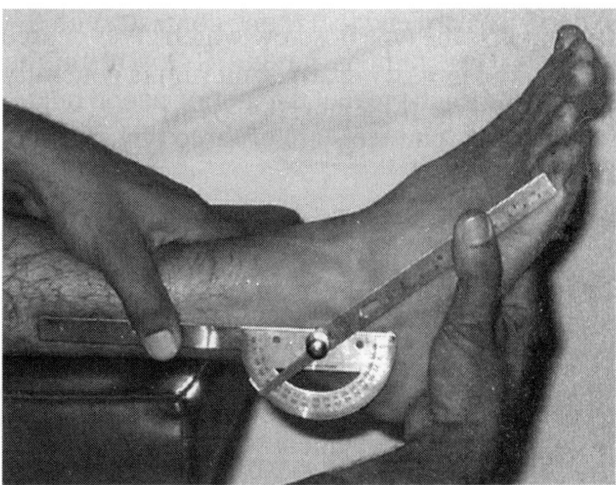

Fig. 6.9: Placement of Goniometer for ankle joint (showing fulcrum on lateral malleolus; stationary arm over the proximal part of the joint and moving arm over the distal part of the joint)

alignment of arms may be vice versa (stationary arm is aligned parallel to the longitudinal axis of the distal segment while moving arm is placed over the proximal segment/part of the joint.

6. After placement of fulcrum, stationary arm and moving arm, the examiner stabilizes the stationary arm with the proximal segment of the joint, while moving arm is held with the distal segment of the joint, ask the patient to move the distal segment of joint in the available range of motion. During motion the arms of the goniometer should be kept with the proximal and distal segment of joint do not allow them to change the position, although slight adjustments are needed to be done. Active and passive ranges are measured.

END FEEL—NORMAL

The feeling which is experienced by the therapist at the end of passive range of motion. The end range of motion of the normal joint is prevented by the soft tissue structures or bones, for example: The normal end of elbow extension is prevented as olecranon process of ulna contacts with the olecranon fossa of humerus, and when joint is extended passively, the hands of the therapist experience hard end feel (bone contacts with the bone). Every joint is having its own unique structures which prevent the motion at end range. Normally end feels are of three types:

1. **Hard**
   - Bone contacting bone, example–elbow extension.
2. **Firm:** Firm as the name suggests, a firm feeling by the hands of the therapist is because of stretching of soft tissue structures (mainly joint capsule, ligaments and muscles) at the end range of movement.
   - i. **Stretching of capsule** example—The anterior joint capsule (MCP) gets stretched and prevents further extension as metacarpophalangeal joints are extended passively.
   - ii. **Stretching of muscle** example—When hip joint is flexed with knee extended, the hamstring muscles get stretched and prevents the further hip flexion.
   - iii. **Stretching of ligaments** example— Supination of forearm places extension in the proximal radioulnar joint, interosseous membrane, oblique cord.
3. **Soft:** Soft tissue approximation mainly because of contact of soft tissues of the proximal and distal segments of the joint (e.g. at end of knee flexion calf muscles contact with the posterior thigh).

Restriction in the range of motion is generally caused by tightness of the soft tissue structures (muscles, ligamentous and joint capsule) or pathological changes in the intraarticular structures of the joint. These pathological changes can change the normal end feel of the joint.

END FEELS—PATHOLOGICAL (by Cyriax, Kalten born and Paris)

Table 6.1: Pathological end feels

	End-Feel	Examples
Soft	Occurs sooner or later in the range of motion that is usual, or in a joint that normally has a firm or hard end feel.	Soft tissue oedema synovitis
Firm	Occurs sooner or later in the range of motion that is usual, or in a joint that normally has a soft or hard end feel.	Increased muscular tonus capsular, muscular, ligamentous shortening
Hard	Occurs sooner or later in the range of motion than is usual, or in a joint that normally has a soft or arm end feel a bony grating or bony block is felt.	Chondromalacia Osteo-arthritis, loose bodies in joint, myositis ossification, fracture
Empty	No real end feel because pain prevents reaching end of range of motion. No resistance is felt except for patient's protective muscle splinting or muscle spasm.	Acute joint inflammation: – Bursitis – Abscess – Fracture – Psychogenic disorder

Precautions and Contraindications

A. Measurement of joint range of motion is contraindicated in case of following conditions:
   1. Joint dislocation
   2. Fracture
   3. Immediate by following surgery of soft tissue structures.

B. Extra precautions should be taken in case of following conditions:
   1. Acute joint inflammation
   2. Osteoporosis
   3. Haemophilia
   4. Haematoma.

Therapeutic Approaches

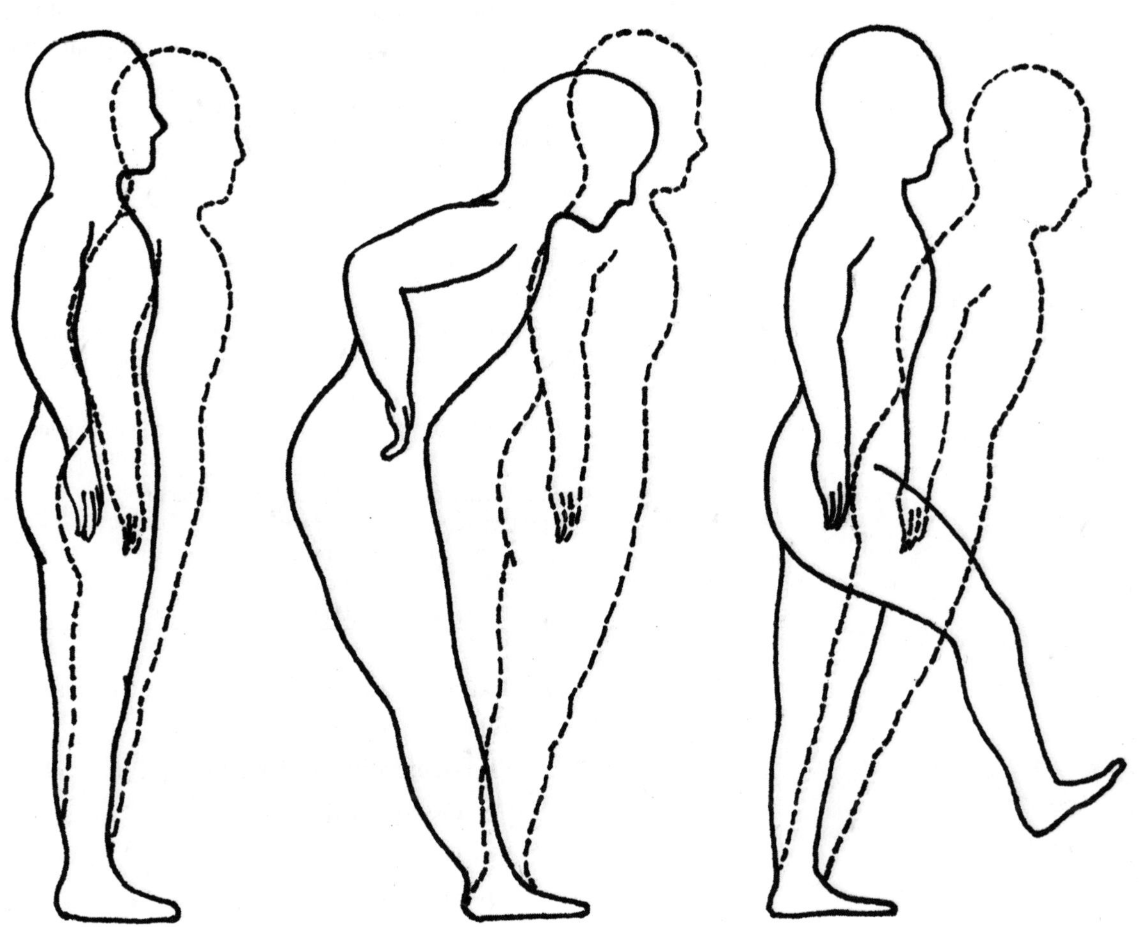

Mobilization of Peripheral Joint

INTRODUCTION

The technique of mobilization is being used from the time of Hippocrates, a physician in the fourth century. For some time in the past these important techniques of mobilization were lost from practice because earlier the use of mobilization technique was passed quietly on empirical evidence of their effectiveness there was no scientific basis for their use.

In late 1700s and early 1800s this influence prevailed and joint manipulation remained in the hands of bonesetters. The bonesetters had no basic knowledge of joint structures and manipulation technique other than their past experience they endorsed upon their knowledge keeping their secret and ordinarily made.

Hutton was the bonesetter who was famous for his free services to the patients, he suffered from serious illness and was treated by Dr. Peter Hood, father of Dr. Wharton Hood. In repayment of treatment, Hutton offered Dr. Peter to teach all techniques, the knack of bonesetting but Dr. Peter Hood did not accept the offer, however his son Wharton Hood accepted the offer and learnt the technique of bonesetting from Hutton. He has written medical book on manipulation which was published in 1870s. In his paper on the same published in 1871 Dr. Hood described Hutton's techniques of spinal and peri-

peral manipulation. The techniques described by Hutton were always at a high velocity thrust and essentially identical to the manipulations used by manual therapists and even some orthopedists and physicians. Hutton had no interest to knowing anatomy, however, he avoided the technique of manipulation of inflamed joint. He employed

Mobilization of Peripheral Joint

INTRODUCTION

The technique of mobilization is being used from the time of Hippocrates, a physician in the fourth century, BC. Some time in the past these important techniques of mobilization were lost from practice because earlier, the use of mobilization techniques was based purely on empirical evidence of their effectiveness, there was no scientific basis for their use.

In late 1700s and early 1800s this influence prevailed and joint manipulation remained in the hands of bonesetters. The bonesetters had no basic knowledge of joint structures and manipulation techniques other than their past experience, they tended to guard their knowledge, keeping their secret among family members.

Then rivalry started between physicians and bonesetters. Thomas who was the son and grandson of bonesetters was one of the physician who spoke against the bonesetters and invented the splint, known as Thomas splint.

Hutten was the bonesetter who was famous for his free services to the patients. He suffered from serious illness and was treated by Dr Peter Hood, father of Dr Wharton Hood. In repayment of treatment, Hutten offered Dr Peter to teach all techniques he knew of bonesetting but Dr Peter Hood did not accept the offer. However his son Wharton Hood accepted the offer and learnt the techniques of bonesetting from Hutten. He has written medical book on manipulation which was published in 1870s. In his paper on the subject, published in Lancet in 1871, Hood described Hutten's techniques of spinal and peripheral manipulation. The techniques described by Hutten were always of a high velocity thrust and essentially identical to the manipulations used by manual therapists and even some orthopedists and physiatrist today. Hutten admitted to knowing nothing of anatomy, however, he avoided the techniques on acutely inflamed joints. He employed his techniques primarily on post-immobilization stiffness, displaced cartilage and tendons and ganglionic swellings.

MOBILIZATION AND MANIPULATION

The articular surfaces of a joint move every day in anatomical and physiological ranges as required by normal activities of daily living. Adhesion formation in the region of joint followed by injury or pathological changes restricts the motion of articular surfaces, subsequently the range of motion decreases, and activities of daily living are compromised. Pain becomes the most dominant problem and because of it patient avoids activities. If condition is not treated at the right time, the joint range of motion is severely restricted and gradually the joint space decreases as well, which is called as fibrous ankylosis. Rehabilitation programme which includes mobilization techniques of the joints has significant effect on restricted joints by breaking up the adhesion formation, subsequently increasing range of motion and joint space as well.

Mobilization

- Mobilization is a passive movement directed at the joint without any high velocity thrust and within the range of motion.

- It is a gentle, coaxing, repetitive rhythmic movement of a joint that can be resisted by the patient. Unlike manipulation, it can be performed over a wide range and can thus involve a series of movements, referred to as stages.

Manipulation

- Manipulation is a high velocity thrust of small amplitude.
- It is a very rapid, passive movement at the end of the range of a joint, is far more forceful than mobilization and can not be controlled by the patient.

EFFECTS OF IMMOBILIZATION ON CONNECTIVE TISSUES

Immobilization and trauma significantly change the histology and normal mechanics of connective tissue.

Macroscopically, fibrofatty infiltrate is evident in the recesses of the immobilized tissues. With prolonged immobilization the infiltrates develop a more fibrotic appearance, creating adhesions in the recesses. These fibrotic changes occur in the absence of trauma. Histologic and histochemical analysis show significant changes primarily in the ground substance, (whose function is to bind the water), with no significant loss of collagen. The changes in the ground substance consist of substantial loss of glycosaminoglycans and water, subsequently the ground substance loses the capacity of hydration. The ground substance also functions to lubricate adjacent collagen fibres and maintain a crucial interfiber distance. *As the ground substance loses this function during immobilization, the collagen fibres approximate too closely, the distance between fibres diminishes, the fibres adhere to one another and form cross links adhesions.* These cross-link create a series of microscopic adhesions that limit the pliability and extensibility of the tissues.

Furthermore because movement affects the orientation of newly synthesized collagen, the collagen in the immobilized joints is laid down in a more haphazard, *"haystack"* arrangement. This orientation restricts tissue mobility, further by adhering to existing collagen fibres.

THE EFFECTS OF MOBILIZATION ON CONNECTIVE TISSUES

Studies suggest that mobility and remobilization prevent the haystack development of collagen fibres and stimulate the production of ground substance. As the movements are employed or connective tissues are mobilized, the ground substance returns to its function (water binding capacity). The rehydration process starts, which diminishes the collagen-cross-links, subsequently new collagen is laid down in a more orderly fashion.

The passive and active range of movements also stretch the macroadhesions formed during the immobilization period, subsequently increasing the extensibility of the tissues.

INDICATIONS FOR JOINT MOBILIZATION AND MECHANISM OF ACTION

1. **Pain:** *The international association for the study of pain* has defined pain as an unpleasant sensory or emotional experience associated with actual or potential damage described in terms of such damage.

   Pain is experienced by an individual as the nociceptor fibres myelinated (A delta) and/or unmyelinated (c fibres) situated in the skin reach the conscious brain followed by injury or strong noxious stimuli.

   Both A delta and C fibres project to the spinal cord where they synapse (both directly or via inter-neurons) with neurons in the dorsal horn of the grey matter. These neuron-transmission cells (or T cells) are either involved in local spinal reflex, or project to higher centers of the nervous system via the spinothalamic tracts, it is therefore T cells that receive nociceptors from the peripheral part relay them to the higher centers.

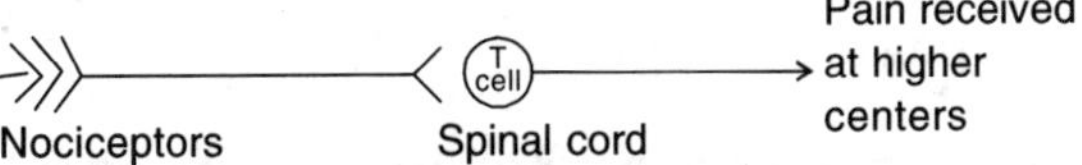

Large diameter myelinated A beta fibres known as pain inhibitors arise from the peripheral part, terminate on T cells through substantia gelatinosa (S.G.) of the spinal cord dorsal horn grey matter.

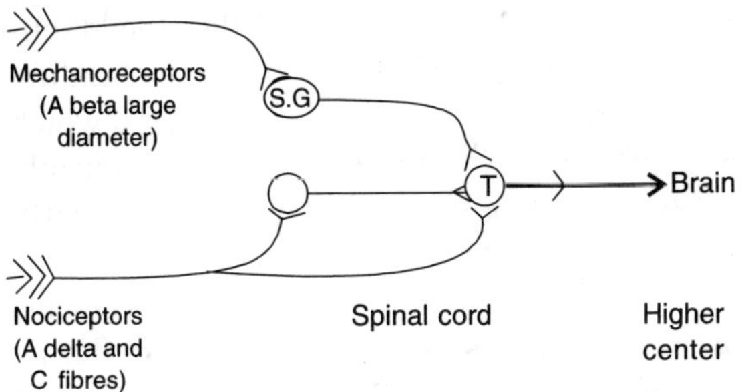

Now T cells receive excitatory input from the nociceptors and inhibiting input from mechanoreceptors through substantia gelatinosa. When nociceptors get excited following an injury, this sensation is relayed from the T cells to the higher centers. If mechanoreceptors also get activated they inhibit the nociceptors at the T cells and prevent the transmission. The inhibitory input caused by activation of the large diameter, mechanosensitive afferents is said to close the gate to nociceptor transmission through the T cells in the spinal cord. This is also known as "Pain Gate Control Theory", which was given by Malzack and Wall in 1965.

Mobilization techniques such as small amplitude oscillatory, translatory, traction and compression are used to activate large diameter, mechanoreceptors (A beta fibres) which increase the amount of inhibition impinging on the T cells in the spinal cord via the cells of the substantia gelatinosa, and ultimately inhibit nociceptors transmission in the spinal cord by closing the gate. Mobilization of joint in grade 1 and 2 activates the A beta fibres and reduces pain (These grades are discussed later in the same chapter).

2. **Muscle spasm:** Muscles guard the joint by preventing the movements in certain painful conditions. Movements are prevented to such an extent which is not necessary at all. Therefore sustained contraction of the muscles for prolonged period of time causes tightness of the muscle fibres which is known as protective muscle guarding or muscle spasm. Joint mobilization such as oscillatory techniques in grade-1 and grade-2 in painfree range of motion allows the muscles to lengthen and prevents muscle guarding or spasm.

3. **Joint stiffness:** Stiffness of the joint is the most common complication following immobilization. Because the collagen fibres approximate too closely, the distance between fibres diminishes, the fibres adhere to one another and form cross link adhesions which prevent the joint to move in full range of motion. The stiffness of the joint depends greatly on the period of immobilization and formation of adhesion between collagen fibres.

Historically use of mobilization was advocated to improve cartilage nutrition by the synthesis of synovial fluid. The ground substance of synovial fluid which is diminished during immobilization process returns to its function as the mobilization of the joint is started. The rehydration process starts and diminishes the cartilage-cross-links, subsequently new collagen is laid down in a more orderly fashion.

The mobilization of the joint also stretches the macroadhesions formed during the immobilization period, subsequently increase the extensibility of the collagen fibres and eventually increase range of motion.

Contraindications of Joint Mobilization

- *Absolute:*
  - Arthrodesis
  - Bony ankylosis
  - Any undiagnosed condition
  - Vertebro bacillary insufficiency (VBI)
  - Rheumatoid arthritic cervical spine
  - Infective arthritis (an acute osteomyelitis)
  - Acute inflammation
  - Malignancy involving the vertebral column.
  - Fractures (Acute)
  - Rupture or tear of ligament or tendon.

- *Relative contraindications:*
  - Metabolic bone diseases, such as osteoporosis, Paget's disease and tuberculosis
  - Joint effusion
  - Hypermobility
  - Rheumatoid arthritis.

Methods of Peripheral Joint Mobilization

- Muscle relaxation techniques
  - Free exercises
  - Hold relax
  - Contract relax
- Muscle stretching techniques
  - Forced passive movements
  - Auto passive stretching or self stretching exercises
  - Mechanical stretching
- Oscillatory techniques
- Sustained translatory joint play techniques.

The Oscillatory Techniques

These techniques are performed in the physiologic range (voluntary movements) or accessory movements (not controlled voluntarily but accompany movements).

Oscillatory techniques are best described by Maitland, who describes oscillations as passive movements to the joint which can be of small or large amplitude and applied anywhere in the range of movement, and can be performed while the joint surfaces are held distracted or compressed. There are four grades of oscillations:

Grade 1 : is a small–amplitude movement performed at the beginning of range.

Grade 2 : is a large–amplitude movement performed within the range, but not reaching the limit of the range.

Grade 3 : is a large–amplitude movement up to the limit of range.

Grade 4 : is a small–amplitude movement performed at the limit of range.

Grade 1 and Grade 2 are used primarily for neurophysiologic effects and do not engage detectable resistance. Grade 3 and Grade 4 are designed to initiate mechanical changes in the tissue and do engage tissue resistance (Fig. 7.1).

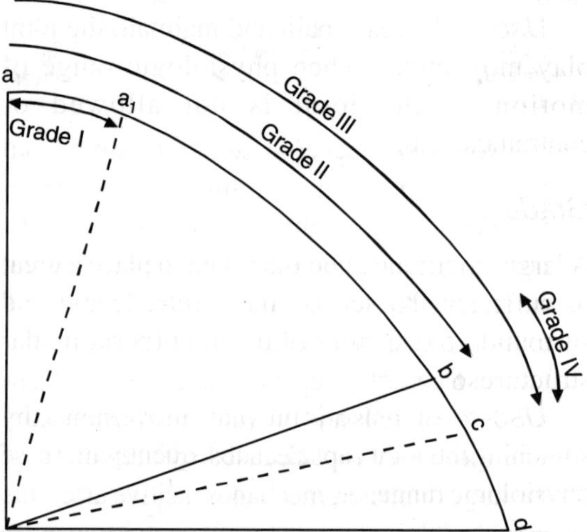

Fig. 7.1: a to d full ROM, a to b available ROM, b to c elastic limit (can be stretched by mobilization), c to d can not be stretched by mobilization, b to d total limited ROM—a to a_1 = Grade I; a to b = Grade II; a to c = Grade III; b to c = Grade IV

Sustained Translatory Techniques

These are the joint play movements which occur between the joint surfaces and are necessary for joint functioning through the full range of motion. These are demonstrated passively but can not be performed voluntarily by the patient. The joint play movements include distraction, sliding, compression, rolling and spinning of the joint surfaces. The term arthrokinematics is used to describe the joint play movements. The sustained translatory techniques are graded as:

Grade I

Small amplitude glide or distraction is applied which does not place any stress on joint capsule. Capsule remains loose.

Use–for relief of pain.

Grade II

Sufficient distraction is applied to glide the joint surfaces to stretch the tissues around the joint.

Use–to decrease pain and maintain the joint play movements when physiologic range of motion of the joint is not allowed or contraindicated.

Grade III

A large amplitude glide is applied to place a great or sufficient stretch on the joint capsule and surrounding structures of the joint (periarticular structures).

Use–to increase joint play movements by stretching the joint capsule, subsequently increase physiologic range.

> *Physiologic movements*–are the movements that the patient performs and controls voluntarily such as–flexion, extension, abduction, adduction, internal and external rotations. The term osteokinematic is used to describe the physiologic movements.
>
> *Accessory movements*–are the movements that occur between the joint surfaces and surrounding tissues and are necessary for

> normal joint functioning through the range of motion. These movements can not be performed or controlled voluntarily but can be performed passively. Accessory movements are categorised into two groups–joint play and component motions.
> a. *Joint play*–occurs between the joint surfaces include distraction or glides, sliding, compression, rolling and spinning of the joint surfaces.
> b. *Component motion*–Accompany active movements such as upward rotation of the scapula and clavicle during the shoulder flexion, and rotation of fibula during active movements of the ankle joint.

PRINCIPLES OF PERIPHERAL JOINT MOBILIZATION

Position of Patient

Position of patient should be comfortable. The proximal part of the joint should be stabilized with the weight of body or by the straps, or the hand of therapist.

Position of Therapist

Position of therapist should be convenient to allow the joint to move. Proper body mechanics are essential in application of mobilization techniques. The desired force and direction of movement can be imparted if therapist applies these from wide base of support (position of stability). Therapist should stand close to the area being mobilized and use weight shifting through legs and trunk to assist movement in the vector of mobilization. The therapist's hands and arms should be positioned to act as fulcrums and levers to fine tune mobilization.

Position of Hands of Therapist

The mobilizing hand should be placed as close as possible to the joint surface and the force applied should be directed at the periarticular tissues. **The stabilizing hand** counter acts the movement of the mobilizing hand by applying an equal but opposite force or by supporting or preventing movement at surrounding joints.

Direction of Movement

Direction of movement during treatment is either parallel or perpendicular to the treatment plane. Treatment plane was described by Kaltenborn as a plane perpendicular to a line running from the axis of rotation to the middle of the concave articular surface. The plane is in the concave partner so its position is determined by the position of the concave bone.

The direction of movement of mobilization should take in account the mechanics of the joint mobilized, the arthrokinematic and osteokinematic impairment of the dysfunction and the current reactivity of the tissue involved.

Glide is applied in the direction in which slide occurs:

a. If the surface of moving bone is convex, slide occurs in the opposite direction of the angular movement of the bone (Fig. 7.2a).

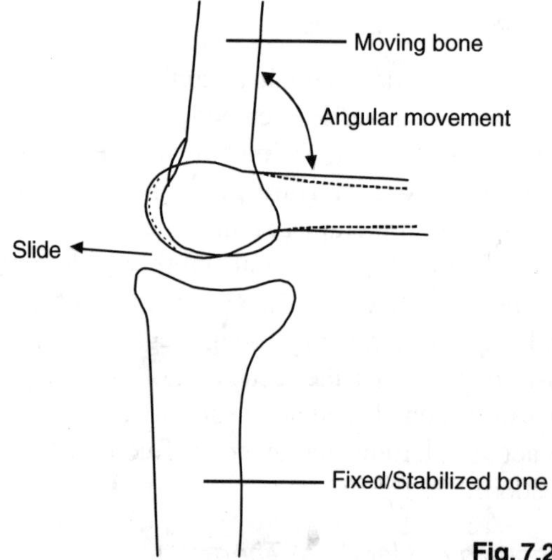

Fig. 7.2a

b. If the surface of the moving bone is concave, sliding occurs in the same direction of angular movement of bone (Fig. 7.2b).

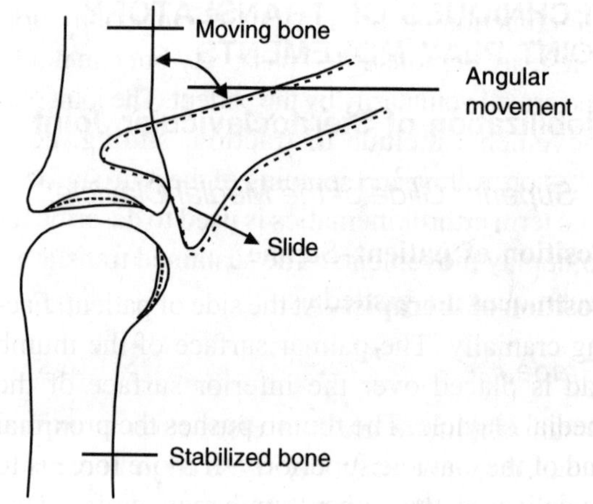

Fig. 7.2b

Intensity and Duration

The several comparative studies (between low load, long duration and heavy load, short duration) have shown that to obtain permanent elongation of collagenous tissues, the long duration with low load mobilization treatment is more effective than short duration with high intensity.

By using sustained translatory techniques the minimum stretch duration should be 6 seconds, however the oscillatory stretch can be applied for 2 to 3 seconds only, every stretch is followed by rest period and several repetitions are performed per treatment session to place effective stretch on joint capsule and surrounding structures of the joint to cause increased extensibility of the collagenous tissues.

Distraction or Traction

It is a separation of the articular surfaces by pulling them apart. Traction places stretch on periarticular structures. This stretching effect on periarticular structures facilitates the movement by lessening resistance between articular surfaces. Therefore, sustained translatory and oscillatory techniques should be performed with the traction. To perform oscillatory mobilization the traction is applied in the form of therapist's hand which can be assisted by belt.

TECHNIQUES OF TRANSLATORY JOINT PLAY MOVEMENTS

Mobilization of Sternoclavicular Joint

1. Superior Glide of the Medial Clavicle:

Position of patient–Supine.

Position of therapist–At the side of patient. Facing cranially. The palmar surface of the thumb pad is placed over the inferior surface of the medial clavicle. The thumb pushes the proximal end of the clavicle superiorly. If more force is to be delivered, then other thumb may reinforce the mobilizing thumb (Fig. 7.3).

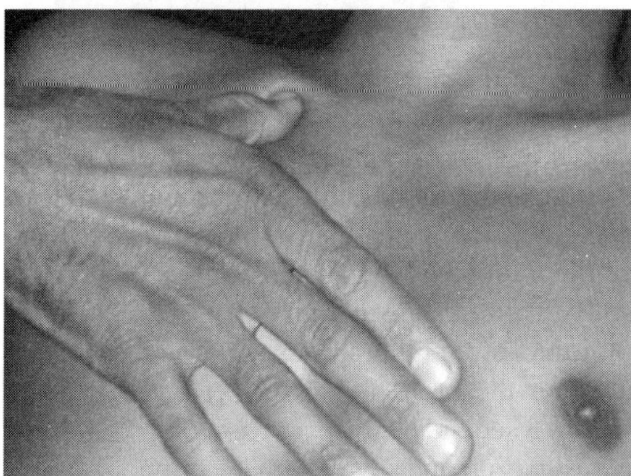

Fig. 7.3: Superior glide of the proximal clavicle

2. Inferior Glide of the Medial Clavicle

Position of patient and therapist remains same as superior glide.

Placement of hand–The palmar aspect of thumb is placed over the superior surface of the medial portion of the clavicle. The medial clavicle is pushed into caudally, more pressure/force can be applied by reinforcing the thumb by other thumb (Fig. 7.4).

3. Posterior Glide of the Medial Clavicle

Position of patient and therapist remains same as superior glide.

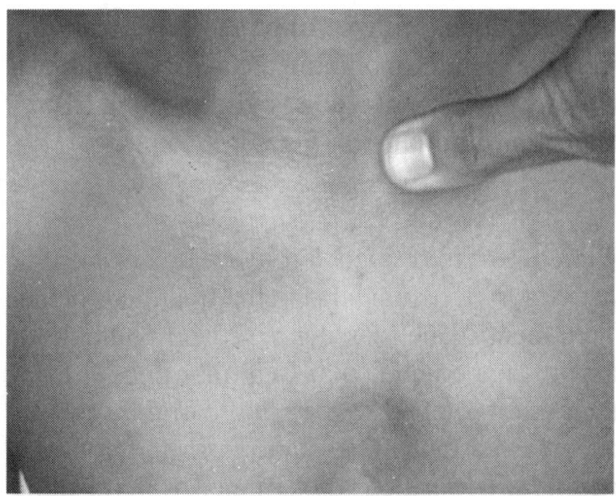

Fig. 7.4: Inferior glide of the proximal clavicle

Placement of hand–The palmar aspect of thumb is placed over the anterior aspect of the medial clavicle. To apply more pressure pisiform aspect of wrist can be placed over the proximal part of clavicle then it is pushed posteriorly (Fig. 7.5).

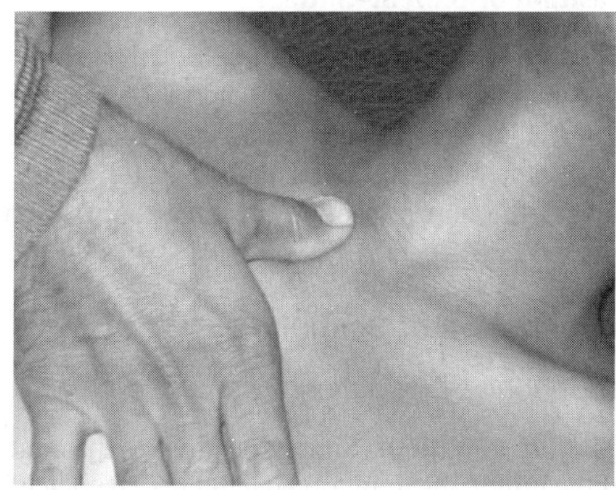

Fig. 7.5: Posterior glide of the proximal clavicle

Mobilization of Acromioclavicular Joint

1. Anterior Glide of the Distal End of Clavicle

Position of patient–Sitting, back is supported with the back rest of chair.

Position of therapist–Stands behind the patient, one hand is used to stabilize the acromion process.

The thumb and fingers of other hand grasps the clavicle. While stabilizing the acromion process distal end of the clavicle is glided anteriorly by the thumb and fingers (Fig. 7.6).

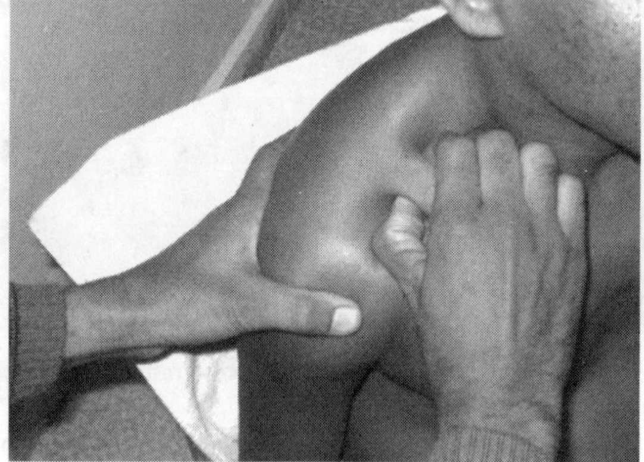

Fig. 7.6: Anterior glide of the distal clavicle

2. Gapping of the Acromioclavicular Joint

Position of patient–Sitting.

Position of therapist–Stands behind the patient. One hand is placed over the spine of scapula, other hand over the distal end of clavicle. The force is applied simultaneously by both hands, pushes the bones in opposite direction to each other (Fig. 7.7).

Mobilization of Scapula

1. Scapular Distraction: Technique-1

Position of patient–Side lying close to the edge of the plinth, the uninvolved hand may be placed under the head, the involved arm rests on the radial side of forearm of therapist with slight abduction.

Position of therapist–Standing in front of the patient, the anterior aspect of the patient's shoulder rests on the therapist's waist. The one hand holds the inferior angle of the scapula while other hand grasps the vertebral border or medial border of the scapula. The therapist leans forward, distracts the scapula away from the thoracic wall, or both hands pull the scapula

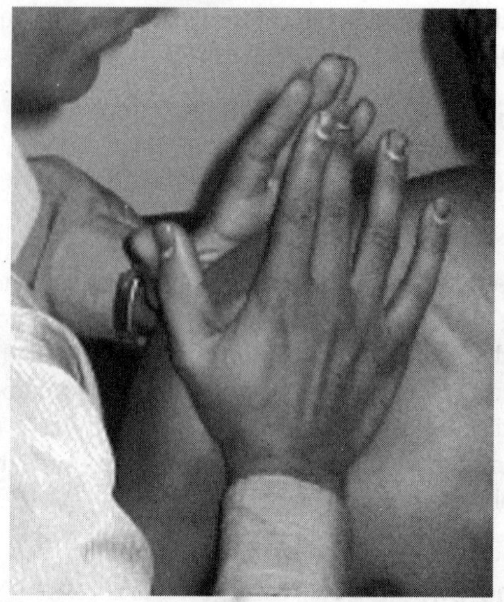

Fig. 7.7: Gapping of the acromioclavicular joint

toward the body away from the thoracic wall (Fig. 7.8).

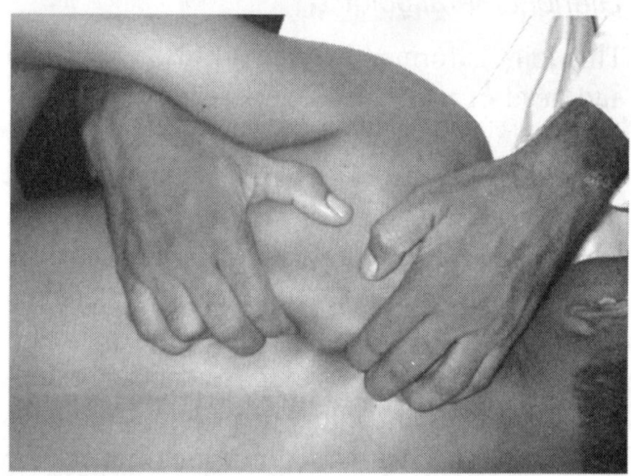

Fig. 7.8: Scapular distraction (Technique-1)

2. Scapular Distraction: Technique-2

Position of patient–Prone.

Position of therapist–At the side of patient, standing with forward bending of trunk. One hand is placed under the head of humerus and other hand under the inferior angle of the scapula. The force is applied simultaneously which lifts the head of humerus and inferior angle of scapula (Fig. 7.9).

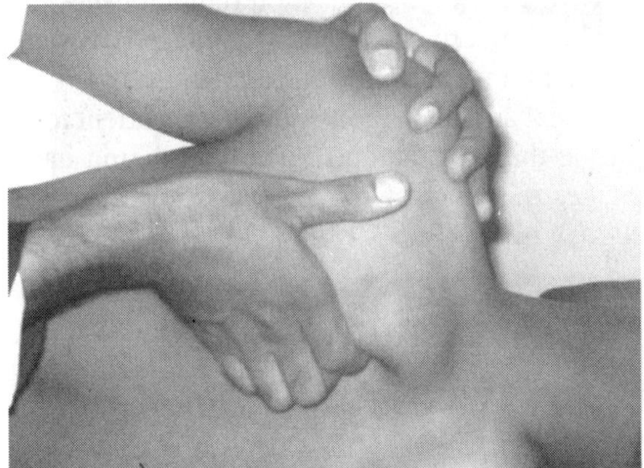

Fig. 7.9: Scapular distraction (Technique-2)

The Shoulder Girdle Complex

The shoulder girdle complex is composed of seven joints, each joint can be mobilized separately.

Glenohumeral Joint

This joint is formed by glenoid fosa of scapula and head of humerus. The head of humerus is glided into the superior, inferior anterior, lateral and posterior direction with respect to the glenoid fossa. The gliding force must be sufficient enough to place stretch on capsule and periarticular structures. The stretch of the capsule is considered on the resistance to the movement. Improper stabilization, wrong direction of movement and excessive force can cause injury to the joint structures. Glide is applied with traction which can also be achieved by using belt.

1. Longitudinal Distraction

Position of patient–Supine, the involved side should be as close as possible to the edge of table. The proximal part of the joint (glenoid fossa of scapula) is stabilized with weight of body (straps can also be used to stabilize the proximal part of the joint).

Position of therapist–At the side of the patient, facing the joint, the mobilizing hand is placed over the shoulder joint and lower hand grasps the distal arm. While maintaining the position the lower hand pulls the arm downward which causes longitudinal traction (Fig. 7.10).

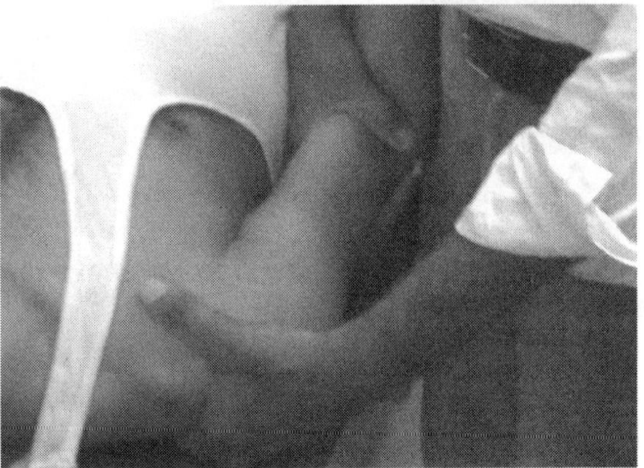

Fig. 7.10: Longitudinal distraction

2. Inferior Glide of Humerus

Position of patient–Supine, shoulder is abducted at 45°. A strap may be used to stabilize the scapula.

Position of therapist–At the side of patient, facing the joint by rotating the trunk. The mobilizing hand is placed over the superior aspect of the head of humerus and an assisting hand holds the arm just above the elbow joint. An assisting hand applies traction by pulling the arm toward the body while mobilizing hand pushes the head of humerus into inferior direction with respect to the glenoid fossa (Fig. 7.11).

3. Superior Glide of Humerus

Position of patient–Supine, arm remains at the side of body or abducted if it is desired to place sufficient stretch on capsule and increase range of motion.

Position of therapist–Standing at the side of patient, mobilizing hand is placed under the axilla

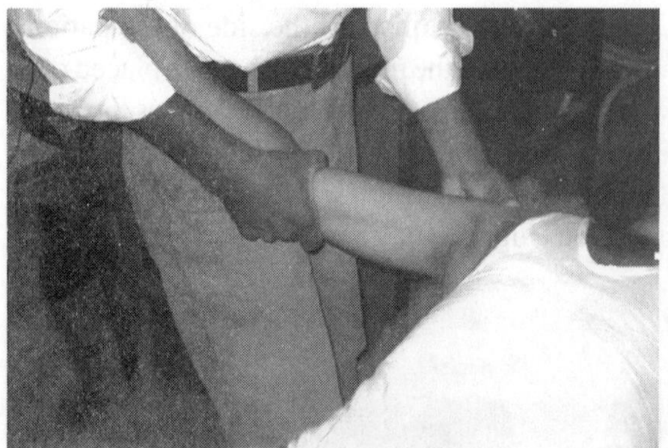

Fig. 7.11: Inferior glide

and assisting hand holds the arm just above the elbow. The mobilizing hand pushes the head of humerus up with mild traction to the lateral side. An assisting hand keeps the arm at the side of body (Fig. 7.12).

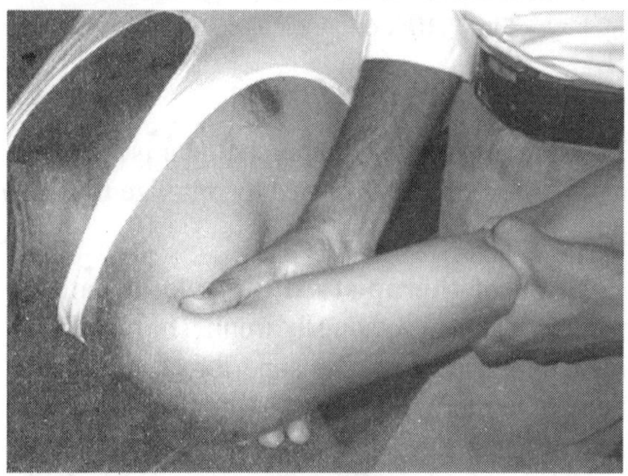

Fig. 7.12: Superior glide

4. Posterior glide of Humerus (Technique 1)

Position of patient–Supine, the shoulder is abducted slightly and elbow is flexed at 90° with palm facing the body of therapist. A wedge or pillow is placed under the scapula. The arm rests on therapist's thigh.

Position of Therapist–Sits or stands at the side of patient, facing the joint with slight rotating the

trunk. The mobilizing hand (fingers are placed on the medial aspect and thumb on the head of humerus, during mobilization thumb pushes the head of humerus posteriorly) is placed over the anterior humeral head while assisting hand holds the distal arm and elbow joint of the patient rests on the thigh of therapist. The mobilizing hand pushes the head of humerus downward to the edge of plinth (Fig. 7.13a).

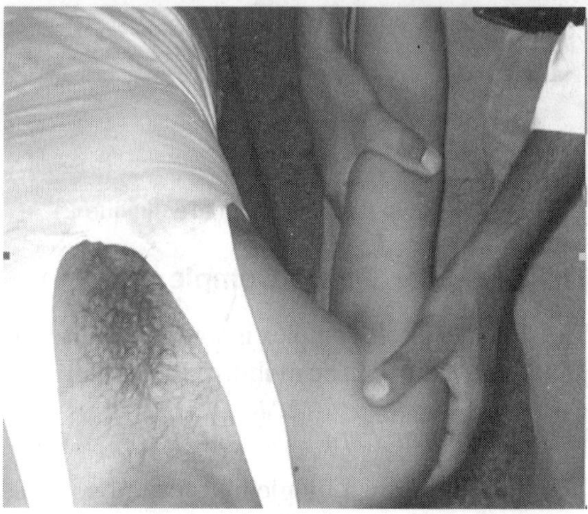

Fig. 7.13a: Posterior glide

5. Posterior Glide (Technique 2)

Position of patient–Supine, shoulder is flexed at 90°, elbow is flexed at approximately 120°, the hand of patient rests on his or her chest. A wedge or small rolled towel may be placed under the scapula which should not prevent the movement of head of humerus.

Position of therapist–Stands at the side of patient facing the joint. A belt is used to apply traction, which passes from the head of humerus to the therapist's waist/buttocks. Therapist places both hands on the elbow and applies traction through the buttocks by taking them away from the table. The humerus is pushed posteriorly by applying a pressure through hands and body. When buttocks are taken away, trunk bends automatically which gives a thrust force to the humerus and causes posterior glide (Fig. 7.13b).

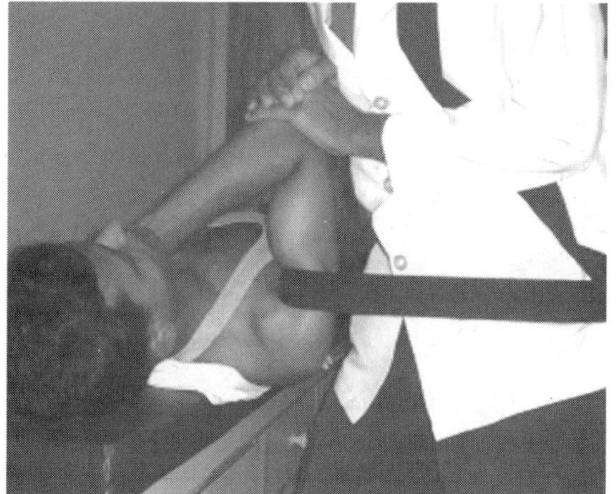

Fig. 7.13b: Posterior glide of head of humerus

6. Anterior Glide

Position of patient–Prone, with the involved extremity as close as possible to the edge of the table. The shoulder should be off the table.

Position of therapist–Stands at the side of patient, facing the joint. The mobilizing hand is placed over the posterior **aspect** of the head of humerus, the assisting hand holds the elbow. Arm of patient rests on therapist's thigh. Assisting hand pulls the arm apart from the plinth and mobilizing hand pushes the head of humerus anteriorly causing stretch to the posterior capsule (Fig. 7.14).

7. Anterior and Posterior Glide of the Head of Humerus

Position of Patient–Supine, the involved extremity's arm rests on plinth and forearm over the chest.

Position of therapist–Sits on chair, facing laterally. The thumbs of both hands are placed over the anterior aspect of humerus. The head of humerus is glided anteriorly by pushing up by the

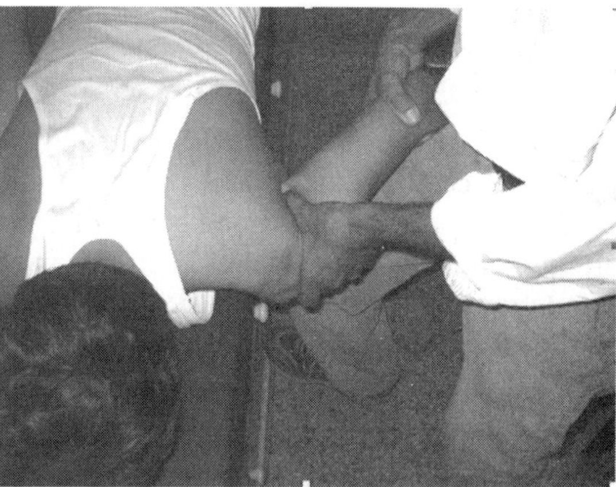

Fig. 7.14: Anterior glide

fingers, the stretched position is held for atleast 6 seconds then released. Now thumbs push the head of humerus posteriorly. These up and down movements of the head of humerus by thumbs and fingers cause anterior and posterior glides alternately (Fig. 7.15).

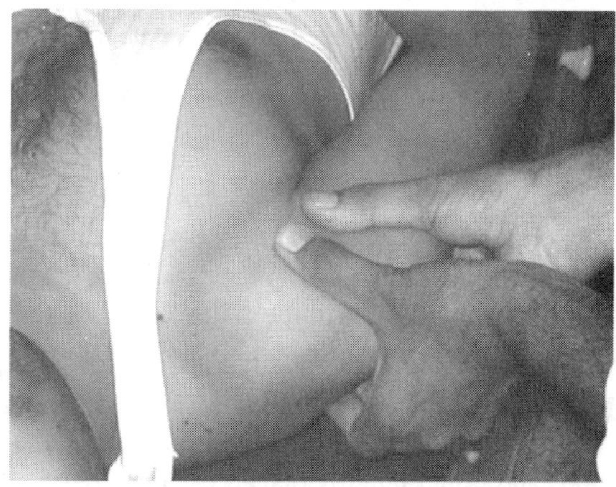

Fig. 7.15: Anterior and posterior glide

8. To improve External Rotation of the Shoulder

To improve external rotation of the shoulder, the joint is placed into abduction and external rotation (extreme ranges/stretched ranges) then head of humerus is pushed inferiorly.

Technique

Position of patient–Supine.

Position of therapist–Standing. The mobilizing hand is placed over the superior aspect of the head of humerus while assisting hand holds the arm just above the elbow joint. The forearm of patient rests on waist of therapist. An assisting hand abducts and externally rotates the arm with traction, while the mobilizing hand glides the head of humerus inferiorly (Fig. 7.16).

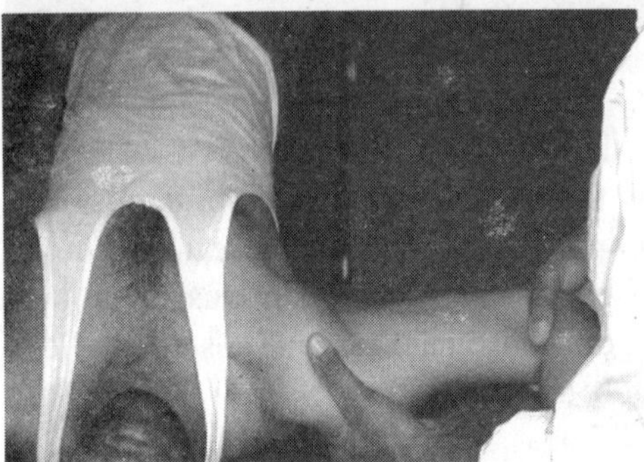

Fig. 7.16: To improve external rotation of the shoulder

Elbow Joint

The Humero-ulnar Joint

1. Joint Logitudinal Traction

Position of patient–Supine with elbow flexed at 90° and forearm supinated.

Position of therapist–Stands by the patient's side. Lower hand grasps the forearm at the wrist joint, and upper hand is placed over the palmer aspect of the proximal forearm (heel of the wrist over the proximal part of the joint while fingers spread distally).

Mobilizing force–While maintaining above position, therapist leans forward and pushes the proximal part of the forearm through the mobilizing hand (upper hand) (Fig. 7.17).

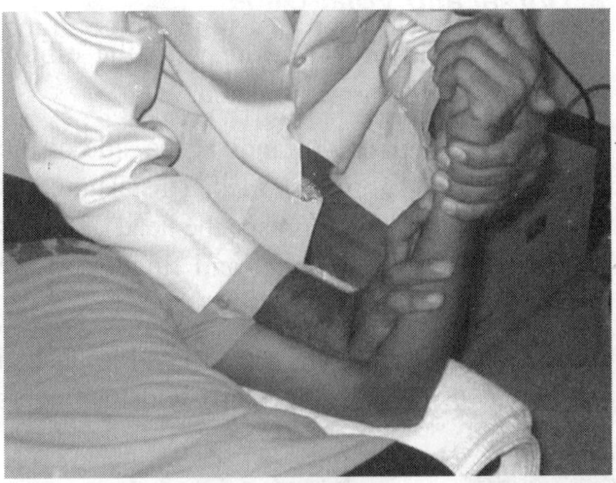

Fig. 7.17: Humeroulnar joint traction

2. Joint Compression

Position of patient–Supine, elbow is flexed at 90° and shoulder is abducted at 90°.

Position of therapist–Standing at the side of the patient upper hand stabilizes the distal part of the elbow joint while lower hand grasps the patient's hand.

Mobilization force–While maintaining above position, the mobilizing hand pushes the hand to the plinth (Fig. 7.18).

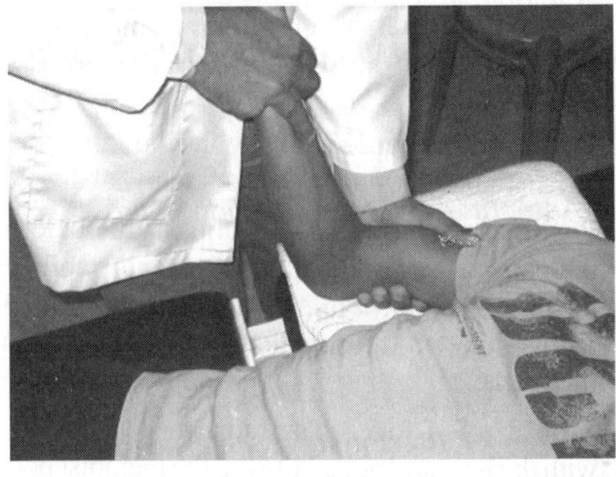

Fig. 7.18: Joint compression (humeroulnar)

3. *Dorsal and Volar Glide*

Position of patient–Supine with the elbow extended and forearm supinated.

Position of therapist–Stands at the side of the patient, one hand grasps the medial distal humerus to stabilize it and other grasps the head of radius (heel on the palmar aspect and fingers on the dorsal aspect).

Mobilization force–The radial head is pushed dorsally with the heel and volarly with the fingers alternately.

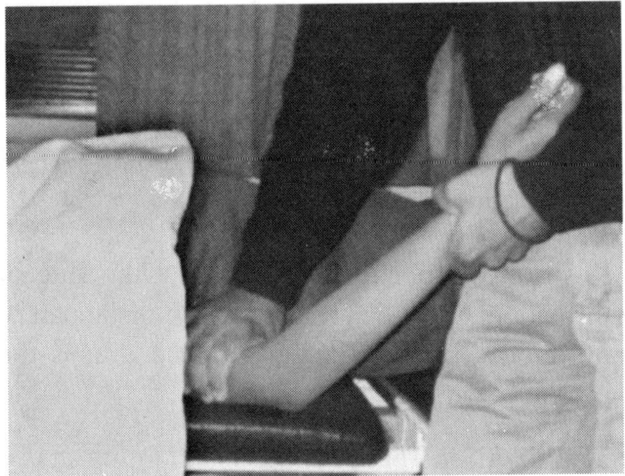

Fig. 7.19: Humeroulnar joint distraction

Radioulnar Joint

1. *Dorsal and Volar Glide of the Proximal Radioulnar*

Position of patient–Sitting with elbow and forearm in mid range and shoulder slightly abducted.

Position of therapist–Standing at the side of the patient facing the joint. One hand stabilizes the proximal ulna while other grasps the head of radius (heel on the dorsal aspect and fingers on the palmer).

Mobilization force–The radial head is pushed with the heel and pulled toward the therapist body alternately (Fig. 7.20).

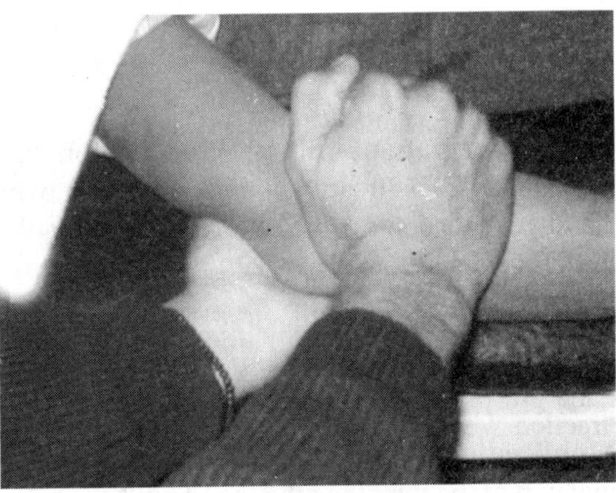

Fig. 7.20: Dorsal and volar glides of the proximal radioulnar joint

2. *Dorsal and Volar Glide of the Distal Radioulnar Joint*

Position of patient–Sitting on stool, forearm rests on treatment table in midprone position.

Position of therapist–Standing at the side of patient one hand grasps the distal ulna to stabilize it and other hand grasps the distal radius (thenar aspect is placed on the dorsal aspect and fingers on the palmar).

Mobilizing hand–While maintaining above position, the distal radius is glided anteriorly with the thenar aspect and posteriorly (volar) with the fingers (Fig. 7.21).

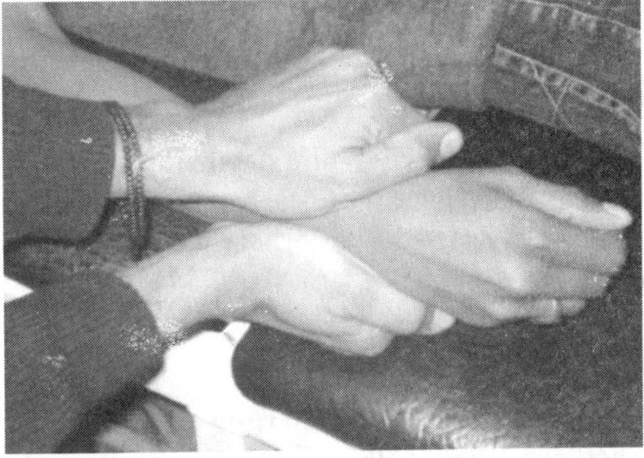

Fig. 7.21: Dorsal and volar glides of the distal radioulnar joint

Wrist Joint

1. Traction

Position of patient–Sitting on stool, forearm pronated rests on treatment table and wrist over the edge of the table, a rolled towel can be placed under the distal forearm.

Position of therapist–Standing, facing the joint, one hand stabilizes the proximal part while other hand grasps the distal part or hand.

Mobilization force–While stabilizing the proximal part of the joint the other hand pulls the hand in longitudinal direction (Fig. 7.22).

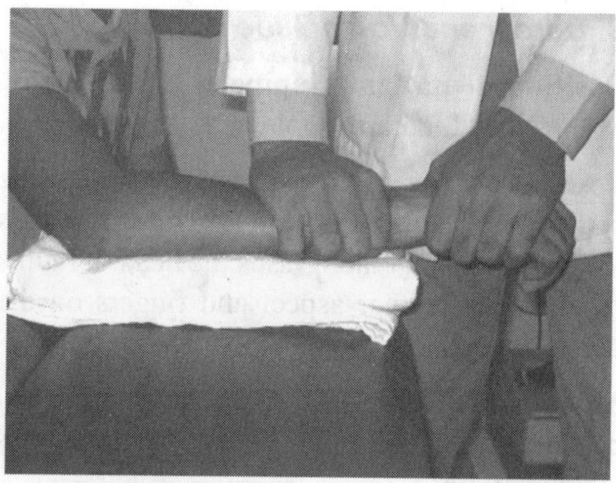
Fig. 7.23a: Wrist joint dorsal glide

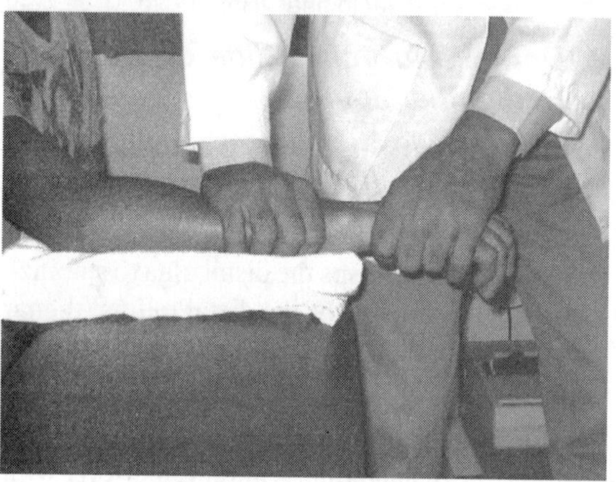
Fig. 7.22: Wrist joint traction

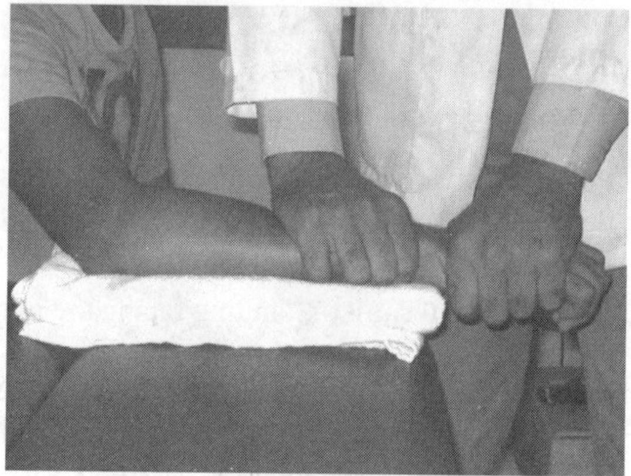
Fig. 7.23b: Wrist joint volar glide

2. Dorsal and Volar Glides

Position of patient, therapist and hands remain same as traction.

Mobilization force–While stabilizing the proximal part of the joint, the distal part is glided posteriorly (Dorsal) and anteriorly (volar) alternately (Figs 7.23a and b).

3. Radial Glide and Ulnar Glide

Position of patient and therapist remain same. Therapist stabilizes the proximal part of the joint with one hand the other hand grasps the distal part of the joint.

Mobilization force–The distal part of the joint is glided alternately toward the radial and ulnar side (Figs 7.24a and b).

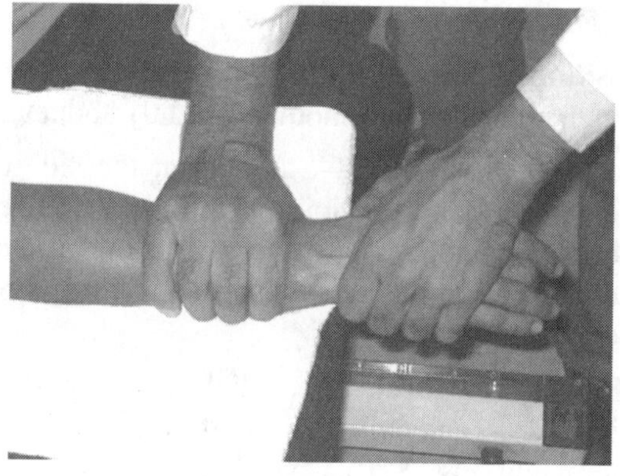
Fig. 7.24a: Wrist joint radial glide

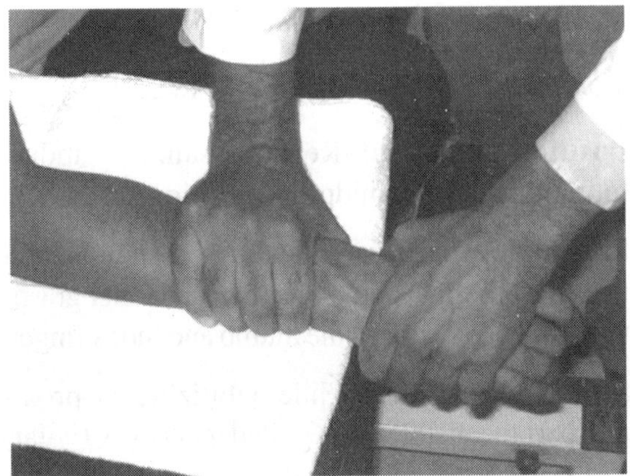

Fig. 7.24b: Wrist joint ulnar glide

Intercarpal Joints

1. Volar Glide

Position of patient–Supine or sitting elbow flexed at 90° and forearm is pronated and rested on treatment table.

Position of therapist–Standing facing the joint, the thumb of one hand is placed over the dorsal aspect of carpal bone which is not being mobilized but proximal to the mobilizing bone. The thumb of other hand is placed over bone which is to be mobilized. Fingers of both hands rest on palmar surface of the corresponding bones.

Mobilizing force–While stabilizing the one carpal bone, the other carpal bone is glided anteriorly (volar) (Fig. 7.25).

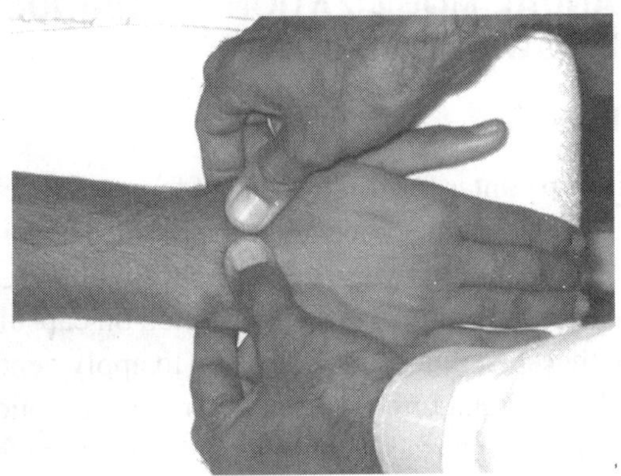

Fig. 7.25: Dorsal glide of intercarpal joint

2. Dorsal Glides

Position of patient–Supine or sitting elbow is flexed at 90° and forearm is supinated.

Position of therapist–Standing, facing the joint, thumb of one hand is placed over the palmer aspect of the bone which is not being mobilized but next to the mobilizing bone and index and middle fingers on the dorsal aspect of the same bone. The thumb of other hand is placed on the palmer aspect of the carpal bone which is to be mobilized and fingers on the dorsal aspect of the same bone.

Mobilization force–The bone which is being mobilized is glided posteriorly (dorsal) (Fig. 7.26).

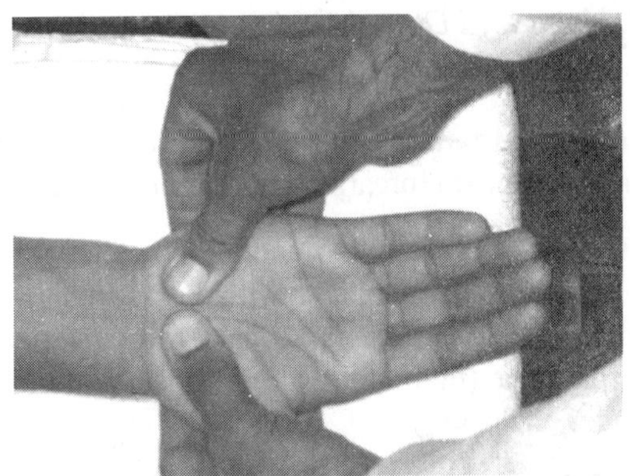

Fig. 7.26: Dorsal glide of intercarpal joint

Carpometacarpal (CMC) Joint

1. Palmar Glide (2nd to 5th finger)

Position of patient–Sitting on stool, hand rests on the treatment table with forearm pronated.

Position of therapist–Standing, facing the joint. The proximal part of the CMC joint which is to be mobilized is stabilized with one hand, and the thumb of other hand is placed over the proximal part of the metacarpal bone, which is to be mobilized.

Mobilization force–While stabilizing the proximal part of the joint the distal part is glided anteriorly (palmar) (Fig. 7.27).

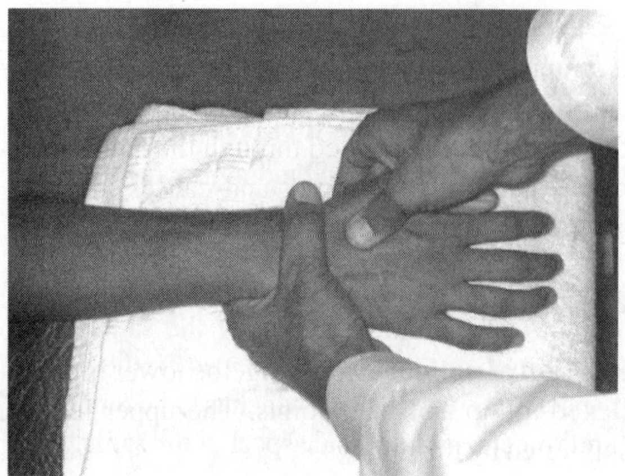

Fig. 7.27: Palmar glide of CMC joint

2. Volar and Dorsal Glide of the Ist CMC Joint

Position of patient–Sitting, hand rests on treatment table with forearm in midprone position.

Position of therapist–Standing facing the joint, the trapezium is stabilized with the one hand and other hand grasps the proximal part of 1st metacarpal bone (thumb on palmer aspect and index finger on dorsal).

Mobilization force–While stabilizing the proximal part of the joint the distal is glided anteriorly (palmar) and posteriorly (dorsal) alternately (Fig. 7.28).

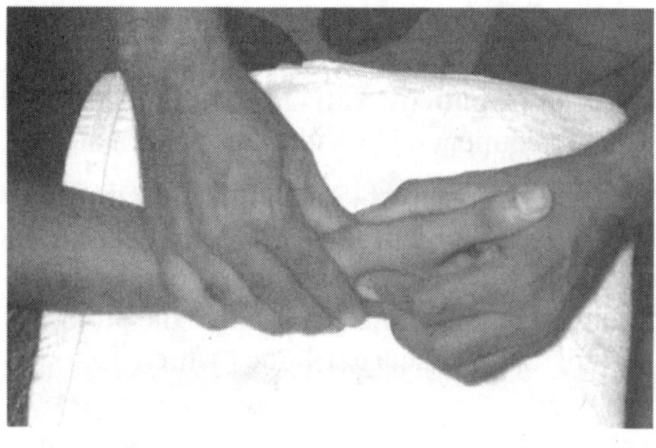

Fig. 7.28: Dorsal and Palmar glide of Ist CMC joint

Metacarpo-phalangeal (MCP) Joint

Volar and Dorsal Glides

Position of patient–Remains same as above, forearm may be in midprone position.

Position of therapist–Standing one hand stabilizes the proximal part of the joint and other grasps the distal part between the thumb and index finger.

Mobilization force–While stabilizing the proximal part the distal part is glided anteriorly (volar) and posteriorly (dorsal) alternately. Each MCP and IP joint can be mobilized by following this maneuver (Fig. 7.29).

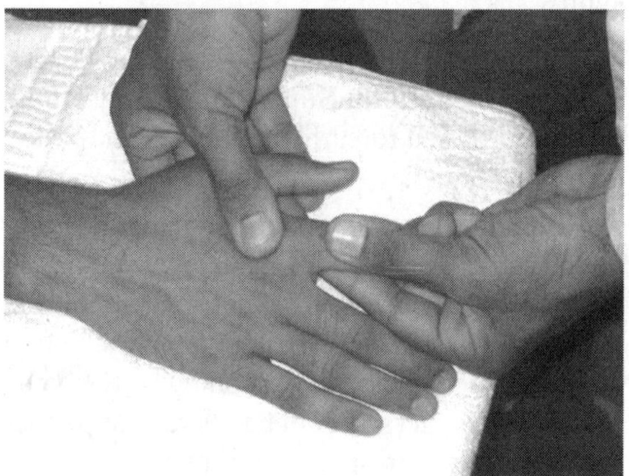

Fig. 7.29: Dorsal and Palmar glide of IInd MCP joint

MANUAL MOBILIZATION TECHNIQUES OF LOWER LIMB JOINT

Hip Joint

The hip joint is formed by head of femur (convex) and acetabulum (concave) of the ilium. The joint is surrounded by large and thick muscles, therefore to achieve effective stretch on capsule, the therapist must concentrate on to apply gentle and significant force. To increase range of motion the articular surfaces are brought to the restricted range and then significant force is applied to cause glide, and stretch the joint capsule which allows the joint to move further.

1. Inferior or Caudal Glide

Position of patient–Supine with hip in resting position with knee extended.

Stabilization–The pelvis is stabilized with the strap or by an assistant.

Position of therapist–Standing at the end of the treatment table. A belt is used to apply longitudinal pressure/force which is wrapped around the waist of the therapist and crosses over just above the ankle joint. The therapist places hands under the belt at the ankle joint as shown in Figures 7.30a and b.

Procedure–While maintaining above position the longitudinal force is applied with hands and the belt as therapist leans backward.

In case of knee joint pain or dysfunction, belt is wrapped around the lower thigh (above patella) and hands are placed under it, the knee is kept flexed. A force is applied through the hands and belt which pulls the femur and causes inferior glide of head of femur.

2. Anterior Glide of the Head of Femur

Position of patient–Side lying, the lower limb is flexed at hip and knee joints. The upper leg is supported by the pillows.

Position of therapist–Standing, facing the anterior aspect of joint. A belt is used, which passes around the upper thigh (neck of femur) and wraps around the waist of therapist. Therapist places one hand over the pelvis and other just above the knee joint.

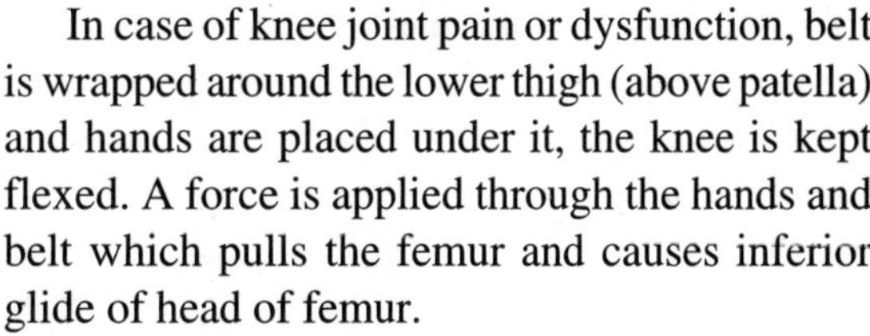

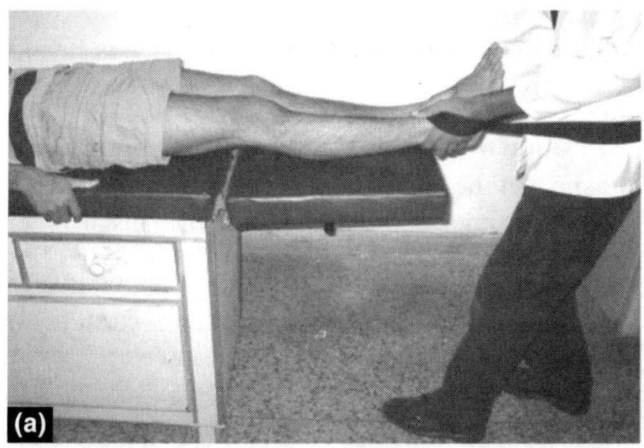

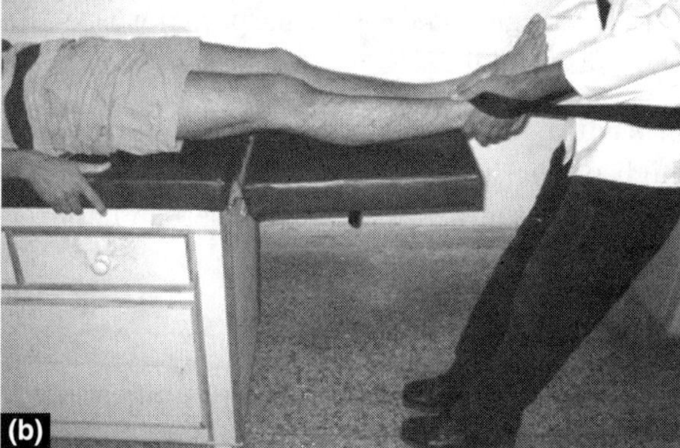

Figs 7.30a and b: Inferior or caudal glide of the femur

Procedure–While maintaining above position, therapist leans backward, which causes anterior glide of the head of femur. Both hands stabilize the pelvis and distal thigh (Fig. 7.31).

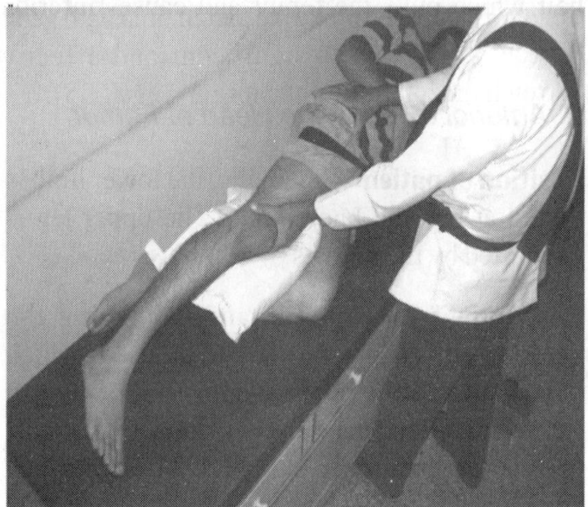

Fig. 7.31: Anterior glide of the head of femur

3. Posterior Glide of the Head of Femur

Position of patient–Side lying, the lower leg is flexed at hip and knee joints, the upper leg (which is being mobilized may also be flexed slightly at hip and knee joints and supported by the pillows.

Position of therapist–Standing, behind the patient facing the posterior aspect (gluteal) of the hip joint. A belt is applied around proximal end of the femur of the patient and wrapped around the waist of therapist. Therapist places one hand over the gluteal region and other on the posterior aspect of the distal thigh.

Procedure–While stabilizing the pelvis and distal thigh by the hands, therapist leans backward, which causes posterior glide of the head of femur (Fig. 7.32).

Knee Joint

The knee comprises of two joints, patellofemoral and tibiofemoral:

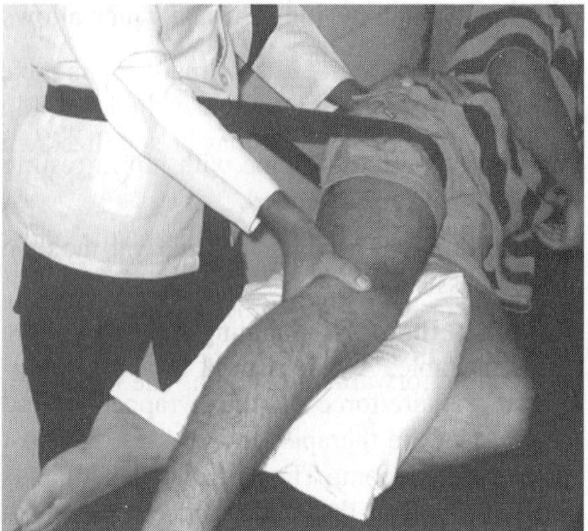

Fig. 7.32: Posterior glide of the head of femur

1. Distraction of Tibiofemoral Joint

Technique No. 1:

Position of patient–High sitting, knee is flexed slightly (45°).

Position of therapist–Sitting, facing the anterior aspect of the joint, one hand grasps the leg above the ankle joint, and other is placed over distal thigh.

Procedure–A downward force is applied gently to place significant and effective stretch on capsule (Fig. 7.33).

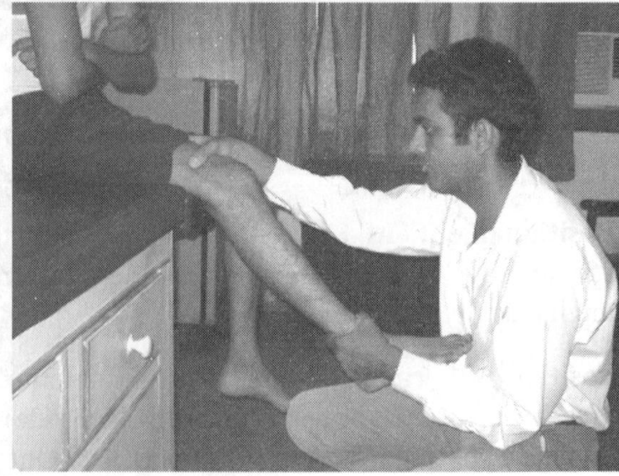

Fig. 7.33: Distraction of tibiofemoral joint

Technique No. 2:

Position of patient–High sitting, knee is flexed at 45°, a wedge is placed under the knee joint. The proximal part of joint may be stabilized with the strap.

Position of therapist–Standing at the end of treatment table, facing the joint (antero–inferior part). Both hands grasp the leg just above the ankle joint, then downward force is applied by leaning forward and bending the knees (Fig. 7.34).

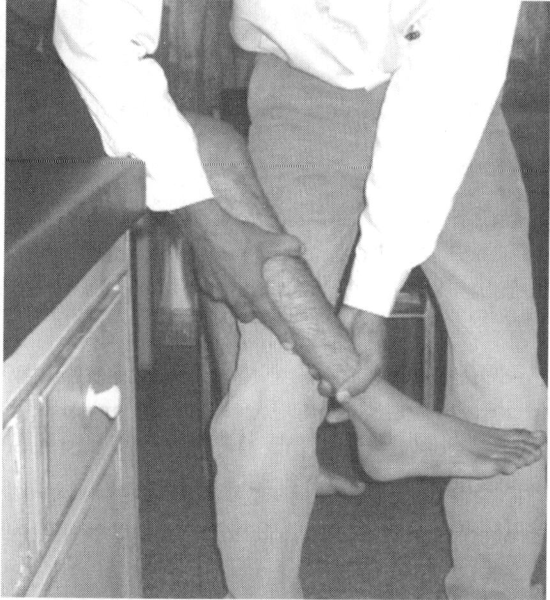

Fig. 7.34: Distraction of tibiofemoral joint

2. Tibiofemoral Joint Anterior Glide

Technique No. 1:

Position of patient–High sitting, knee flexed at 25°, a wedge is placed under the popliteal fossa, thigh may be stabilized with straps.

Position of therapist–Sitting, facing the anterior aspect of the joint. The ankle joint (involved side) is placed between the knees of therapist. One hand is placed over the knee joint and other grasps the lower leg. A belt is used which passes through posterior aspect of the knee and then waist of therapist.

Procedure–While maintaining above position, the therapist pulls the proximal part of tibia with gentle force which places significant and effective stretch on anterior joint capsule (Fig. 7.35).

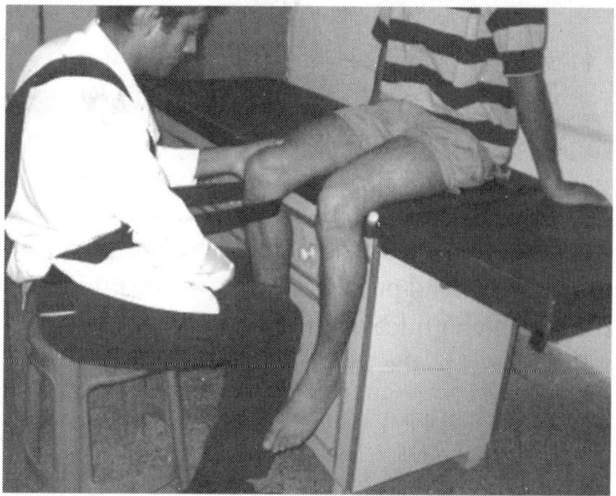

Fig. 7.35: Anterior glide of the proximal tibia

Technique No. 2:

Position of patient–Supine, knee is flexed at 45°, the foot rests under the therapist's thigh.

Position of therapist–Sitting on treatment plinth, grasps the proximal tibia (fingers placed on posterior aspect and thumbs on tibial tuberosity).

Procedure–While maintaining above position, a gentle force is applied to pull the upper end of tibia toward the body (Fig. 7.36).

Technique No. 3:

Position of patient–Prone, knee is flexed at 25°. A wedge or small towel may be placed under the knee joint.

Position of therapist–Standing, facing the joint. The mobilizing hand is placed on the posterior aspect of the tibia and an assisting hand grasps the leg at the ankle joint to maintain the flexion.

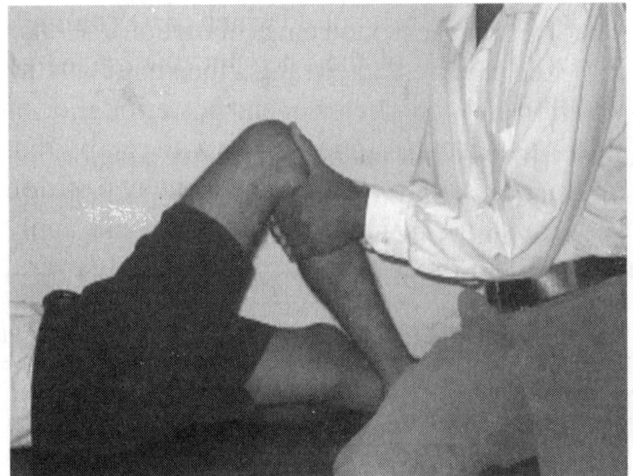

Fig. 7.36: Anterior glide of proximal tibia

Procedure–While maintaining above position, mobilizing hand pushes the tibia with significant force, which glides the tibial condyles anteriorly with respect to the femoral condyles (Fig. 7.37).

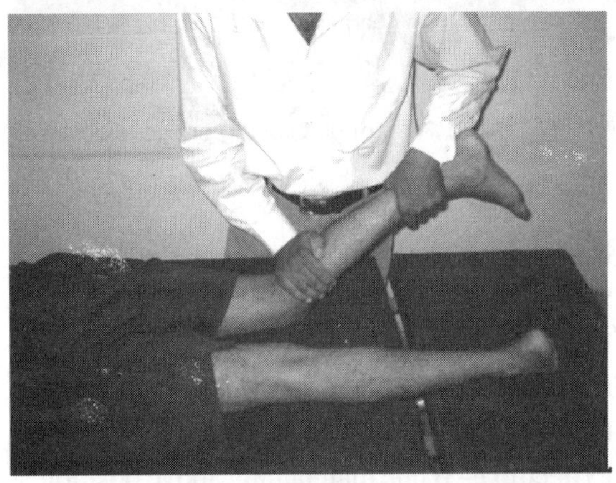

Fig. 7.37: Anterior glide of proximal tibia

3. Tibiofemoral Joint Posterior Glide

Technique No. 1:

Position of patient–High sitting, knee is flexed.

Position of therapist–Sitting, facing the anterior aspect of the joint, the ankle joint (involved side) is placed between the knees of therapist.

Procedure–While maintaining above position, the proximal end of tibia is pushed posteriorly by

the thinar aspect of the hand. Force should be sufficient enough to glide the tibia posteriorly. Excessive force can damage the ligament and capsule (Fig. 7.38).

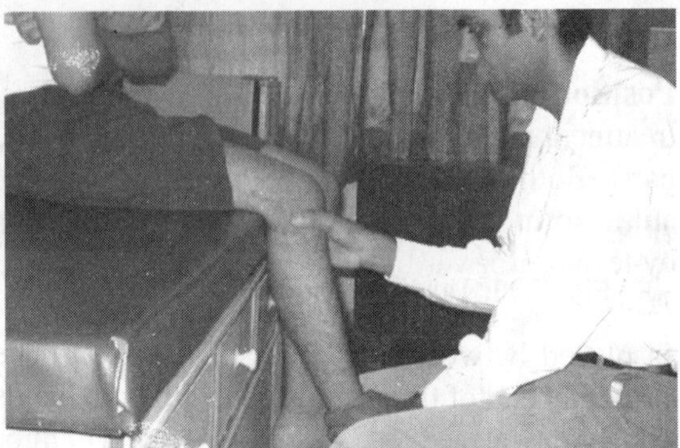

Fig. 7.38: Posterior glide of proximal tibia

Technique No. 2:

Position of patient–Supine, knee is flexed at 25°, the heel rests on treatment table and toes on therapist's waist (A paper can be placed between toes and therapist's body).

Position of therapist–Standing at the end of treatment table, leans forward and grasps the upper end of tibia (fingers placed on posterior aspect and thumbs on tibial tuberosity).

Procedure–While maintaining above position, therapist pushes the upper end of tibia with the thumbs and thenar aspect of hands. The force is transmitted through the body by leaning forward, It should be gentle and sufficient enough to cause posterior glide of the tibia (Fig. 7.39).

4. Antero–Posterior Glide of the Tibia

Technique 1:

Position of patient–High sitting, knee is flexed at 25°, a wedge is placed under the popliteal fossa, thigh may be stabilized with straps.

Position of therapist–Sitting, facing the anterior aspect of the joint. The involved side ankle joint

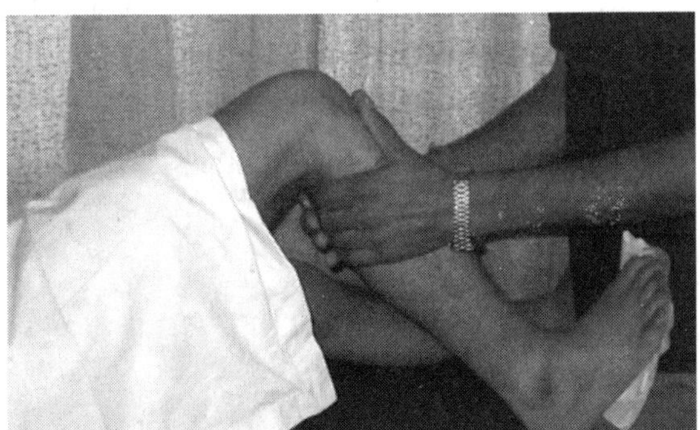

Fig. 7.39: Tibiofemoral joint posterior glide

is placed between the knees of therapist. The proximal end of tibia is grasped with both hands (fingers are placed on posterior aspect and thumbs on tibial tuberosity).

Procedure–Therapist pulls the tibia forward then holds it for some time then releases the force gradually and pushes it posteriorly, and again holds it for sometime and releases the force gradually. It includes one cycle (anterior and posterior glides), (every cycle is followed by rest period. Generally to achieve good results and cause sufficient stretch on joint capsule, prolonged stretching of capsule is more effective) (Fig. 7.40).

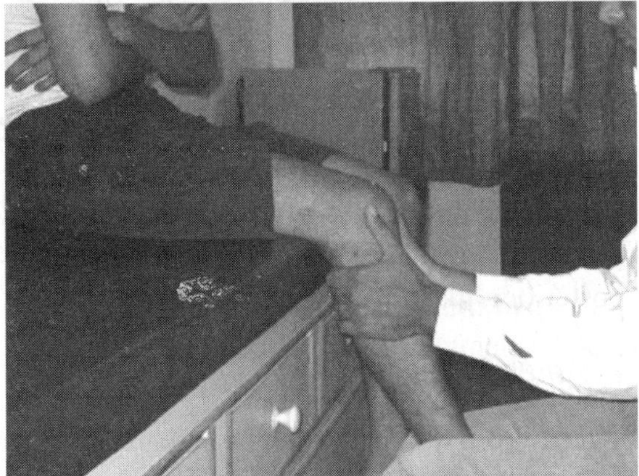

Fig. 7.40: Anterior posterior glide of proximal tibia

Technique No. 2:

The antero–posterior glides can also be performed in same position as in anterior glide of tibiofemoral joint, technique no. 1.

*To increase flexion range of motion, the knee is flexed to its restricted range, then maintain the position and apply anterior and posterior glide of the tibia. After 10–15 repetition with rest period, again flex the knee joint to its next position (progression), maintain the position and apply glides. The procedure can be repeated several times to place sufficient stretch on joint capsule and periarticular structures.

Patello–Femoral Joint

1. Inferior Glide of the Patella

Position of patient–Supine, knee is extended.

Position of therapist–Standing, facing the anterior aspect of the joint. A web space (formed by thumb and index finger) is placed over the superior border of the patella.

Procedure–Patella is pushed inferiorly, parallel to the tibia. If patella is being pressed instead of pushing inferiorly, no inferior glide will be caused, therefore to glide it should not be pressed. To apply more force the mobilizing hand can also be reinforced by an assisting hand (Fig. 7.41).

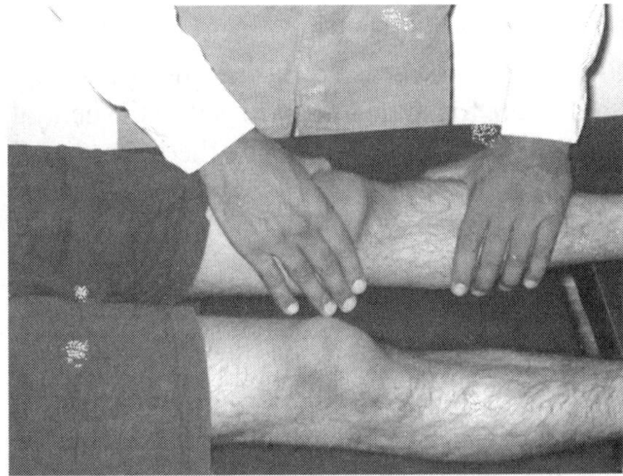

Fig. 7.41: Inferior glide of the patella

2. Superior Glide

Position of patient–Supine, knee is extended.

Position of therapist–Standing, facing lateral aspect of the joint, patella is placed between the thumb and fingers (web space).

Procedure–The patella is pushed up, parallel to the femur (Fig. 7.42).

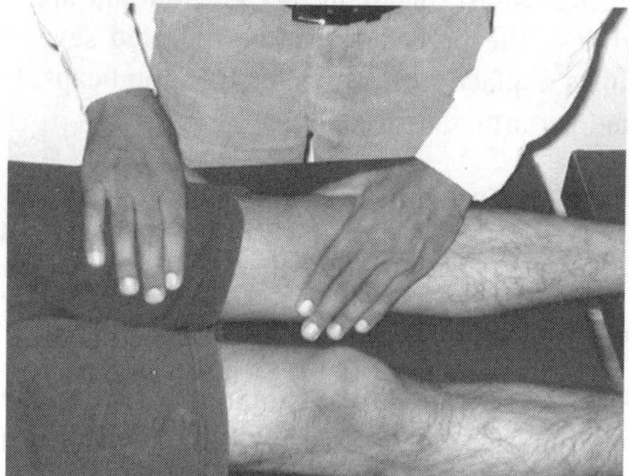

Fig. 7.42: Superior glide of the patella

3. Supero–inferior Glide of the Patella

Position of patient–Supine with knee extended.

Position of therapist–Standing or sitting, facing anterior aspect of the joint. The superior border of the patella is grasped with the web space of the one hand while other hand is placed over the inferior border of patella.

Procedure–Lower hand pushes the patella up, holds there for some time brings it to the neutral position, then push it down by the upper hand. The superior and inferior glide is followed by rest period.

4. Medio–Lateral Glide of the Patella

Position of patient–Supine, knee is extended.

Position of therapist–Standing or sitting, facing the joint. The thumbs of both hands are placed over the medial aspect of the patella and fingers are placed over the lateral aspect of the patella.

Procedure–The thumbs push the patella laterally while fingers pull the patella toward the body alternatively (Figs 7.43a and b).

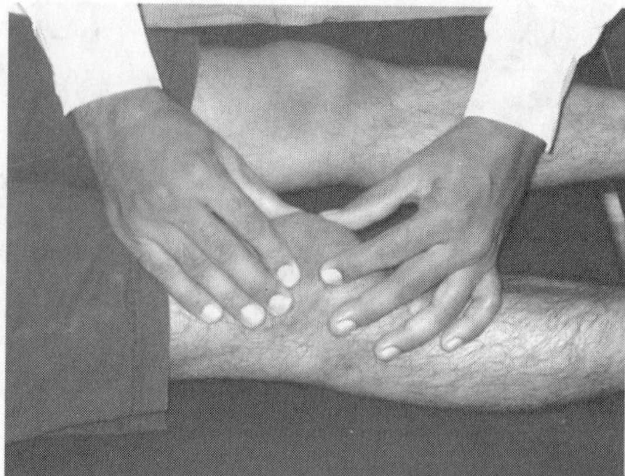

Fig. 7.43a: Medial glide of the patella

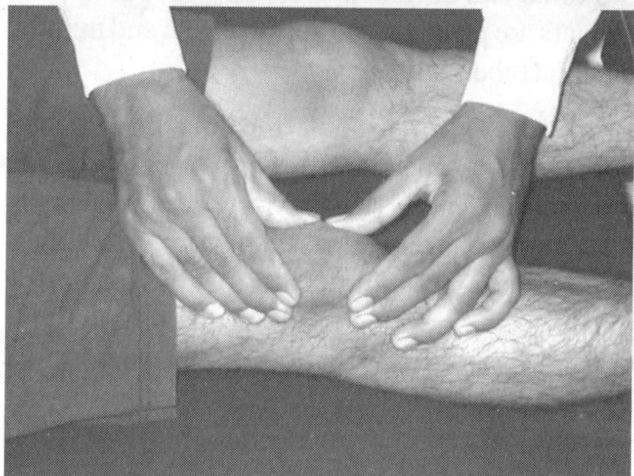

Fig. 7.43b: Lateral glide of the patella

Superior Tibiofibular Joint

1. Posterior Glide

Position of patient–Side lying, lower limb is flexed at hip and knee joints.

Position of therapist–Sits in front of the patient, tip of the thumb or pisiform aspect of heel is placed over the fibular head.

Procedure–The posterior pressure is exerted against the head of fibula through thumb or heel (Figs 7.44a and b).

2. Anterior Glide

Position of patient–Side lying, the upper leg is flexed slightly at hip and knee joint, a pillow may

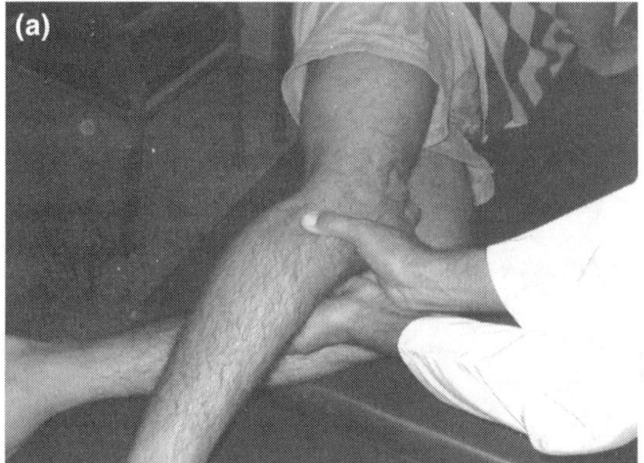

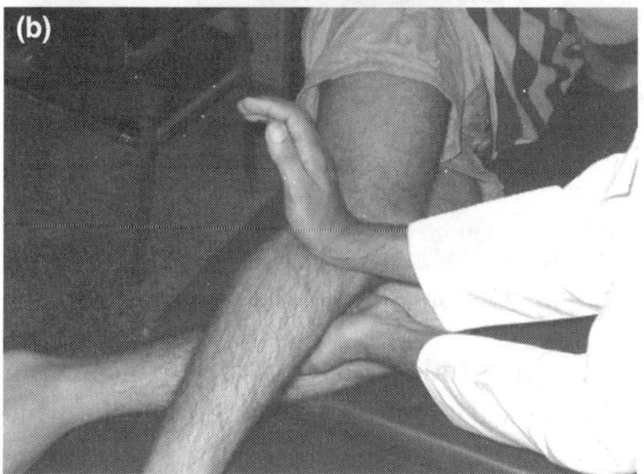

Figs 7.44a and b: Posterior glide of proximal fibula (superior tibiofibular joint)

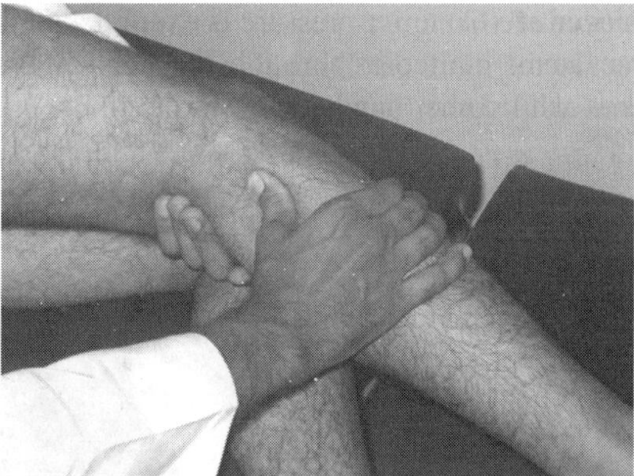

Fig. 7.45: Anterior glide of the proximal fibula

Position of therapist–Standing at end of treatment table. The heel of one hand is placed over anterior aspect of the lateral malleolus. The other hand grasps tibia at medial malleolus between the heel and fingers to stabilize the tibia.

Procedure–A posterior pressure is exerted against the lateral malleolus through the heel of one hand while other hand stabilizes the tibia (Fig. 7.46).

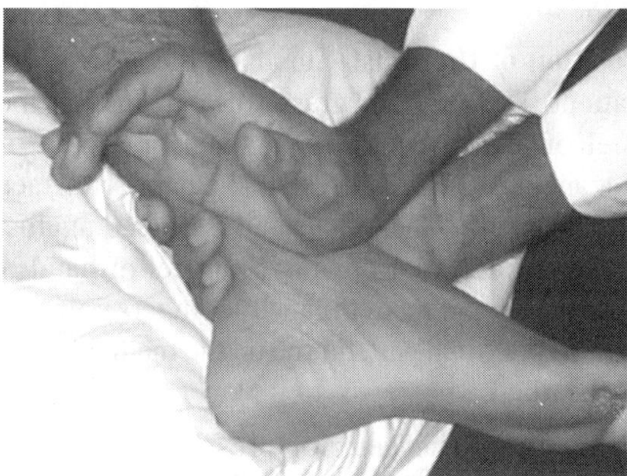

Fig. 7.46: Posterior glide (inferior tibiofibular joint)

be placed under upper knee joint, lower limb rests on the plinth.

Position of therapist–Stands behind the patient, the thumb or heel of one hand is placed over the posterior aspect of the fibular head, fingers rest on the anterolateral aspect of knee joint. The other hands grasps the tibia from medial side to stabilize it.

Procedure–The anterior pressure is exerted against the head of fibula through thumb or heel of stabilizing hand (Fig. 7.45).

Inferior Tibiofibular Joint

1. Posterior Glide

Position of patient–Side lying, the ankle rests on pillow.

2. Anterior Glide

Position of patient–Side lying, the ankle joint rests on pillow.

Position of therapist–Stands at the side of leg. The heel of upper hand is placed against the posterior border of the lateral malleolus.

Procedure–Anterior pressure is exerted against the lateral malleolus through the heel of one hand while other hand stabilizes the tibia (Fig. 7.47).

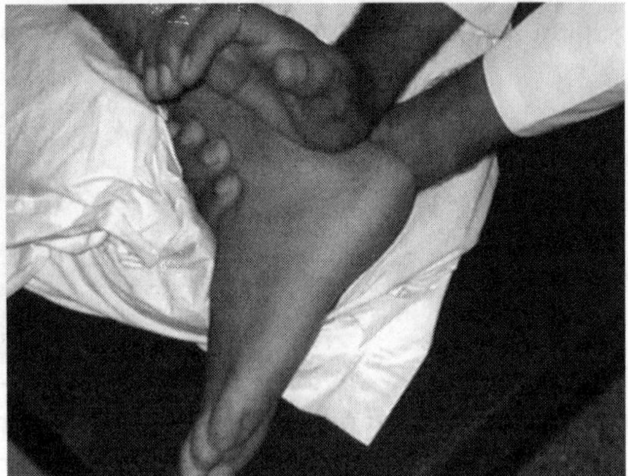

Fig. 7.47: Anterior glide (inferior tibiofibular joint)

Ankle Joint

1. Anterior Glide

Position of patient–Prone lying with knee flexed at 90°.

Position of therapist–Stands at the side of the patient. The one hand grasps the calcaneum (the heel of hand is placed on posterior aspect of calcaneum and fingers rest on the palmar surface of calcaneum. The other hand is placed against the anterior border of tibia (the heel of hand is over the lower end of tibia while fingers pointing toward proximal part, thumb on the medial aspect of the tibia).

Procedure–The anterior pressure is exerted against the calcaneum through the upper hand while lower hand stabilizes the tibia (Fig. 7.48).

2. Posterior Glide

Position of patient–Prone lying with knee flexed at 90°.

Position of therapist–Stands at the side of the patient. One hand grasps the distal part of the

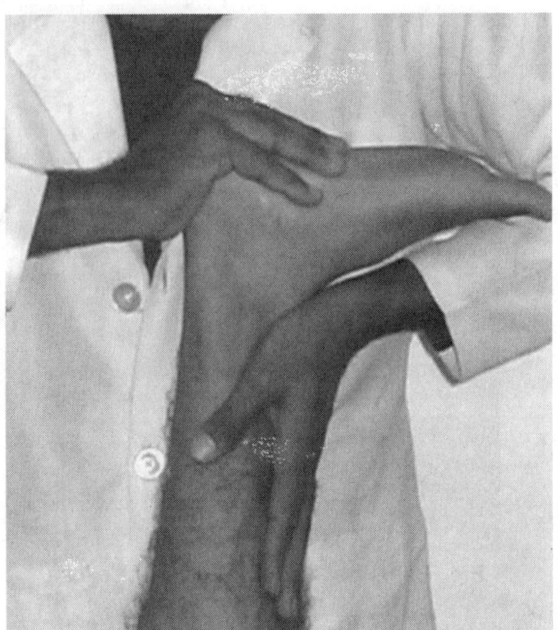

Fig. 7.48: Anterior glide of the ankle joint

ankle joint (Index finger rests on the medial malleolus and thumb on the lateral malleolus while web of the 1st interosseous on the neck of the talus. The other hand holds the tibia to stabilize it (thenar and hypothenar aspect on the lateral side and fingers on the antero-medial aspect of tibia).

Procedure–The pressure is exerted through the web of upper hand while lower hand stabilizes the tibia (Fig. 7.49).

3. Ankle Joint Compression

The patient is placed in prone position with knee flexion. The therapist stands at side of the patient, places both hands on the plantar surface of the heel. Therapist may flex his knee joint and place it on the plinth so that the anterior leg of patient rests on the inner aspect of the therapist's thigh. This is because it stabilizes the leg and controls the force. Therapist applies compression force to the ankle joint through the shoulders by leaning forward (Fig. 7.50).

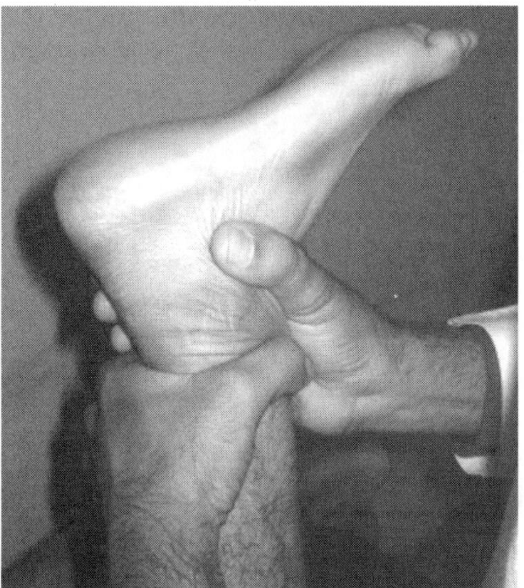

Fig. 7.49: Posterior glide of the ankle joint

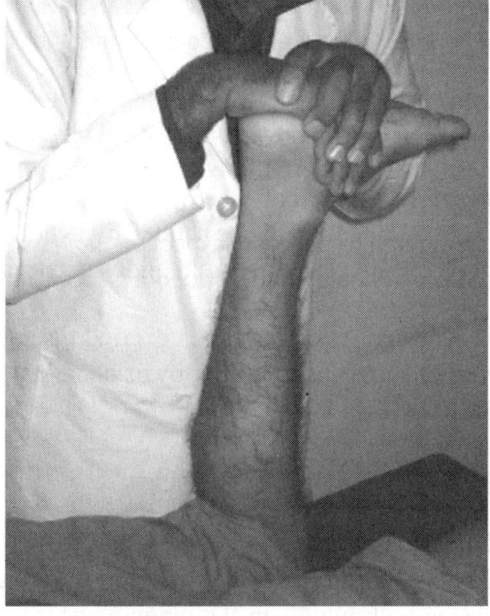

Fig. 7.50: Ankle joint compression

Ankle joint traction: The patient is placed in prone position with the leg flexion. The therapist stands at the side of leg, grasps the distal part of ankle joint with both hands and places his knee joint (proximal part of the leg) over the posterior aspect of the patients thigh to stabilize the knee joint.

While maintaining the position therapist lift the talus towards the ceiling with both arms.

During the traction and compression of the ankle joint, repeated stress comes on the joint, so if patient is having any ailment the techniques should be performed gently or avoided (Fig. 7.51).

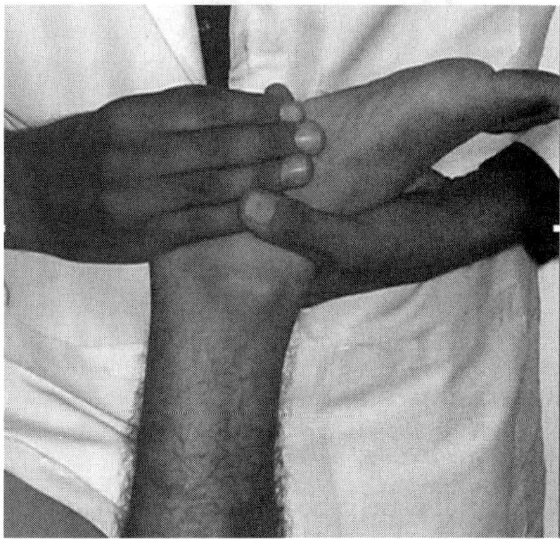

Fig. 7.51: Ankle joint traction

Inter-Tarsal Joints

To perform *anterior and posterior* glides of tarsometatarsal joints the therapist should have knowledge of surface anatomy of the each tarsal bone so that appropriate placement of thumbs and fingers can be achieved satisfactorily.

Posterior Glide

Position of patient–Supine lying, with hip and knee flexion.

Position of therapist–At the end of the couch, facing the joint. The thumbs of both hands are placed over the dorsal aspect of tarsal bone which is being mobilized.

Procedure–The posterior pressure is exerted by the thumbs to cause posterior glide of tarsal bone. During posteriorly directed force, fingers do not exert any pressure.

All tarsal bones can be glided by placing the thumbs and fingers over them separately (Fig. 7.52).

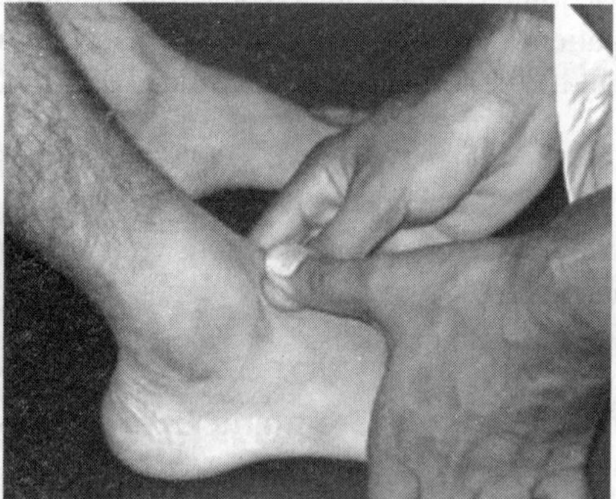

Fig. 7.52: Posterior glide of intertarsal joints

Intermetatarsal

Antero-Posterior Glide

Position of patient–Supine lying, the ankle joint remains out of the edge of treatment table.

Position of therapist–Stands at the side of patient's leg, facing the dorsal aspect of foot. The thumbs of both hands are placed over the dorsal aspect of the two adjacent metatarsal bones and fingers are over the plantar aspect of the corresponding metatarsal bones.

Procedure–One hand stabilizes the one metatarsal bone, while other hand applies anterior glide (by the thumb) and posterior glide (by the fingers of same hand), alternately.

For example—To mobilize the 1st metatarsal bone (anterior and posterior glide) the 2nd metatarsal bone is stabilized by one hand while other hand glides the I metatarsal bone in anterior and posterior direction (Fig. 7.53).

1st MTP joint: The proximal segment of the joint is stabilized with one hand while other hand

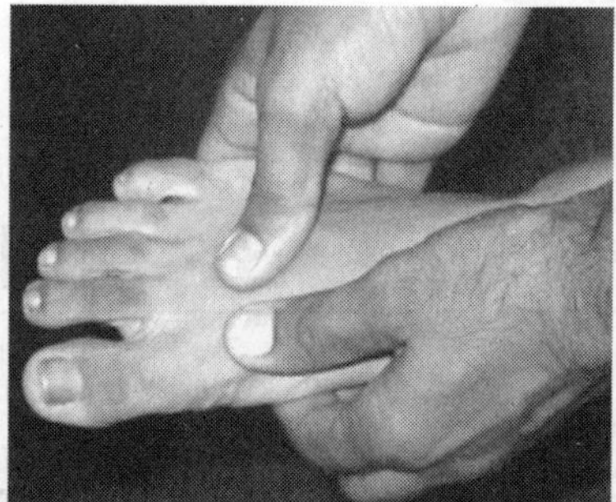

Fig. 7.53: Anterior posterior glides of inter-metatarsal joints

grasps the distal and glides it anteriorly and posteriorly (Fig. 7.54).

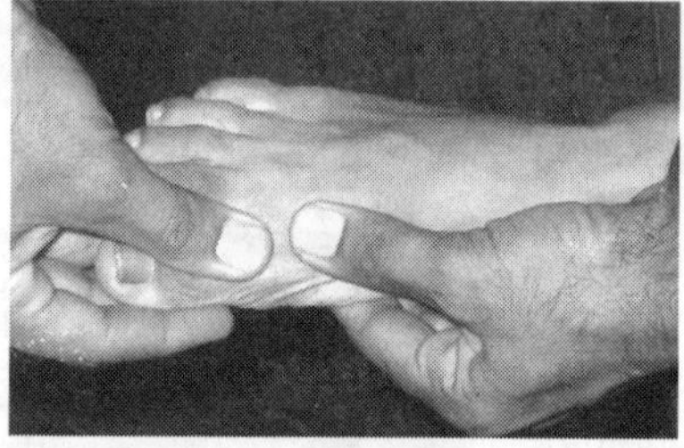

Figs 7.54: Dorsal and palmar glide of Ist MTP joint

2nd MTP joint: The proximal segment of the joint is stabilized with one hand while other hand grasps the distal segment and glides it anteriorly and posteriorly (Fig. 7.55).

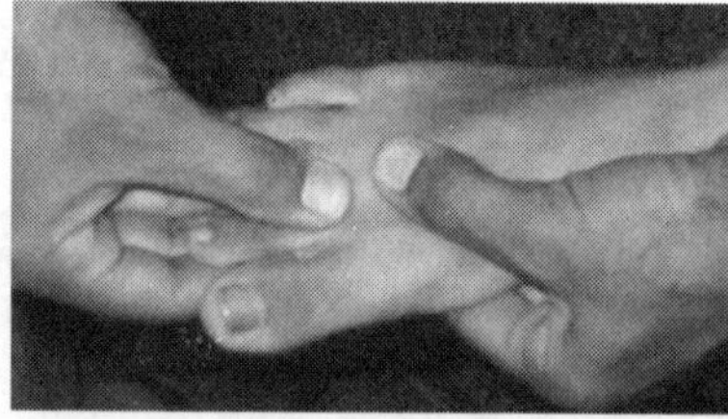

Figs 7.55: Dorsal and palmar glide of 2nd MTP joint

Interphalangeal Joints

The proximal part of the joint is stabilized with the assisting hand and distal segment is moved anteriorly and posteriorly, by the mobilizing hand.

CHAPTER-8

Breathing Exercises

INTRODUCTION

Exercises which are given to strengthen the respiratory muscles (Diaphragm, accessory costal and apical muscles) to maintain or increase the range of expiration and inspiration.

INDICATIONS OF BREATHING EXERCISES

1. Acute respiratory distress.
2. Chronic obstructive pulmonary disease (COPD), Asthma, Bronchiectasis..
3. Pneumonia.
4. Nervous system deficits or trauma which cause weakness of respiratory muscles:
   - High spinal cord injury.
   - Acute, chronic or progressive myopathic or neuropathic diseases.
5. Ankylosing spondylitis.
6. Scoliosis, kyphosis which affect the respiratory function.
7. Stress.

Goals of Breathing Exercises

1. Improve ventilation.
2. Increase the effectiveness of the cough mechanism.
3. Improve the strength and endurance of respiratory muscles.
4. Maintain or improve chest and thoracic mobility.
5. Prevent pulmonary impairments.
6. Promote relaxation.
7. Maintain or improve the lung volumes and capacities.
8. To prevent atlectasis.

Classification of Breathing Exercises

Breathing exercises are classified on the basis of their locations:

1. Costal breathing
   a. Apical
   b. Upper costal
   a. Lower costal.
2. Diaphragmatic breathing exercise.
3. Glossopharyngeal breathing.
4. Pursed lip.
5. Pacebreathing.

It is very essential to understand that exercises can be given to patient at clinic or taught to patient so that he or she can learn and perform at home as prescribed by therapist. Whenever breathing exercises are taught following points should be kept in mind:

1. Position of patient.
2. Position of therapist's/patient's hands (placement of hands).
3. Resistance during expiration/inspiration.
4. Assistance during expiration or inspiration.

The best starting positions for these exercises are crook half-lying, crook lying and half lying.

1. Apical Breathing Exercise

Position of patient: Crook lying, crook half lying, or half lying, adequate pillows can be placed under the knees, back and neck. Patient should be

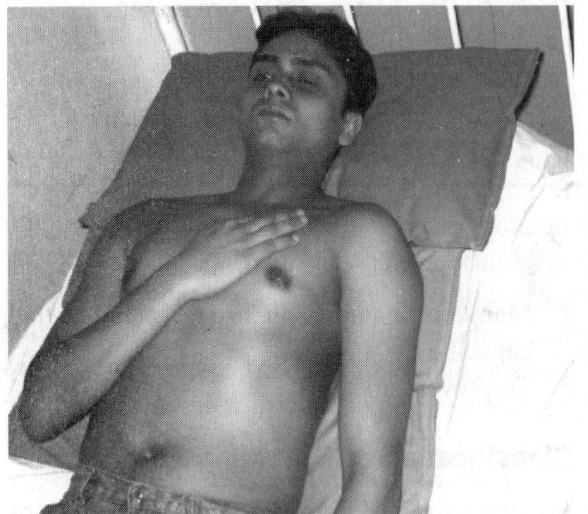

Fig. 8.1: Apical breathing—self resistance with the fingers

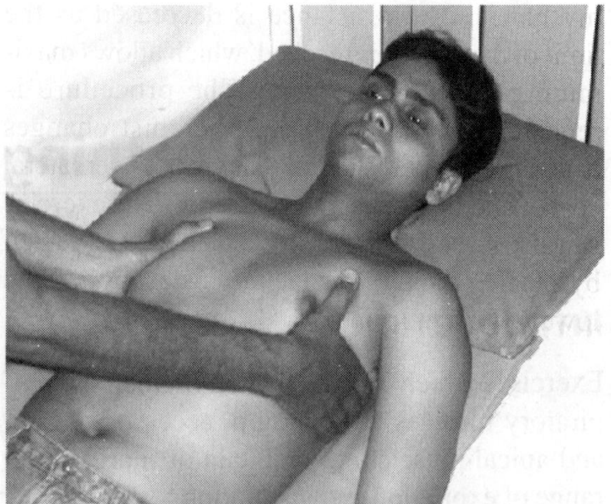

Fig. 8.2a: Upper lateral costal breathing

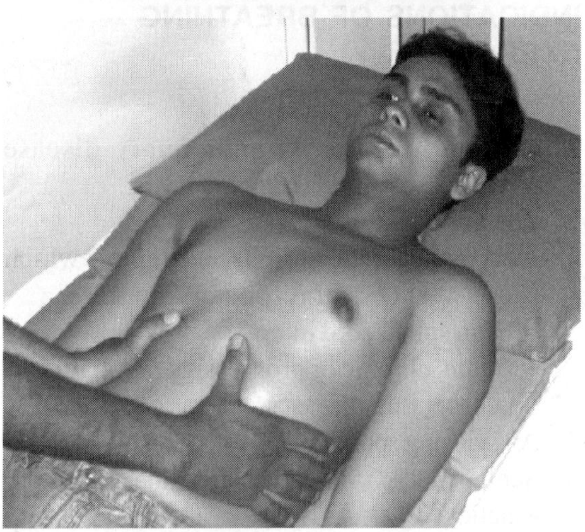

Fig. 8.2b: Lower lateral costal breathing

instructed to relax other muscles (shoulder girdle, lower limb and abdominal muscles).

Position of patient's hand: The fingers or the palm of patient rests over the clavicle with adduction of the fingers (Fig. 8.1).

Resistance

The patient is instructed to 'blow' as he breathes out the therapist applies pressure against the chest. At end of expiration therapist maintains pressure and asks the patient to breathe in under my hand and allow the chest to expand against the hands. Therapist decrease resistance as the limit of chest expansion is reached which allows maximum expansion to occur. The procedure is repeated for several repetitions. The exercise can be performed by patient himself or herself at home by placing the hand(s) over the apical part (clavicle) and applying resistance during inspiration and expiration as advised by therapist.

2. Costal Breathing

I. Upper lateral and lower costal

Position of patient: Crook lying, crook half lying, or half lying, adequate pillows can be placed under the knees, and upper back. Patient should be instructed to relax abdominals, shoulder girdle and lower limb muscles (Figs 8.2a and b).

Position of therapist: Patient turns his or her neck to the opposite of therapist. Therapist uses both hands and places over the upper lateral costal and lower lateral costal.

Resistance: The therapist instructs the patient to blow. As patient breathes out therapist applies pressure and at the end of expiration therapist maintains it and asks patient to breathe in against my hands. The resistance is decreased as the limit of expansion is reached, which allows maximum expansion to occur. The procedure is repeated several times and therapist changes hands from upper lateral costal to the lower lateral costal, and repeats same procedure. The exercise can also be performed by patient himself or herself by placing hands over lateral costal (upper and lower) (Figs 8.2c and d).

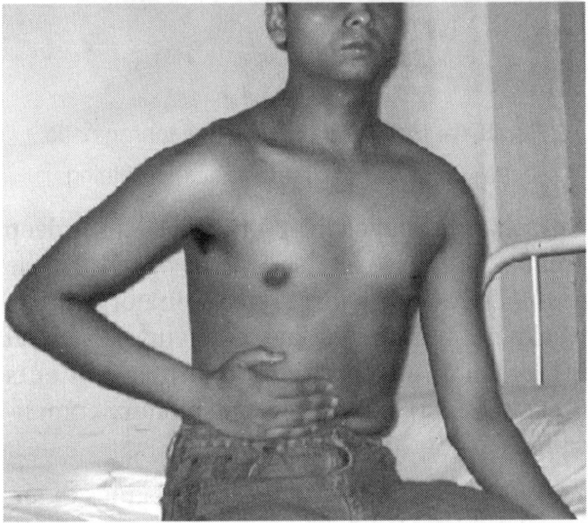

Fig. 8.2c: Self resistance unilateral lower costal breathing with whole hand

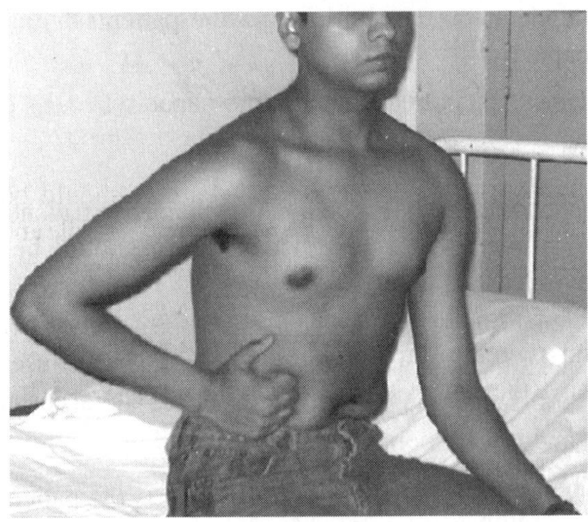

Fig. 8.2d: Self resistance unilateral lower costal breathing with the back of the fingers

II. Posterior basal costal breathing

Position of patient: Arm lean forward crook sitting.

Position of therapist's hand: Heels of hands rest on lateral to the rib angles (Fig. 8.3) fingers lie along the line of the eighth, ninth and tenth ribs, and thumb is just below the scapula. Therapist asks patient to breathe out and applies pressure and at the end of expiration therapist maintains pressure and asks patient to breathe in and applies resistance against inspiration. The resistance decreases as the limit of expansion is reached, which allows maximum expansion to occur.

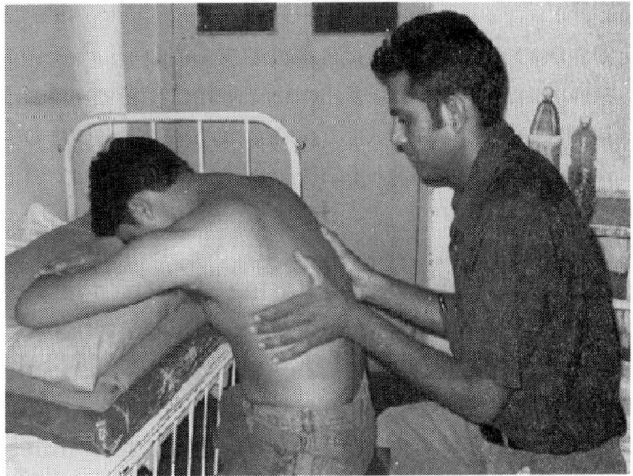

Fig. 8.3: Arm lean forward crook sitting posterior basal breathing–therapist resisting

3. Diaphragmatic Breathing

Diaphragmatic breathing is the most common form of breathing which has to be caught to a patient to improve the efficiency of ventilation, decrease the work of breathing and improve gas exchange and oxygenation. This exercise helps to strengthen the diaphragm muscle (Figs 8.4a and b).

Position of patient: Crook half lying, adequate pillows are placed under the knees and upper back. The patient is instructed to relax the shoulder girdle and upper chest muscles.

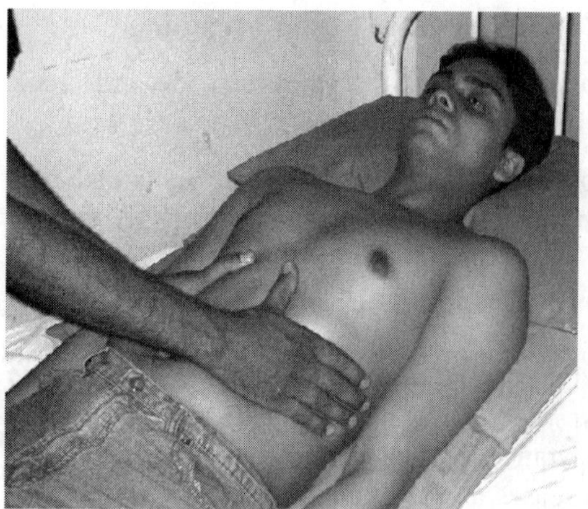

Fig. 8.4a: Diaphragmatic breathing

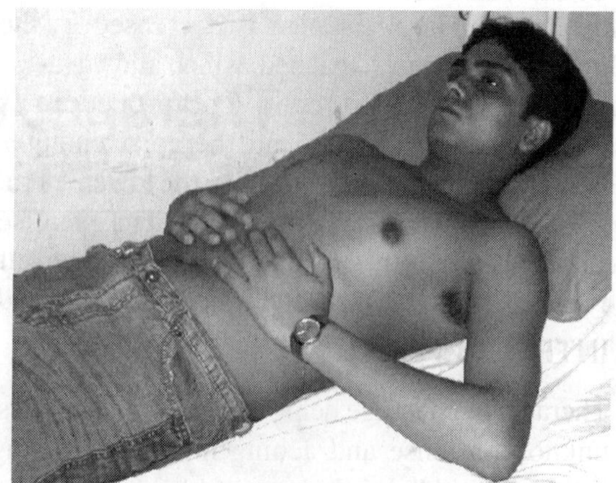

Fig. 8.4b: Half lying practicing diaphragmatic breathing

Position of therapist's hands: Over the rectus abdominals just below the anterior costal margin. The patient is then instructed to breathe out by asking him to blow gently. This will ensure an expiratory action and he is made aware of the inward movement of the costal margins. The therapist applies gentle pressure at the end of expiration and asks patient to breathe in against my hands. The therapist decreases the pressure as the limit of abdominal expansion is reached to its limit. If the diaphragm is being used in its middle inner range the costal margin will separate whereas the intercostal (central epigastric) area will swell slightly. But if the diaphragm is contracting in its outer range the abdominal wall will bulge slightly. The pressure which is applied during inspiration by therapist depends on the strength of diaphragm and therapist should allow diaphragm to contract as much as possible by decreasing resistance. The pressure may be increased after some time as diaphragm gets strengthened. The pressure may also be applied by patient himself or herself by placing hands over the rectus abdominals below the anterior costal margin.

Glossopharyngeal Breathing

The exercise is basically given when there is severe weakness of respiratory muscles and patients who have difficulty taking in a deep breath. Initially exercise was designed for the postpolio patients with severe respiratory muscle weakness, but now-a-days is having beneficial effect on high spinal cord injury patients (Quadriplegia) and prevents respiratory complications to develop.

Technique: After taking in several gulps of air, mouth is closed and air is pushed back and traps it in the pharynx. The air is forced into the lungs when the glottis is opened. This increases the depth of the inspiration and the patients' vital capacity.

Uses: To increase inspiratory capacity.

Pursed-lip Breathing

Procedure: The procedure is explained to patient very well that forceful expiration should be avoided.

The patient is placed on suitable position, then instructed to breathe in slowly and deeply then have the patient slowly purses the lips and exhale.

Uses:
- COPD.
- Dyspnea.
- Atelectasis
- Bronchiectasis.

CHAPTER-9

Therapeutic Massage
(Soft Tissue Manipulation)

INTRODUCTION

Therapeutic massage helps to smooth away stress, unknotting tense and aching muscle, relieving headache and helping sleep problems.

History

The word massage comes from the Greek *masso* meaning to kneed. In classical Greek culture, massage flourished. The physician, Aesculapius, was known as the God of healing in Greek mythology because of his use of massage in healing. Hippocrates (460-377 BC), known as the father of medicine, described the benefits of using oils and massage on joints.

In the Greek countryside, the ruins of healing centres such as Epidourous can be seen today.

In the ancient Roman massage was the part of daily life.

The Traditional Chinese Medicine (TCM) includes various components of massage (Chi Gong exercises, herbals, acupuncture, and massage).

Sanskrit word *makeh* means to press softly. In India, rubbing was used in connection with religious ceremonies, cleaning rituals developed into a form of medicine known as Ayurvedic Medicine.

Development

History shows that although the early Egyptians made reference to the benefit of massage but the Chinese were among the first to recognize its healing value at around 3000 BC. Roman and Greek philosophers and physicians prescribed it both for its restorative powers after battle and for general preservation of the body and mind. Although Roman believed in its curative powers.

Ling (Per Hinrik Ling 1776-1839) was a Swede who travelled to China and returned with a detailed insight into their techniques. *From there he developed his own system of massage based on a variety of movements.* The practical knowledge of massage gradually spread all over the world. Today the massage is established on the basis of its movements or strokes but in many ways the technique of massage remain same as those early Swedish massage. The benefit of massage is being explored by various medical and non-medical professionals worldwide.

Definitions

The term is used to designate certain manipulations of the soft tissues of the body; these manipulations are most effectively performed with the hands and are administered for the purpose of producing effects on the nervous, muscular, and respiratory systems and the local and general circulation of the blood and lymph (beard).

Manoeuvers performed by the hands of a therapist on the skin of a patient and through the skin on the subcutaneous tissues. Massage manipulations may be stationary or progressive; they may be variable in intensity of pressure exerted, surface area treated and frequency of application (Boni and Walthard, 1956).

Massage is the scientific manipulation of the soft tissues of the body, as apart from mere rubbing (Prosser, 1941).

PHYSIOLOGICAL EFFECTS

It is very important for the clinician to understand how the body reacts or responses to the different strokes of soft tissue manipulation (STM) techniques. Any form of STM technique, applied on the tissues causes several physiological changes on the different systems of the body. The body responses to massage in two ways:

1. Mechanical response and
2. Reflexive response.

Mechanical Response

It refers to the direct effects/influences of STM on the soft tissues being manipulated. Every stroke of soft tissue manipulation technique causes mechanical response. The examples of mechanical response are—increasing blood circulation, reducing swelling and breaking up of scar tissues.

Reflexive Response

It refers to the indirect effects/influences of soft tissue manipulation techniques on tissues. Neural mechanisms are influenced by manual intervention on the tissue. The process is centered on the inter-relationship of the peripheral (cutaneous) and central nervous systems their, reflex patterns and multiple pathways. The reflex effect of massage is perhaps more significant than its mechanical action. The reflexive responses are such as increasing the diameter of blood vessels, reducing blood pressure and general relaxation.

A massage response can be primarily mechanical or reflexive in nature but both responses are closely related and often occur simultaneously. Reflex responses to STM frequently occur due to mechanical stimulation of nerve receptors.

1. *Cardiovascular*
   - Increases blood circulation
   - Decreases blood pressure
   - Release of histamine and acetylcholine cause dilatation of the blood vessels.
   - Removes metabolic waste products and nutrients.
   - Stimulates vasomotor nerves.
   - Increases systolic stroke volume
   - Decreases heart rate
   - Increases RBCs, WBCs, Platelets
   - Decreases ischaemia.

2. *Lymph and lymphatic system*
   - Decreases lymphedema (swelling)
   - Strengthens immune system
     Clears away debris, fat and unwanted substances.

3. *Skin*

   The sebaceous glands are situated in the skin, these glands get stimulated when the skin is rubbed, and secrets the sebum which improves the skin condition, texture, and tone. The superficial effleurage on face causes tone up the face.

   The superficial blood vessels (arterioles and capillaries) get dilated as they are massaged and increase the local blood circulation.
   - Keeps the skin healthy
   - Increase insensible perspiration
   - Increases vasomotor activity
   - Decreases formation of superficial keloids and excessive scar formation.

4. *Nervous system*

   The sensory receptors situated in the skin, gets stimulated as the skin is pressed, rubbed, squeezed or touched. The information about the type of stimuli is sent to the brain, and makes the brain aware of the stimuli.

   The strokes of massage such as superficial effleurage, superficial vibration, superficial friction and shaking soothen the nervous system and causes sedative effect.

   The strokes of STM such as deep effleurage, Tapotement, Petrissage (deep), deep transverse friction having stimulating effect on nervous system (These strokes are discussed later in the chapter).

The afferent (sensory) neuron transmits information from the tissues and organs of the body to the central nervous system (CNS).

The efferent (motor) neuron transmits information out from the CNS to effector cells (muscle on gland) which receives and reacts to the impulse in following ways:

- Stimulates and soothes the nervous system.
- Releases endorphin, enkephalins, and other pain reducing neurochemicals.
- Stimulates parasympathetic nervous system and promotes relaxation, decreases insomnia and improve sleeping pattern.
- Decreases stress related hormones such as nor-epinephrine and cortisol.
- Increases in dopamine and serotonin levels.

5. *Muscular system*

1. Increases extensibility of muscle fibres
2. Decreases stiffness
3. Breaks adhesion formation between muscle fibres
4. Decreases muscle spasm
5. Increases muscular relaxation
6. Increases blood circulations.

Classification of Massage (Table 9.1)

1. Effleurang
2. Petrissage
3. Tapotement
4. Friction
5. Vibration
6. Shaking.

Clinicians Preparation of Materials for Treatment

Room

The room in which therapeutic massage has to be applied should be free from all sort of noises (telephone, traffic etc). The room should not have bright lights. Curtain should be used to avoid sunlight.

Table 9.1: Classification of therapeutic massage

Effleurage	1. Superficial	
	2. Deep	
Petrissage	1. Kneeding	: Palmer kneading
		: Finger pad kneading
		: Thumb pad kneading
		: Knucle kneading
		: Reinfinforced kneading
	2. Picking up	
	3. Wringing	
	4. Skin rolling	
Tapotement	1. Clapping	
	2. Beating	
	3. Hacking	
	4. Pouding	
Friction	1. Superficial	
	2. Deep	: Deep Transverse Friction (James Cyriax)
		: Circular Deep Friction
Vibration		
Shaking		

Treatment Plinth

It is an essential tool in the practice of massage. The dimensions of the table should be at least 28×72 inches and adjustable for height to accommodate for various needs. It should be solid and firm. Adjustable head support may also be added (Figs 9.1a to c).

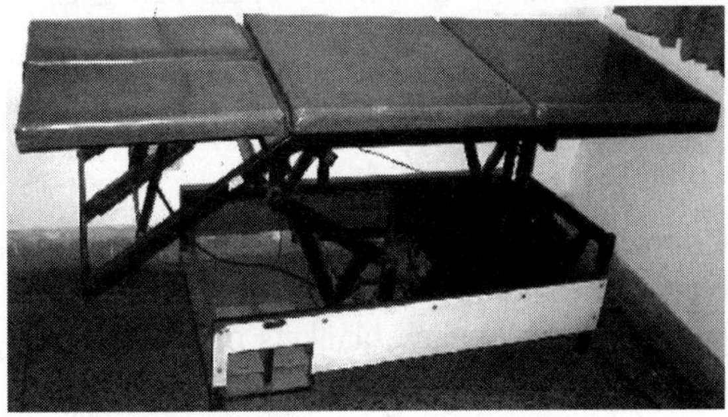

Fig. 9.1a: Treatment plinth

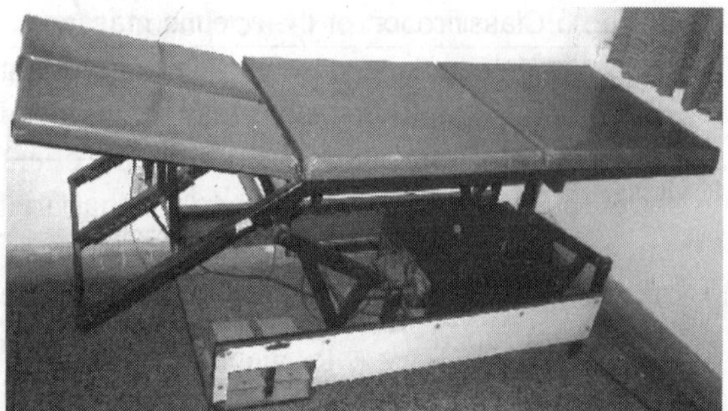

Fig. 9.1b: Inclined treatment plinth (adjustable head support)

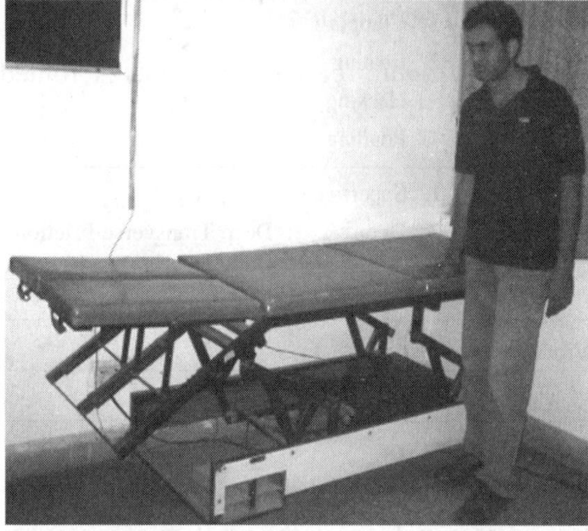

Fig. 9.1c: Measurement of treatment plinth shown by therapist by placing the hand on the plinth with dorsiflexion of wrist (ideal height)

Supports

Towels, pillows of various sizes, bed sheets, wedges; commercially available bolsters etc. can be used to provide support.

Linen

Cotton material is preferred. All linen should be bleachable. Pillow covers, small and large size towel, bed sheets and blankets one among the common linen supply.

Lubricants

The purpose of lubricant is to reduce the friction and control the amount of drag and glide between therapists hand and patient's body. Lubricants are also helpful in preparation of subcutaneous tissue. but their use should be done as and when need arises. Following lubricants are mainly used in practice:

Oils

It is one of the commonly used lubricant vegetable oil such as olive, coconut, almond etc. are considered to be more nutritious for skin as compared to mineral oil. Unabsorbed oil should be wiped from the client's skin by using tissue paper or small towel.

Creams–are thicker suspension. They lie somewhat between oil and lotion in terms of their rate of absorption. They promote glide or they may contain sticky ingredients like lanolin and bee wax that reduce glide helps in dragging the skin of the client.

Powder–used for gliding and also when patient refuse to use oil. It is also preferred for lymph drainage technique.

Positioning and Draping the Client during Treatment

Positioning—It depends upon the aim of treatment, the parts to be assessed or treated, client's preference and comfortability. Prone lying, supine, sidelying, seating, seated inclined and long-sitting are commonly used.

Positions for various muscles:
i. *Prone position*—Recommended position for treatment of:
   • Posterior neck muscles.
   • Upper and Lower back muscles.
   • Gluteal region.

- Back of thigh and leg
- *Position can also be used for following muscles*
    - Latissimus dorsi
    - Rhomboid
    - Trapezius
    - Spinal extensors
    - Gluteus maximus
    - Hamstrings
    - Triceps surae
    - Foot intrinsics.

ii. *Supine position*—Recommended for all muscles of head and neck, pectoralis, arm, abdominal, quadriceps and anterior compartment of leg.

iii. *Sidelying*—Scalenes, Rotator cuff, pectoralis minor, serratus anterior, abdominals, quadratus lumborum, intercostals, gluteus medius and minimus, iliotibial tract, peronei, adductors of the hip and triceps surae.

iv. *Seated upright*—Upper trapezius.

v. *Seated inclined*—Muscles of the posterior aspect of the head and neck.
    - Muscles of the upper back.
    - Muscles of posterior aspect of the upper arm.

Draping

Draping should place the client in safe, warm and comfortable position to receive the desired massage. It should maintain the boundary between the client and therapist in all practice settings including training setup. It sets a symbolic and an actual boundary hence therapist must make draping comfortable, yet precise and secured when exposing the clients body for treatment purposes.

Undraping Rules

- One part should be undraped at a time.
- Undrape only those area which has to be treated.
- Gluteal cleft, perineum, genital and female breast should not be undraped.

The female breast may be exposed if massage is clinically indicated by taking prior consent from the client. Similarly pelvis may be undraped by taking prior consent and informing the client about the importance of massage for that area (such as in labor/delivery).

- Infants under the age of two years may be treated undraped.
- Students must practice the draping technique repeatedly and extend appropriate respect to each other during classroom practice.

Draping Techniques

i. *Undraping the female torso*—A folded towel is placed on top of the sheet over the breasts. The client holds the edge of the towel while the clinician withdraw the sheet from under the towel. The towel is tucked under the torso or arms then the abdomen is exposed from xiphoid process to the anterior superior iliac spine.

ii. *Undraping the anterior leg*—After exposing and lowering the leg the extra sheet is gathered between the legs. The extra sheet is then pulled underneath the exposed leg back toward the side of the table. Here the sheet is securely anchored by the weight of the leg. The top edge of the drape can be tucked under the gluteal at the level of greater trochanter or the edge can be rolled higher to expose the anterior superior iliac spine and tucked under the lower back.

iii. *To expose the top leg in sidelying*—Fold the posterior portion of the sheet forward, more as much of the extra sheet as possible out of the way in a superior direction.

Edge of the drape is pulled back under the leg. The leg to be exposed is now surrounded by drape. The outer leg is not exposed at any tissue during the procedure. Again move as much of the extra sheet as possible out of the way in a superior direction. Keep it tight to the leg, gradually pull the drape upto the thigh.

Finally pull the superior edge of the drape toward the groin, toward the glutetral cleft and roll it over the iliac crest. It takes practicenar to get this draping tight and secure. A pillow may be kept under the knee for support.

iv. Undraping the torso in prone.
   – The back is exposed to the level of posterior superior iliac spine.
   – The drape is securely tucked.
   – The arms of client may be kept either on the sides overhead.

Clinicians Posture, Alignment and Body Mechanics During Treatment

Effectiveness of massage technique is also depends on the therapist's correct use of his feet, leg, pelvis, respiratory apparatus (as in most of shoulder girdle), shoulder, elbow and of course hands. The following general principles of body mechanics should be applied during STM techniques:

i. Posture is aligned as upright as possible except during the controlled transfer of body weight.

ii. Both feet remain in contact with the floor.

iii. Therapist must bend his knee to reduce vertical distance between himself and client instead of bending trunk.

iv. Similarly therapist must reposition his leg or shift his weight onto his forward leg rather than by bending at the waist or reaching excessively.

v. The therapist orients his navel area toward the body segment of the client being treated.

vi. Use body weight to increase pressure instead of muscular force.

vii. Therapists joints are positioned as close to neutral as possible rather than being loaded while they are in a closed-packed position.

viii. Therapist should change his posture frequently by to avoid undue mechanical stress on his body.

ix. Therapist should also avoid unwanted static contraction. Hand muscles must be elongated after few grasps during the massage technique.

x. Therapist should control the amount of his body weight that is being transferred to the client, precisely and continuously.

STROKING AND EFFLEURAGE

The movement of both stroking and effleurage are so similar that they can be discussed together. Even some authors use the term stroking and effleurage interchangeably.

- *Mennel* has not used the effleurage in his classification, he classified stroking into superficial and deep.
- *Despard*—He used both stroking and effleurage, according to him, the direction of stroking and effleurage remains same (centripetal) but the pressure in stroking is vigorous and in effleurage varies from superficial to deep according to condition.

- *Hoffa* used light pressure at the beginning of the stroke manipulation, increases it over the fleshy part of the muscles and decreases it again at the end of stroke.
- *Ling* said pressure of effleurage varies from the lightest touch to one of considerable force.
- *Murrel* and *Kleen* said that it varies.
- Different authors have different opinions but conclusion is that the stroking and effleurage may be used to produce similar reflex effects, so this book follows the convention used in many texts, and explains that effluerage constitutes pressures from superficial (light) to deep

and produces the similar physiological effects such as stroking. In other words the stroking movements are the part of effleurage movements.

EFFLEURAGE

Definition

It consists a long, soothing, stroking movements performed by palmar aspect (over the large area) or fingers (over the small area) of one or both hands.

- Effleurage is used to start off any type of massage, soothing the nerve endings and again at the end of massage. It means every soft tissue manipulation technique starts and ends with the effleurage

Classification of Effleurage

- Superficial Effleurage, and
- Deep Effleurage.

Superficial Effleurage

Procedure: The technique may be performed by single or both hands. The hand(s) should be as relaxed as possible, fingers and thumb may be abducted but not so widely that hand becomes tense. Minimal palmar or radial deviation of wrist is used to enable to conform to local body contours. While maintaining above position, the hands are placed over the patient's body.

Superficial Effleurage (Longitudinal Stroke) for Back Region

Position of patient: Prone lying, the whole back should be exposed fully. An extra care should be given in case of female patient.

Position of therapist: Standing at the side of patient, with one foot slightly behind but in line with the other. This position allows therapist to shift the body weight forward and backward.

Lubricants: Talcum, oil.

Procedure: The talcum or oil is poured over the whole back to avoid friction and uneven strokes. The both hands are placed on the lower back region (one hand on either side of the spine) and the hands are kept relaxed throughout the movement. Both hands move longitudinally from just above the sacrum to the lumbar, thoracic and axilla. As the hands move from sacrum a mild pressure is applied through the hands by shifting the body weight forward on the front leg (slight flexion of the chephalad knee joint). As soon the hands approach an upper thoracic region, are slide toward the axilla and pressure is released gradually. After completing stroke at the axilla hands are returned back to the original position from axilla to the lateral wall of the thorax. When hands return, pressure is not applied but fingers maintain contact with the skin through the return stroke. Again the hands are positioned on the lower back region and prepares for another stroke. Several similar strokes are performed on the back to achieve effective results. Every stroke of effleurage should be in steady rhythm and may take 6 seconds. This technique of effleurage is known as longitudinal effleurage on back (Figs 9.2a to d).

Reverse Longitudinal Stroke of Superficial Effleurage

Position of patient—Prone lying.

Position of therapist—Standing at the head, end of the treatment table.

Lubricants: Talcum, oil.

Procedure—Both hands are placed over the upper back (one on either side of the spine). The fingers and thumbs are kept closed. Both hands are moved with little pressure to the lower back. The pressure is applied through the hands by leaning forward. As soon as hands approach the lower back, they slide toward the groin (inguinal lymph nodes) and pressure is released gradually. After finishing stroke at groin region, both hands

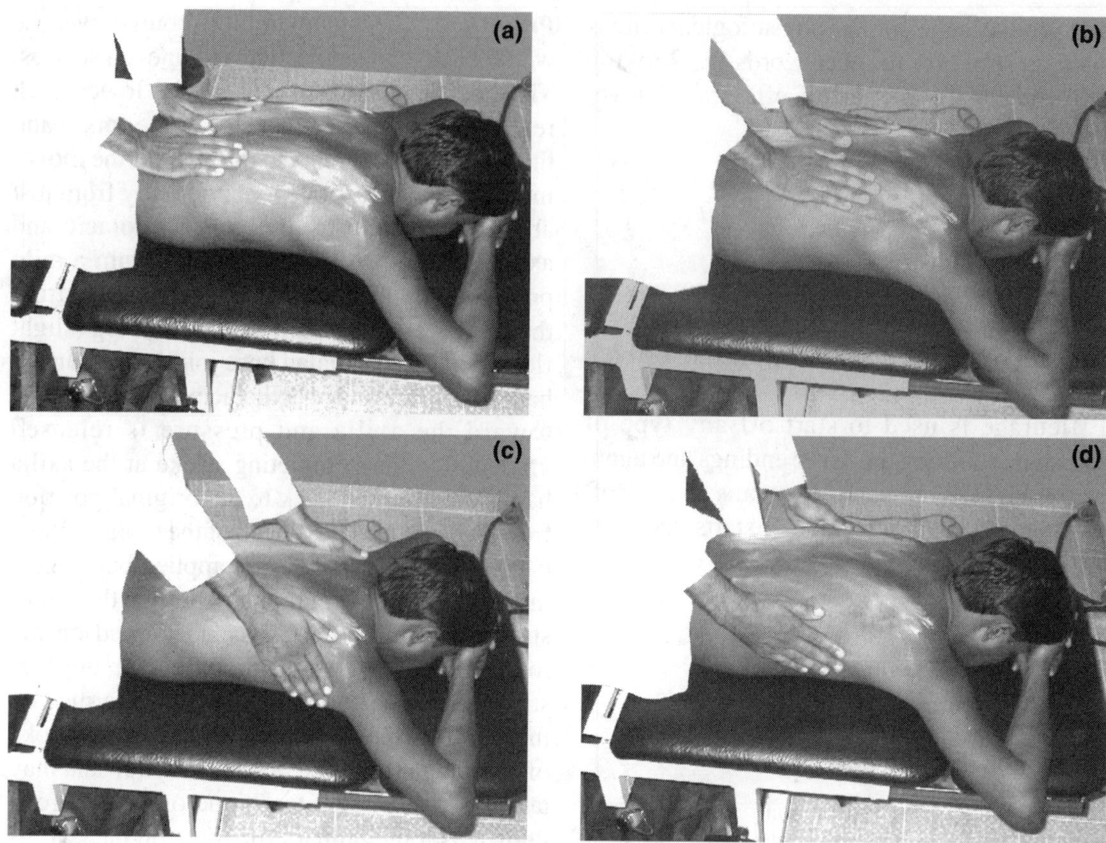

Figs 9.2a to d: Superficial effleurage (Longitudinal stroke)—(a) Initial, (b) Mid position, (c) End position, and (d) Return stroke

return from groin to the lateral border of the trunk (one hand on either side), shoulders then toward the upper back. During return stroke pressure is not applied but fingers maintain the contact with the skin. When return stroke approaches the upper back from the groin, the direction of fingers remain same (pointing in a caudal direction) but the thumbs opened out away from the fingers. The hands are again placed on upper back and prepare for next stroke (Figs 9.3a to d).

Five to ten repetitions of strokes are performed. Repetition of strokes may increase if these are performed over large muscles.

When superficial effleurage is performed on extremities (U/L or L/L), the proximal part of the limb is massaged first then the distal part of the limb, and the direction of movement should be from distal to proximal part.

The purpose of effleurage is to drain the fluid, so the strokes of effleurage are performed from distal or proximal part to the lymph nodes, from these it is taken out to the heart, thus the effleurage helps reducing the swelling or effusion.

Deep Effleurage

The wrist is maintained in neutral position (no radial or ulnar deviation). If more pressure is required the dorsal surface of hand or wrist is reinformed by the other hand. Mainly its strokes are circular, parallel to the long axis of muscle or muscle group may also be performed on whole back region.

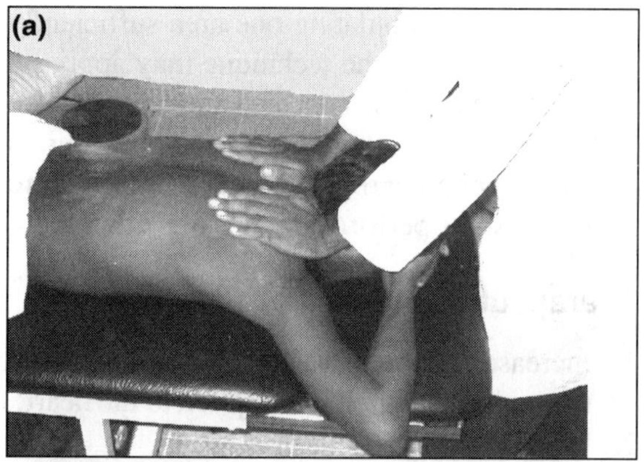

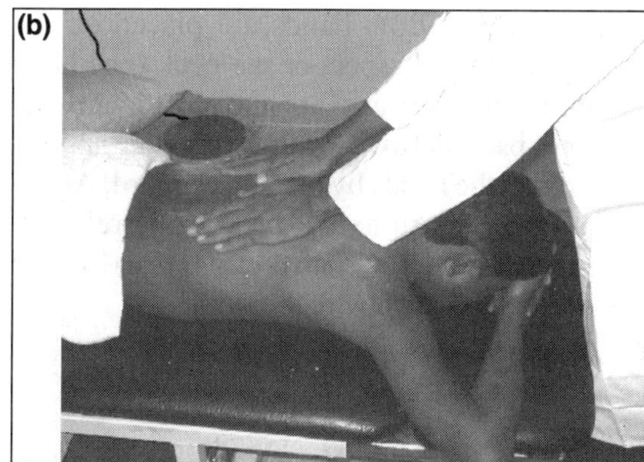

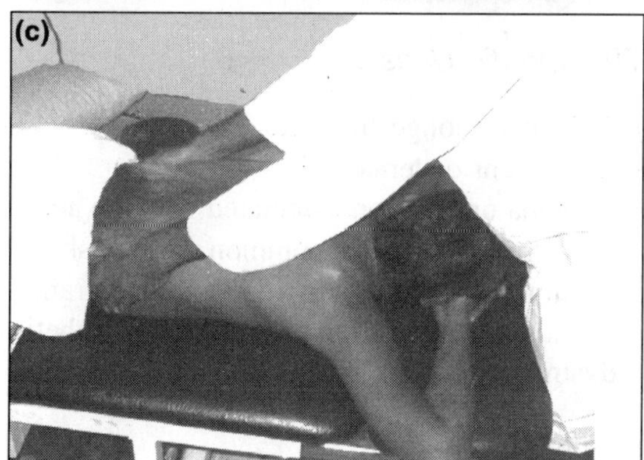

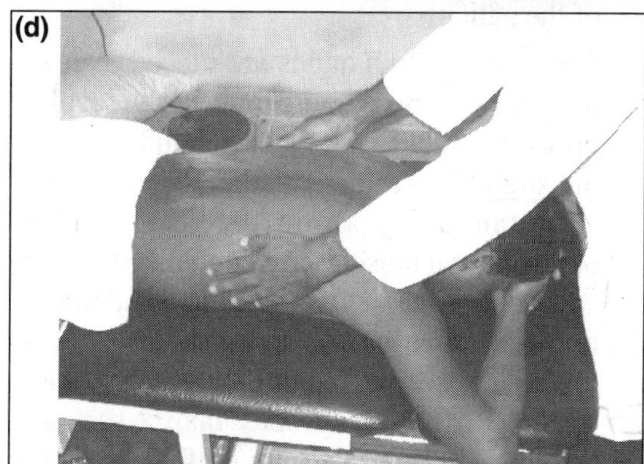

Fig. 9.3a to d: Superficial effleurage (Reverse longitudinal stroke)—(a) Initial stroke, (b) Mid stroke, (c) End stroke, and (d) Return stroke

Procedure

The pressure and return stroke combine to form circles that are oriented along or across the fibres in the different muscle layers. Most often the long axis of the stroke run parallel to the long axis of the body segment or muscle to which the technique is being applied, especially when significant pressure is requested.

A. *On whole back region:* The position of patient and therapist remains same as longitudinal superficial effleurage.

   Lubricants—Talcum or oil.

   Procedure—The procedure also remain same as longitudinal superficial effleurage, but in the technique more pressure is applied than the previous techniques. To apply more pressure one hand may be re-inforced by other hand. The one hand is placed over the lower back region and reinforced by the other hand. The pressure is applied as the hand starts moving from lower back to the upper back. As soon as hands approach the upper back they are slide laterally to the axilla and pressure is released gradually. After completing the stroke the hands are returned to the lower back from axilla to the lateral border of trunk. Again hand is placed on lower back, reinforced by other hand and prepares for next stroke. Several similar strokes are performed.

B. *On neck and upper back:*

   Position of patient—Prone lying.

   Position of therapist—Standing at the head, end of the treatment table.

Procedure—Both hands are placed on the postero-lateral aspect of the neck (one hand on either side) and are moved toward the upper back and axilla with the pressure applied through the hands by leaning forward. As the hands approach axilla, pressure is released gradually and hands are return for next stroke with little contact with the skin.

C. *Deep effleurage with thumbs: (on back)*

Position of patient—Prone lying.

Position of therapist—Standing at the side of the patient.

Procedure—Both hands are placed over the muscle which is being manipulated. The pressure is applied through the thumbs by leaning slightly forward. The thumbs are moved simultaneously along the long axis of paravertebral muscles in a cephalad direction with slight lateral curve. The hand and fingers may also move with the thumb but pressure is applied only by the thumb. The length of each stroke is 5 cm which may take 2 seconds. Several similar strokes are performed on the same muscle unless satisfactory effect is achieved. An indicator that the tissues are treated sufficiently is a feeling of sinking in with the thumbs. This 'giving' of the tissues however is not quickly accomplished, sometimes not at all. Overtreating an area can cause hypersensitivity. If the strokes are performed too quickly and deeply the tension in the muscle tissue may increase.

After manipulating one area sufficiently and effectively the technique may apply on another adjacent area and muscles can be manipulated to the thoracic region as far as the lower border of the scapula. The procedure may also be performed with single thumb.

Therapeutic Effects of Effleurage

1. Increases lymphatics and venous return from the region to which it is applied to the heart.
2. Dilates the superficial arterioles.

Therapeutic Uses

- Lymphatic congestion
- Dependent oedema
- Oedema or effusion associated with the acute and subacute phase of common musculoskeletal injuries such as bursitis, sprains, strains, dislocation, separation and reflex sympathetic dystrophy (RSD).

Cautions

- Acute cardiac conditions.
- Congestive heart failure.

Contraindication

- Acute orthopaedic injuries
- Newly forming scars
- Infected area
- Hypo and hyperthermia
- Open wound, burn and ulcers.

Table 9.2: Difference between superficial and deep effleurage

	Superficial effleurage	*Deep effleurage*
Contact	Whole relaxed palmar surface of hand	Whole relaxed palmar surface of hand often reinforce on the wrist or proximal forearm, sometimes thumb
Pressure	Light	Light to heavy
Engages	Skin, superficial fascia	Muscles and associated tissues
Direction	On limbs-centripetal, on torso-towards axillary or inguinal lymph nodes	Circular, parallel to the long axis of muscle or muscles group
Rate	5-50 cm/sec	10-25 cm/sec
Duration	2 min or longer	20-60 sec or more

PETRISSAGE

Petrissage is derived from French word *Petrir* means knead.

Definition

It is a technique of soft tissue manipulation which includes various types of strokes in which tissues are compressed, lifted, squeezed and released with varying amount of pressure, drag and glide. Various types of strokes are performed to mobilize skin, subcutaneous tissues and deep structures like muscles.

Classification

1. Kneading
2. Picking up
3. Wringing and
4. Skin rolling.

Kneading

Kneading is a manipulation in which muscles and subcutaneous tissues are alternately compressed and released. The movement takes place in a circular motion which is divided into two phases pressure and release. During the pressure phase of each stroke, the hand(s) and skin move together on the deeper structure and during the release phase, the hand glides smoothly over the skin.

Direction of strokes: The basic direction of each stroke is circular.

Techniques

The stroke of kneading are performed in a circulator manner:

The hand or tip of fingers move over the underlying structures with the skin during the one half circle (⊃) which is also known as pressure phase, after pressure phase, the pressure is released and the hand(s) glides smoothly over the another half circle (⊂) which is known as release phase and after performing stroke in full circle the stroke is repeated on adjacent area (Fig. 9.4).

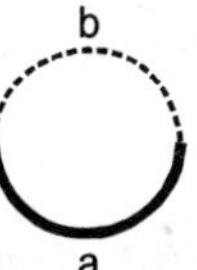

Fig. 9.4: Kneading—a-pressure phase (∪), and b-release phase (⌢)

Rate of Movement

The both pressure phase and release phase should be completed in 3-4 seconds.

Pressure

The pressure is applied during half of the circle but how much pressure will be delivered by the hands or fingers of therapist depends on the parts or structure which is being treated. The delicate structures like face and dorsum of hand require minimal pressure. More pressure can be delivered by using both hands on the back, thighs and calf muscles. The therapist should take an extra precautions while performing the strokes on geriatric patients on osteoporotic bones.

Classification of Kneading

As it is already mentioned that in kneading tissues are alternately compressed and released by using single or both hands. It is therefore kneading is classified on the basis of the part of hand which is used to deliver the pressure, example—when the whole palm of hands are used to deliver the pressure, this kneading is named as palmar kneading. Following kneadings are clinically used:

- Palmar or compression kneading
- Finger pad kneading
- Thumb pad kneading
- Kunckle kneading

- Reinforced kneading
- Squeeze kneading.

Palmar ("compression", "circular", "flat handed" or "whole handed) kneading" is performed over large areas. Back, thigh, calf, arms and gluteal region. The whole palm is used to direct the pressure upward and inward in a circular motion and the skin moves with hand(s) over the underlying structures. Pressure is applied during half of circle and released during another half of circle and than repeated on the adjacent area.

Finger Pad Kneading

This kneading stroke is used to deliver pressure over the small area. The pads of one or more finger tips are placed over the target structure and movement is performed in a circular manner which includes pressure and release phase. Finger pad may be performed by single or both hands, when it is performed with both hands, the movements of hands take place opposite to each other (Fig. 9.5).

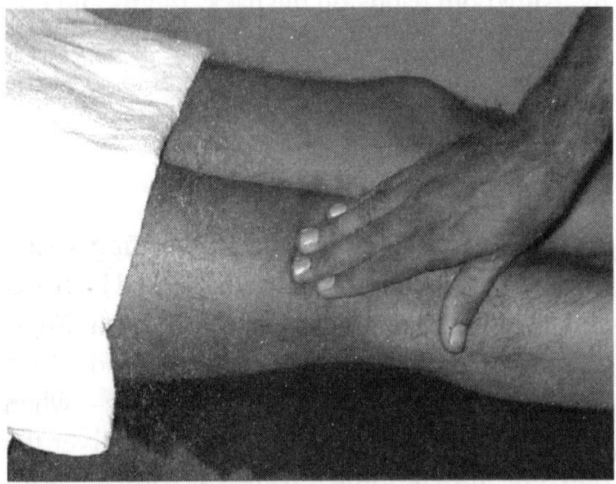

Fig. 9.5: Finger pad kneading

Uses of Finger Pad Kneading

Useful in tendinitis, fibromyalgia and muscles spasm.

Thumb Pad Kneading

It is performed on small areas (wrist, ankle, elbow joint and face). The pressure over the tissues are applied by the pad of one or both thumbs. The basic direction of movement is circular which includes pressure and release phase. Thumbs of both hands are used to work side by side (Fig. 9.6).

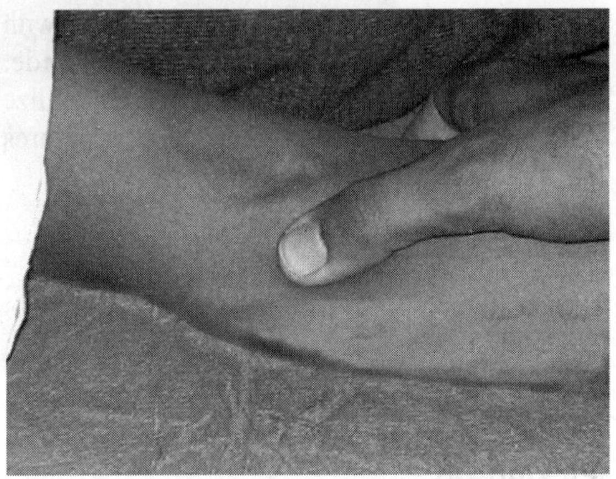

Fig. 9.6: Thumb pad kneading

Knuckle Kneading

It is also performed on small areas. The pressure is applied over the tissues by knuckles (dorsal surface) of the middle or proximal phalanges (Fig. 9.7).

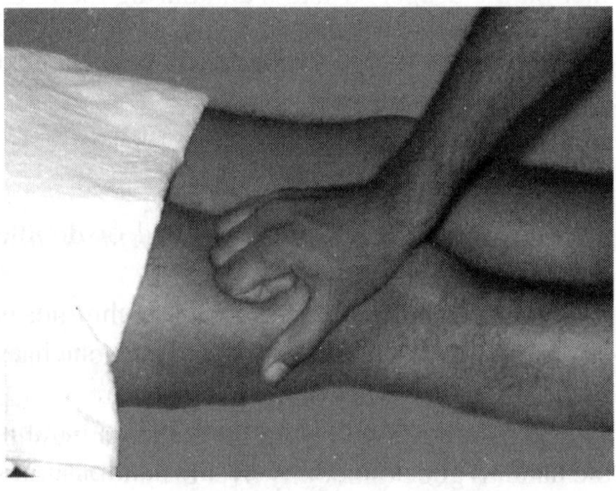

Fig. 9.7: Knuckle kneading

Reinforced Kneading

To deliver more pressure, an extra effort is required for the effective treatment (Fat patients) by placing other hand over the hand which is being used to deliver pressure (Fig. 9.8).

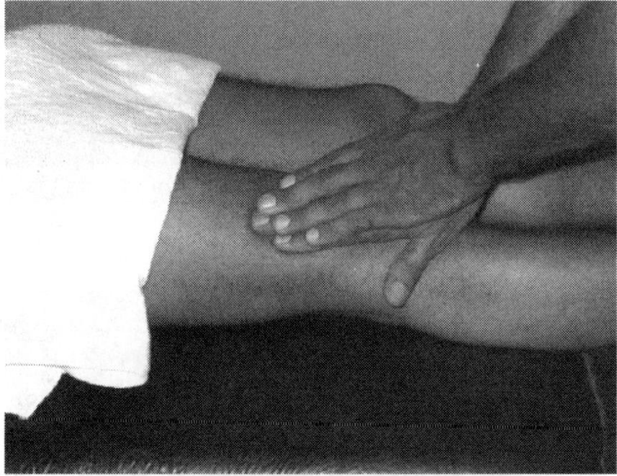

Fig. 9.8: Reinforcement Kneading

Picking Up

The skin, subcutaneous tissues and muscles are grasped and lifted away from the underlying structures and then squeezed and released—The sequence of picking up may be followed as:
- Step 1—Compression of tissues/gliding.
- Step 2—Skin, subcutaneous tissues and muscles are grasped, lifted and squeezed.
- Step 3—Compression is released and hand(s) are placed on adjacent area to start the next stroke of picking up.

Technique

Picking up either be single handed or double handed.

One handed picking up: This technique is performed on smaller body segments such as arms, forearms and calf muscles.

Position of hand: The thumb of the hand is abducted, fingers are adducted and hand assumes in a C-shape position (Figs 9.9a to c).

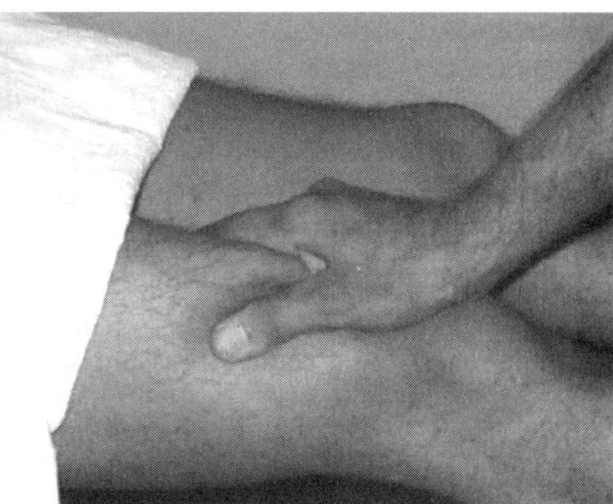

Fig. 9.9a: Picking up of quadriceps muscles

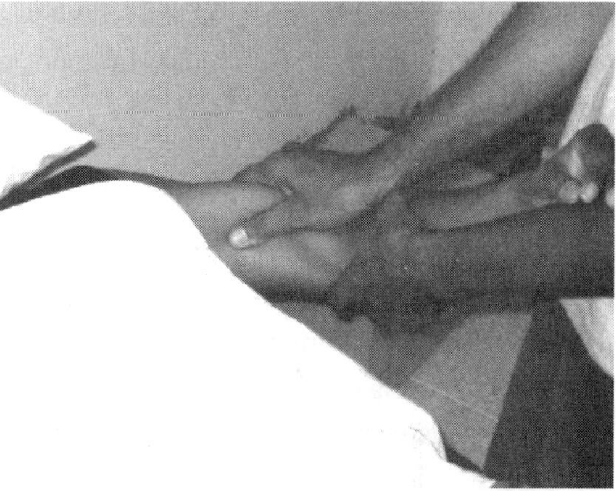

Fig. 9.9b: Picking up of elbow flexors

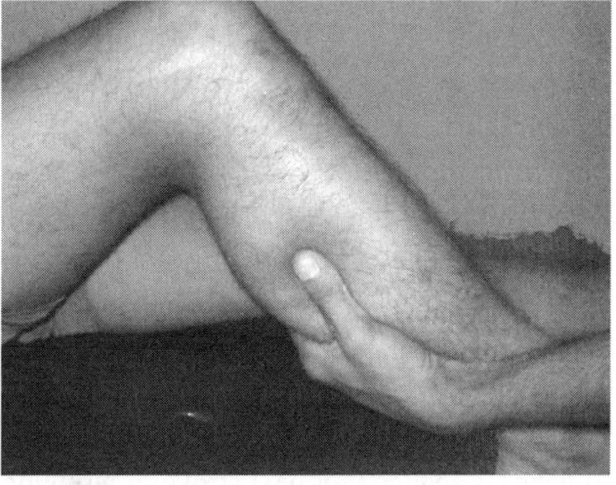

Fig. 9.9c: Picking up of gastrosoleus muscles

Procedure

While maintaining the C-shape position, hand is placed on the part to be treated and tissues are grasped between the thumb and fingers then lifted away from the underlying structure by using the extension of the wrist. Then tissues are squeezed between thumb and fingers and in the final stage of picking up tissues are released. Hands again assume in a C-shape position for next stroke in an adjacent part.

Wringing

The skin with muscles are grasped, lifted and squeezed alternately by both hands in opposite direction to each other.

Procedures

Position of hands same as in picking up both hands are placed on the skin across the long axis of muscles. The skin with muscles grasped between the thumb and fingers then lifted away from the underlying structures (Fig. 9.10a), in the next step of wringing the tissues are pulled toward the therapist's body by pulling the fingers of one hand, and at the same time the thumb of other hand pushes the tissues away from the therapists body and tissues assume in a S-shape position (Fig. 9.10b). In the next step the fingers and thumb move in opposite direction to each other and the tissues assume again in S shape position (Fig. 9.10c). So in one cycle of wringing tissues assume in S shape position for two times. Several repetitions of wringing may be performed on same tissues if required. In the final step of wringing the tissues are released by both hands and position of hands is changed for next stroke of wringing in an adjacent part.

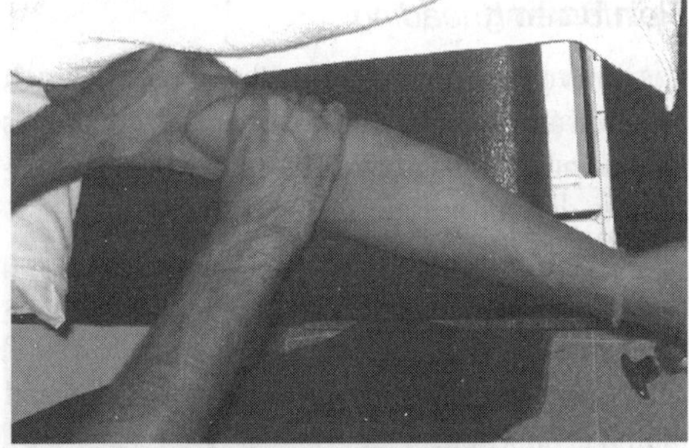

Fig. 9.10a: Wringing of elbow flexors (initial)

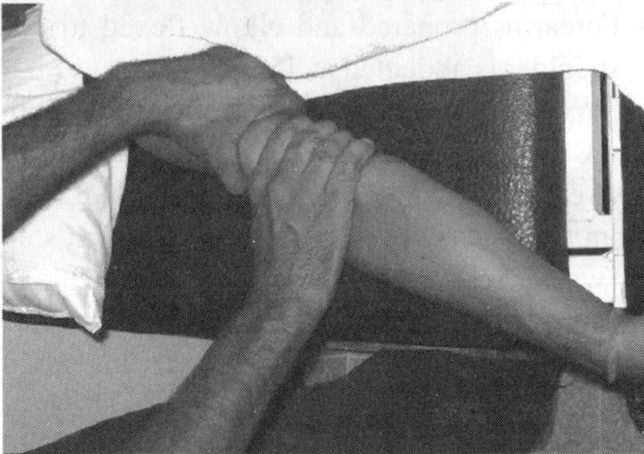

Fig. 9.10b: Wringing of elbow flexors (mid position)

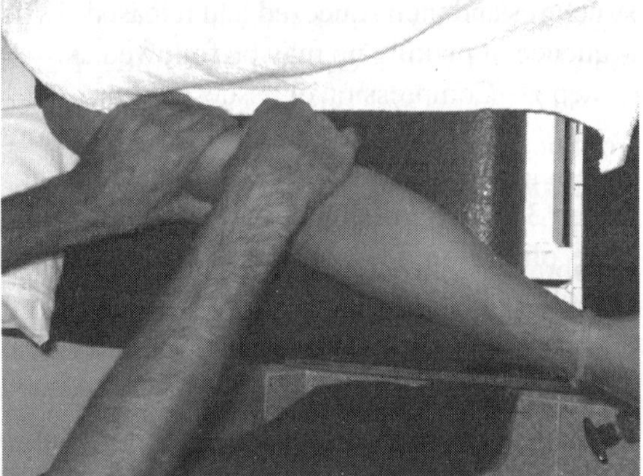

Fig. 9.10c: Wringing of elbow flexors (end position)

Direction of movement: Thumb of one hand and fingers of other hand work opposite to each other along the long axis of the muscle fibres.

Rate of movement: Four to six inch per second, rate may decrease on smaller muscles.

Skin Rolling

It is a soft tissue manipulation technique in which the skin and subcutaneous tissues are rolled over the underlying structures (muscles).

Procedure

Position of hands—using the action of lumbricals the metacarpo-phalangeal joints are flexed at 90° and interphalangeal (IP) joints kept extended and thumb is opposed.

- Wrists are slightly extended.
- Forearms pronated and elbow flexed to 90° shoulder is abducted at 45°.

While maintaining above position the both hands are placed over the skin. The skin is grasped between the thumb and fingers and lifted away from the underlying structures. In the next step of wringing the fingers of right hand move forward and grasp the skin, the thumb of the same hand drags and draws the skin to the fingers. In the next step while maintaining the position of right hand the fingers of left hand move forward and grasp the skin while the thumb of same hand drags and draws the skin to the fingers. It is therefore in this technique the fold of skin between thumb and fingers can be maintained from one part to the other part.

Example—On upper back fold of skin can be maintained between the fingers and thumb from vertebral column to the rib cage and from lumbar to the thoracic spine (Figs 9.11a and b).

Therapeutic Effects of Petrissage

1. Dilatation of capillaries and arterials increase the blood supply and promote resolution of inflammatory processes of skin and subcutaneous tissues.
2. Increases extensibility and elasticity of skin and subcutaneous tissue.
3. The blood supply of muscles increases, which eliminates the waste metabolic products, thus:

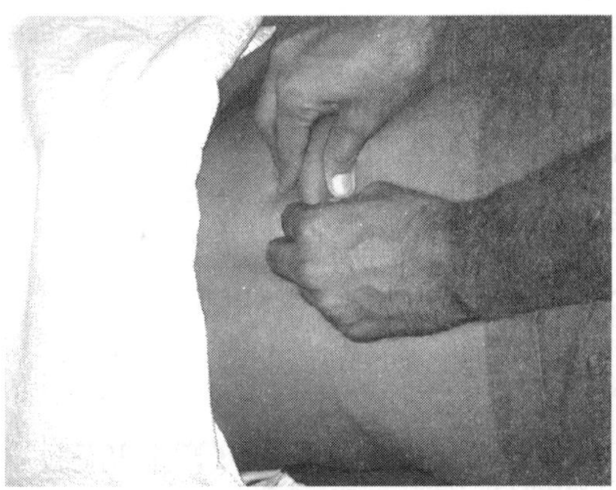

Fig. 9.11a: Skin rolling, from lumbar to thoracic spine

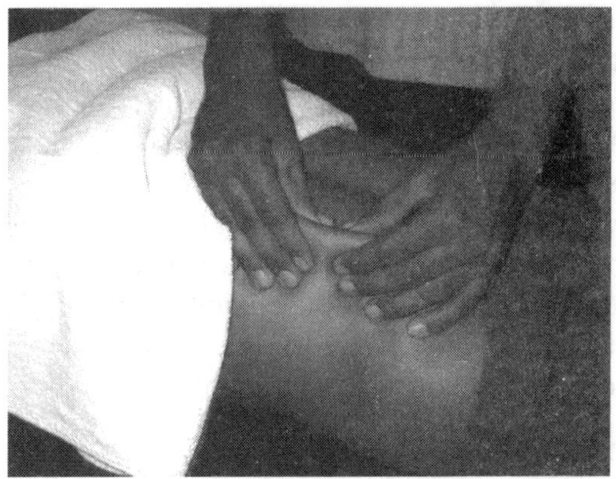

Fig. 9.11b: Skin rolling, from vertebral column to the rib cage

- Relaxes the muscles.
- Increases flexibility of muscles.
4. Increase lymphatic blood flow.

Therapeutic uses of Petrissage

1. To increase extensibility and mobility of connective tissues.
2. To reduce anxiety, stress and improve relaxation.
3. To alleviate the behavioural symptoms of depression hyperactivity.
4. To increase joint range of motion (ROM).
5. To mobilize skin and subcutaneous tissues.
6. To decrease chronic oedema.
7. To decrease pain during labour.

The observed positive effect of petrissage on pulmonary conditions such as asthma, chronic obstructive pulmonary disease (COPD) and cystic fibrosis may be as a result of the combined effects of decreased anxiety and increased chest wall mobility, following petrissage manipulations.

Contraindications

- Acute inflammation.
- Infection.
- Confirmed or suspected thrombosis and thrombophlebitis.
- Extra care should be taken if patient is (i) suspected osteoporotic (ii) taking anticoagulants.
- Malignant disease.
- Acute musculo-skeletal injuries, fracture, muscle strain, ligaments sprain.

TAPOTEMENT OR PERCUSSION

Tapotement is a technique of soft tissue manipulation in which the part which is being treated strikes repeatedly by the various modified positions of hand(s). In all tapotement movements the fingers, hands and wrists should be as relaxed as possible. Tapotement strokes are fast, precision action, bringing one hand quickly after the other into contact with the patient's body. After few strokes of tapotement the clinician must ask the patient whether the pressure which is being delivered by hands is comfortable or not.

Classification of Tapotement

1. Clapping
2. Beating
3. Hacking
4. Pounding.

Clapping (Cupping)—Clapping is a soft tissue manipulation technique of tapotement in which the patients body (skin) is struck alternately by cup shaped hands. To achieve cup shaped position of hands the metacarpo-phalangeal joints (MCP) are flexed at 45°, interphalangeal joints are kept in neural position (extended) wrist should be as loose as possible (Fig. 9.12).

Technique: The cup shaped hands strike alternately over the posterior chest wall and lateral surface of the rib cage by using the alternate flexion and extension of the wrist joints. It is performed rapidly with coordinated hands and

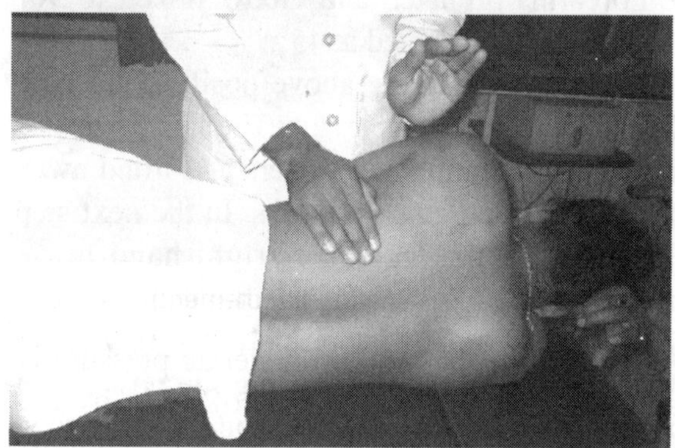

Fig. 9.12: Clapping (cupping)

pressure should be light. To achieve light pressure the movements (flexion and extension) should be taken place at the wrist joints and elbows remain almost at full extension.

Uses of clapping: It is performed on posterior chest wall and lateral rib cage to loosen the secretin or drains the fluid from lungs. Therefore, it is important for the clinician to place the patient in appropriate position which helps to drain the fluid while performing clapping. The technique should be followed by postural drainage positions.

- It is also performed on larger muscles group to mobilize and achieve stimulating effect.

Beating—Beating is a soft tissue manipulation technique of tapotement in which the patients skin is struck by the dorsal aspect of the fingers heel of one or both hands.

Technique: The hands are positioned in a loose fist and tissues are struck by dorsal aspect of the fingers and heel of hand. Beating is a single or double handed technique. When it is performed by both hands, the hands strike the tissues alternately (Fig 9.13).

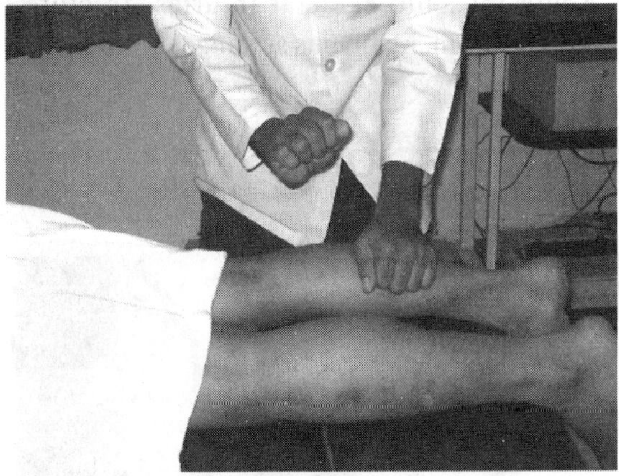

Fig. 9.13: Beating (tapotement)

Pressure: The mild to moderate pressure is applied according to the part of body by the flexion and extension of wrist joints, the elbow joints, remain almost in extension.

Uses of beating:
- To mobilize the muscles
- To stimulates the skin and subcutaneous tissues.
- To mobilise the joints like lumbosacral junction.

Hacking—Hacking is a soft tissue manipulation technique of tapotement in which the tissues are strike alternately by the medial edges and dorsal aspects of the fingers in rapid succession to create a strong stimulating effect.

Technique: The fingers and wrists of clinician should be as relaxed as possible. The repetitive supination and pronation take place at the forearm with slight radial and ulnar deviation at wrist joint. The therapist flexes the elbows and abducts the shoulder joints. The ulnar border of the hand and little finger strike the patient's body at the same time the medial and dorsal edge of other fingers also strike on skin on each other sequentially which causes an audible sound. The technique is performed on long axis of fleshy muscles with single hand or both hands repeatedly (Figs 9.14a and b).

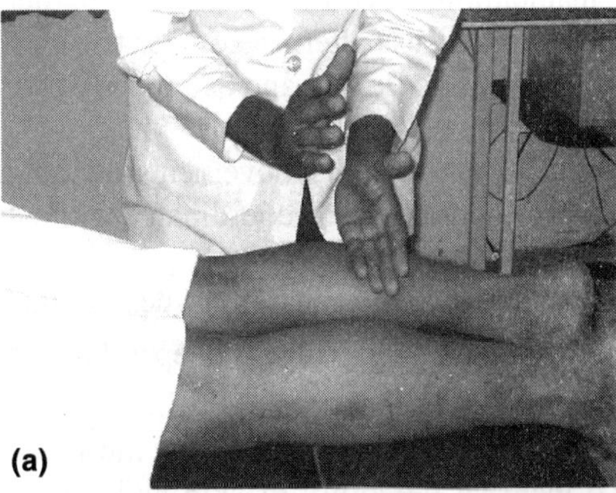

(a)

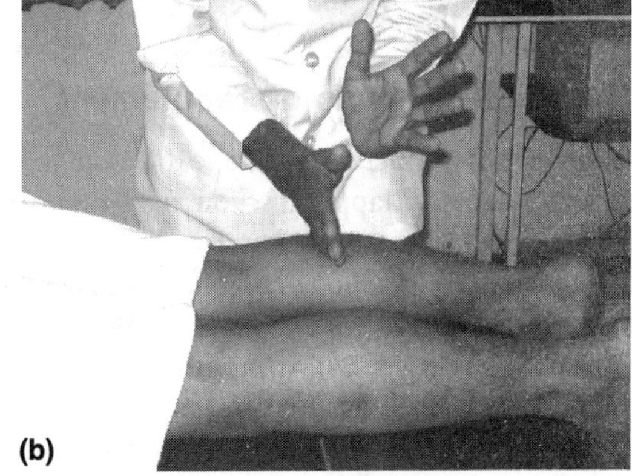

(b)

Figs 9.14a and b: Hacking

Rate of movement: The clinician needs more practice to learn this technique before administrating on the patient's body. The smooth coordinated movements are performed as fast as possible.

Pressure: There is no pressure other than the weight of the relaxed fingers striking the skin surface in rapid succession.

Uses:
- To stimulate the skin and subcutaneous tissues.
- To mobilize the muscles.

Pounding—is the soft tissue manipulation technique of tapotement in which the tissues are strike or percuss alternately by the ulnar border of the hands.

Technique: The clinician loosely clench the fist, but keeps the wrists as relaxed as possible. While maintaining this position the ulnar border of both hands percuss alternately over the long fleshing muscles by flexion and extension of the wrist joints (Fig. 9.15a and b).

Rate of movements: The movements are rapid but should be controlled and coordinated without thumping the patient's skin/body.

Pressure: The pressure is delivered by the ulnar border of the hand which is deeper than the hacking.

Uses: To mobilize the large fleshy muscles.
• To increase flexibility of skin and subcutaneous tissues.

Therapeutic Effects of Tapotement

Various forms of percussion have different therapeutic effects. Clapping when performed on posterior chest wall and lateral wall it mechanically looses the secretion or mucus from the lungs and facilitates airways clearance while hacking stimulates sensory nerve endings and causes contraction of the muscles.

In cardio-pulmonary physiotherapy, percussion is combined with postural drainage and is followed by or alternately with vibration of rib cage.

Contraindications

• Rib fractures.

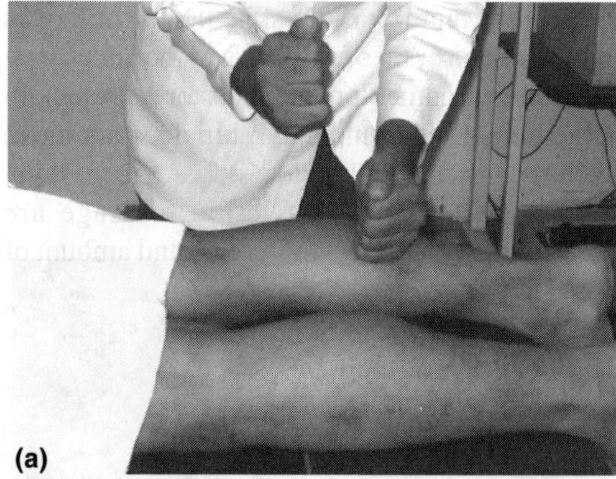

(a)

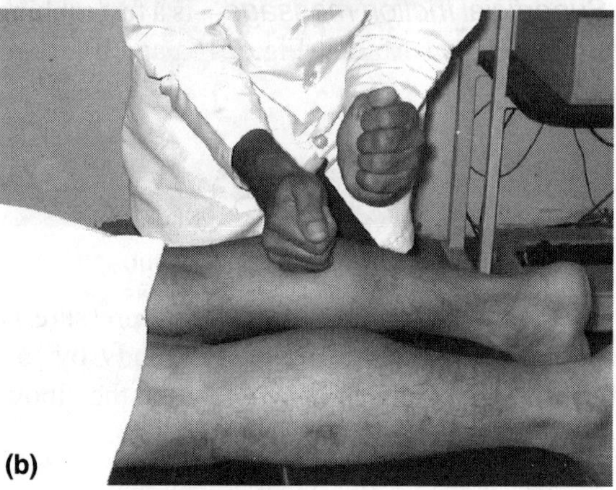

(b)

Figs 9.15a and b: Pounding

• Untreated tension pneumothorax.
• Confirmed or possible coronary thrombosis.
• Pulmonary embolism.
• Unstable cardiac condition.
• Spastic muscles.
• Acute traumatic oedema.
• Cancer or tumors.

FRICTION

Friction is derived from Latin word frictio, which means to rub.

It involves brisk, repetitive, specific, compressive strokes which are delivered by hand, tip of fingers, or thumb on the skin. The skin moves with the hand or tip of fingers over the underlying structures (ligamentous, tendons or muscles). In superficial friction massage skin does not move with the hands.

The techniques of friction massage are classified on the basis of direction and amount of force that is applied.

Classification

1. Superficial friction massage.
2. Deep friction massage.

Superficial friction massage—is a fast rubbing of the body's surfaces (Fig. 9.16a and b).

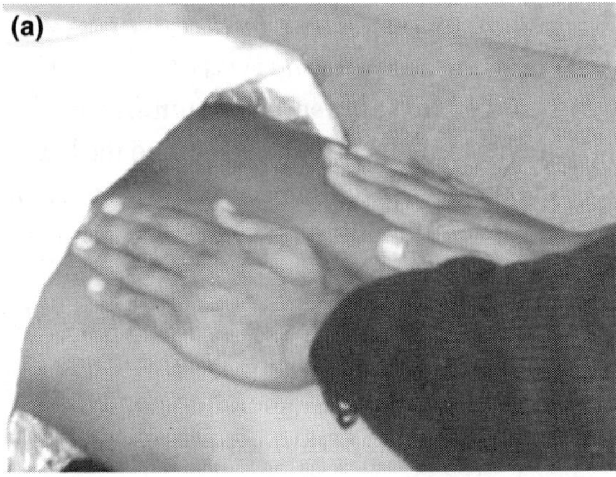

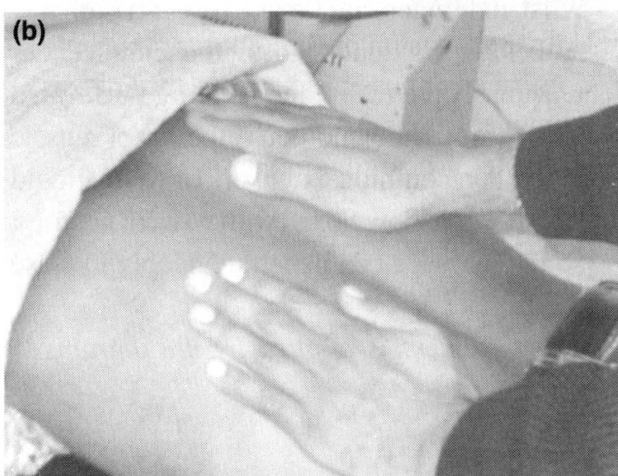

Figs 9.16a and b: Superficial friction massage

Technique: This requires thin use of a lubricant (an amount of lubricant depends on body's

hair and speed of movement). The both hands with fingers and thumb adducted placed over the skin and move simultaneously in opposite directions over the skin. The movements are taken place in the shoulder joint and elbow, while dragging the hands over the skin no movements are taken place at wrist and hand and these should be as relaxed as possible for better strokes.

Deep friction massage—is a small, repetitive localised, deep penetrating stroke performed by the tip of fingers, thumb or olecranon process of elbow in a circular or transverse manner on the muscles, ligaments, tendons. The tip of fingers, thumb or olecranon process move with the skin over the underlying structures (muscles, ligamentous and tendon). The strokes of deep friction massage are similar to kneading strokes of petrissage but differ on the basis of length, direction, pressure, and are performed across the connective tissue fibres.

Classification of deep friction massage:
A. Transverse friction.
B. Circular friction.
A. **Transverse friction**–also known as cross fibres friction, deep transverse friction and cyriax friction (Figs 9.17a to e).

Technique: The technique varies slightly from condition to condition but the principles remain same.

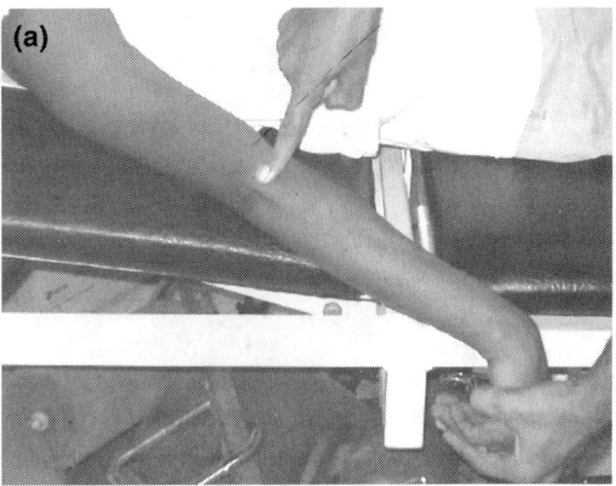

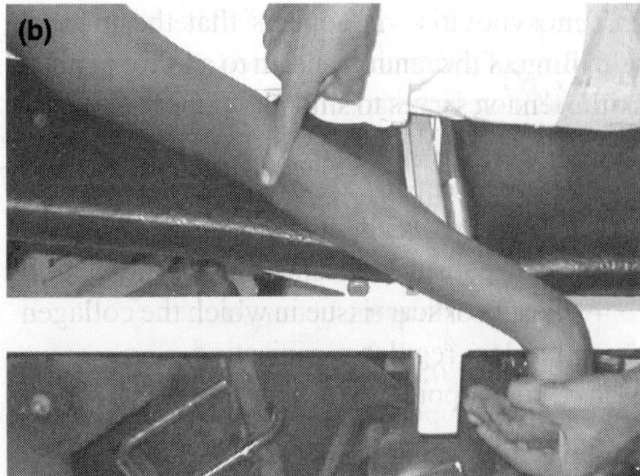

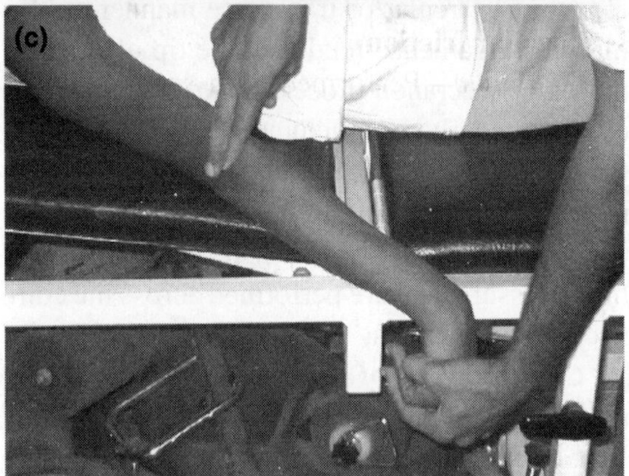

Figs 9.17a to c: Deep transverse friction massage (a) Initial position—over tendons of extensor communis, (b) End position—over tendons of extensor communis and (c) Reinforcement—over tendons of extensor communis

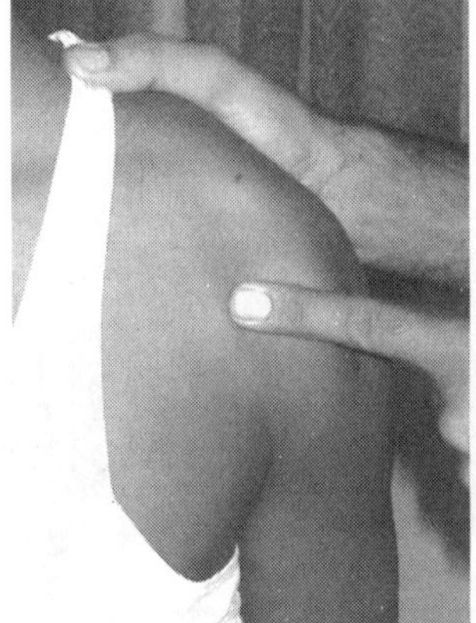

Fig. 9.17d: Deep transverse friction massage over tendon of superaspinatus

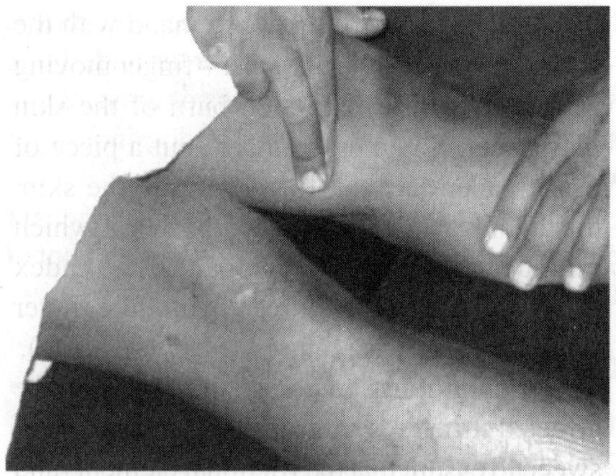

Fig. 9.17e: Deep transverse friction massage over medial collateral ligament of left knee joint

1. *Treatment part must be brought within reach of the therapist's finger:* For instance, in supraspinatus tendinitis the patients arm must be placed behind the back. This brings the tendon out of the acromion which would otherwise shield the entire structure.

2. *The tissue to receive the massage should be in appropriate tension (except muscle belly):* For intance in lateral epicondylitis if the technique is performed on tendon, then wrist and fingers are flexed, forearm pronated and elbow is extended to put the tendon under tension. If the technique is being performed over the musculotendinous junction or muscle belly then common extensors of wrist should be relaxed (elbow flexed with wrist in neutral), so the massage can penetrate deeply to tease the fibres apart.

3. *The treatment is applied by the therapist's finger tips.*

Procedure:

• The tip of finger (index) is placed on the skin (area to be treated), the finger tip moves with the skin over the underlying structures. The technique is to move the whole hand with the patient's skin and the therapist's finger moving as one, otherwise a friction burn of the skin may occur. Some practitioners put a piece of tissue paper between fingertips and the skin, this avoids the burn and absorbs sweat which might otherwise cause slippage. The index finger can also be reinforced by middle finger if more pressure is required (Figs 9.17a to c).

- The friction must be across the fibres of the affected structures with sufficient amplitude of sweep to ensure that the frictional element (and not the pressure) is paramount.
- The strength (pressure) of massage depends on the stage of the lesion. In acute cases it is given extremely gently and in chronic cases with greater rigour.
- *Duration of treatment:* Varies from condition to condition ranging from 5 min to 20 min. The technique is performed at a rate of 2-3 cycles per second for 5-6 minutes in the first treatment session and increases by 2-3 minutes per session with an upper limit of 15-20 minutes.

  Some discomfort may be caused during first few minutes which can be minimised by a gentle start. **If there is continuous discomfort massage should be stopped immediately.**
- The treatment is directed on alternate days for 6 to 12 session although it depends on severity of symptoms.

Deep transverse friction massage on following conditions/structures:

1. Muscular lesions—The massage breaks down the adhesions formed by the scar tissue between individual muscle fibres.
2. Muscle tendon—The scar is eroded by the abrasive action (Fig. 9.17d).
3. Ligamentous lesions—The formation of adhesions during the period of healing is prevented by moving the ligament over the bone in limitation of its normal behaviour (Fig. 9.17e).

4. Tenosynovitis—It appears that the manual rolling of the tendon sheath to and fro against the tendon serves to smooth off the roughened surfaces.

   Uses:
   - Tendinitis/Tendentious.
   - Joint capsule adhesion.
   - Fascia or scar tissue in which the collagen has less regular organisation.
   - Trigger points.
   - Fibrosis.
   - Ligamentous injuries.

B. Circular friction

Technique—Performed with second, third and fourth digit or thumb. The tip of thumb or fingers are placed over the exact location of the affected structure and moved with the skin over affected structures in a circular direction.

To apply significant pressure the index finger can be reinforced by the middle finger. The technique is performed at a rate of 2 to 3 cycles per second for 5 to 6 minutes in the first treatment session and increases by 2 to 3 minutes per session with an upper limit of 15 to 20 min per session.

Indications:
- Tendinitis
- Fascitis
- Ligamentous injuries
- Trigger points

VIBRATION

Vibration is a soft tissue manipulation technique in which fine shaking strokes are performed over the patients body by single or double hands.

Basic technique—To perform vibration technique single or both hands are placed over the patient's body, then rhythmic, vibrating strokes are delivered from in and out, up and down manner. When technique is performed on the lateral and posterior chest wall to loosen lung secretions, strokes should be delivered during the expiratory phase of the respiration (Fig. 9.18).

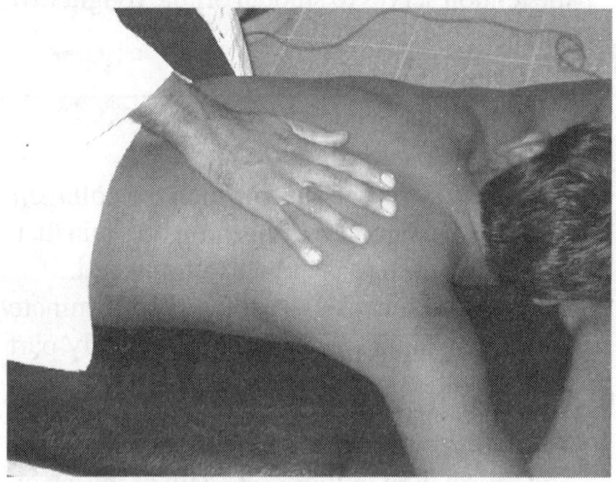

Fig. 9.18: Vibration on posterior chest wall

Indications

1. Chronic obstructive pulmonary disease (COPD)
2. Before and after operation to clear the secretion from lungs
3. To reduce chronic oedema.

Contraindication

1. Severe rib fractures
2. Hyper reflexia
3. Acute pulmonary embolism
4. Hyper tension
5. Spasticity.

SHAKING

Shaking is a soft tissue manipulation technique in which rhythmic, shaking strokes are delivered over the patient's body, by single or both hands.

Basic technique—Shaking technique can be performed with single or both hands (Fig. 9.19).

i. *On lateral or posterior chest wall*— one or both hands are placed over the patient's body (lateral or posterior chest wall, hands should be as relaxed as possible and the

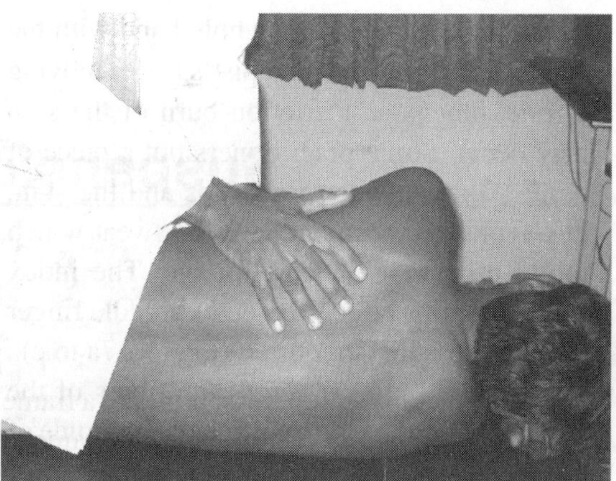

Fig. 9.19: Shaking on lateral costal chest wall with both hands

palmar surface of hand should contact the surface. A relaxed hand that produces minimal tissue compression will result in the freest tissue excursion. A fine rhythmic, shaking strokes are delivered by the hand(s) from side to side or up and down during the expiratory phase of respiration to drain the secretions from lungs.

ii. *On muscles*—One or both hands are placed on the surface wrist remain relaxed as the hand moves back and forth rhythmically, perpendicular to the long axis of the limb to produce waves of tissue motion, that moves along the long axis of the muscle.

Indications

– To loosen the adherent mucus secretion from the lungs.
– To alter the resting muscle tone through stimulating of complex proprioception reflexes.

Contraindication

– Acute muscular injury
– Muscle spasm
– Hyperreflexia
– Spasticity
– Severe rib fractures.

CHAPTER-10

Suspension Therapy

INTRODUCTION

Suspension therapy is the exercise unit or a frame which is also known as "Guthrie Smith" frame in which muscles are strengthened by using ropes, pulleys, and slings (Fig. 10.1).

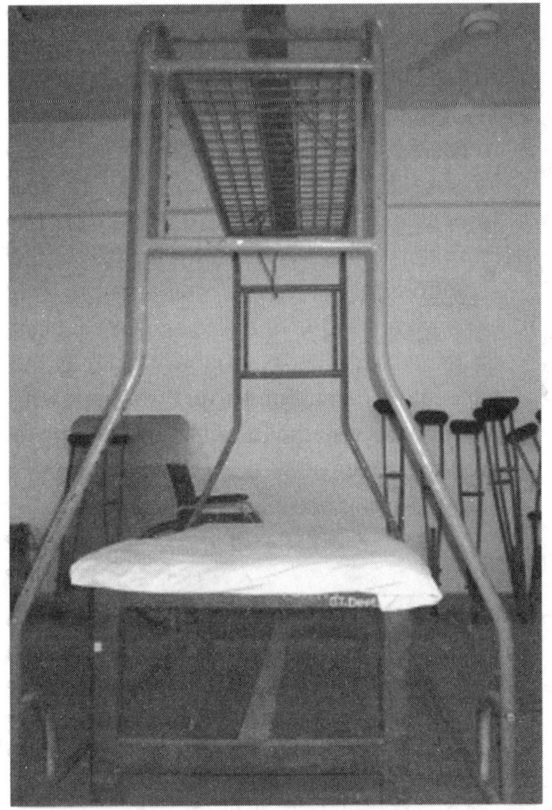

Fig. 10.1: Guthrie smith frame

The effect of suspension on movement from the resting position is similar to that of an inclined re-education board which supports the limb during movement up the incline but differs from it in that, in suspension friction is virtually eliminated.

Suspension functions as not only to eliminate frictional resistance from the moving body part but also promotes a feeling of weightlessness such as experienced by buoyancy in the hydrotherapy pool.

Uses

It is mainly used to allow the muscle to contract actively in the gravity eliminated position or against gravity and subsequently improve the muscle strength, joint range of motion and decrease the pain and muscle spasm.

Types of Suspension

Axial Fixation

The fixation point for all ropes which are attached with the slings to support the moving limb is located immediately above the centre of the moving joint. This type of suspension allows maximum movement of the joint to occur as the limb moves parallel to the floor.

Example of axial fixation—To strengthen the gluteus medius and minimum (hip abductors) the point of fixation is positioned or placed immediately above the anterior marking of the centre of the hip joint. The ropes positioned at the fixation point are attached with the slings at the knee and ankle joints (Fig. 10.2).

Vertical Fixation

The fixation point for all ropes is located over the center of gravity of the moving segment. The

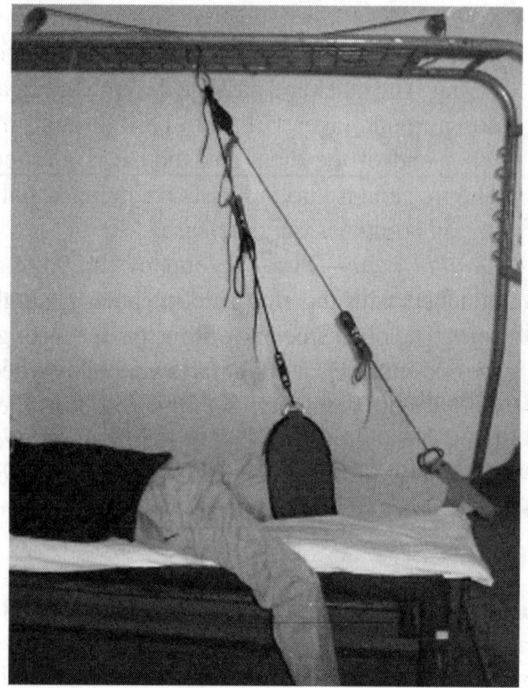

Fig. 10.2: Axial Fixation (axial line from fixation point to hip joint)

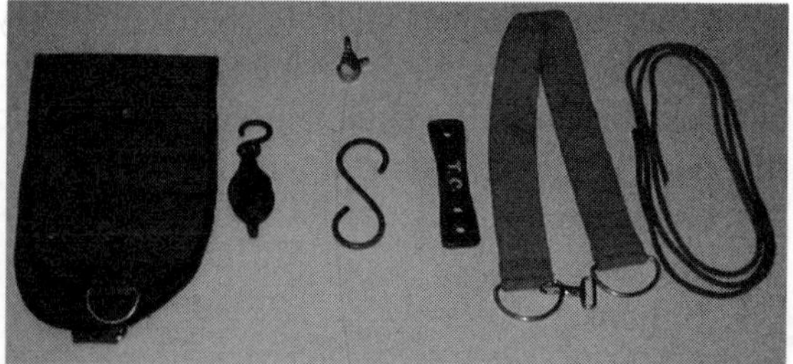

Fig. 10.3a: Devices used in suspension therapy

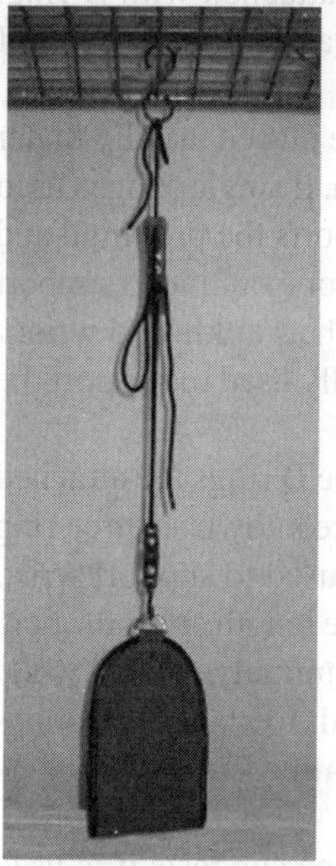

Fig. 10.3b: Pulley rope with single sling

vertical suspension is used primarily for support and usually the movement is in small range. To achieve the required outcomes (range of motion and strength) it is often combined with axial fixation.

Pendular Suspension

It is a type of suspension in which the axis of axial suspension is changed to apply resistance to the moving limb. The axis is shifted away from the axial fixation of the hip joint (e.g. patient lies in side lying the axis of the suspension is shifted posterior to the hip joint to strengthen the flexors of the hip joint).

DEVICES USED WITH SUSPENSION THERAPY (Figs 10.3a to d)

Clips and Hooks—The clips are used to attach the ropes with the slings while hooks are suspended on the suspension unit (fixed point)

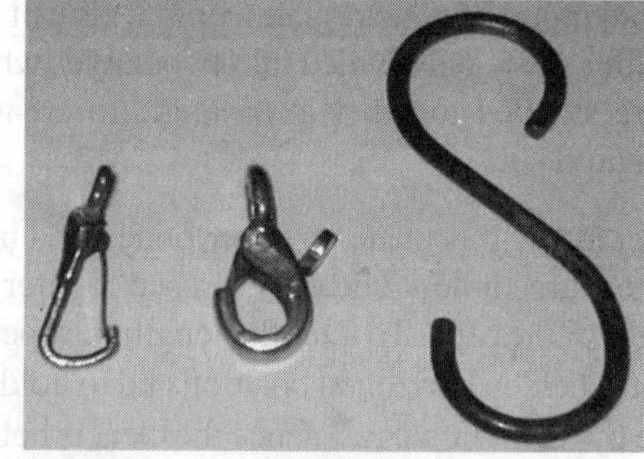

Fig. 10.3c: Carabine clip (left), Dog clip (middle), S-hook (right)

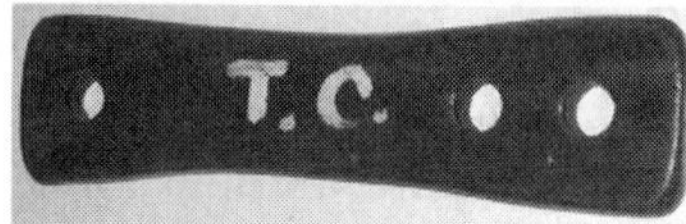

Fig. 10.3d: Cleat

with one end and other end is attached with pulley or rope, generally an 'S' shaped hook is used. The either end of 'S' hook is used according to the fixed point. Common clips and hooks are:

    Carabine clip

    Dog clip

    'S' hook.

Slings—These are used mainly to support the limbs, and the each end is attached with D ring. Slings are made up of canvas. Common types of slings are as follows:

- *Single slings*—These are placed usually under the joints to support them. If single sling is used as figure of eight it supports the proximal and distal parts of the joint (for example to support the peripheral joints such as ankle and wrist).
- *Double slings*—Generally used to support the trunk and pelvis.
- *Three ring slings*—Three D rings are attached with the sling so these are known as three ring slings. These slings are used to support wrist, hand, ankle and foot. The length around 71 cm and width 3-4 cm is commonly used. Two D rings attached at both ends to make two loopes and one D ring is at the centre which is attached to the dog clip.
- *Head sling*—As the name suggests it is used to support the head. The central part of the sling splits and divided into two halves which are stitched together at an angle to create a central slit.

The cleat—It is made up of a wooden and have two or three holes. The cleat is used to alter the length of the rope. To alter the length of rope the cleat is held in horizontal position and to hold the rope by its frictional resistance the cleat is held in oblique position.

The Supporting Ropes

The ropes can be used in three arrangements as follows:

- *Single rope*—It is tied at one end at which it is hung up. This end may tie with the 'S' hook or D ring. The other end passage through the cleat, dog clip and takes U turn to pass through the other end of the cleat and then it is knotted. The free end is knotted in such a manner that a tug on it enables quick release.
- *Double rope*—The one end of the rope is attached with the ring or clip same as single rope. The other free end of rope passes through the one end of cleat, rounds a lower pulley wheel (the wheel is attached with the dog clip) then back through the other end of the cleat over the wheel of an upper pulley. The rope then passes down again through the centre hole of the cleat where it is finally knotted.

  Double rope is used to suspend the pelvis, thorax, and both thighs.
- *Pulley rope*—The one end of the rope is attached with the dog clip or D ring at the sling. The other free end of the rope passage up over the wheel of a pulley then down through one end of the cleat and through the dog clip of the sling. Finally it takes U turn to the other end of the cleat where it is knotted. This type of rope is used for three dimensional movements of a limb i.e. abduction or adduction with flexion or extension and medial or lateral rotation.

SUSPENSION THERAPY FOR THE LOWER EXTREMITY

The Hip

- Flexion and Extension
- Type of suspension—Axial

The patient is placed in side lying, the lower leg or unaffected leg is flexed at hip and knee joints. For axial fixation, the 'S' hook is fixed immediately over the hip joint on which two ropes are suspended. The two slings at knee and ankle joint are attached with the D rings and then dog clips and ropes (Figs 10.4a to c).

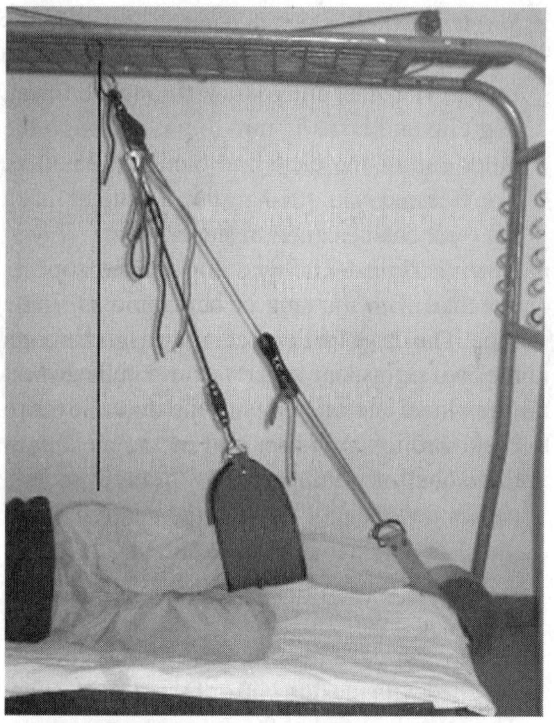

Fig. 10.4a: Hip joint in neutral position

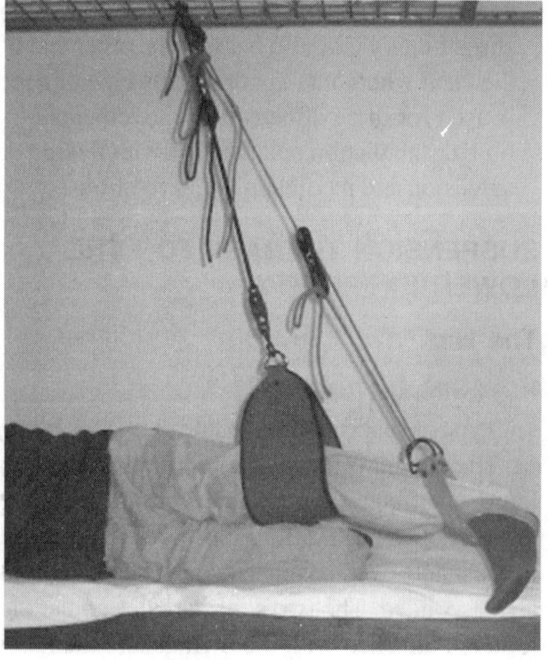

Fig. 10.4b: Hip joint in flexion

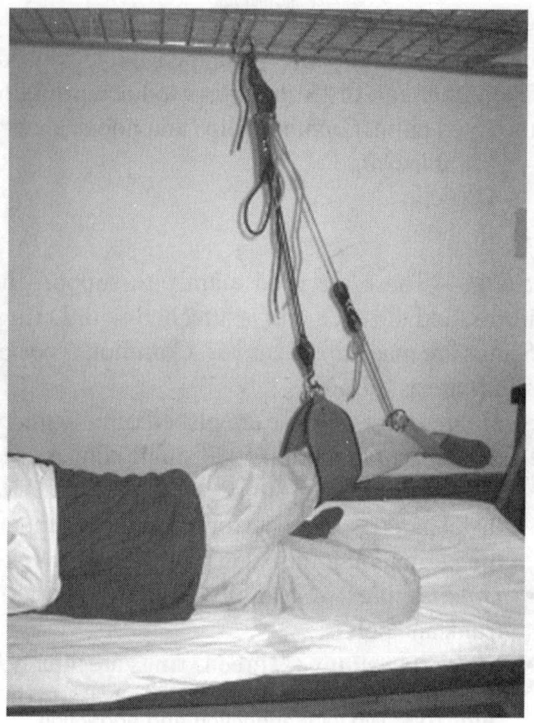

Fig. 10.4c: Hip joint in extension

The length of ropes is altered by the movements of the cleat until the limb is lifted horizontal. The patient is then allowed to move the joint in flexion or extension.

- *Abduction and Adduction*

- *Type of Suspension—Axial*

The patient is placed in supine lying the unaffected extremity is abducted at hip joint and flexed at knee joint, the foot is placed on stool. The placement of 'S' hook, ropes and slings remain same as flexion and extension (immediately over the hip joint) (Fig. 10.5).

The length of ropes is altered by the movements of the cleat until the limb is lifted horizontal. The patient is then allowed to move the hip joint in abduction and adduction.

- *Flexion and Extension*

- *Type of Suspension—Vertical*

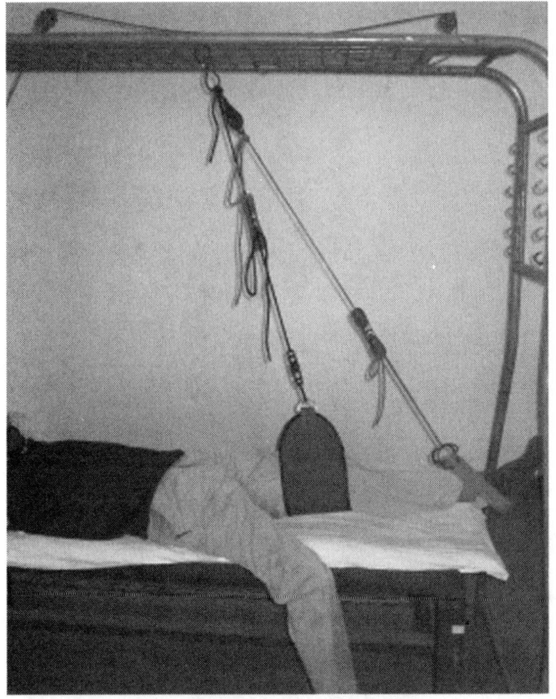

Fig. 10.5: Hip joint abduction and adduction

The patient is placed in side lying, the lower unaffected extremity is flexed at hip and knee joints.

The 'S' hook is placed immediately over the center of gravity of the thigh, and is attached with rope than the sling of the knee joint. As vertical fixation is often combined with axial fixation, therefore one 'S' is also placed just above the hip joint and is attached with rope. The three ring sling supports the foot and ankle and its centre ring is attached with the rope. The length of rope is altered by the movement of the cleat until the limb comes in horizontal line than patient is allowed to move the joint in flexion and extension.

- *Abduction and Adduction*

- *Vertical Fixation*

The patient is placed in supine position, the unaffected limb is abducted at hip and flexed at knee joint, the foot is placed on the stool and rest

of procedure remains same as above flexion and extension.

The Knee

- Flexion and Extension
- Axial Fixation

The patient is placed in sidelying, the lower most leg is flexed slightly at hip and knee joint, one or two pillows are placed between the thighs. The 'S' hook is placed immediately over the knee joint. Two slings, one single to support the lower thigh or knee and one three ring sling to support the foot and lower leg may be used. The slings are attached with the ropes, then ropes are attached with the 'S' hook (Figs 10.6a and b).

The limb is lifted up until it comes in horizontal line and then patient is allowed to move the knee joint.

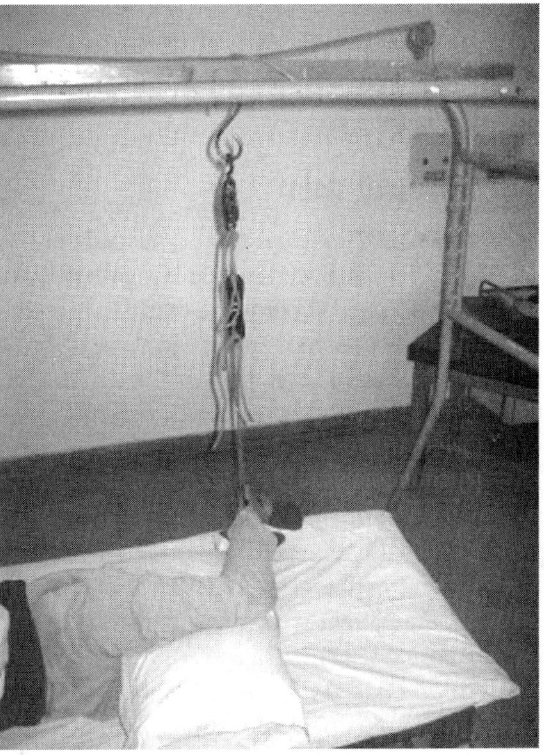

Fig. 10.6a: Knee flexion

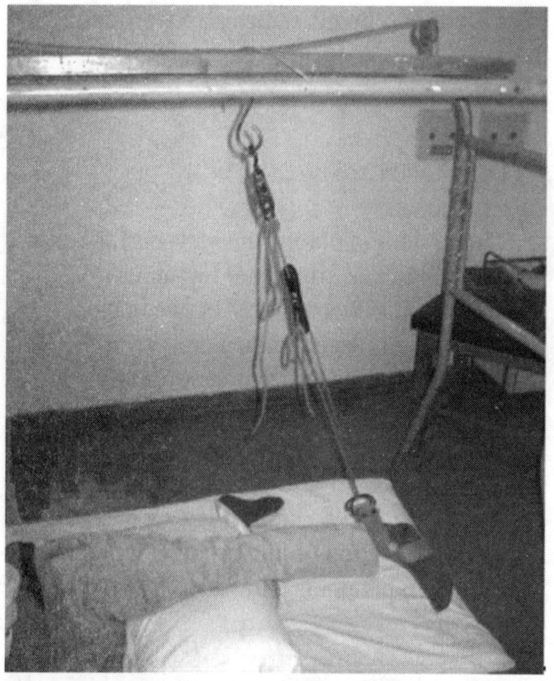

Fig. 10.6b: Knee extension

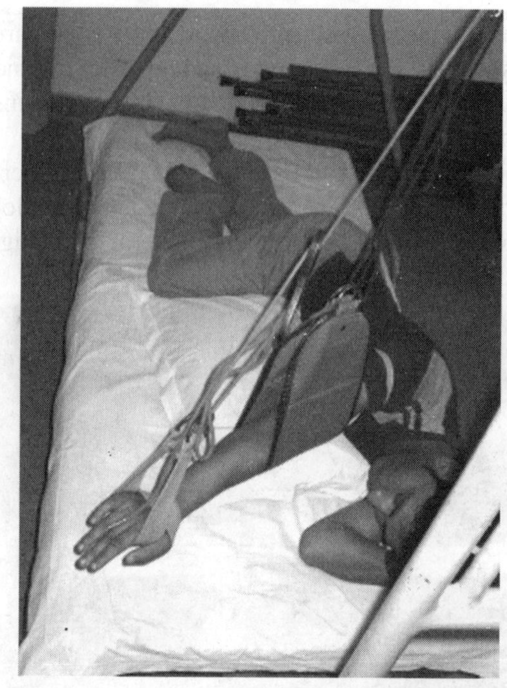

Fig. 10.7a: Shoulder flexion

SUSPENSION THERAPY FOR THE UPPER EXTREMITY

The Shoulder Joint

• *Flexion and Extension* (Axial suspension)

The patient is placed in side lying on pillows and body is turned slightly and chest rests on the pillows, so that the movement can be performed in scapular plane. The 'S' hook is fixed immediately over the glenohumeral joint. Two slings, one single sling to support the elbow and one three ring sling to support the hand and wrist, are used. The slings are then attached to the ropes. The length of ropes is changed by altering the position of cleat and as the arm comes in the plane of scapula, the patient is asked to perform flexion and extension (Figs 10.7a and b).

• *Abduction and Adduction* (Axial suspension)

The patient is placed in supine lying, one or two pillows may be placed under the scapula. The 'S' hook is placed immediately over the

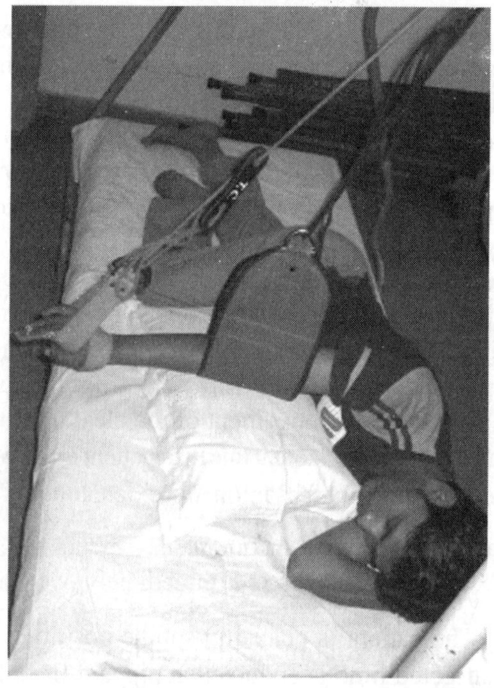

Fig. 10.7b: Shoulder extension

glenohumeral joint from which two ropes are suspended. Two slings as in shoulder flexion and extension are used. Rest of procedure remains same as above.

The abduction and adduction may also be performed in prone to see the movement of scapulo-thoracic joint as well as glenohumeral joint (Fig. 10.8).

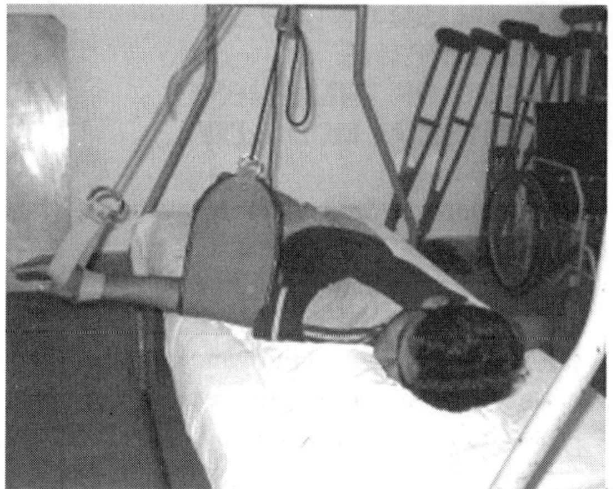

Fig. 10.8: Shoulder abduction and adduction

The Elbow Joint

- *Flexion and Extension in Lying*

- *Axial Fixation*

The position of patient remains same as in shoulder abduction and adduction. the 'S' hook is fixed at just above the elbow joint. Single sling is used to support the distal arm and three ring sling to support the wrist and hand. The flexion and extension is performed as the elbow comes horizontal in the shoulder line.

Flexion and Extension in Sitting

Patient sits on chair and shoulder is abducted at 90°. One 'S' hook is fixed immediately over the elbow joint for axial fixation. Single sling which is attached with axial fixator is used to support the distal arm and three ring sling which is attached with 'S' hook is to support the wrist and hand

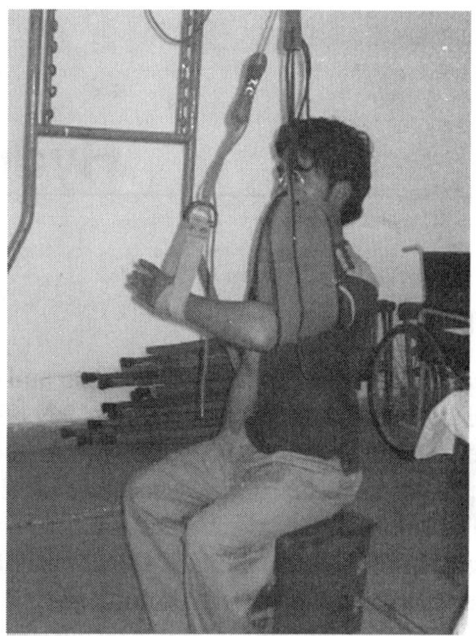

Fig. 10.9a: Elbow flexion

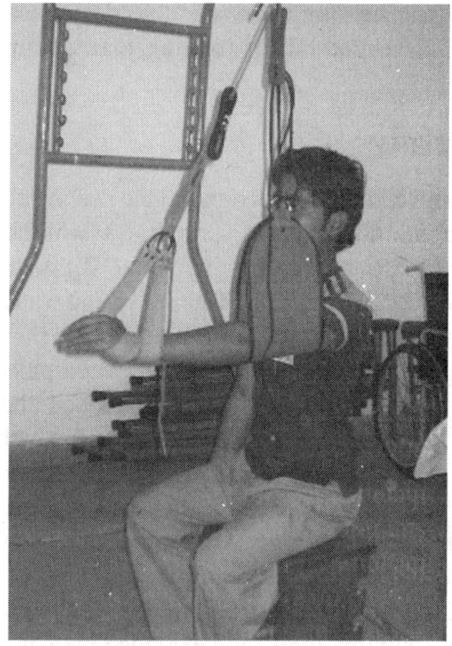

Fig. 10.9b: Elbow extension

(two ring sling may also be used). The arm is lifted up till it comes in horizontal line and then patient is instructed to move the elbow joint (Figs 10.9a and b).

CHAPTER-11

Hydrotherapy

INTRODUCTION

Hydrotherapy is the use of water to heal and ease a variety of ailments. It is the most beneficial system of resting normal functions in the body, which is employed to help balance the metabolism.

The benefits of 'water healing' or hydrotherapy have been recognised for thousands of years. In Europe, where hydrotherapy is especially popular, there are numerous health spas and health facilities for all types of 'water cures'.

Water healing is one of the oldest, cheapest and safest method for treating many common ailments.

HISTORY

Ancient civilization recognised the healing power of natural hot and cold springs. Back in the 4th century BC the greek physician Hippocrates prescribed bathing and drinking spring water for its therapeutic effects. The greeks were the first to appreciate the relationship between physical and mental well being. They developed centres near springs and rivers using them for bathing and recreation. The Romans built outstanding communal baths because they believed in the value of hot springs. The baths were centres where intellectual, recreational activities, health and hygiene were pursued. Around AD 339 some baths (built by greek, and extended by Romans) were used solely for healing purposes and treatment was indicated first of all for symptoms of rheumatic disease, paralysis, and the *effects of injuries.*

RATIONALISM OF USE OF WATER FOR THE PURPOSE OF TREATMENT AS A PHYSICAL MODALITY

Water produces several effects on the body, when the body is immersed in the water:

i. *Buoyancy*—There is the upward force in the water which works against the gravity. The force of gravity and buoyancy balance each other and minimises the muscular effort which is required during standing. The effect of Buoyancy reduces the weight and stresses on weight bearing joints.

These effects of water (reducing the muscular effort and weight on weight bearing joints during standing) help to improve the balance and coordination of paraplegic or paralytic patients, as well as painful weight bearing joints.

ii. *Hydrostatic pressure* is the pressure exerted by the water on the immersed body. According to Pascal's law, when a body part is immersed in the water a pressure is exerted equally at any level in a horizontal direction. This pressure is exerted by the water on all surfaces of the body when it is at rest at a given depth.

The hydrostatic pressure increases with depth and with the density of the fluid (the density of the water increases with the depth). Therefore standing and walking in the water is having greater importance to decrease edema. For example when the person is standing in the water, the distal part of an extremity is lowest in the water, therefore, the pressure gradient between the surface and deeper water favors reduced accumulation of fluid (edema) in distal parts of an extremity. Studies of head-out immersion in thermoneutral (35°C) suggest that there is increase in venous return from the periphery to the central body and shift of fluid from the interstital space to the capillary.

Recently full body (head-out) immersion is recommended as a treatment for "diuretic-resistant" edema in patients with cirrhosis and nephrosis.

iii. *Hydrodynamic pressure*—Kolb explains it as the pressure caused by movement of either the object or the water is called as hydrodynamic pressure. When the person walks in the water the resistance is encountered and demand is made on the walking muscles. The faster one walks, the more resistance is encountered and the more demands are made on the walking muscles.

Hydrodynamic pressure provides resistance against the movements of limbs, therefore, resistance is used to strengthen the weak muscles.

iv. *Turbulence*—It is defined as "the velocity at a given point varies erratically in magnitude and direction". The movements of the limbs in the water moves the water in circular patterns creates small whirlpools or eddy currents and turbulence. Movement through turbulent water or against the current than through calm water encounters greater resistance which requires more muscular effort.

The combined effects of buyancy and hydrostatic is helpful in balancing the body in the water. The pressure supports the body all around to an equal degree in the horizontal direction while buyancy maintains the vertical position.

PHYSIOLOGICAL EFFECTS OF TEMPERATURE

If the temperature of water which is more than the temperature of the body-causes several physiological changes in the body. The normal temperature of the skin and subcutaneous tissues is 33°C and the internal body temperature is 37°C.

The living tissues of body are affected by temperature in two fundamental ways:

1. The direct effect of temperature on body such as—increase metabolic rate, increase collagen tissue extensibility and decrease viscosity.
2. The changes occur in the body to regulate the temperature and protect the tissues from damage, such as—vasodilatation and increase in fluid exchange across capillary walls and cell membranes.

1. *The direct effect of temperature on tissues (body):*
   a. *Increase metabolic activity*—Metabolic activities are the series of chemical reactions which increase as temperature increases and decrease with a fall of temperature. An appropriate rise in temperature increases all cell activities including cell motility and synthesis and release of chemical mediators.

   Excessives temperature (above 45°C) of the body causes so much protein, cell and tissue destruction. If the temperature of body rises by 1°C it increases 13% metabolic activities.
   b. *Decrease viscosity*—The resistance to flow blood in a vessel depends directly on the viscosity of the fluid and inversely on the fourth power of the radius of the vessel.

   As the temperature rises, the blood vessels get dilated and allow the viscosity of fluid to fall down to normal level.

Collagen Tissue Changes
- Mason and Rigby (1963) found in their study that collagen melts at above 50°C temperature.

- Lehmann *et al.* (1970) have found that if the temperature of collagen rises within therapeutic range (40°C to 45°C), the extensibility of collagen increases.

  (To break the adhesion or stiffness of the joint the collagen tissues are stretched simultaneously when they are heated at therapeutic temperature).

2. *Changes occur in the body to regulate the temperature:*

   a. *Nerve Stimulation*—As the temperature of skin rises, the receptors which are situated in the skin get stimulated and send information to the higher centers (Thalamus) to control the temperature. *Counter-irritant mechanism*—Gammon and Starr (1941) stated that an afferent nerve fibres get stimulated by heat are having analgesic effect by acting on the gate control mechanism in the same way as the mechano-receptors.

   b. *Vasodilatation*—An axon reflex triggered by stimulation of polymodal receptors is an important cause of the vasodilation; in this mechanism only the peripheral branches of the afferent nerve fibres are involved. The vasodilatation which is followed by rise of temperature of the skin helps to circulate/distribute an additional heat around the body and protects the skin. The subcutaneous tissues and fat do not conduct the heat effectively to the deeper structures. Therefore dilatation of capillaries and arteriovenous conduct/distribute the heat through the blood to other parts of the body, and protect the tissues from heat.

Uses of Hydrotherapy

1. Relieves pain and muscle spasm.
2. Maintains range of motion.
3. Strenghens weakened muscles.
4. Muscle re-education.
5. Improves balance and co-ordination.
6. Facilitates weight bearing activities.
7. Reduces mental and physical tension.
8. Decreases infection.
9. Increases healing process of soft tissue injuries and musculoskeletal disorders.
10. Increases extensibility of scar tissues by relaxing the collagen fibres.

RISKS, CAUTIONS AND CONTRAINDICATIONS OF HYDROTHERAPY

Risks

Persons with impaired temperature and sensation are at the risk of scalding or frostbite at temperature extremes.

Cautions

- When conditions persistent or recurrent.
- Pregnancy.

Contraindications

- Severe peripheral and vascular disease.
- Haemorrhage.
- Skin infections such as tinea pedis and ringworm.
- Vesicular skin conditions.
- Diabetes—Avoid application of hot water to feet or legs.
- Multiple sclerosis.
- Patients with incontinence of bowel and bladder and Patients with indwelling catheters.
- High and low blood pressure.
- Diarrhoea.
- Patient with blood borne infections—HIV and HBV that have open lesions or lesions which produce exudate or blood.

TECHNIQUES OF HYDROTHERAPY

Several techniques are used to treat the different ailments.

Common Techniques

- Foot baths.
- Sitz baths, contrast sitz baths.
- Body wraps.
- Contrast baths—alternating hot and cold.
- Moist heat.
- Hubbard's tank.
- Hydrotherapy pool.

Foot Baths

Cold Foot Bath

Indications:
- Varicose veins.
- Headache.
- Low blood pressure.
- Sweaty feet.
- Contused ankle.
- Circulatory problems.

Precautions: This type of treatment is best avoided by people who suffer from:
- Cold feet, very high blood pressure.
- Irritable bladder, urinary tract infection.
- Vascular occlusion.
- Diabetes.

Technique: A small tub is used, water is filled to the level of calf muscles. The temperature of water should not exceed to 18°C. Feet are placed into cold water. The feet are taken out when the water is no longer perceived as being particularly cold.

If a large size of tub is used then patient can walk in water (walking stroke-like on a non-slip mat, placed under the water).

Warm Foot Bath

Indications: Cold feet, start of a common cold for relaxation.

Precautions: Varicose veins, lymphostasis or edema.

Technique: A small tub may be used. The tub is filled with water at body temperature (around 97°F). Feet are immersed in a foot bath (tub) and hot water is gradually added till it reached to the 103-104°F. Temperature of tub is maintained at this level and procedure should last 10-15 minutes. The procedure can be repeated daily. Although the temperature of tub and how long treatment (treatment sessions) will be given depends upon the condition which is being treated.

Sitz Baths

Indications:
- Piles and anal fissure.
- Difficulty in voiding the bladder, an irritable bladder.
- Inflammation or infection of the prostate.
- Preparation for pregnancy.

Precautions: Hemorrhoids

Technique: A small tub is filled with hot water at body temperature, patient sitz in the water then warm water is added till the temperature of water reached to 103-104°F. Treatment lasts for 15-20 minutes (Piles and fissures). Although the temperature and duration of treatment depends on conditions.

Piles and fissures require 103-104°F for 15-20 minutes per session.

Body Wraps

Wrap is primarily used as supportive measure for treating fever and local inflammation. For the purpose of treatment hot wraps and cold raps are basically used. The treatment period lasts around 45 to 60 minutes sometimes upto three hours. The patient lies on comfortable position then a linen cloth is moistered with cold or hot water. The cold water wraps are advised for pyrexia and hot packs are for respiratory diseases. They are wrapped properly around the part which is being treated. The patient is wrapped in a blanket or another cloth and should rest for 45-60 minutes.

Indications:

* *Cold wraps:*
  – Rheumatoid arthritis, Pyrexia.
* *Hot wraps:*
  – Rheumatoid arthritis, ankylosing spondylitis.
  – Osteoarthritis.
  – Bronchitis, lung disease, neuralgia.
  – Prostatitis, vaginitis, inflammation in the pelvic cavity.

Contrast Bath

Alternating application of ice and heat is referred to as contrast bath therapy. This technique is directed in the treatment of distal extremities to improve the circulation and decrease swelling or oedema.

Method: Two containers are used one is filled with cold water (10°C to 18°C), and the second with warm water (38°C to 44°C). The containers should be large enough to enable immersion of the extremity to cover at least the level of the injury.

The extremity is immersed in the warm water for 10 minutes and then in the cold water for one minute. The extremity is returned to the warm water for 4 minutes and the cycle continues for 30 minutes, with the last immersion in the warm water. Although these specific times do not have to be followed, the generally accepted hot and cold ratio is 3 : 1 or 4 : 1.

This treatment method is having lack of scientific supports. It is hypothesized that the technique is used to stimulate local circulation in the treated extremity and to a lesser extent, to increase circulation in the contralateral extremity.

Moist Heat

"Hydrocollator" Packs: The commercial hydrocollator pack or hot pack is one of the most ways to deliver superficial moist heat. Generally these packs contain hydrofolic substance, such as silica gel or betonite, encased in channeled canvas covers. The silicate gel has the capacity to absorb large quantities of water. The packs are immersed in hot water which is maintained at 80°C. When the packs are removed from the hot water they carry considerable amount of thermal energy, absorbed during immersion. After removing they are wrapped in dry terry towelling (6-8 layers) and applied directly to the part being treated for 20-30 minutes.

Hubbard Tank: Named after the engineer who designed it, is a large tank with a shape that resembles a keyhole. The tank is designed in such a way that a person can abduct his legs and arms in supine position. It is 8 feet long tank with 6 feet wider at one end and 4 feet wider near the other end. The 6 feet wider end enables a supine person to fully abduct the arms and 4 feet wider end allows the legs to abduct. At mid-side the width narrows to 36 inches enabling the therapist to get closer to the patient.

The tank can be used as hot or cold thermal modality and transfers heat primarily by convection

Hydrotherapy Pool or Unit

Different size, shape and depth of hydrotherapy unit is installed in physiotherapy department according to the number and different conditions of patient. Three types of hydrotherapy pool are commonly constructed in physiotherapy department:

1. Below ground.
2. Below ground deck level.
3. Semi-raised or raised.

Below ground pool with or without deck level is generally advised to construct.

* *The size of pool:* In the daily physiotherapy practice the size of pool should not smaller than of the 9.24 meter (30 feet) by 4.57 meter (15

feet). This size of pool provides a good working size for approximately 8 people at a time and can be used for most of rehabilitation activities.

- *The shape of pool:* Rectangular shape of pool is strongly advised.
- *Depth:* The depth varies from .84 meter to 1.42 meter.
- *Floor of pool:* Generally two type of floors are used (i) uniform (ii) stepped floor. Stepped floor is having advantages of providing several depth. To avoid fear of stepped floor, the edge of each step must be clearly marked.
- *Steps:* To lead into the pool kinner and Thomson (1983) suggested that the steps should have following dimensions:
  - i. Riser (height of step) 150 mm
  - ii. Depth 300 mm
  - iii. Width (distance between two railings) 600 mm.

The patient may also be shifted into the pool by hoists (mechanical hydrolytic and electrical).

The assistive equipments used in hydrotherapy unit:

- Handrails.
- Turbulence.
- Underwater jets.
- Floats.
- Parallel bars.
- Strolls of varying heights (railing) etc.

The Temperature of Water

The temperature of water depends upon patient to patient. Different authors have suggested different temperature for hydrotherapy unit ranging from 28°C to 37°C but the temperature of pool should be kept between 34 and 35°C in winter and 31°C and 33°C in summer.

Although temperature of water will depend upon the condition to be treated. For example if the purpose of treatment is to relax muscles (decrease spasticity) as in spastic paralysis a high temperature from 98° to 100°F is most suitable.

Ventilation

The temperature of air of the hydrotherapy unit should be slightly lower than that of the temperature of water to allow gently cooling. The temperature of air of pool is kept at 25°C.

Changing Room

The air temperature of changing room should be 4°C lower than the temperature of air and it is kept at 21°C.

Preparation of patient before treatment in pool:

- Patient should be examined thoroughly and should not have any disease which is contra-indicated for hydrotherapy.
- Treatment should not be given immediately after meals, nor is it wise to give them too long after meals.
- The patient should be asked to empty his or her bladder before immersion, since a warm bath often has a diuretic action.
- The patient should be asked to put on shorts or in the case of female patients a proper bathing suit is given.
- Before entering into to the pool patient is asked to take bath.
- Non ambulatory patients are transferred into the pool with a manually or electrically or hydroulically operated hoist.
- The ambulatory patients walk down the steps of the pool, supporting themselves with the handrails.

Oxford Scale for Muscle Power Modified for Water

This scale is used to test the power of muscles in water but it is limited to the assessment of muscles which retain little power but good range of movement (Skinner and Thomson, 1983).

The scale of muscle power of land is graded from 0 to 5 with 0 (zero) equalling no contraction, and 5 as normal. In water the scale commences at 1 and continues to 5 but it must be recognized that grade 5 in water is not normal as such function cannot be tested there (Skinner and Thomson, 1983).

The scale of muscle power modified for water:
1. Contraction with buoyancy assisting.
2. Contraction with buoyancy counter balanced and contraction against buoyancy.
3. Contraction against buoyancy at speed.
4. Contraction against buoyancy and light float.
5. Contraction against buoyancy and heavy float.

EXERCISES IN HYDROTHERAPY POOL

1. Relaxation exercises.
2. Strengthening exercises.
3. Stretching exercises.
4. Mobility, functional control and balancing exercises.
5. Gait training.

Relaxation Exercises

Indications

- Muscle spasticity
- Muscle spasm

The most important use of hydrotherapy pool is to treat the neurological and orthopaedic ailments or diseases. In neurological patient's spasticity is the hurdle for the patient which prevents the patient to perform voluntary movements. Spasticity is the sustained contraction of muscle or group of muscles which is one of the dominant clinical feature of the upper motor neuron lesion. To reduce the spasticity of muscle the temperature of water is kept around 34 to 35°C. Slow, rhythmical passive movements are given to spastic group of muscles in the water. Temporarily reduction of spasticity allows the patients to contract the antagonistic muscles and patient performs voluntary movements. If patient starts voluntary movement of the muscles antagonistic to spastic muscles, resisted movements should be started to strengthen the antagonistic muscles.

Muscle Spasm

To reduce the muscle spasm temperature is maintained at 34-35°C. The hold relax and contract relax exercises are the best exercises to reduce the muscle spasm in water.

Strengthening Exercises

These exercises are most commonly carried out in the hydrotherapy pool. The starting position of each exercise is important as on this will depend whether the movement has buoyancy either assisting, supporting, or resisting. Buoyancy resisted exercises are generally advised to strengthen the muscles. Standing, sitting, kneening and lying are the main starting positions for buoyancy resisted exercises. The therapist must explain the nature of exercise or movement and verbal commands are given to the patient to perform the movement in desired range.

Functional Controlling and Balancing Exercises

Indications

- Paralytic patients such as:
  1. Paraparesis
  2. Quadriparesis
  3. Cerebral palsy
  4. Hemiparesis.

Principles

(i) The upward force in the water which works against the gravity reduces the weight stresses on weight bearing joints in standing, (ii) The force of gravity and buoyancy balance each other and minimise the muscular efforts in standing, (iii) The water provides resistance against the movements of body and extremities—all these three functions of water make the patient stand up more comfortably in the water than in the land.

Stabilization

Therapist stabilizes the pelvis and trunk.

Exercises

Lifting one hand in the air then other hand and then both hands. Patient learns these exercise and after few sessions of treatment improves his balance and coordination. Now therapist removes the stabilization and allows the patient to stand up without support and does the exercises. Exercises such as—bending trunk forward, backward, sideward are added later on with the little stabilization of pelvis. As patient improves balance and coordination all these exercises are allowed to perform without the stabilization of pelvic and trunk.

Lower limb exercises such as place the limb forward, backward and sideward, lift it up with flexion of hip and knee and hold for count of 10. Bend the both knees then extend them.

- Every new exercise should start with the little support provided by therapist.
- The repetition of exercises should increase gradually as the balance and coordination develops.
- The temperature should be maintained at 32-33°C. If patient is having spasticity, to decrease the spasticity initially temperature may be kept at 34-35°C but during exercises temperature is kept low.
- Whole treatment session should not last for more than 15 to 20 minutes.

Gait Training Exercises

When patient starts standing up without the support of therapist, then patient is instructed to place the one leg forward, emphasis should be given to place the heel first then foot. Patient shifts the weight of body on the forward placed limb and then contralateral limb is allowed to swing.

Railing may also be used in the pool for support. All support (railing and therapist) may be removed as patient starts walking independently.

CHAPTER-12

Relaxation

INTRODUCTION

Relaxation may be defined as a state in which muscles are free from tension or are in the normal physiological state. This is accompanied by a feeling of diminished consciousness of the external world, drowsiness, passivity, and focussing of the attention on feeling of internal well being *(Rosa 1976)*.

Muscle Tension

Normal muscle is never free from tension even when the person is in fully relaxed state. This tension in the muscle is known as physiological muscle tone/tension which is provided or maintained by the intrafusal muscle fibres.

There are two types of muscle fibres in a muscle, extrafusal and intrafusal. Contraction of extrafusal muscle fibre causes increase in muscle tension or tone, and movement occurs at the joint. The tone of extrafusal fibres decreases when they come to the original position or resting state from contracted state. Therefore the tone of extrafusal fibres keeps changing. The tone of intrafusal muscle fibres do not change during the voluntary movement and at the resting state. These are the muscle fibres whose tone remains constant during the activities and at the rest and their fibres provide firmness and maintain the muscle tone/tension during resting state.

There are some abnormal conditions in which the tone of muscle fibres increases as the response of trauma, stress, head injury, stretching of muscle fibres and pathological diseases.

Response of the Body to Stress (Mental and Physical)

Stress is a physiological response to a stimulus, some stress is necessary for an individual to function normally, a mild level emotional arousal produces alertness and the nervous system needs a certain amount of stimulation to function properly. To the some extent stress is an appropriate and necessary response that enables individual to cope with life's challenge *(Kim Jones and Barker)*.

Schmidth (1988) states that arousal may be considered as a neutral state that it represents the amount of effort that an individual applies to an action. Stress and motivation represents different types of arousal and are considered to have directional components—stress usually being considered as negative and motivation as positive.

Mental attitudes such as fear, anger and excitement give rise to a general increase in muscular tension which serves a useful purpose by preparing the muscles, for rapid or forceful action *(Dina Gardiner)*.

Different authors have different opinions on stress but when stress exists or persists for longer period of time it changes the behaviour of the person and there is alteration in posture, which causes tension in the muscles. Such types of individuals must need relaxation exercises to remove the mental as well as physical stress.

Pathological Tension in the Muscles

Every muscle of the body is supplied by the nerve via spinal reflex arc, spinal cord to higher motor centres (brain). Lesion in the pathway above the nucleus of anterior horn cell of spinal cord causes sustained contraction of muscle fibres (spasticity or rigidity). Local relaxation techniques such as passive movements are used to decrease the spasticity temporarily. Inflammatory, degenerative conditions of the joint, local trauma or injury to the muscles can cause protective muscle guarding (increase tension in the muscles). Hold-relax/contract-relax (for decreasing muscle spasm) can be used to reduce the increased tension of the muscles.

Indications of Relaxation

1. Acute neuro-muscular hypertension.
2. Chronic neuro-muscular hypertension.
3. States of fatigue and exhaustion.
4. States of debility.
5. Various pre-operative and post-operative conditions.
6. Sleep disturbance.
7. Spasticity.
8. Arthritis and related conditions.
9. Bell's palsy.
10. Burns (Post burn contractures).
11. High blood pressure.

Physiological Manifestation of Relaxation

1. Decrease heart rate.
2. Decrease blood pressure.
3. Decrease O_2 consumption.
4. Decrease CO_2 production and excretion.
5. Decrease blood cholesterol and lactate.
6. Decrease tension of muscle.
7. Decrease metabolic rate.
8. Peripheral vasodilatation.
9. Increased peripheral temperature.
10. Pupil constriction.
11. Increase saliva output.
12. Increase digestive activity.
13. Increase urine output.

Relaxation Techniques

- Local relaxation
  - Therapeutic massage *(Discussed in Ch-9)*
  - Passive movements *(Discussed in Ch-3)*
  - Muscle energy techniques *(Discussed in Ch-20)*
  - Hold relax
  - Contract relax
- General relaxation
  - Contrast method
  - Reciprocal inhibition.
- Other relaxation techniques.

Local Relaxation

Therapeutic massage: It is the technique which is used to improve the blood circulation and remove waste products from the target area. After performing few strokes of massage, the extensibility of the scar tissue/spasmodic muscle increase and patient feels relaxed.

Passive movements: More beneficial to stretch the muscles, when it is performed on particular muscle or group of muscles followed by *hold relax* or *contract relax.*

- **Hold relax:**

  Indications: This technique is especially used when the patient has no movement because of pain or muscle spasm.

  Briefly it consists of different episodes of isometric contraction.

  The muscle or group of muscles which are said to be antagonistic to the movement do not allow the joint to move because of spasm. To overcome this problem the resistance is applied to a muscle or group of muscles which are in tension. Then patient is asked to hold this position unless therapist responses 'Relax' or 'let go'. The position is maintained for 6 sec or when the therapist feels that the patient has reached the limit of his potential contraction, he grasps the limb firmly, but comfortably and at the same time tells the patient to 'relax' or 'let go' and allow a period of time at least as long as or perhaps longer than the time to build up the maximum contraction.

For example: Spasm in the shoulder adductors can prevent the shoulder abduction. Resistance is applied to adductors of the shoulder joint.

Spasm in the shoulder adductors can prevent the abduction of the shoulder joint, because when patient attempts to abduct the shoulder joint stretching in the spasmed muscles (adductors) causes pain and thus limits to further abduction.

The procedure is as follows:

1. Therapist grasps the elbow joint firmly but comfortably (Fig. 12.1a).
2. The shoulder is abducted slightly by the therapist passively, till the patient complains no pain.
3. Patient is instructed to adduct the shoulder joint (try to take it to the chest) against the resistance.
4. Therapist maintains the position (isometric contraction) while patient is engaged with contraction of adductors for six seconds and then instructs the patient to relax the adductors (relaxation period should be more than six seconds) (Fig. 12.1b).

• Therapist again abducts the shoulder joint and finds increase in the range of motion and abducts the shoulder joint till the patient complains no pain, and the position where patient complains pain, grasps the arm at the elbow joint firmly but comfortably and repeats the same steps from 1 to 4. The several isometric contractions can be held at different positions as the range increases (Fig. 12.1c).

• The main purpose of this exercise is to relax the muscles and increase the range of motion.

• **Contract relax:**

Indications: This technique may be used when a patient has a small range of motion and then

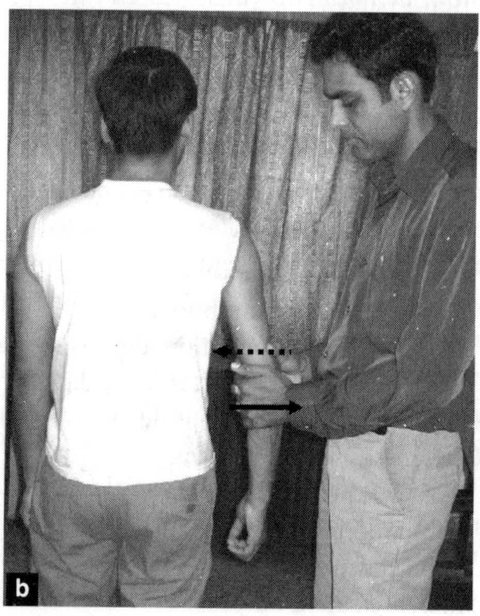

Figs 12.1a and b: Hold relax—(a) Initial position and (b) Dotted arrow shows contraction of shoulder adductors and black arrow shows resistance by therapist

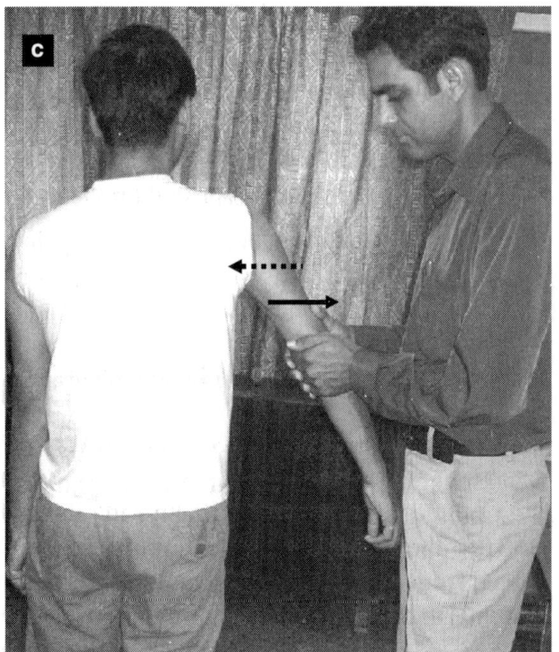

Fig. 12.1c: Hold relax (next angle for hold relax) dotted arrow shows contraction of shoulder adductors and black arrow shows esistance by therapist

is prevented from moving further by the spasm of the muscles which are antagonist to the movement.

Technique: The patient is asked to move the joint in painfree range, this range may also be achieved by passive movement the therapist grasps the limb and patient is then asked to make a small strongly isotonic resisted contraction back to the original position. At the end of the movement the part is grasped firmly, but comfortably and the patient is told to relax. The period of relaxation should be of adequate time (Figs 12.2a and b).

The next painfree range should again be attempted with passively or actively. Gain in ROM may be found and a further contract relax should now allow a small range movement which should not return the limb to the original position, but should be less than the total range (the arm

should not return each time to the original position in which the limb was resting).

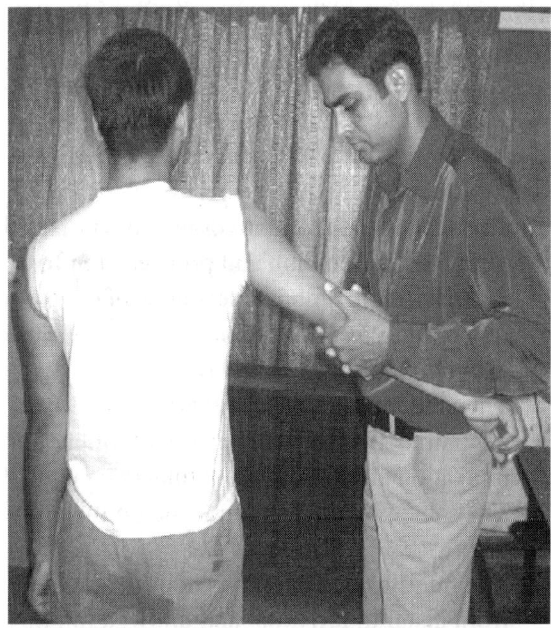

Fig. 12.2a: Contract relax (initial position)

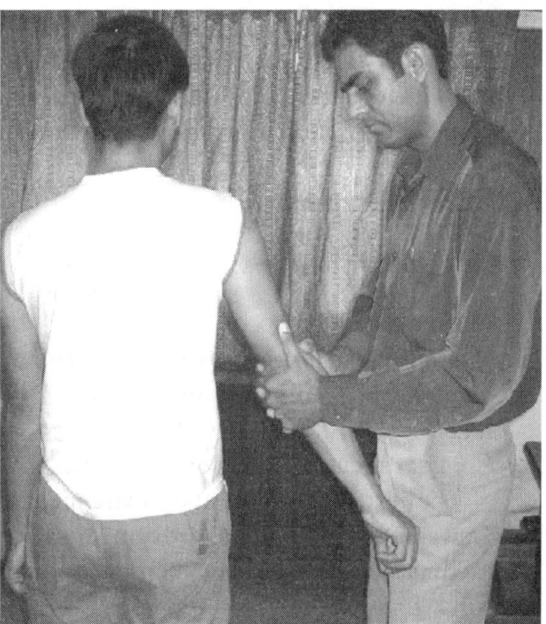

Fig. 12.2b: Contract relax (end position)

General Relaxation

Contrast method (Progressive muscular relaxation):
The physiology of this method is that a strong contraction of a muscle is followed by an equal relaxation of the same muscle (Excitation = Inhibition).

Technique

1. The relaxation technique commences from the distal part of the limb and proceeds to proximal part of the limb in a sequence of contraction of muscles. The therapist commands the patient to contract and relax.
2. Then the muscles of whole limb are allowed to contract from distal to proximal and go for relaxation phase from proximal to distal.
3. The same procedure is repeated on the other limb.
4. The muscles of both limbs contract together from distal to proximal and allowed to relax from proximal to distal.
5. Procedure is repeated in the same manner on upper extremity.
6. Both upper and lower extremity muscles are allowed to contract from distal to proximal and asked for relaxation from proximal to distal.

For Upper Extremity

Command the patient to:

i. Make a fist and relax.
ii. Contract wrist flexors or extensors and relax.
iii. Contract elbow flexors or extensors and relax.
iv. Contract shoulder adductors and relax.

   The muscles of whole upper extremity are contracted simultaneously from distal to proximal and allowed to relax from proximal to distal.

Command is given as follows:

i. Make a fist, contract wrist flexors or extensors, elbow flexors, and shoulder adductors.
ii. Relax the shoulder muscles, elbow flexors, wrist extensors or flexors and hand muscles.

The same procedure is repeated on the other upper extremity.

For Lower Extremity

Command the patient to:

i. Contract dorsiflexors or plantar flexors and relax.
ii. Contract the quadriceps or hamstrings and relax.
iii. Contract the gluteus maximum and relax.

Then the muscles of the extremity are contracted from distal to proximal and relaxed from proximal to distal.

Command the patient as follows:

1. Contract the plantar flexors or extensors.
2. Contract the knee extensors.
3. Contract the hip extensors.
4. Relax the hip extensors.
5. Relax the knee extensors.
6. Relax the plantar flexors or extensors.

The same procedure is repeated on the other lower extremity.

The technique is then performed on both L/L and U/L muscles simultaneously.

Command the patient as follows:

1. Contract the dorsiflexors or plantar flexors, hand and wrists muscle.
2. Contract the knee extensor and elbow flexors.
3. Contract the hip extensor and shoulder adductors.
4. Relax the hip extensor and shoulder adductors.
5. Relax the knee extensor and elbow flexors.
6. Relax the dorsi or plantar flexors, hand and wrist muscles.

Reciprocal Inhibition Method

The physiology of this method is when agonist muscles are contracted, their antagonistic muscles get relaxed reciprocally and equally to the contraction of the agonist muscles.

> Contraction of agonist muscles = Reciprocal inhibition or a relaxation of antagonistic muscles

In some circumstances it would be difficult to allow the contraction of the tensed or spasmed muscles because of pain. It is therefore in order to decrease the muscle spasm the agonistic muscles are allowed to contract isometrically to cause relaxation of the tensed muscles.

> Agonistic muscle(s) = opposite to tensed muscles

For example: To relieve the tension of elbow flexors, the extensors of elbow are allowed to contract. The contraction of elbow extensors causes relaxation of the elbow flexors reciprocally and equally to the contraction of the agonist muscles (extensors).

Other Relaxation Techniques

1. *Mental imagery:* is a relaxation method in which the patient is instructed to imagine himself in a place associated with pleasant memories. For example—sitting at beach, greenry, lake etc. Such images allow the patient to enter a relaxed state. This type of relaxation is useful in reducing stress or anxiety related tensions.
2. *Autogenic training:* In this technique patient learns to monitor level of body functions such as blood pressure, muscle tension etc. (usually by using biofeed back equipment) and then try to relax himself by do not letting bodily functions crossing the limits.
3. *Yoga and Meditation:* These are two very commonly used techniques in Indian system. In India these techniques have been used since centuries. Now scientific proof has also been made this two techniques are also very useful in making mental as well as physical relaxation.
4. *Music therapy:* Research studies have shown that appropriate music causes calming and relaxing effect. Soft, low noise, instrumental music can be used for relaxation.
5. *Pet therapy:* It has been seen people who have pets are less suffered from hypertension and other cardiac problems. Having pet is a good option to reduce day to day stress.
6. *Creational activities:* such as dance swimming etc. can also be utilized as mode of relaxation.
7. *Social modality:* Family and friends should be valued as they are like shock absorber of once daily life event which helps in maintain mental relaxation.

CHAPTER-13

Stretching Techniques of Soft Tissue Structures

INTRODUCTION

In activities of daily life we do activities like combing, dressing, putting on shoes etc. without facing any problem because our soft tissue structures (muscles, ligaments, tendons, joint capsule, fascia and skin) provide full range of motion in the joint to perform the activities. Soft tissue structures can tighten due to internal or external injuries which restrict the joint motion, and is known as hypomobility of the joint, that causes difficulty to perform the activities. Therefore the tighten structure requires stretching to bring it into normal functional capacity.

Some professionals like gymnasts, dancers move their joint beyond the normal range of motion as their soft tissue structures allow the joint to move beyond the range of motion. This is because these professionals start stretching of the soft tissue structures from childhood which is required for their profession. It is known as hypermobility.

Stretching is a general term used to describe any therapeutic technique which is used to increase the flexibility of soft tissue structures and subsequently improve ROM by elongating or lengthening the soft tissue structures which are responsible for hypomobility of the joint.

Effects of Prolonged Immobilization on Muscles

Immobilization of a muscle for a prolonged period of time deteriorates the contractile properties and decreases the number of myofibril, resulting in atrophy of muscle. The atrophy of the muscle depends on the duration of immobilization which ranges from as little as few days to a week. The longer the duration of immobilization, the greater the atrophy of muscle fibres.

Lieber suggests the most important factors in atrophy from decreased use to be the degree of immobilization (i.e. number of joints crossed), followed by the degree of change to normal function. For example when knee and ankle joints are immobilized the calf muscles atrophy occurs greatly. The atrophy of the soleus (static postural muscle) is greater than the gastroenemius (relatively lower use muscle).

Atrophy occurs quickly and more extensively in tonic (slow–twitch) postural muscle fibres than in phasic (fast–twitch) fibres.

The atrophy of muscles also greatly depends on the positions of muscles during immobilization.

The muscle which is immobilized in a lengthened position shows less atrophy than when immobilized in the shortened position.

The profound effects of immobilization on muscles are—decreased cross sectional size of muscle fibres, deterioration in the motor unit recruitment and absorption of sarcomeres. All these above changes lead to decrease in the overall length of the muscle fibres which is the most important cause of the hypomobility of the joint.

Purpose of Muscle Stretching

The main purpose of stretching is to lengthen the muscle and increase the extensibility of the muscle fibres subsequently increasing the range of motion, by breaking up adhesions which are formed between the muscle fibres.

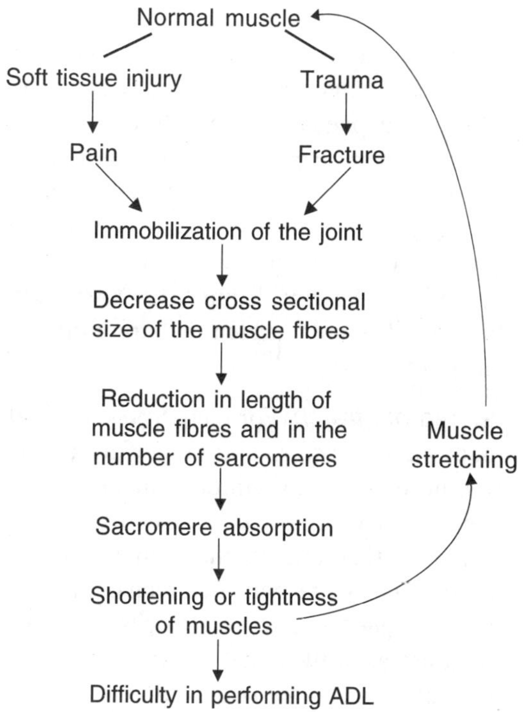

Effects of Prestretching

It has been demonstrated in amphibians and in humans that a muscle performs most work when it shortens immediately after being stretched in the concentrically contracted state than when it shortens from a state of isometric contraction (Cuillo and Zarins, 1983). This phenomenon entirely depends on the elastic energy stored in the series elastic component during stretching and energy stored in the contractile component.

Neurological Changes in the Muscle to Stretch

As the muscle is stretched the sensory receptors (composed of intrafusal muscle fibres) located in the central portions of muscle spindle called the nuclear bag and nuclear chain, get stimulated and sends information about the intensity, velocity and duration of stretch to the CNS via primary (type Ia) and secondary (type II) afferent fibres. These fibres facilitate the contraction of intrafusal and extrafusal fibres respectively and inhibit the contraction of antagonistic muscle fibres. Excessive tension caused by active contraction or passive stretching is controlled by Golgi Tendon Organ (GTO), situated near the musculotendinous junctions which wraps around the ends of the extrafusal fibres of a muscle, and transmits afferent stimuli via type IIb fibres. Therefore, golgi tendon organ is a protective mechanism that inhibits tension in the muscle, and the effect is known as autogenic inhibition.

The Physiological Changes in the Muscles to Stretch

The deep sensory receptors, muscle spindles and Golgi tendon organs (GTO) located in muscle are the responsible structures for the changes due to the stretch.

The muscle spindles are of two types, intrafusal and extrafusal, located in a parallel arrangement to the muscle fibres. The intrafusal muscle spindles are further classified into primary and secondary, which respond to changes in the rate of muscle lengthening and actual amount of lengthening.

The GTO is located at both the proximal and distal tendinous insertion of the muscle. These organs get excited during the muscle stretching and function to monitor tension within the muscle. They also are considered to provide a protective mechanism by preventing structural damage to the muscle in situations of extreme tension. Therefore when the parallel and series elastic components get stretched during active contraction or passive stretching, tension is produced within the muscle, the GTO prevents the passive over stretch of contractile elements, thereby lessening the danger of muscle injury.

Indications of Stretching

- Muscle spasm/guarding
- Muscle tightness.

- Muscle spasticity.
- Muscle rigidity.
- Skin and fascia tightness/post burn stiffness.
- Joint capsule tightness/stiffness.
- Fibrous ankylosis of a joint.

Contraindications of Stretching

- Acute inflammation
- Muscle strain
- Ligament sprain
- Muscle rupture
- Muscle tear
- Fracture
- Subluxation or dislocation of the joint
- Ligament injuries (acute)
- Myositis ossificans (common in elbow joint)
- Within three weeks of tendon transfer
- Following the surgical reconstruction of ligaments or tendons (wait for at least three weeks or green signal from surgeon).
- Severe osteoporotic changes (osteomyelitis, tuberculosis) stretching may be done with extra precaution.

Difference between Muscle Tightness and Muscle Contracture

See Table 13.1 for the difference.

Parameters of Soft Tissue Stretching

1. Intensity of stretch.
2. Speed of stretch.
3. Frequency of stretch.
4. Duration of stretch.

1. *Intensity of stretch:* The force which is applied to stretch the soft tissue structures is termed as the intensity of stretch. The intensity of stretch depends on the soft tissue structure which is being stretched. For example—to stretch the trapezius muscles, less intensity of stretch is required than the gastrocnemius. The general rule of intensity to stretch the soft tissues is to be low. Though an experienced therapist can only stretch the structure with an optimal intensity.

2. *Speed of stretch:* For the purpose of treatment the exercise should be performed in a smooth, slow and rhythmical manner. High speed of exercise can cause increase in stretch reflex and further tension in the muscles which prevents stretching of muscles. A slow speed stretch is also easier for the therapist as well as patient to control and prevent injury to the stretched structures. In addition a slow speed stretch affects the viscoelastic properties of connective tissues making them more compliant.

3. *Frequency of stretch:* It refers to the number of sessions per day or week. The frequency of stretch depends on the severity and underlying cause of tightness of the soft tissue structures. Structures immobilized for long period of time, often require more frequent treatment twice or thrice daily while those structures immobilized for short period of time require only twice or thrice a week.

Table 13.1: Difference between muscle tightness and muscle contracture

Muscle tightness	*Muscle contracture*
Muscle tightness includes decrease in the length of the muscle and its fibres and in the number of sarcomeres in series within myofibrils as the result of sarcomere absorption. If this state of muscle can be lengthened or elongated by passive stretching is termed the muscle tightness.	Muscle contracture also includes the same physiological changes like muscle tightness but these changes occur severely and decreases the length of muscle permanently which causes deformity at the joint and cannot be stretched by passive stretching and require surgical intervention to elongate the muscle fibre/length.

4. *Duration of stretch:* The structures are held at the stretched position for a sufficient period of time with an optimal intensity to lengthen the soft tissue structures, so that they do not go back to the original position. The length of time a stretch must be held to facilitate muscle flexibility remains a point of disagreement among clinicians. Lantell G *et al.* state that a low load prolonged stretch (15-30 sec) is more effective and that there does not appear to be any advantage to hold the stretch longer than 15-30 seconds.

STRETCHING TECHNIQUES

It has already been mentioned that stretching means elongation of soft tissue structures (especially muscles). To achieve good results it is very essential to apply superficial heat *modalities* or *active contraction* (hold relax, contract relax exercise) to warm up the muscle prior to stretching. The studies show that if hold relax or contract relax is followed by stretching it provides very good results. Though the selection of stretching exercise entirely depends on the tightened structure which is being treated. There are some common stretching techniques which are frequently used to stretch the soft tissue structures.

1. Passive stretching—static and intermittent.
2. Active stretching (Self or auto stretching).
3. Isometric stretching.
4. Dynamic stretching.
5. PNF stretching.
6. Ballistic stretching.

1. Passive Stretching

It is the manual technique which is performed by the hands of therapist. The tightened structure are stretched beyond the available range of motion but within anatomical range in a smooth, rhythmic manner. The stretched structures are held at the end of range for some time and released gradually to the normal position, which *consists one cycle of stretching.* Several cyclic stretchings are performed per treatment session. This whole procedure is known as intermittent passive steching of soft tissue structures.

Generally at the end of range the skeletal structures are held for 5-10 seconds in intermittent passive stretching. But if the tightened structure is held for more than 15 seconds to minutes then it is called as *static passive stretching.* The stretched structure can also be held from almost an hour to several days or weeks by using the mechanical device.

Agonist Contraction with Passive Stretching

It is a type of passive stretching where patient is asked to contract the agonist muscle during stretching, the tightened muscle will reflexively relax and make muscle elongation easier. Some clinician refers to it as a term of neuromuscular inhibition. While patient contracts the muscle, the therapist passively stretches the antagonistic muscles.

2. Active Stretching (Self or Auto Stretching)

It is a type of stretching in which a person/patient is taught the stretching exercise which is performed by himself or herself without assistance from therapist.

Technique: Patient should choose a comfortable position as therapist advises. During the stretching the patient is taught to relax the antagonistic muscles and allow the tightened muscle to stretch fully.

For example: To stretch the hamstrings and extensors of lower back the patient is advised long sitting position and allowed to touch the toes with the fingers without flexing the knees.

3. Isometric Stretching

It is a type of static stretching of muscles which does not allow the joint to move during the contraction. Resistance is applied against active contraction of the muscle or group of the muscles in the isometric manner. The use of isometric stretching is one of the fastest ways to increase flexibility and is much more effective than either passive stretching or active stretching alone. Isometric stretching also helps to develop strength in the "tensed" muscles (which helps to develop static-active flexibility), and seems to decrease amount of pain usually associated with stretching.

4. Dynamic Stretching

It involves moving parts of body and gradually increasing reach, speed of movement, or both. Dynamic stretching consists of controlled leg and arm movements performed within the limit of range of motion. It improves dynamic flexibility and is quite useful as part of warm up for active or aerobic workout.

The dynamic stretching differs from ballistic as ballistic stretching forces a part of the body beyond its range of motion in a bouncy or jerky manner.

5. PNF Stretching

It is not really a type of stretching but is a technique of combining passive stretching and isometric stretching in order to achieve maximum static flexibility.

In PNF stretching, first muscle(s) is allowed to contract isometrically against the resistance then is stretched passively.

Hold relax—The most common PNF stretching technique is the hold relax. In first step of this technique muscle is taken passively in extreme stretched position and then patient is allowed to contract the stretched muscle isometrically for 6-10 seconds. In the last step patient is instructed to relax the muscle gradually, and as the patient relaxes the muscle, therapist stretches the muscle passively into extreme range in the smooth and controlled manner. Several repetitions may be performed.

Isometric contraction → Passive stretching
= Hold relax stretching

Hold-relax-contract—It is the type of PNF stretching which involves isometric contraction of the both agonist and antagonistic muscles. In the first step of this technique an agonist muscles are allowed to contract isometrically against resistance for 6-10 seconds, then patient is asked to relax the agonist muscle. In the last step of the repetition as the patient relaxes the agonist muscle, the therapist commands the patient to contract antagonistic muscles against the hand. The position of hand should be in such a manner that it applies resistance to agonist and antagonistic muscles without changing its position.

Isometric contraction of agonist →
Isometric contraction of antagonistic =
Hold-relax-contract stretching

Hold-relax-swing—This technique actually involves the use of dynamic or ballistic stretching in conjunction with isometric stretches. The technique is very risky and is successfully used only by the most advanced athletes and dancers that have managed to achieve a high level of control over their muscle stretch reflex.

The hold relax swing constitutes, initially isometric contraction for 6-10 seconds which is immediately followed by ballistic stretching.

Isometric contraction → Ballistic stretching
= Hold-relax-swing

Hold-relax-bounce—This is the PNF stretching technique which is very similar to hold relax swing and involves the use of dynamic or ballistic stretching in conjunction with static and isometric stretching.

Both hold relax swing and hold relax bounce stretching techniques should not be performed by any person or even professional athlete under guidance of therapist as the techniques involve quick stretching. Both techniques have the greatest potential for rapid flexibility gains, but only performed by people who have a sufficiently high level of control of the stretch reflex of the muscles which are being stretched.

6. Ballistic Stretching

An athlete uses the momentum of a moving body or limb in an attempt to force it beyond its normal range of motion. This is stretching or "warming up", by bouncing into a stretched position, using the stretched muscle as a spring which pulls out of the stretched position (e.g. bouncing down repeatedly to touch the toes).

It is a type of passive stretching which involves quick, forceful, intermittent stretch with high speed and high intensity stretching of muscles and tissues through bobbing or bouncing movements involving active antagonist muscle contractions. This type of stretch can elongate muscles and subsequently increase range of motion in young, healthy patients but is associated with higher rates of microtrauma and injury. Ballistic stretching is generally viewed as inappropriate for the sedentary or elderly patients with musculoskeletal pathology or chronic condition (Fig. 13.1).

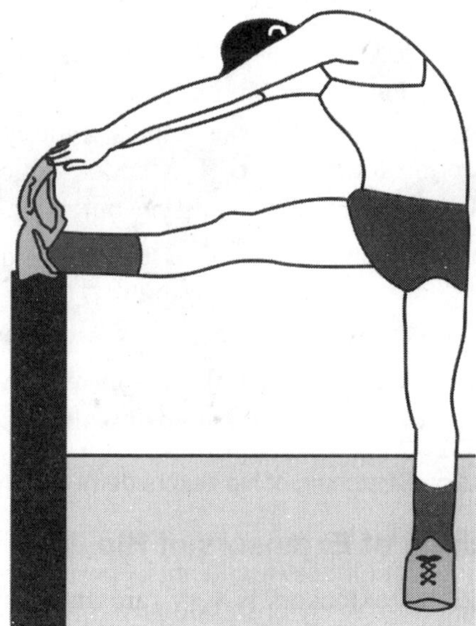

Fig. 13.1: Ballistic stretching

Technique of Passive Stretching

Position of patient and therapist should be comfortable. Every stretching exercise requires suitable and comfortable position of the patient. Though the position varies from athletes to the persons with health related problems. Athletes do not require specific position to stretch the muscle because of flexibility.

For example: A 65-year-old lower back problem patient requires long sitting position to stretch the hamstrings as well as back extensors to avoid further strain of the lower back region which already has pathological changes. While a 25 year athlete can stretch the muscle in standing by touching the toes with fingers.

The proximal part of the joint should be stabilised but the muscle which is being stretched should not be stabilised or compressed by straps. The patient is asked to relax the muscle and not allow the tightened muscle to contract. The therapist holds the distal part of the limb where the muscle attaches, and moves the limb slowly, smoothly and in a controlled manner through the available range of motion.

After a repetition of intermittent passive stretching the structure may come back to the original position (*tightened position*) so number of repetitions are performed, so that the structure should not go back to the tightened position and remain stretched even after releasing the intensity of stretch.

In mechanical static stretching where tightened muscles are held in elongated position for an hour to days, after releasing the intensity the structures do not tightened the position and remain stretched.

- Stabilisation of the proximal part of the joint can be achieved by body weight.
- The intensity, speed duration and frequency of stretching exercise should be optimal and do not cause any injury to the other structures as well.

- *Emphasis* should be given on warming up the tissues with mild heat or gentle rhythm activities, such as cycling, push ups, jogging etc.
- The movement should be carried out in the anatomical range of motion to avoid any injury to other structures.

LOWER EXTREMITY MUSCLES STRETCHING

Iliacus and Psoas Major

Position of patient-prone:

A. *In prone lying*—Therapist places one hand on the gluteal region to stabilise the pelvis, other hand grasps the knee joint. The leg of the patient rests on the therapist chest and shoulder. The therapist extends the hip joint by pulling the knee joint upward. The joint is kept in stretched position for brief time of period then the stretched muscles released to the starting position, several repetitions are performed to bring the effect of plasticity (Fig. 13.2a).

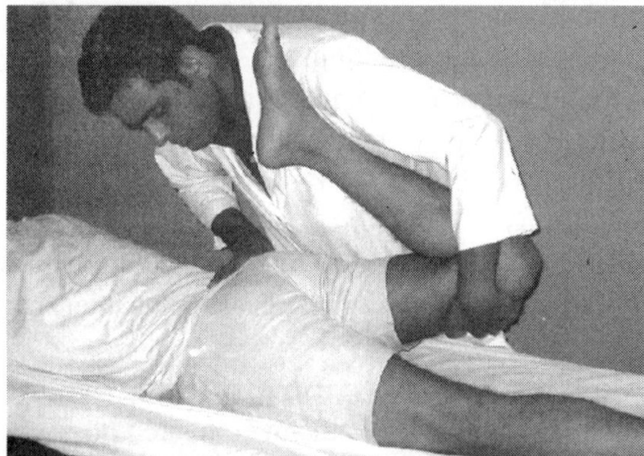

Fig. 13.2a: Stretching of hip flexors (right side)—Prone (Complete flexion of knee joint should be avoided as it causes tension in the quadriceps and restricts hip extension)

The tightness of iliopsoas is very common in patient with below and above knee amputations where limb is kept in flexed (elevated) position to avoid oedema.

B. *In supine lying*—Therapist stands at side of patient places upper hand on the flexed knee and lower hand on the left knee. While stabilizing the right knee joint, therapist flexes the left hip and knee joints (Fig. 13.2b).

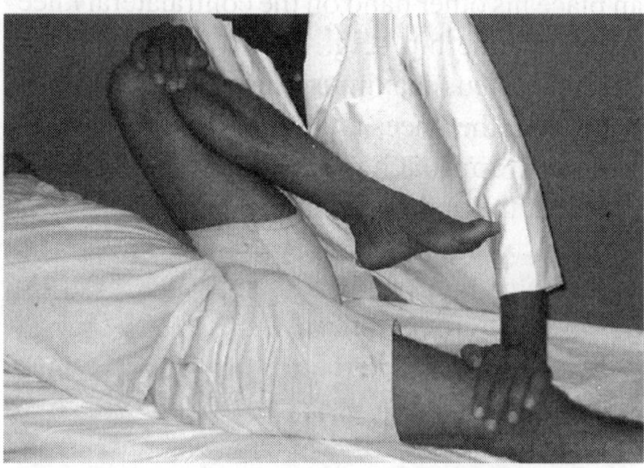

Fig. 13.2b: Stretching of hip flexors (right side)–Supine

C. *In side lying*—Therapist stands behind the patient, places one hand on the pelvis to stabilize the trunk and grasps the knee joint with other hand. The leg of patient rests on the therapist forearm. While stabilizing the pelvis and trunk therapist extends the hip joint. Avoid excessive lumbar lordosis during stretching (Fig. 13.2c).

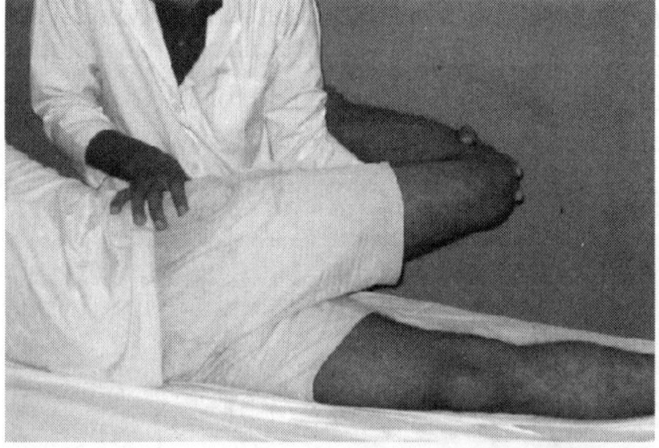

Fig. 13.2c: Stretching of hip flexors (left)–Side lying

Stretching of Extensors of Hip Joint

Tightness of extensors is very rare and easy to stretch.

Position of patient-supine—The therapist stands at the same side of the affected muscle. The knee is grasped with the hand and hip is flexed at the point where restriction starts, stretches the muscle by bringing the knee joint to the chest, the therapist can place his other hand on the contralateral knee to stabilize the hip (Fig. 13.3a). To stretch the bilateral gluteus maximus muscles the therapist grasps both the knees and brings to the chest, as the knees approaches chest overpressure is applied at the end range.

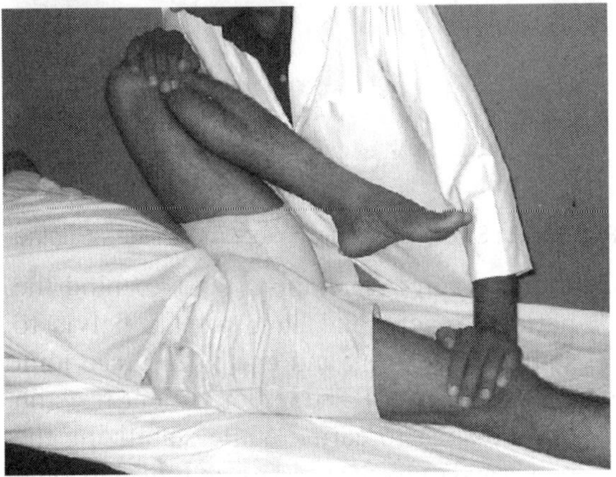

Fig. 13.3a: Stretching of left hip extensors

Self stretching of the gluteus maximus (knee to chest)—Position of patient-supine lying. The patient flexes the hip and knee joint gradually toward the chest where it is held for 10-15 seconds and then released (Fig. 13.3b).

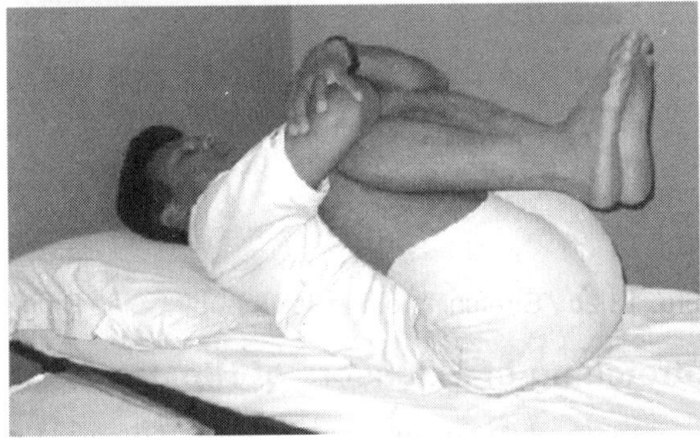

Fig. 13.3b: Self stretching of hip extensors

Adductors of Hip Joint

Position of patient-supine—The unaffected leg may be stabilised with the straps or hand of therapist stabilizes the pelvis. The therapist grasps the knee joint of affected side (the calf muscles rest on the forearm of the therapist) while maintaining the above position he abducts or pulls the leg toward his body (Fig. 13.4a).

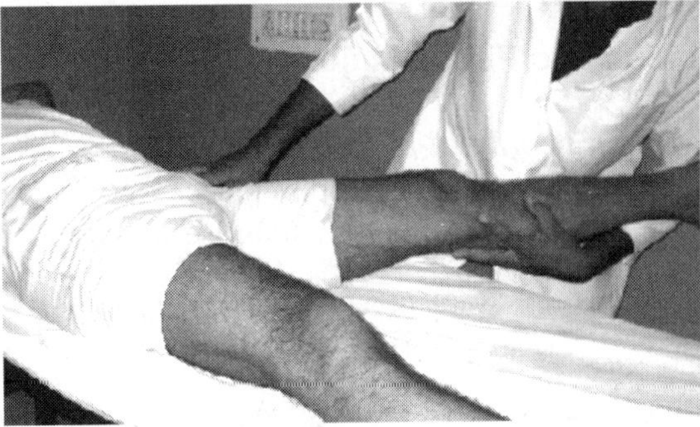

Fig. 13.4a: Stretching of hip adductors (left side)

Self stretching of adductors of hip joint—Position of patient-standing in front of wall. The patient holds the grill or wall with both hands and gradually slides the both feet apart (abduction) (Fig. 13.4b).

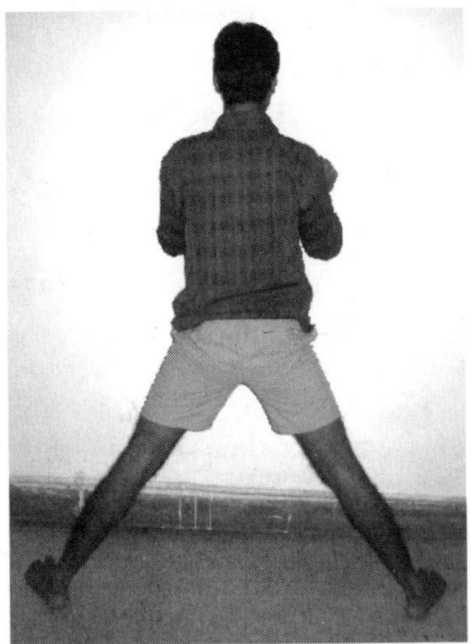

Fig. 13.4b: Adductors self stretching—Legs slide apart from each other while holding the grill or wall

Alternative technique of adductors: The patient is placed in supine position with flexion of the both knees. Therapist stands at the feet of the patient, and grasps the both knees the patient is instructed to relax the muscles and then knees are taken apart, this position is used to stretch the adductors of cerebral palsy children.

Hamstring Muscles

Position of patient-supine—The contralateral leg is stabilised with the straps to avoid lifting or therapist places one hand on the thigh of patient to stabilise the limb, the posterior aspect of the lower leg of the affected side is placed over the shoulder of therapist. While keeping the knee joint straight, the therapist flexes the hip joint by using the body motion (Fig. 13.5a).

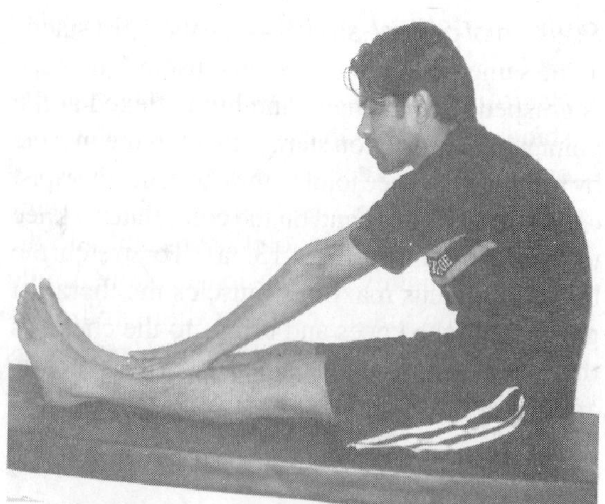

Fig. 13.5b: Self stretching of hamstrings (bilateral)

gets tightened when the plaster of paris applied to immobilise the fractured bone (Fig. 13.6a).

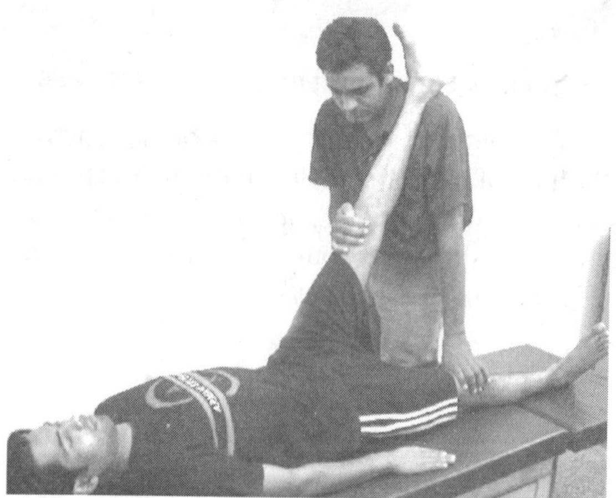

Fig. 13.5a: Stretching of left hamstrings

An autostretching or self stretching of Hamstring muscles: Position of patient— Long sitting on plinth or couch. The patient flexes the trunk and touches the knee joints with hands. The hands are further slide down the leg with the flexion of hip joint. During sliding of hands down the leg patient should emphasis more on hip flexion rather than trunk flexion (Fig. 13.5b).

Rectus Femoris

It is a prime mover of the knee extention which

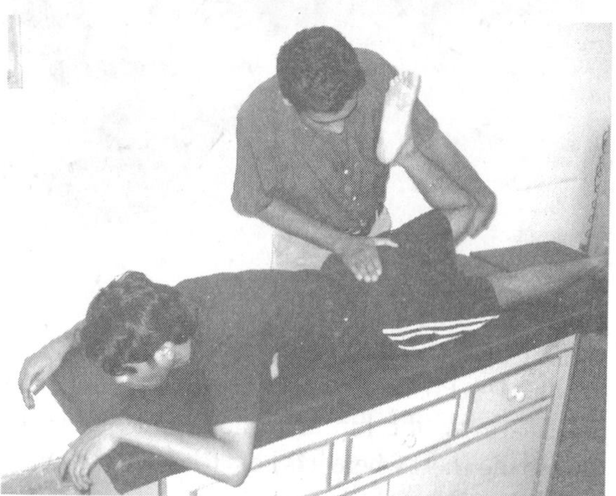

Fig. 13.6a: Stretching of right rectus femoris

Position of patient prone—The knee joint is flexed beyond 90°. Therapist places one hand on the gluteal region to stabilize the pelvis and stop lumbar lordosis, another hand is used to grasp the knee joint, the anterior aspect of leg rests on the forearm of the therapist, which helps to keep the knee joint flexed. While maintaining the above position the therapist extends the hip joint. Discomfort in the anterior thigh indicates stretching of rectus femoris.

Self stretching of quadriceps muscles (Rectus femoris):

- *Position of patient-standing*—The patient stands in front of table and holds the table with one hand. The knee (stretching side) is flexed and the ankle joint is grasped with the same side of hand. The hip joint is brought into the neutral or slightly in extension position. A mild pain in the anterior of the thigh indicates stretching of the quadriceps muscles or rectus femoris (Fig. 13.6b).

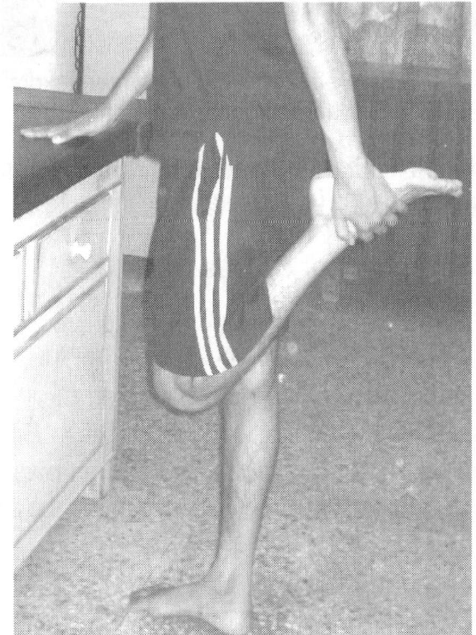

Fig. 13.6b: Self stretching of left rectus femoris

Tensor Fascia Latae (TFL)

The position of patient—Side lying, the affected limb is placed upper, the lower most (contra-lateral) limb is flexed at hip and knee joints to widen the base of support. The therapist places one hand over the iliac crest to stabilise the pelvis and other hand grasps the knee joint, the leg of the patient rests on the forearm of the therapist. While maintaining above position the therapist adducts, extends and rotates the limb laterally to stretch the TFL and holds the stretched TFL for some time then releases. Several repetition are

performed (Fig. 13.7a). The procedure is also known as reverse Ober test.

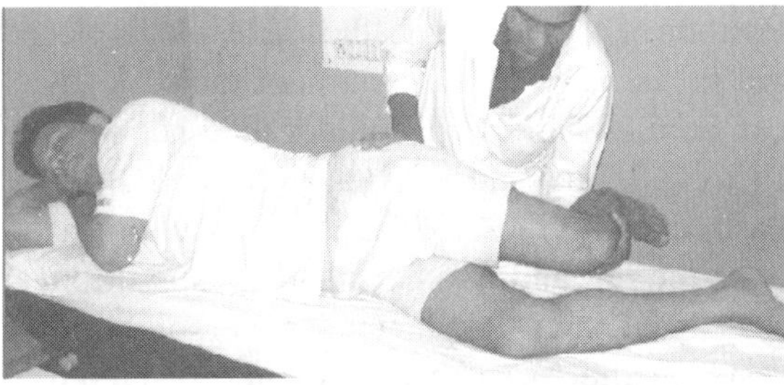

Fig. 13.7a: Stretching of tensor fascia latae

Self stretching of TFL—(Figs 13.7b and 137c).

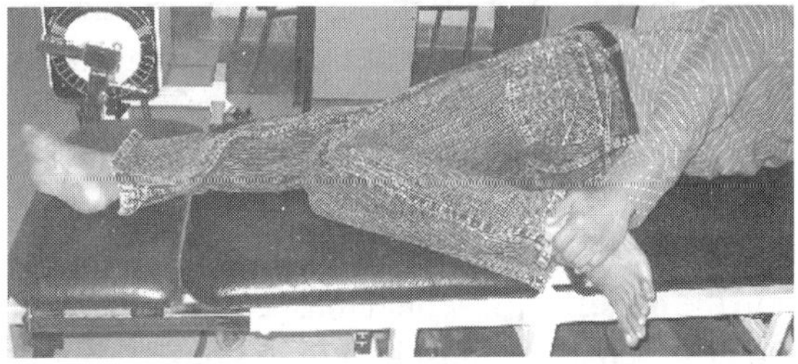

Fig. 13.7b: Self stretching of TFL—Position of patient sidelying, the involved leg is flexed at knee joint and patient grasps the ankle joint. In the next procedure the hip joint is extended and is allowed to adduct, It is known as self-Ober stretch

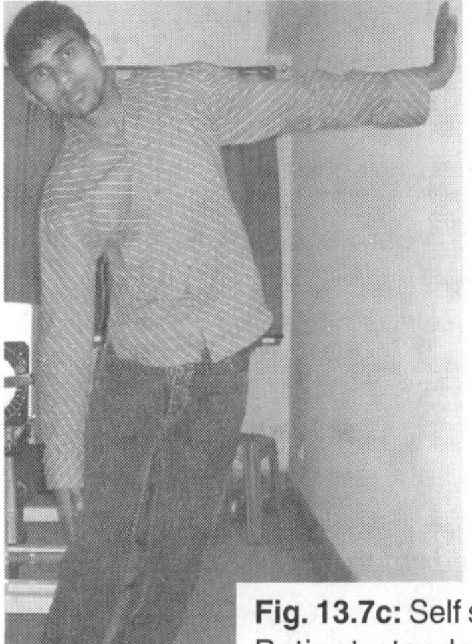

Fig. 13.7c: Self stretching of TFL— Patient stands and places one hand on the wall, the involved leg is closer to the wall. Patient slides the contralateral hand down the leg

Tendo Achilles (Gastrocnemius and Soleus)

Position of patient-supine, the ankle joint is placed out of the edge of the treatment table. A towel can be rolled and placed under the knee joint to flex it slightly and facilitate the stretching of gastrocnemius muscle. Therapist places one hand over the leg and another hand grasps the heel (calcaneal part), the plantar aspect (sole) of foot rests on the forearm of the therapist. While maintaining the above position the therapist pulls the heel into the dorsiflexion, at the same time forearm also transmits the force to the plantar aspect into the dorsiflexion, the force must be able to cause movement at the ankle joint to get effective results. Sometimes movement occurs at the metatarsal joints only and therapist understands that TA is getting stretched. To stretch the TA the heel should be held firmly and pulled into the dorsiflexion which must cause tension in the gastrocnemius muscle (Fig. 13.8a).

Self Stretching of Gastrosoleus Muscle

The patient stands in front of wall. The forefoot of involved leg is placed on the wooden board/ stool and a stretch is applied by delivering the weight of body. A mild pain may be felt in the posterior leg during extreme dorsiflexion of the

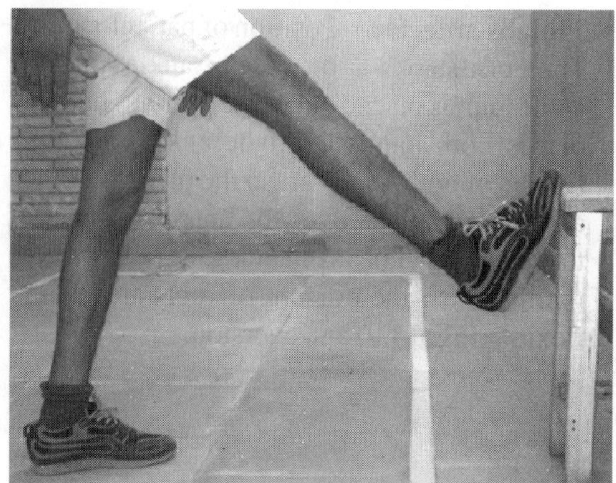

Fig. 13.8b: Self stretching of plantar flexors (Gastrosoleus)

ankle joint which indicates stretching of gastrocnemius muscle (Fig. 13.8b).

Self Stretching of Soleus Muscle

In standing position the forefoot is placed on the stool (this places the knee joint at 90° flexion). The patient may place both hands on the flexed knee joint. A stretch is applied by shifting the body weight on the flexed knee joint. Patient may feel mild pain during extreme dorsiflexion of the ankle joint (Fig. 13.8c).

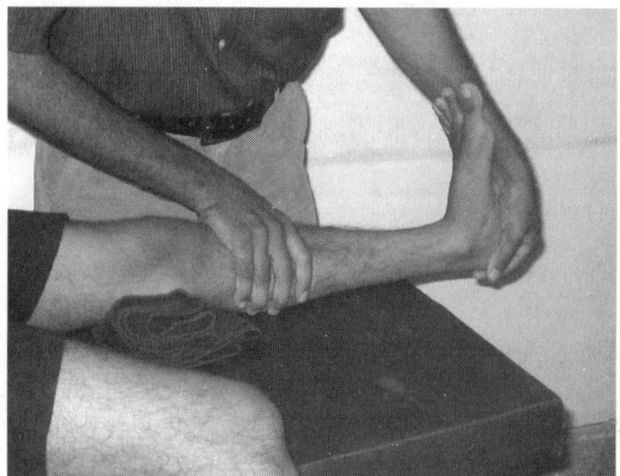

Fig. 13.8a: Stretching of plantar flexors (Gastrosoleus)

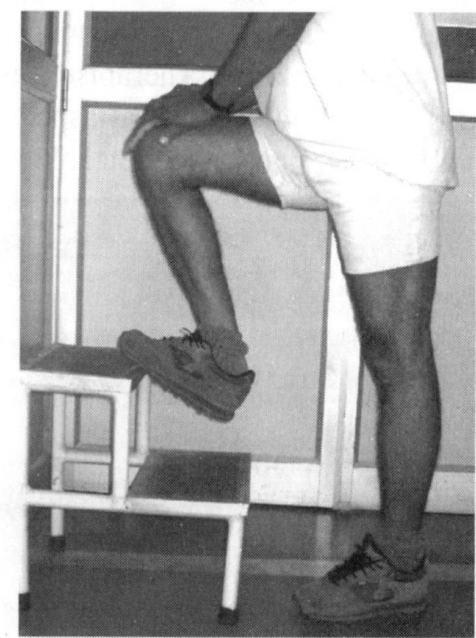

Fig. 13.8c: Self stretching of plantar flexors (Soleus)

- **Tibialis anterior**—Position of patient-supine. Therapist stands at the side of ankle joint the ankle joint is placed out of the plinth. Therapist places both hands over the ankle joint, the fingers of both hands grasp the plantar surface and thumbs place over the anterior aspect of the forefoot. While maintaining the position both thumbs push the dorsum of foot into plantar flexion (Fig. 13.9) and eversion.

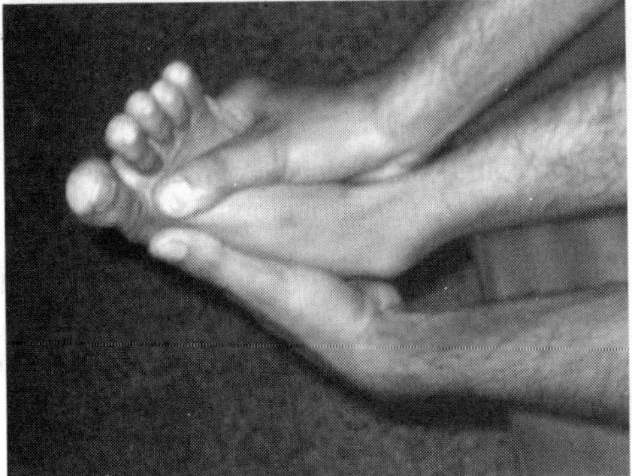

Fig. 13.9: Stretching of tibialis anterior

- **Peroneus Longus and Brevis**—The position of patient and placement of hands remain almost same as tibialis anterior. Therapist pushes the dorsum of foot into plantar flexion and inversion (Fig. 13.10).
- **Tibialis posterior**—Position of patient remain same as tibialis anterior. Therapist grasps the heel with one hand and lateral aspect of the forefoot by other hand, and then ankle joint is

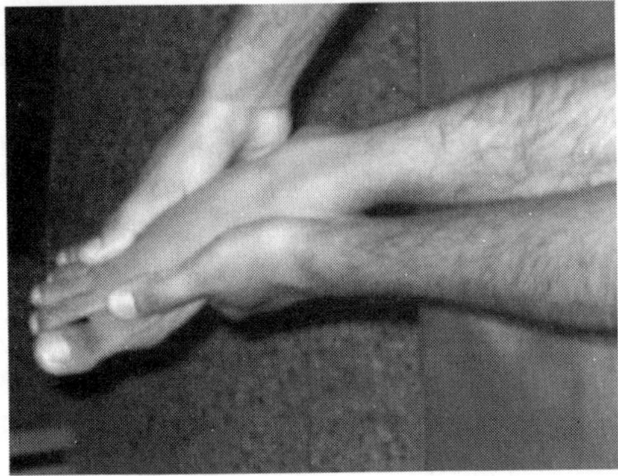

Fig. 13.10: Stretching of peroneus Longus and Brevis

pushed into the dorsiflexion and eversion (Fig. 13.11).

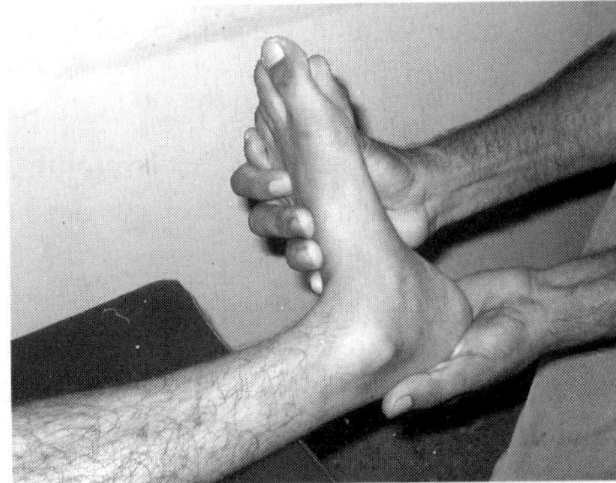

Fig. 13.11: Stretching of tibialis posterior

- **Peroneus tertius**—Position same as tibialis anterior. Therapist pushes the foot into dorsiflexion and inversion.
- **Extensor Hallusis Longus, extensor digitorus Longus and Brevis**—Position of patient remains same, the therapist places fingers over the toes and then pushes the toes into plantar flexion. An individual muscle may be stretched by pushing the individual toe (Fig. 13.12). Plantar flexion of ankle adds more stretching.

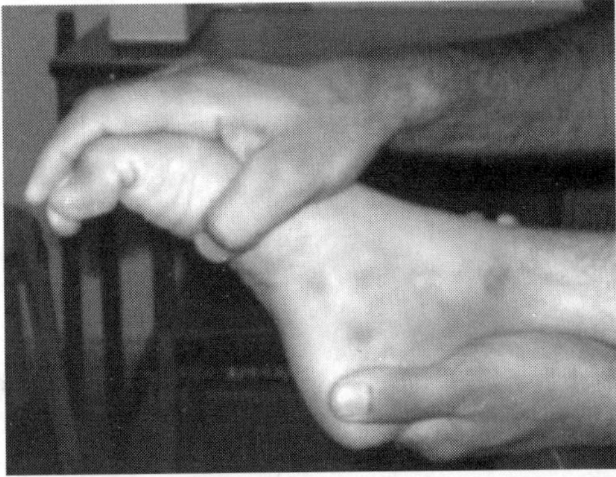

Fig. 13.12: Stretching of extensor Hallucis Longus, extensor digitorum Longus and Brevis

- **Flexor Hallucis Longus, flexor digitorum Longus and Brevis**—The patient is placed in prone or supine position with the ankle joint out of the treatment plinth. The therapist places fingers over the plantar aspect of the toes. The ankle joint may remain at neutral position or slightly in dorsiflexion and the therapist pushes the toes into extension (Fig. 13.13a). The procedure is also used to stretch the plantar fascia.

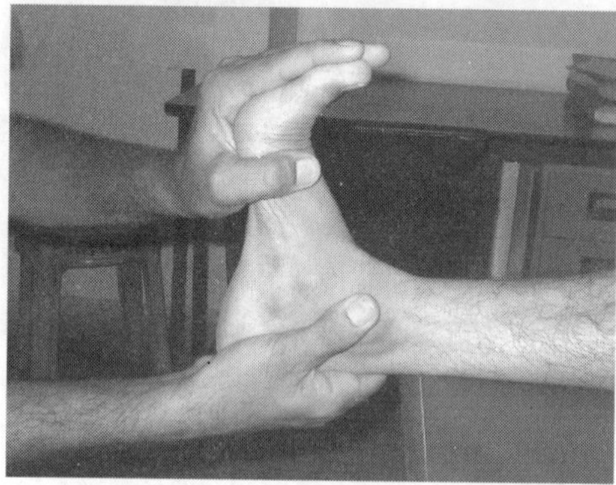

Fig. 13.13a: Stretching of Flexor Hallucis Longus, Flexor Digitorum Longus and Brevis

- **Plantar fascia**—The maneuver is the same as the flexors of the toes but can also be performed in many ways. The patient sits with the knee flexed and heel rests on the plinth. The patient places the fingers over the plantar surface of the toes and gently extends toward the leg (dorsiflexion of the MTP joints (Fig. 13.13b).

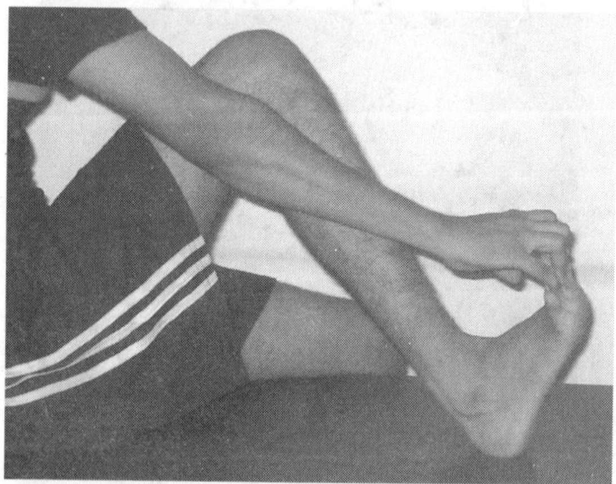

Fig. 13.13b: Stretching of plantar fascia

- *Alternative plantar fascia stretch*—The patient kneels with the toes curled up under the feet (MTP joint extension). The buttocks are

gently lowered to the heels until a mild tension is felt in the bottom of the feet. Patient holds the position for 30 seconds and repeats five times per session (Fig. 13.13c).

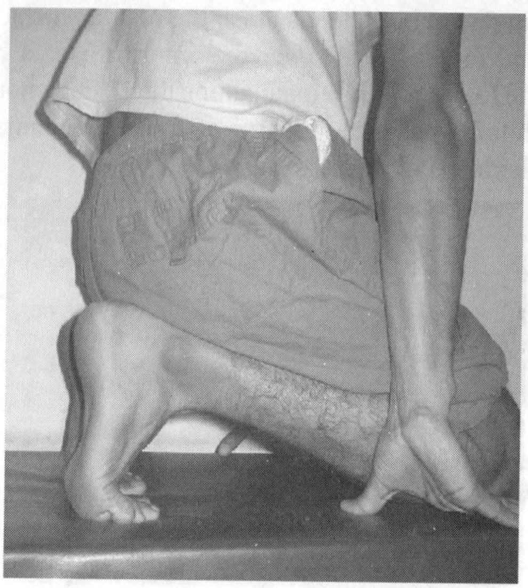

Fig. 13.13c: Plantar fascia stretching—Patient kneels with the toes curled up under the feet

- **Piriformis muscle**—The patient is positioned in sidelying with the treatment side uppermost. The hip joint is flexed at 90° with adduction and medial rotation. The lower limb may be flexed at hip and knee joints (Fig. 13.14a).

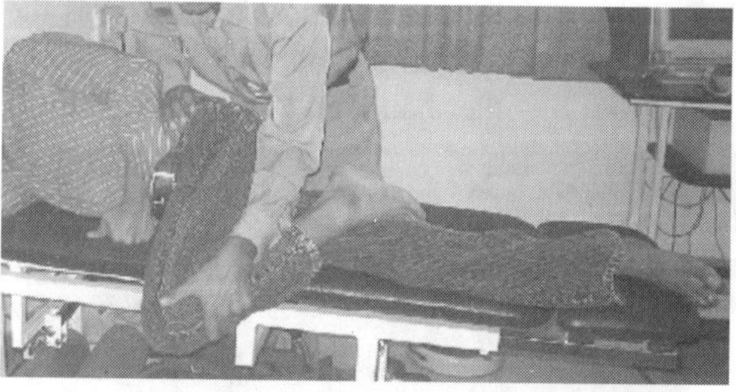

Fig. 13.14a: Stretching of piriformis

- Alternative position for piriformis muscle—The patient lies in supine position, therapist stands at the side of the patient and places one hand over the pelvis to stabilize it. The therapist grasps the knee joint and flexes it with the hip joint, as the hip approaches 90° of flexion therapist adducts it with medial rotation (Fig. 13.14b).

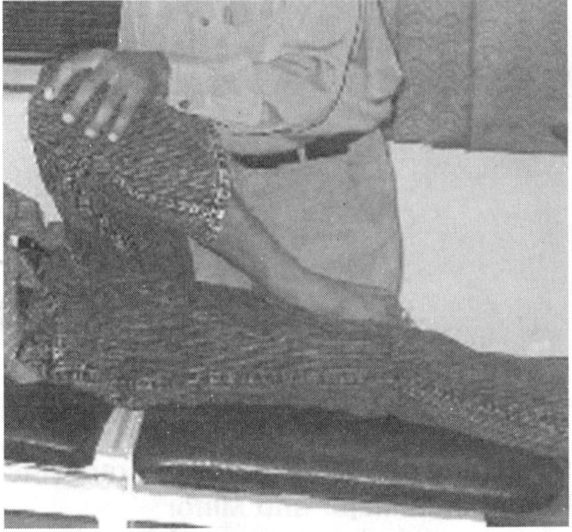

Fig. 13.14b: Stretching of piriformis (alternate)

Self stretching of piriformis muscle: The position of patient is side lying. The patient places the hand on the lateral aspect of the knee joint and then flexes the hip joint at 90° with adduction and medial rotation. The lower limb may be flexed at hip and knee joints (Fig. 13.14c).

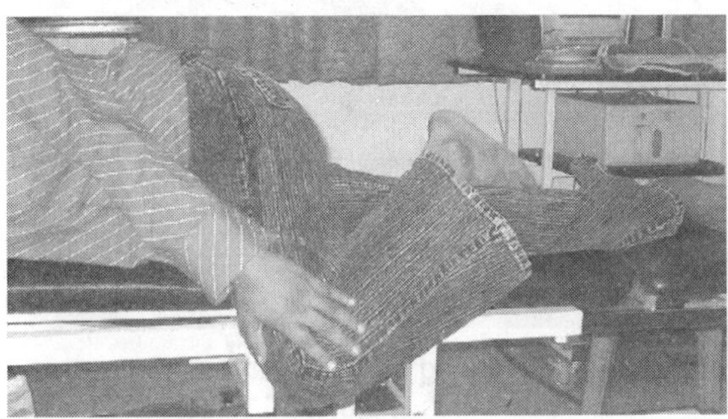

Fig. 13.14c: Self stretching of piriformis

TRUNK AND UPPER EXTREMITY MUSCLE STRETCHING

Lower back extensors: Position of patient-high sitting—while maintaining the position the patient flexes the lumbar spine by trying to touch the

shoulders to the knees. Therapist pushes both shoulders to the knees (Fig. 13.15a).

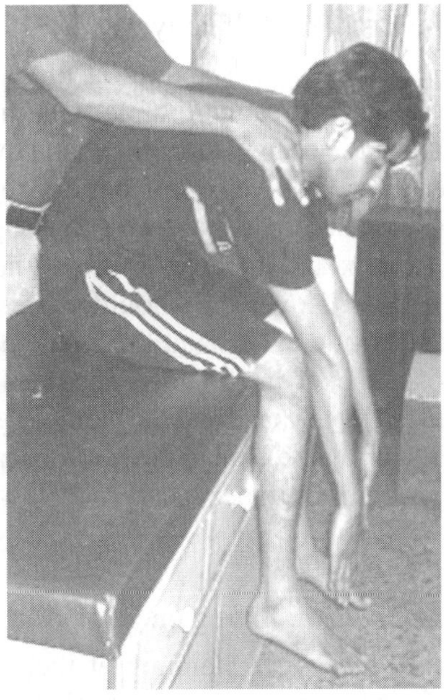

Fig. 13.15a: Stretching of lower back extensors

Self stretching of extensors of back: The procedure remains same as above (the technique is performed without the assistance of therapist) (Fig. 13.15b).

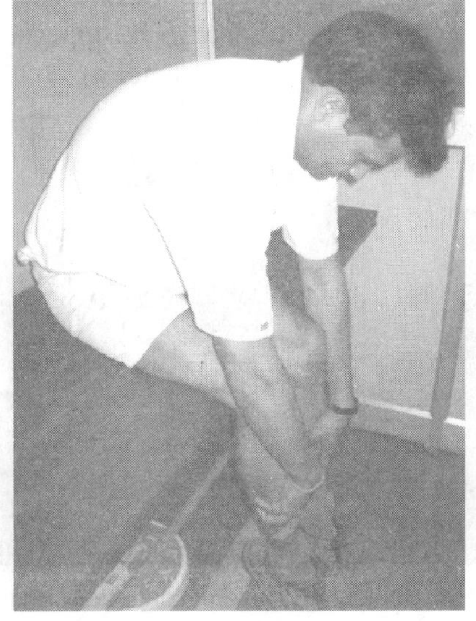

Fig. 13.15b: Self stretching of lower back extensors

Stretching of Levator Scapulae and Trapezius (Upper fibres)

Position of patient: Supine lying.

Position of therapist: Standing at the head of patient or end of treatment table. One hand is placed under the occiput and other hand over the shoulder joint. The vertex of patient rests on therapist's waist. A paper or towel can be placed between vertex and therapist's waist. The hand which is placed over the shoulder, pushes it downward, while other hand flexes the neck to the opposite side of the shoulder. The side flexion is carried out by the hand and the therapist's body together. It brings tension in the levator scapulae and upper fibres of trapezius.

Alternate Position

Position of patient: Sitting on stool.

Position of therapist: Standing at the back of patient, facing posterior aspect of neck. One hand is placed over the shoulder (same side of the muscles being stretched), the other hand is rest on the head (palmar surface of hand on the vertex and fingers on the temporal aspect of the same side). While maintaining the position of hands, therapist depresses the shoulder by one hand, and simultaneously flexes the neck to the opposite side by the other hand (Figs 13.16a and b).

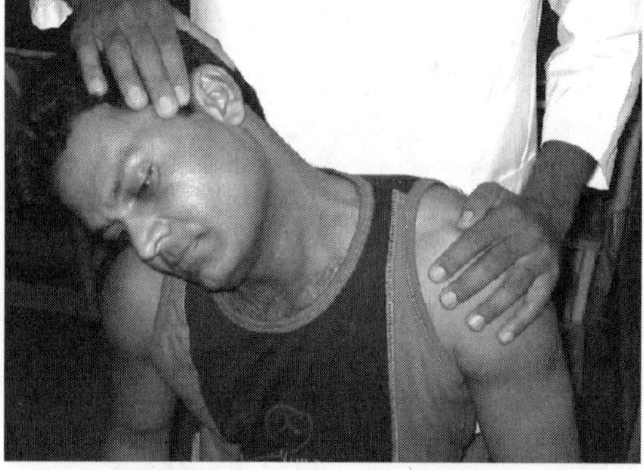

Fig. 13.16a: Stretching of levator scapulae, and trapezius upper fibres (opposite side flexion of the neck)

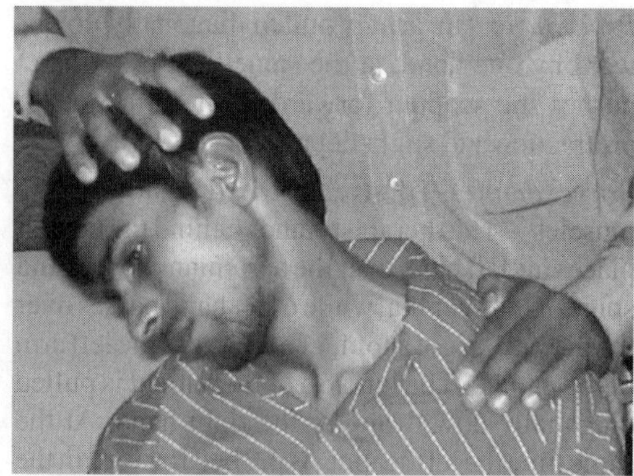

Fig. 13.16b: Stretching of levator scapulae (opposite side flexion and rotation of the neck)

Stretching of Middle Fibres of Trapezius, Rhomboids Major and Minor

Position of patient: Sitting on stool.

Position of therapist: Standing behind the patient facing the back of shoulder (Fig. 13.17).

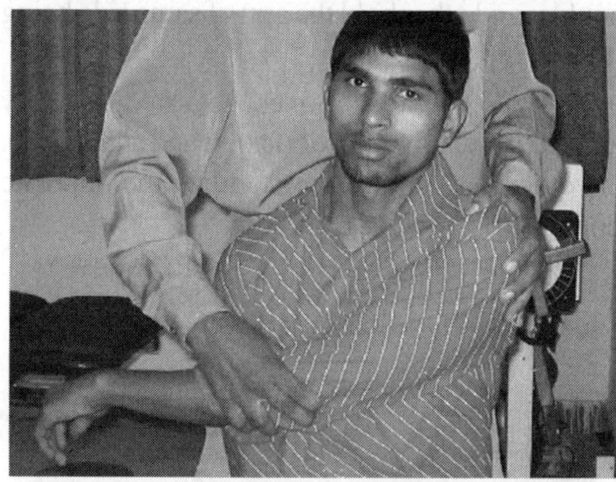

Fig. 13.17: Stretching of middle fibres of trapezius, rhomboids major and minor

One hand is placed over the acromion process and spine of scapula and other hand passes over the shoulder and grasps the arm of the same side of the muscle being stretched.

Stabilization: The trunk of the patient rests on the therapist's thigh which stabilizes the trunk to prevent rotation.

Procedure: The arm is pulled diagonally downward by one hand, at the same time other hand pushes the scapula forward in the direction of protraction and slight depression.

For example: To stretch the left side of the muscles—The therapist stands behind the patient places his left hand over the acromian process and spine of left scapula, while other hand passes over the patient's right shoulder and grasps the left arm of the patient. The left arm of the patient is pulled diagonally downward by the right hand. At the same time the left scapula is pushed forward in the direction of protraction and slight depression.

Stretching of Lower Fibres of Trapezius

Position of patient: Patient sitting on stool.

Position of therapist: Standing at the back of the patient.

Placement of hands: One hand on the opposite shoulder and other hold the arm of same side being stretched.

Procedure: Therapist moves the arm diagonally upward (in the direction of flexion and adduction). The other hand is used to stabilize the opposite shoulders (Fig. 13.18).

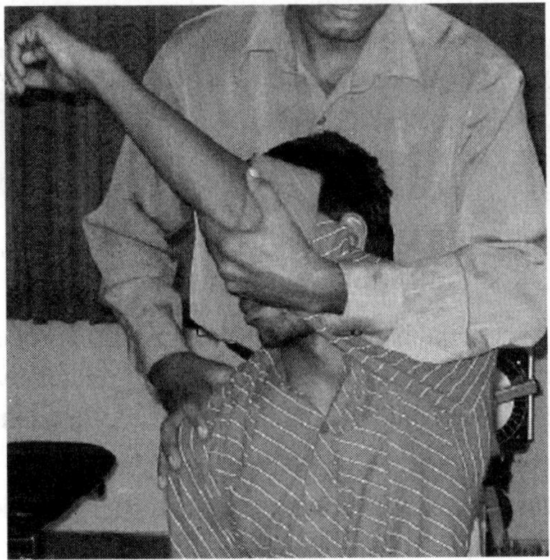

Fig. 13.18: Lower fibres of trapezius

Stretching of Pectoralis Major

Position of patient: Sitting on stool.

Position of therapist: Standing behind the patient.

Placement of hands: Therapist holds the hand of patient with one hand and other hand stabilizes the shoulder (Fig 13.19a).

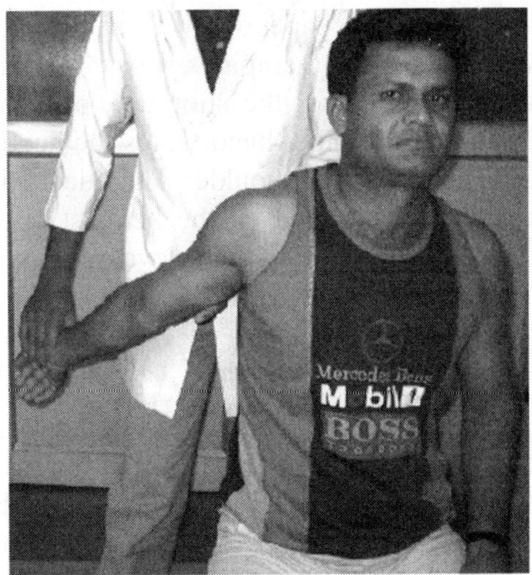

Fig. 13.19a: Stretching of pectoralis major (upper fibres)

Procedure:

i. For upper fibres (clavicular) therapist horizontally abducts the arm as much as possible while stabilizing the opposite shoulder.

   Therapist then comes back to the starting position; extends the shoulder completely by taking the arm in backward direction. (The upper 2 methods stretch almost all upper fibres).

ii. For lower fibres (sternal) therapist takes the arm diagonally upward (Fig 13.19b).

Stretching of Supra Spinatus Muscle

Position of patient: Standing.

Position of therapist: Standing at the back of patient, facing the posterior aspect of shoulder joint. One hand holds the patient's hand, while other hand grasps the patient's elbow.

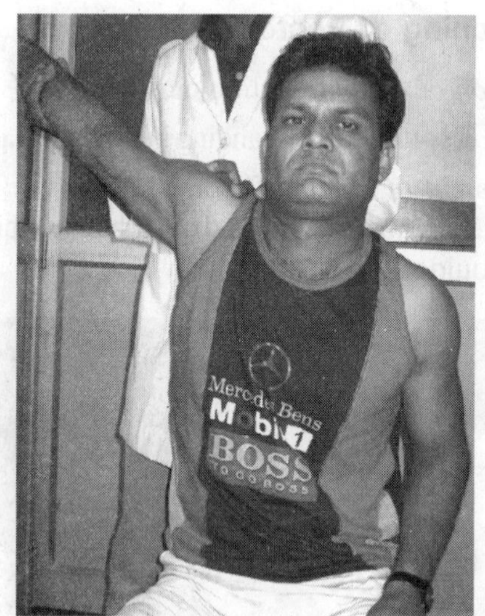

Fig. 13.19b: Stretching of pectoralis major (lower fiber)

Procedure: The therapist extends and internally rotates the shoulder joint passively and flexes the elbow joint, so that forearm of patient rests on his back. While maintaining the position the therapist pushes the elbow toward the midline by both the hands. The elbow which rests on patient's back, remains flexed at 80-90°. The procedure may also be repeated on high sitting or supine (Fig. 13.20).

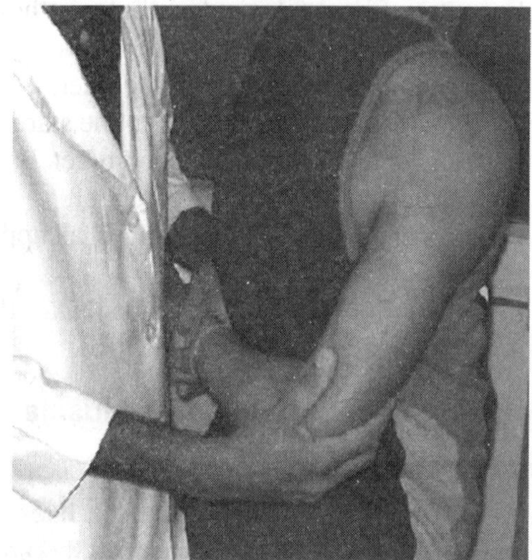

Fig. 13.20: Stretching of supraspinatus in standing position

Stretching of Subscapularis

Position of patient: Supine.

Position of therapist: Standing at the side of patient, facing the shoulder joint. One hand grasps the elbow while other grasps the wrist joint.

Procedure: The shoulder is abducted at 90° and elbow is flexed at 90°. While maintaining the position, the shoulder is rotated laterally by taking the hand up (toward the head) (Fig. 13.21).

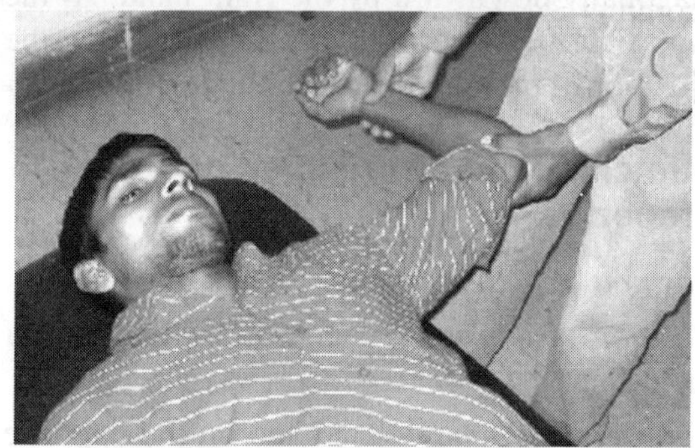

Fig. 13.21: Supine, therapist laterally rotates the shoulder

Stretching of Infraspinatus and Teres Minor

Position of patient and therapist: Same as stretching of subscapularis.

Procedure: The shoulder is abducted at 90° and elbow is kept at 90° flexion. While maintaining the position the shoulder is rotated medially, by taking the hand toward the waist (Fig. 13.22).

Stretching of Latissimus Dorsi

Position of patient: Supine lying.

Position of therapist: Standing at the side of patient, facing the joint. One hand is placed over the lateral border of scapula while other hand grasp the elbow joint.

Procedure: The upper hand abducts the shoulder with external rotation, while lower hand stabilizes the scapula. The lower hand should not press the

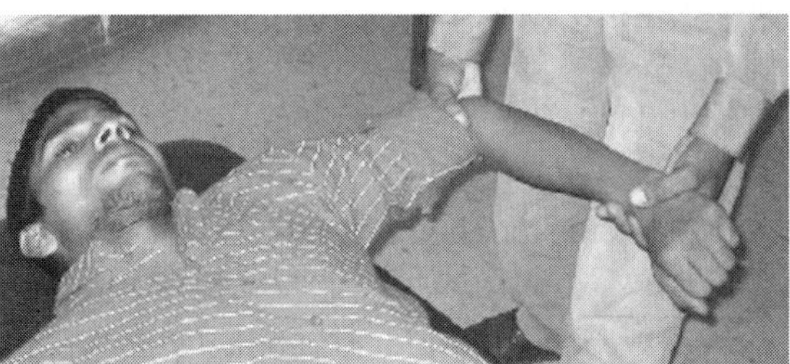

Fig. 13.22: Stretching of infraspinatus

scapula tightly, as latissimus dorsi might get compressed (Fig. 13.23).

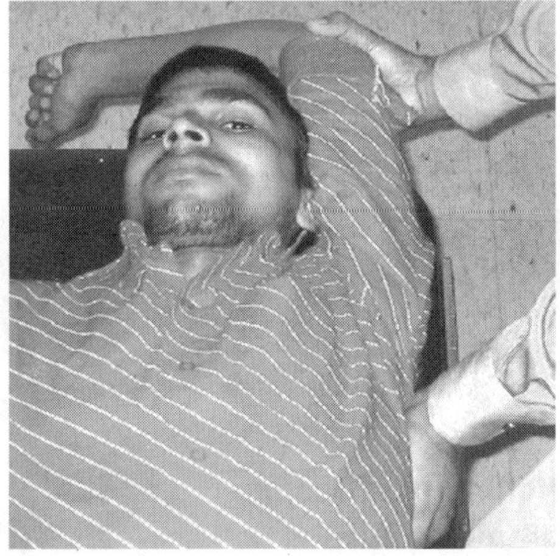

Fig. 13.23: Stretching of latissimus dorsi

Alternate Method of Latissimus Dorsi

Position of patient: Standing.

Position of therapist: Standing behind the patient, one hand is placed over the waist opposite to the side of muscle being stretched and the other grasp the arm.

Procedure: The upper hand of therapist abducts the shoulder with elbow 90° flexion. Then flexes the trunk towards opposite side by pushing the arm. At the same time the other hand stabilizes the trunk (or facilitates the trunk bending) by counterbalancing the weight of the body. Further stabilization at the pelvis is given by therapists thigh on the side of stretching (Fig. 13.24).

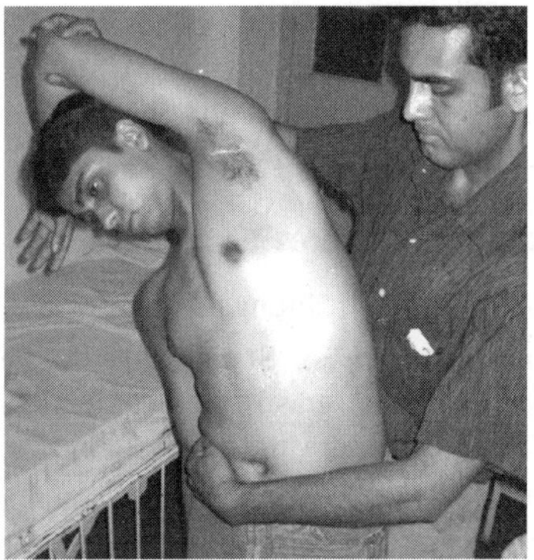

Fig. 13.24: Stretching of latissimus dorsi

For example: To stretch left latissimus dorsi, therapist places his right hand on arm and left hand on the opposite waist. Therapist uses his left thigh to stabilize patient's pelvis from left side (procedure is followed as above).

Stretching of Elbow Flexors

Position of patient: Standing.

Position of therapist: Standing behind the patient. One hand is placed at the elbow joint and other hand grasp the forearm at the wrist joint. (Forced passive stretching of elbow flexors may cause myositis ossification, therefore extra care should be taken to avoid complication, specially in children) (Fig. 13.25).

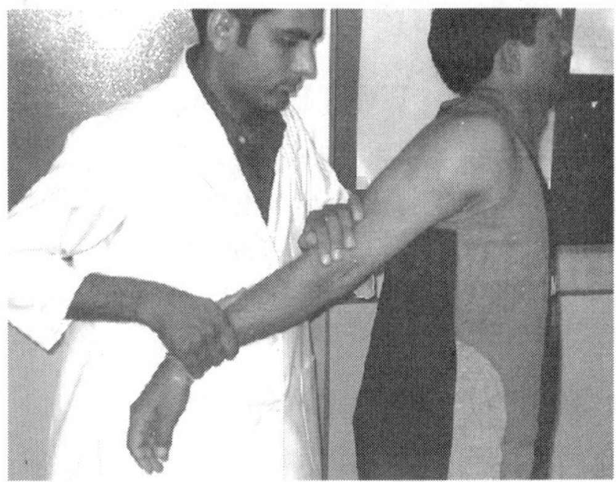

Fig. 13.25: Stretching of biceps

Procedure: The therapist extends the shoulder joint with elbow flexion. In the next step of technique the therapist extends the elbow joint gradually.

Stretching of Elbow Extensors

Position of patient: Sitting on chair or standing.

Position of therapist: Standing at the side of patient. One hand grasps the proximal part of elbow while other grasps the wrist joint.

Procedure: The therapist flexes the shoulder joint (full flexion) at 180° with elbow flexion at 90°. In the next step therapist flexes the elbow joint passively (Fig. 13.26).

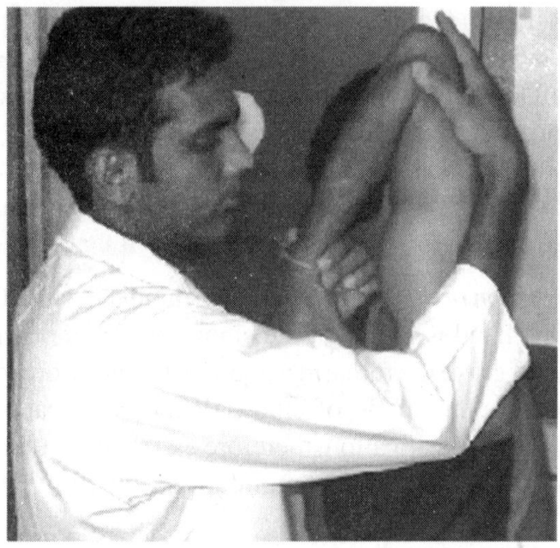

Fig. 13.26: Stretching of triceps

Stretching of Wrist Extensors

Position of patient and therapist: Any comfortable position. The therapist stabilizes the forearm by one hand, while other hand grasps the hand and flexes the wrist joint passively to stretch the extensors (Fig. 13.27).

Stretching of Wrist Flexors

Position of patient and therapist: Remains same as wrist extensors stretching. Therapist's one

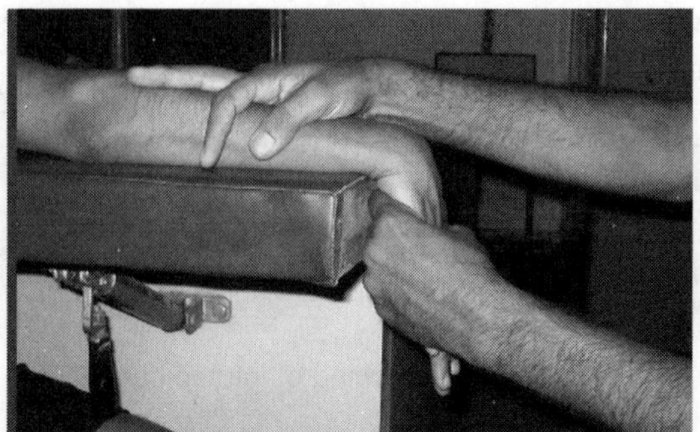

Fig. 13.27: Stretching of wrist extensors

hand stabilizes the forearm and other hand grasps the hand.

Procedure: While stabilizing the forearm by one hand the other hand passively extends the wrist joint (Fig. 13.28).

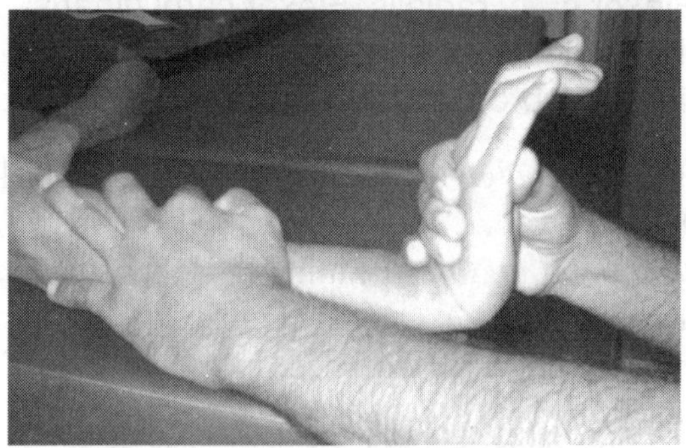

Fig. 13.28: Stretching of wrist flexors

Stretching of Common Extensors (Extensor carpi radialis longus, Extensor carpi radialis bravis, Extensor carpi ulnaris, Extensor digitorum/communis)

Position of patient: Sitting on chair, arm rests on table, and wrist out of the edge of the treatment table.

Position of therapist: Sitting in front of patient (across the table). One hand stabilizes the elbow joint, and other hand grasps the hand of patient.

Procedure: While stabilizing the elbow joint by one hand, the other hand flexes the fingers and wrist joint. In the next step the forearm is pronated and elbow is extended (Fig. 13.29).

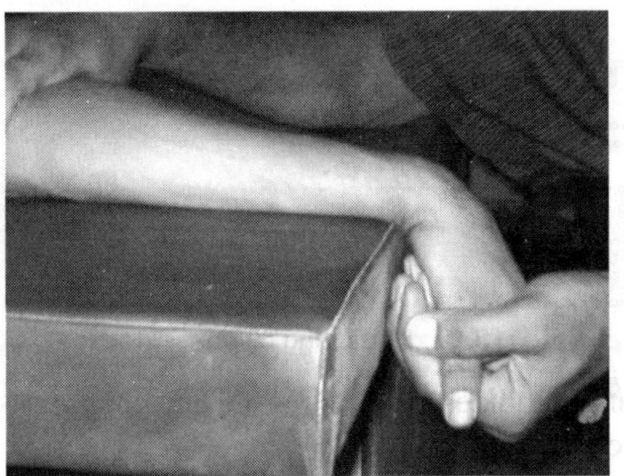

Fig. 13.29: Stretching of wrist common extensors

Stretching of Wrist and Finger Flexors
(Flexor carpi radialis, Flexor carpi ulnaris, Flexor digitorum superficialis, Flexor digitorum profundus)

Position of patient: Sitting on chair, arm rests on table.

Position of therapist: Sitting in front of patient (across the table). One hand grasps the forearm while the fingers of other hand rest on the patient's fingers.

Procedure: Therapist extends the wrist and four fingers (Fig. 13.30).

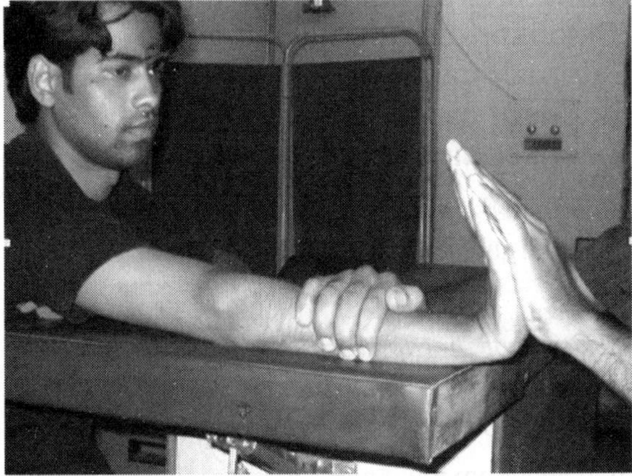

Fig. 13.30: Stretching of wrist and finger flexors

Stretching of Intrinsic Muscles of Hand (Lumbricals and Interossei)

Position of patient: Sitting on chair, arm rests on table.

Position of therapist: Sitting in front of patient (across the table). One hand stabilizes the wrist with fingers. The other hand grasps the finger to be stretched.

Procedure: Therapist flexes the PIP joint and hyper extends the MCP joint with one hand while stabilizing wrist and metacarpal with other hand.
   For all fingers together.

Position of patient: Same.

Position of therapist: Same.

Therapist flexes proximal interphalangeal (PIP) joints of all fingers and hyperextends the MCP joints with one hand while stabilizing the wrist and metacarpal with other hand.

Procedure: Therapist flexes all the PIP joints and hyperextends the MCP joints with one hand while stablizing metacarpals with other hand.

Alternative position for Lumbricals and interossei: The therapist places his/her fingers over the dorsum of the patient's fingers, the tip of the therapist fingers rest on the MCP joints or proximal phalanx. In the first step therapist flexes the PIP and DIP and then hyperextends the MCP joints. The position is maintained for 10-15 seconds (Fig. 13.31).

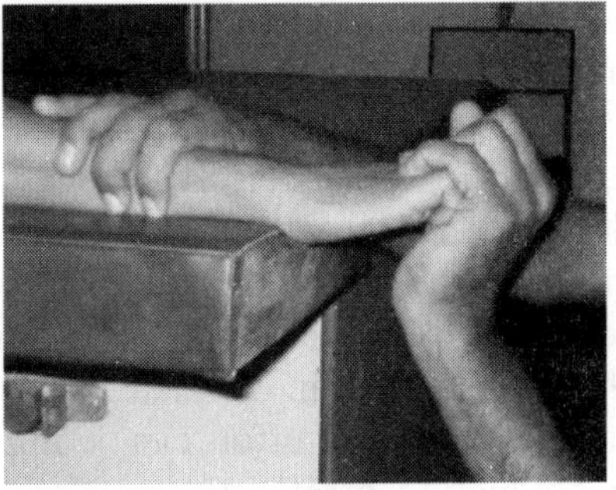

Fig. 13.31: Stretching of lumbricals

CHAPTER-14

Proprioceptive Neuromuscular Facilitation (PNF)

INTRODUCTION

In 1940s, Dr Kabat was the first man who has given the name of proprioceptive facilitation, then in 1956, Ms Voss (Physiotherapist) added the neuromuscular to Dr Kabat's proprioceptive facilitation, and given the name of PNF (Proprioceptive Neuromuscular Facilitation).

- Proprioception—Means stimulation within tissues.
- Neuromuscular—Pertaining to nerves and muscles.
- Facilitation—Makes response easy.

Therefore techniques of PNF may be defined as methods of promoting or hastening the response of the proprioceptors.

Normal Neuromuscular Mechanism

Normal neuromuscular mechanism is capable to produce efficient and purposeful functional movements and activities of daily living without facing any problem.

Deficient Neuromuscular Mechanism

The response of normal neuromuscular mechanism may be limited as a result of trauma, disease of the nervous system and musculoskeletal system, thus the voluntary effort becomes unable to produce the efficient and purposeful functional movements. Therefore by administering the PNF techniques the response of deficient neuromuscular mechanism can be made easy so that the weakened voluntary effort can be improved for the production of effective, efficient and purposeful functional movement.

PROPRIOCEPTIVE NEUROMUSCULAR FACILITATION PRINCIPLES

PNF is a philosophical approach or concept of treatment. Its underlying philosophy is that all the human being including those with disabilities, have untapped existing potential.

1. The treatment approach is always positive, reinforcing and using that which the patient can do on a physical and psychological level. The normal neuromuscular response of an individual is limited to its physical ability, inherent and previously learned neuromuscular responses. However, untapped neuromuscular response may be shown during stressful episodes. Not only that but also the neuromuscular response may be enhanced through environmental influences and voluntary decisions. Based on this philosophy that the individual has untapped neuromuscular potential, the therapist always strives to treat functions, motivates patient to achieve higher levels, and use the patients strength to minimize the weakness.
2. The primary goal of treatment is to help patients achieve their highest level of functions.
3. PNF is an integrated approach; each treatment is directed at a total human being, not at a specific problem or body segment.

The PNF patterns are performed according to the normal development process. Development of motion occurs first in the head and neck, then in the trunk and finally in the extremities. Hence, PNF patterns are strived to the head and neck movements first as they influence the movements of the body. In the next step the patterns are performed on the trunk as it provides foundation of the body. As soon as the patient achieves motor control over the head neck and trunk, the PNF patterns are performed on the extremities to improve their functions.

Mass movement patterns performed in spiral and diagonal patterns closely resemble the movements used in sports and in activities of daily living (ADL). The spiral and diagonal character is in keeping the spiral and rotatory characteristic of the skeletal system of bones and muscles and the ligament structures. This type of motion is also in harmony with the topographical alignment of the muscles from origin to insertion and with the structural characteristic of the individual muscles.

Patterns of Motion

The patterns of motion are mass patterns means during the normal functional activity (to place a specific demand) number of movements occur sequentially from distal part of the limb to the proximal and this activity requires shortening and lengthening of many muscles in varying degrees.

It is also keeping with Beevor's axiom that the brain knows nothing about the individual muscle action but knows only of movements.

Diagonals

There are two diagonals for each major parts of the body (the head and neck, upper trunk and lower trunk and extremities). It is important to know that the PNF patterns are performed in spiral and diagonal patterns because of the topographical alignment of the muscles from origin to insertion and with the structural characteristic of the individual muscles.

Each diagonal is made up of two patterns which are antagonistic to each other.
- Diagonal$_1$ (D$_1$) is made up of two patterns–flexion and extension.

- Diagonal$_2$ (D$_2$) is made up of two patterns–flexion and extension.

Motion Components

It means the movements which take place during the pattern. Each spiral and diagonal pattern is composed of three motion components with respect to all the muscles of action participating in the movement.

These three motion components are as follows:
1. Flexion or Extension.
2. Adduction or Abduction.
3. Internal or External rotation.

BASIC PROCEDURES

Agonists and Antagonists

When muscles contract toward their shortened state the resulting pattern is termed as agonistic pattern. On the contrary when the muscles contract towards their lengthened state, the pattern is called antagonistic pattern.

Indications for patterns:
- Passive ROM.
- Free, active, guided active and resistive range of motion.

Traction and Approximation

Traction and approximation are used to *stimulate proprioceptors within* and *around* the joint such as *Ligaments, cartilage,* capsule etc. Approximation are used to facilitate co-contraction around the joint, while traction is used to increase ROM. Both of these techniques are contraindicated in acute conditions.

Normal Timing

It is the sequence in which the participating muscles in any motor activity contract to carry on coordinated and purposeful movements.

Normally rotation pattern is the movement which is initiated first and then other patterns occur from distal to proximal, if this rotation is blocked other components of motion is not possible.

Stretch Stimulus

The contraction of muscle or group of muscles can be increased if they are stretched before allowing them to contract. Therefore, to achieve more contraction an agonist group of muscles is placed in a lengthened state then a stretch stimulus is given immediately. After stretch stimulus patient is commanded to contract the muscles (agonist muscles). For example to achieve more contraction of wrist and finger extensors, these group of muscles are given a stretch stimulus and then immediately after that, they are allowed to contract. In PNF all group of motion components are given a stretch stimulus.

The rotation component receives first and last consideration since it is the rotatory component that elongates the muscles in a given pattern. After rotation component the stretch stimulus is given from distal to proximal motion components.

Stretch Reflex

The stretch reflex is given to increase the voluntary contraction of agonist muscles and subsequently the strength. Use of stretch reflex aids the patient with intact innervation to learn and perform the patterns with greater ease.

The difference between stretch stimulus and reflex—In stretch stimulus a gentle stretch is given with low intensity to agonist muscles, while stretch reflex includes a sudden or quick stretch with more intensity which is followed by voluntary contraction of the agonist muscles.

All the motion components (agonist muscles) are placed in an extreme lengthened position then a quick stretch reflex is elicited manually by taking the part past the point of tension. All the components should receive stretch reflex specially proper rotation. To be certain that stretch reflex and contraction of agonist muscles are synchronized, the patient is commanded as "Now push" or pull. This warns the patient to be prepared to attempt the motion.

Manual Contact

The placement of the hands of therapist on the patient's limb or body is termed as manual contact.

Appropriate placement of hands facilitates the contraction of agonist muscles. Hands should always be placed over the agonist muscles. When the hand is placed over the patient's skin, it causes tactile stimulation and facilitates the contraction of the underlying muscles or group of muscles. For example—If the finger extensors are the agonist muscles therapist should place hand over the dorsum of the hand to apply resistance. If the therapist places hand on the palmar aspect of the patient's hand (over the antagonists) the tactile stimulation on palmar surface causes contraction of the finger flexors which decreases the contraction of extensors of the fingers.

When patterns are performed on patient passively, the therapist may place hand on the antagonist muscles as it is difficult to perform without it. For example—If patient has spasticity in flexor group of muscles of the upper limb and cannot extend the fingers voluntarily then therapist places the tip of fingers on the palmar aspect of patient's finger tips and extends the fingers during the pattern. Here therapist must make efforts to contact the palmar surface of the patient's hand as minimal as possible.

Command and Communication

Patient makes little effort or does not take interest to perform the patterns. Therefore the biggest job of therapist is to make the patient interested and allow him to participate voluntarily in PNF patterns. This can be achieved by giving an adequate command and appreciate his voluntary efforts during the pattern. There are three types of basic commands: (i) Verbal (ii) Visual (iii) Tactile.

1. *Verbal command:* Tone of voice may influence considerably the quality of response. A tone of voice should be appropriate according to the contraction required. When maximal stimulation of active motion is required a strong, sharp command is given. It simulate a stress situation. A moderate tone of voice should be used when the patient is responding with his best effort. If patient is having musculoskeletal problems such as pain and inflammation the

commands should be soft tone of voice. The verbal command is given as "Push", "Pull", "Hold" and "Relax or Let go". The command "Hold" is given during isometric contraction. The "Push" or "Pull" are given during isotonic contraction of muscles while "Relax" or "let go" used for relaxation.

2. *Visual command:* This type of command is particularly useful in children who do not follow the verbal command. Attractive things or objects are placed in the space/air at different positions (in which the patterns are performed). A child is frequently led to perform by enticing him or her to look at object and his hand tries to follow the direction of object. Several repetitions may be performed in the same manner.

   A visual command is also useful in an adult to make him understand by demonstrating the direction of pattern, if patient finds difficulty to perform the movement in desired direction.

3. *Tactile command:* The therapist places the hand on the agonist muscles and commands the patient by scratching the skin or applying pressure over it. The rubbing and pressing cause tactile stimulation and facilitate the contraction of agonist muscles. Applying pressure or touching the skin also helps to contract the muscle in the desired diagonal.

Line of Movement

The patterns are performed in a diagonal direction from their completely lengthened position to the complete contracting state. The diagonal direction allows the muscles to contract maximum from their fully stretched state.

PNF PATTERNS FOR UPPER EXTREMITIES (Table 14.1)

The PNF patterns in upper extremities are performed in spiral and diagonal manner.

Upper extremities consist two diagonals and each diagonal is made up of two patterns (Flexion, and extension). So there are four patterns and two diagonals in upper extremities.

- Diagonal$_1$—D$_1$ Flexion, D$_1$ Extension
- Diagonal$_2$—D$_2$ Flexion, D$_2$ Extension.

Table 14.1: Upper extremity

Diagonal	Pattern	Motion components
D$_1$	Flexion	Shoulder—Flexion, adduction and external rotation. Elbow—May remain flexed or extended. Forearm—Supination. Wrist—Flexion and radial deviation. Fingers—Flexion and adduction. Thumb—Flexion and adduction.
	Extension	Shoulder—Extension, adduction and internal rotation. Elbow—May remain flexed or extended. Forearm—Pronation Wrist—Extension and ulnar deviation. Finger—Extension and abduction. Thumb—Extension and abduction.
D$_2$	Flexion	Shoulder—Flexion, abduction and external rotation. Elbow—May remain flexed or extended. Forearm—Supination. Wrist—Extension and radial deviation. Finger—Extension and abduction. Thumb—Extension, adduction and external rotation of the first metacarpophalangeal joint.
	Extension	Shoulder—Extension, adduction and internal rotation. Elbow—May remain flexed or extended. Forearm—Pronation. Wrist—Flexion and ulnar deviation. Finger—Flexion and adduction. Thumb—Opposition, adduction and internal rotation of the first metacarpophalangeal joint.

Common points (important) for upper extremities D$_1$ and D$_2$ patterns:

- Shoulder flexion and extension are combined with adduction and abduction.
- External rotation is consistent with flexion.
- Internal rotation is consistent with extension.
- Supination of the forearm and radial deviation of the wrist are combined with flexion and external rotation of the shoulder.

- The pronation of the forearm and ulnar deviation are combined with extension and internal rotation.
- Flexion with adduction of the finger occurs with flexion of the wrist and adduction of the shoulder.
- Extension with abduction of the fingers occur with wrist extension and shoulder abduction.
- Adduction of the thumb is consistent with external rotation and flexion of the shoulder.
- Adduction of the thumb is consistent with external rotation and extension.
- Flexion of the thumb is consistent with adduction of the shoulder.
- Extension of thumb is consistent with abduction of the shoulder.
- Distal joints (Hand and Wrist)–The motions are consistent with proximal components.

D_1 Flexion Pattern

Motion components:

Shoulder	–	Flexion, adduction and external rotation
Elbow	–	Flexion or extension
Forearm	–	Supination
Wrist	–	Flexion and radial deviation
Fingers	–	Flexion and adduction
	–	Rotation toward radial side
Thumb	–	Flexion with adduction and external rotation of the first metacarpal joint.

Free Active Motion

Position the patient in standing. This pattern is performed by the patient without the help of therapist. The pattern starts from extreme lengthened position of the agonist to shortened state. Commands may be given as follows:

i. Look at your hand, place it behind your body away from the midline (in extreme lengthened position of gonists) (Fig. 14.1a).

ii. Close the hand and turn it outward (external rotation of the shoulder) (Fig. 14.1b).

ii. Pull it up across the midline, to the opposite shoulder (Fig. 14.1c).

Facilitation and Reinforcement

Patient is positioned in supine lying. Therapist places both hands over agonist muscles (one hand over the arm and other over the hand). The extremity is placed in extreme lengthened position. A stretch reflex is given by applying a sudden stretch of the agonists and at the same time patient is commanded to contract the agonists and perform the pattern as demonstrated. As patient starts moving the extremity therapist applies resistance. Therapist must use an appropriate verbal command such as push my both hands in the direction of your opposite shoulder. The proximal joints are

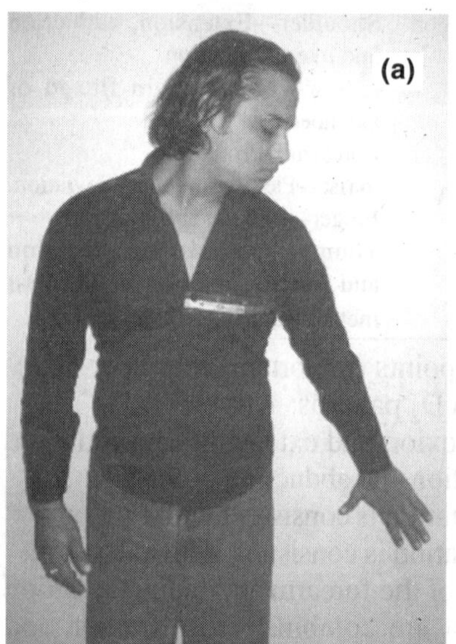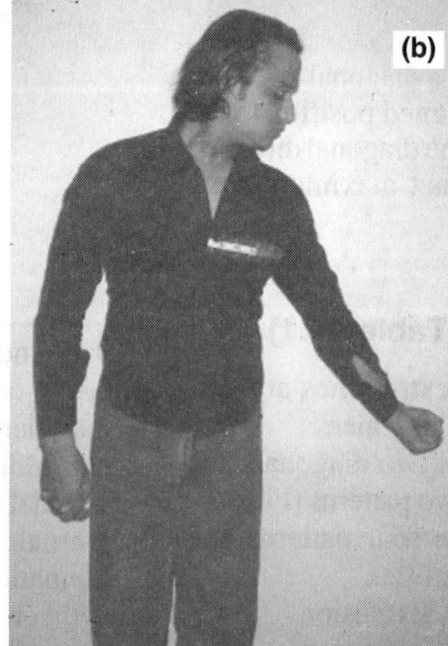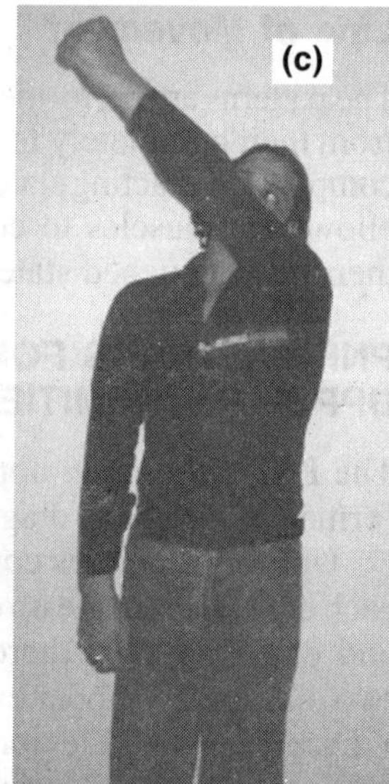

Figs 14.1a to c: D_1 flexion pattern (free active motion)

given more resistance than distal joints and weaker distal components are guided through their optimal range of motion in accordance with normal timing. This pattern is used to strengthen the muscles if they have fair voluntary control (Figs 14.2a to c).

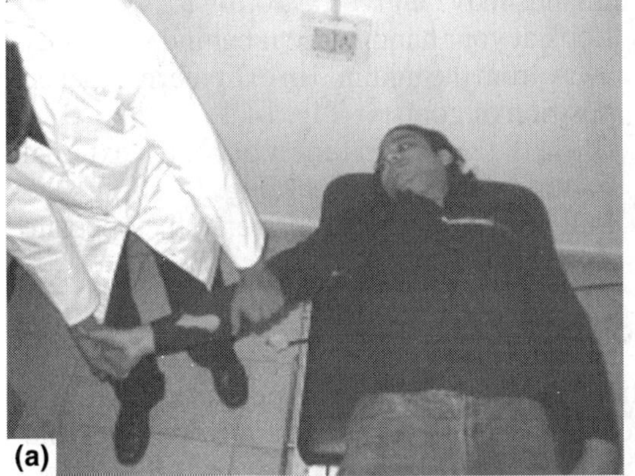

(a)

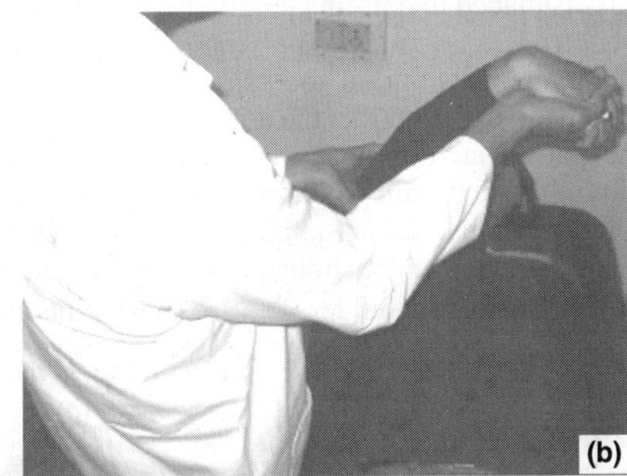

(b)

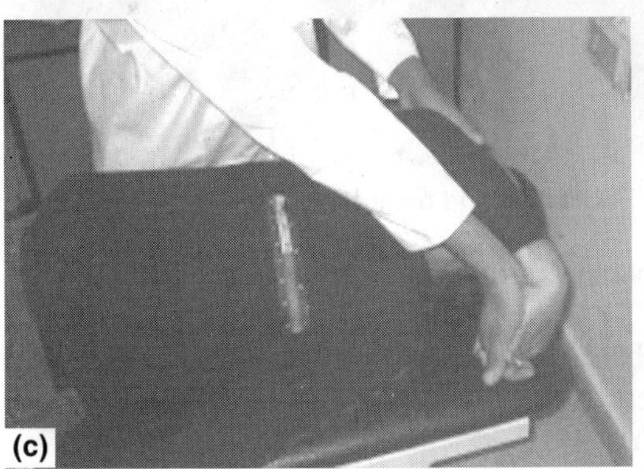

(c)

Figs 14.2a to c: D_1 flexion pattern (facilitation and reinforcement)

D_1 Extension Pattern

Motion components:

Shoulder   – Extension, abduction and internal rotation
Elbow   – Flexion or extension
Forearm   – Pronation
Wrist   – Extension, ulnar deviation
Fingers   – Extension and abduction
    – Rotation toward ulnar side
Thumb   – Palmar abduction with abduction and internal rotation of the first metacarpal.

Free Active Motion

The position of patient remains same as D_1 flexion pattern. All agonist muscles are placed in an extreme lengthened position (end of D_1 flexion pattern). The patient is asked to take the hand down to the opposite hip joint (diagonally) and point the fingers downward with palm facing backward. An extremity is taken in an extreme shortened position of the agonist muscles.

Commands may be given as follows:

i. Look at your hand place it up across the midline (in extreme lengthened position of the agonists muscles).
ii. Now open your hand
iii. Now push it down, away from the midline (Figs 14.3a to c).

Facilitation and Reinforcement

Patient is positioned in supine lying. Therapist stands at the same side of the extremity and places both hands on the agonist muscles at the elbow and dorsal aspect of the wrist. Agonist muscles are placed in extreme lengthened position then a stretch reflex is given which is synchronized by the contraction of agonist muscles. Patient is instructed to move the limb to the opposite hip joint (diagonally). The resistance is applied by the hands through the range of motion (from extreme lengthened state to the extreme shortened state of

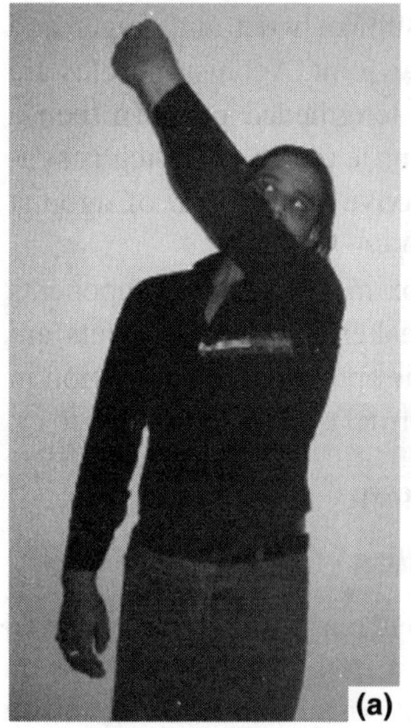 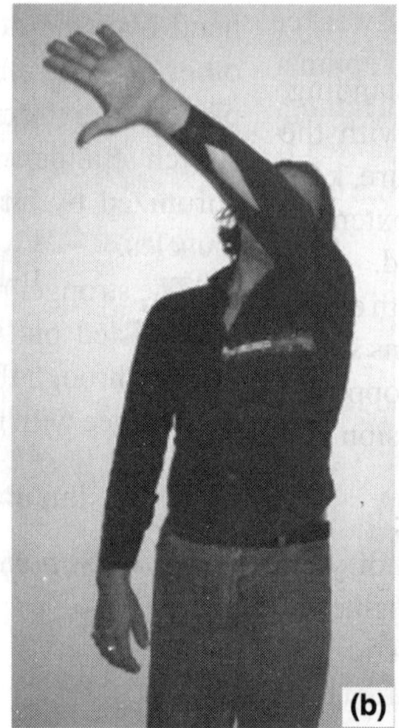 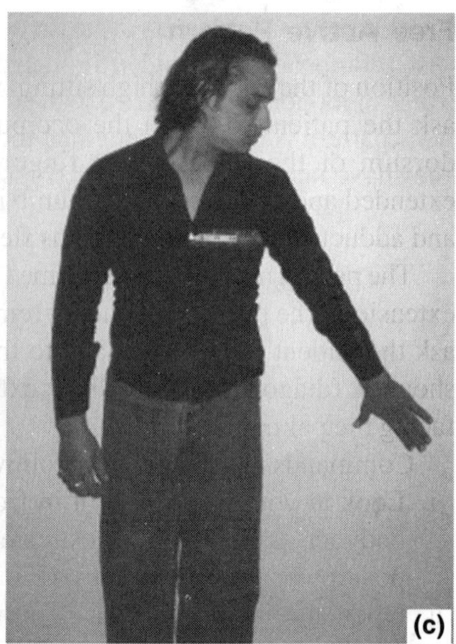

Figs 14.3a to c: D_1 extension pattern (free active motion)

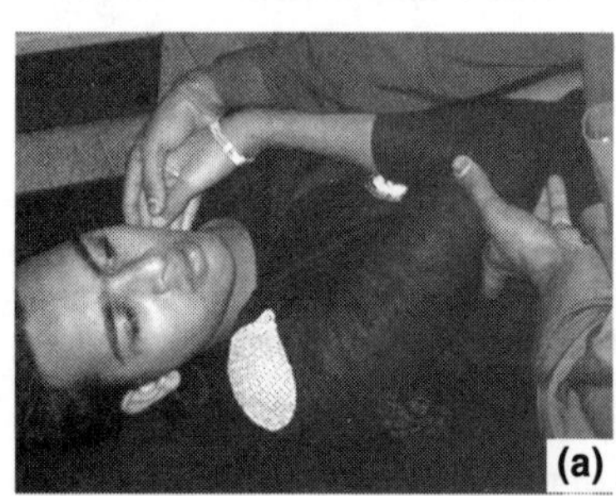 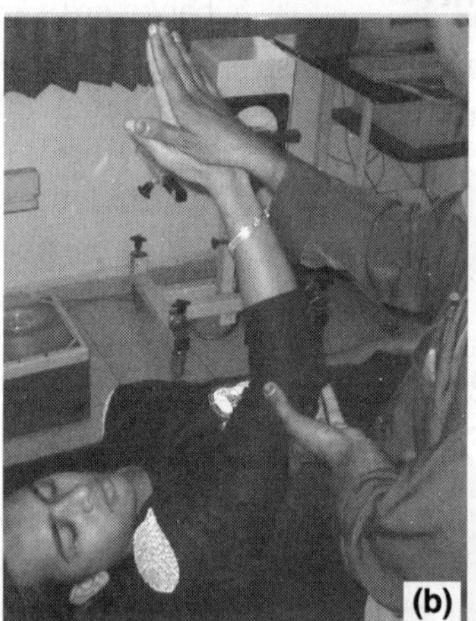 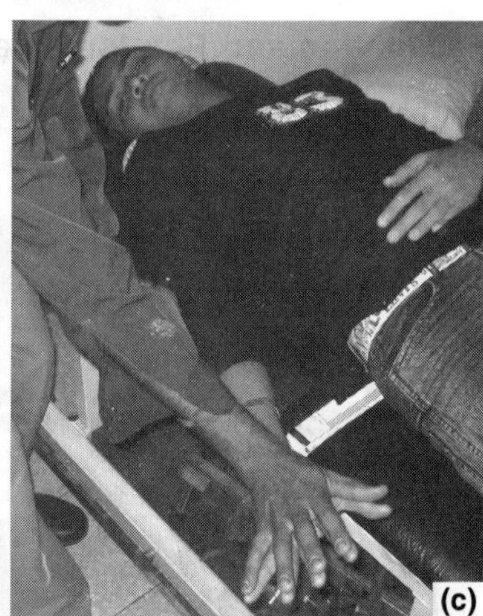

Figs 14.4a to c: D_1 extension pattern (Facilitation and reinforcement)

agonist muscles). The stronger proximal and distal components are resisted but weaker distal components are guided through their optimal range of motion in accordance with normal timing (Figs 14.4a to c).

D₂ Flexion Pattern

Motion components:

Shoulder	– Flexion, abduction and external rotation
Elbow	– Flexion or extension
Forearm	– Supination
Wrist	– Extension and radial deviation
Fingers	– Extension and abduction
Thumb	– Extension, adduction and external rotation of the first metacarpal joint.

Free Active Pattern

Position of the patient is high sitting or standing, ask the patient to touch the occiput with the dorsum of the fingers. The fingers are kept extended and abducted while thumb is extended and adducted. The elbow remains flexed.

The pattern may also be performed with elbow extension. The position of patient remains same, ask the patient to take the hand to the opposite shoulder (diagonally) with elbow extension and facing the palm up.

Commands may be given as follows:

i. Look at your hand place it in front of your body across the midline (in extreme lengthened position of agonist muscles) (Fig. 14.5a).
ii. Open the hand and turn it outward (Fig. 14.5b).
iii. Pull it up away from the midline (Fig. 14.5c).

Facilitation and Reinforcement

The patient is positioned in supine lying. Therapist places both hands on the agonist muscles (one hand over the dorsum of wrist and finger and other over the elbow joint. Agonist muscles are placed in extreme lengthened position then a stretch stimules or reflex is given which is synchronized by an active contraction of agonist muscles.

The stronger proximal and distal components are resisted but weaker distal components are guided through their optimal range of motion in accordance with normal timing (Figs 14.6a to c).

D_2 Extension Pattern

Motion components:

Shoulder	– Extension, adduction and internal rotation
Elbow	– Flexion or extension
Forearm	– Supination
Wrist	– Flexion and ulnar deviation
Fingers	– Flexion and adduction
Thumb	– Flexion, abduction and internal rotation of the first metacarpal joint.

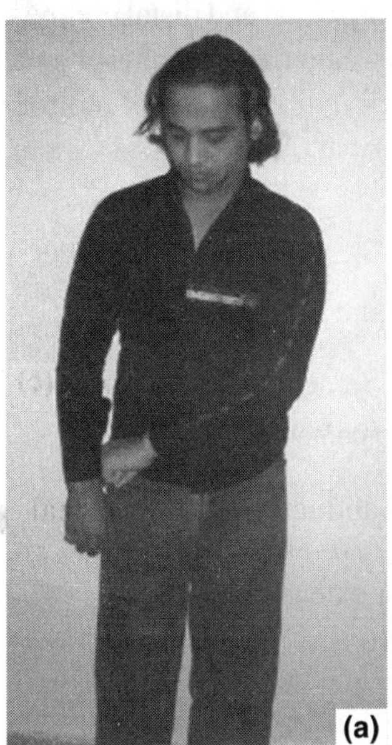
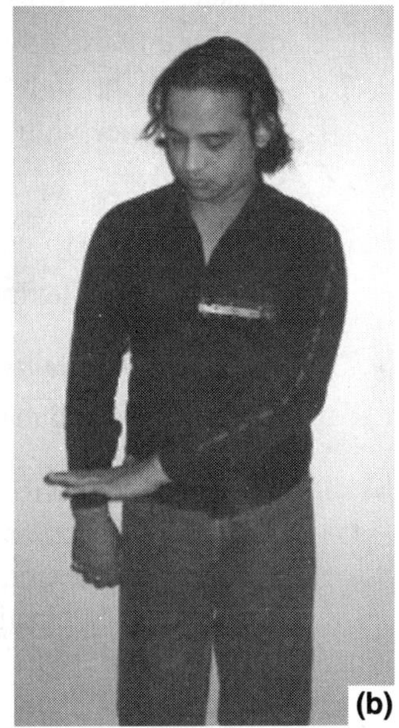
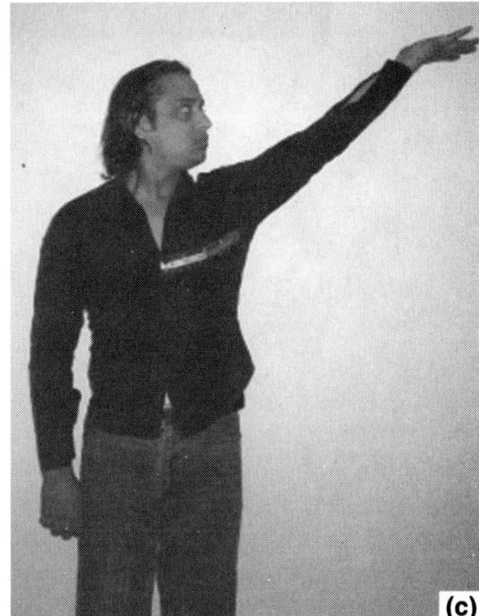

(a) (b) (c)

Figs 14.5a to c: D_2 flexion pattern (free active motion)

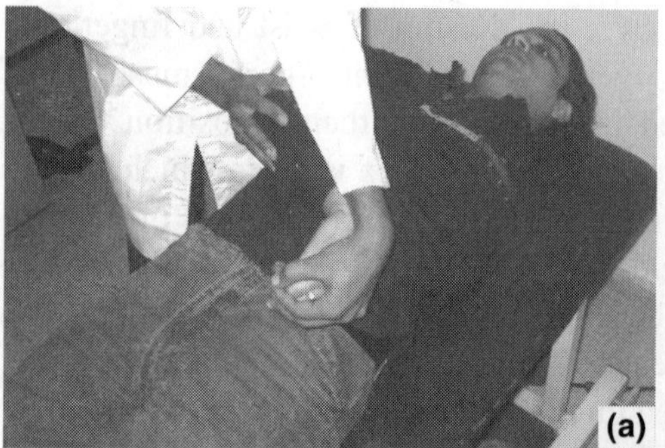

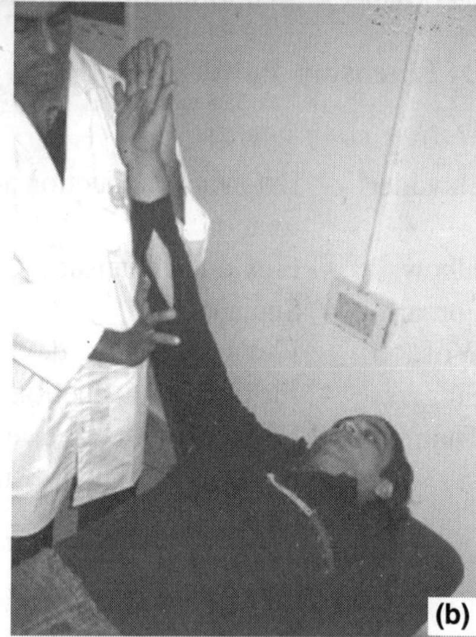

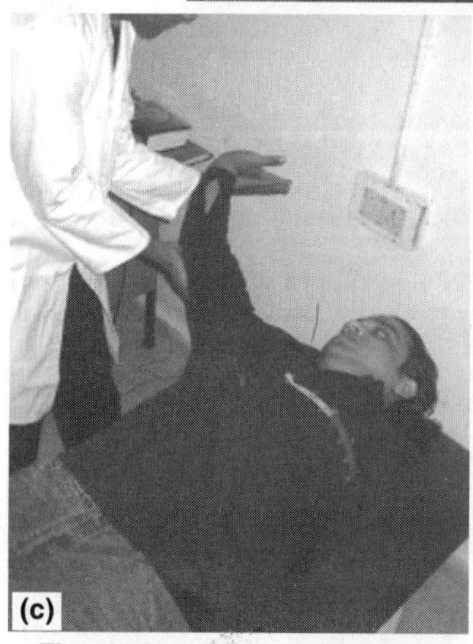

Figs 14.6a to c: D$_2$ flexion pattern (facilitation of reinforcement)

Free Active Pattern

This is the reverse of the D$_2$ flexion pattern. The patient is positioned in high sitting or standing. An agonist muscles are placed in extremely lengthened state and patient is commanded to take the extremity to the opposite buttock (diagonally).

Commands may be given as follows:

i. Look at your hand place it up away from the midline (in an extreme lengthened state of agonist muscles).
ii. Now close your hand and turn it inward.
iii. Pull it down across the midline in front of your body (Figs 14.7a to c).

Facilitation and Reinforcement

The patient is positioned in supine lying, therapist stands at the same side of the shoulder joint and places both hands over the agonist muscles (one over the elbow and other over the palmer surface of the hand) the extremity is placed in extreme lengthened position, a stretch reflex is given which is synchronized by an active contraction of agonist muscles. The stronger proximal and distal components are resisted but weaker distal components are guided through their optimal range of motion in accordance with normal timing (Figs 14.8a to c).

Diagonal – D$_1$
Pattern – Flexion and Extension

Motion components: Same as D$_1$ Flexion and Extension.

Position of the patient–Standing.

Position of the therapist–Standing in front of patient.

Commands are given as follows:

1. Look at your hand, place it behind your body away from the midline, in extreme lengthened position.

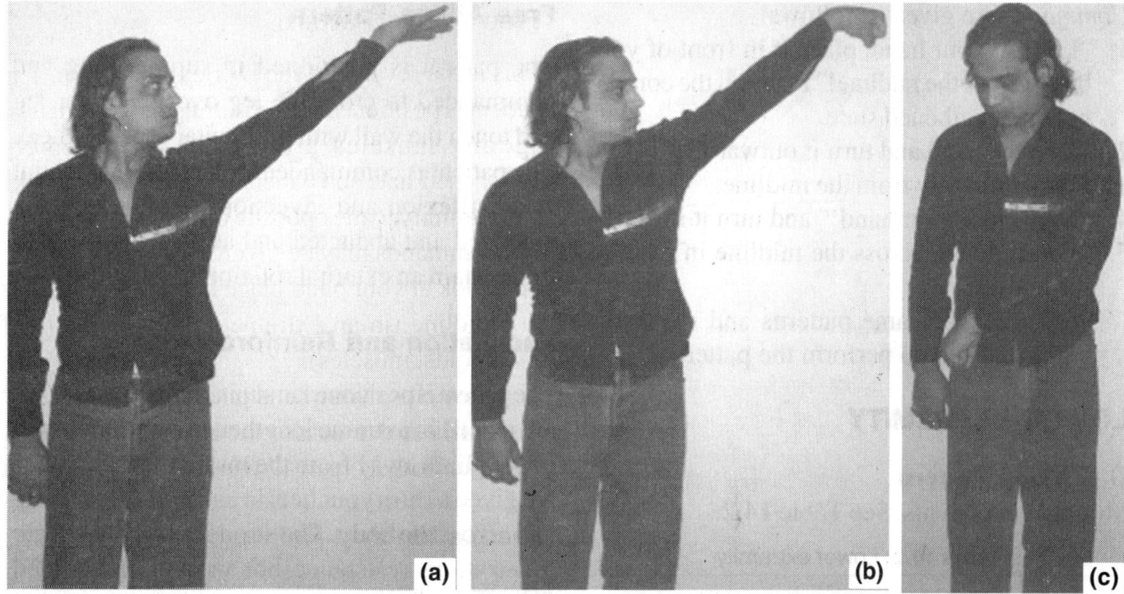

Figs 14.7a to c: D_2 extension pattern (free active motion)

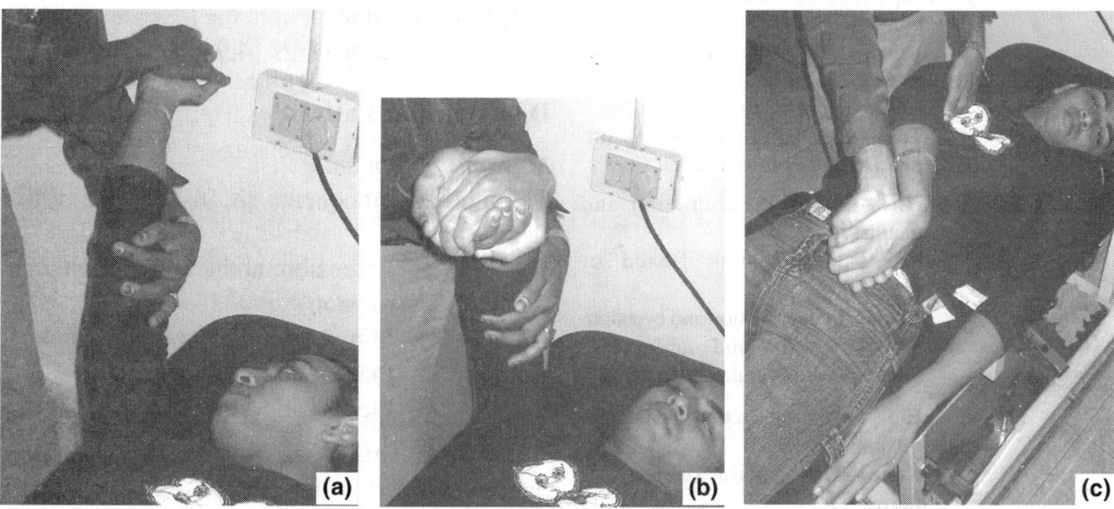

Figs 14.8a to c: D_2 extension pattern (Facilitation and reinforcement)

2. "Close the hand! and turn it outward!"
3. Pull it up across the midline.
4. "Now open your hand!"
5. Push it down, back to your body away from the midline.

    Repeat the same patterns and speak the command as you perform them.

Diagonal   – D_2
Pattern   – Flexion and Extension
Motion components: Same as D_2 Flexion and Extension.
Position of the patient–Standing.
Position of the therapist–Standing in front of the patient.

Commands are given as follows:

1. "Look at your hand, place it in front of your body across the midline!" Place all the component in lengthened state.
2. Open the hand and turn it outward.
3. Pull it up! away from the midline.
4. "Now close your hand!" and turn it inward.
5. "Pull it down, across the midline in front of the body!"

Repeat the same patterns and speak the command as you perform the pattern.

LOWER EXTREMITY

D$_1$ Flexion Pattern

Motion components. See Table 14.2.

Table 14.2: Lower extremity

Diagonal Pattern		Motion components
D$_1$	Flexion	Hip—Flexion, adduction and external rotation. Knee—May remain flexed or extended. Ankle—Dorsiflexion and inversion. Toes—Extension with abduction, rotation of toes toward tibial side.
	Extension	Hip—Extension, abduction and internal rotation. Knee—May remain flexed or extended. Ankle—Planter flexion and eversion. Toes—Flexion and adduction, rotation toward fibular side.
D$_2$	Flexion	Hip—Flexion, abduction and internal rotation. Knee—May remain extended or flexed. Ankle—Dorsiflexion and eversion. Toes—Extension with abduction, rotation toward fibular side.
	Extension	Hip—Extension, adduction and external rotation. Knee—May remain flexed or extended. Ankle—Planter flexion and inversion. Toes—Flexion with adduction rotation toward tibial side.

Free Active Pattern

The patient is positioned in supine lying and commanded to cross the leg over the other leg and touch the wall with the plantar aspect of heel. The patient is commanded to keep the ankle joint at dorsiflexion and inversion. The toes remain extended and abducted and away from the wall to maintain an external rotation of the hip joint.

Facilitation and Reinforcement

The patient is positioned in supine lying, the agonists are placed in extreme lengthened position (lower of the plinth away from the midline). Commands are given as turn your heel in and pull your foot up and across the body. The stronger component are given more resistance but weaker are guided through their optimal range of motion in accordance with normal timing. The ankle is kept at dorsiflexion and inversion, the toes are at extension and abduction (Figs 14.9a to f).

D$_1$ Extension Pattern

Motion components:

The motion components are just reverse of the flexion pattern.

Hip	– Extension, abduction and internal rotation
Knee	– May remain flexed or extended
Ankle	– Planter flexion and eversion
Toes	– Flexion and adduction

Procedure: This is the reverse of D$_1$ flexion pattern and performed as opposite to that (Figs 14.10a to c).

D$_2$ Flexion Pattern

Motion components:

Hip	– Flexion, abduction and internal rotation
Knee	– May remain extended or flexed
Ankle	– Dorsiflexion and eversion
Toes	– Extension with abduction

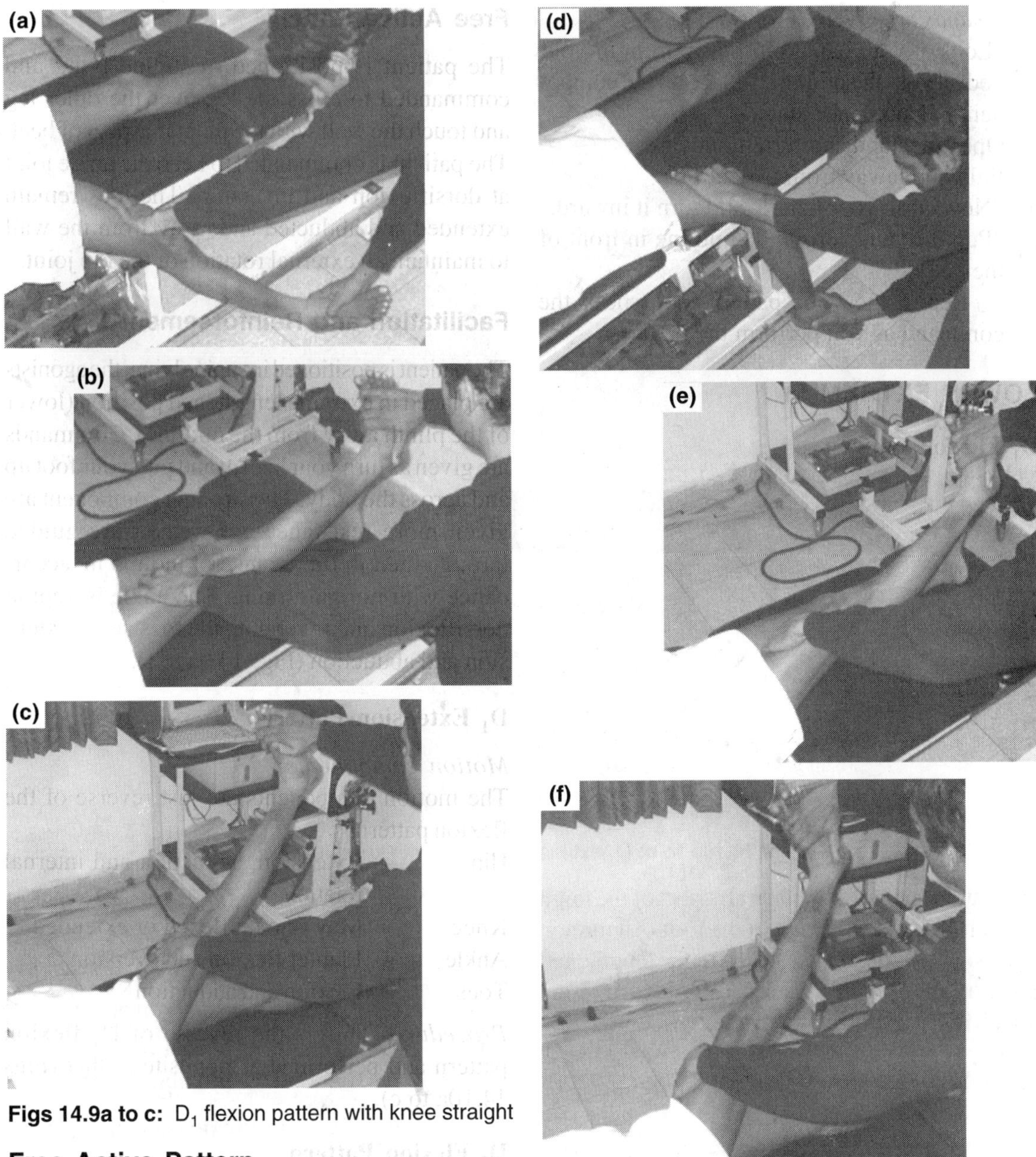

Figs 14.9a to c: D_1 flexion pattern with knee straight

Free Active Pattern

The patient is positioned in supine lying and agonists are placed in extreme lengthened position then commands are given as turn your heel outward and pull the limb up away from the midline as far as possible. The ankle is kept at dorsiflexion and eversion, toes are at extension and abduction.

Figs 14.9d to f: D_1 Flexion pattern with knee flexion

Facilitation and Reinforcement

The patient is positioned in supine lying, therapist stands at the same side of the limb and places

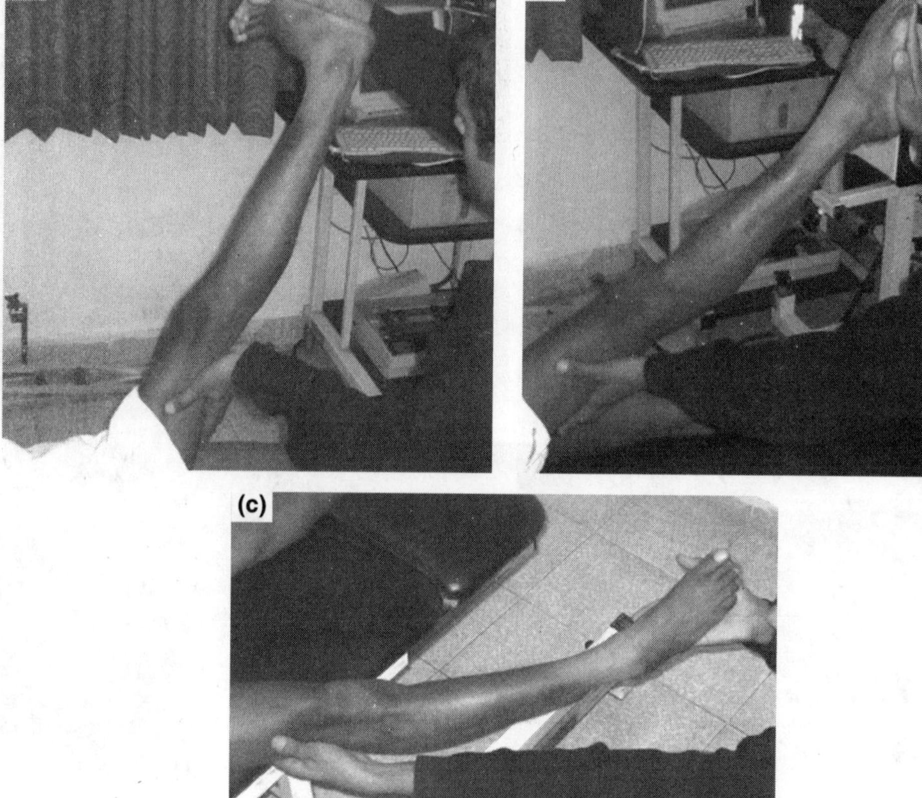

Figs 14.10a to c: D_1 extension pattern with knee extension

one hand over the anterolateral aspect of the thigh and other over the dorsum of the foot. All motion components are placed in extreme lengthened position and are given a stretch stimulus or reflex which is synchronized with an active contraction. Therapist commands the patient to push the hands and take the limb up across the midline. All stronger proximal and distal components are resisted but weaker distal components are guided through their optimal range of motion in accordance with their normal timing (Figs 14.11a to c).

D_2 Extension Pattern

Motion components: The motion components are just reverse of the flexion pattern of Diagonal D_2.

Hip	– Extension, adduction and external rotation
Knee	– May remain extended or flexed
Ankle	– Planterflexion with inversion
Toes	– Flexion with adduction
	– Rotation toward tibial side.

Diagonal (D_1) Flexion and extension pattern with knee straight

Motion components: Same as D_1 Flexion and D_1 Extension.

Position of the patient–Standing.

Position of the therapist–Standing in front of the patient.

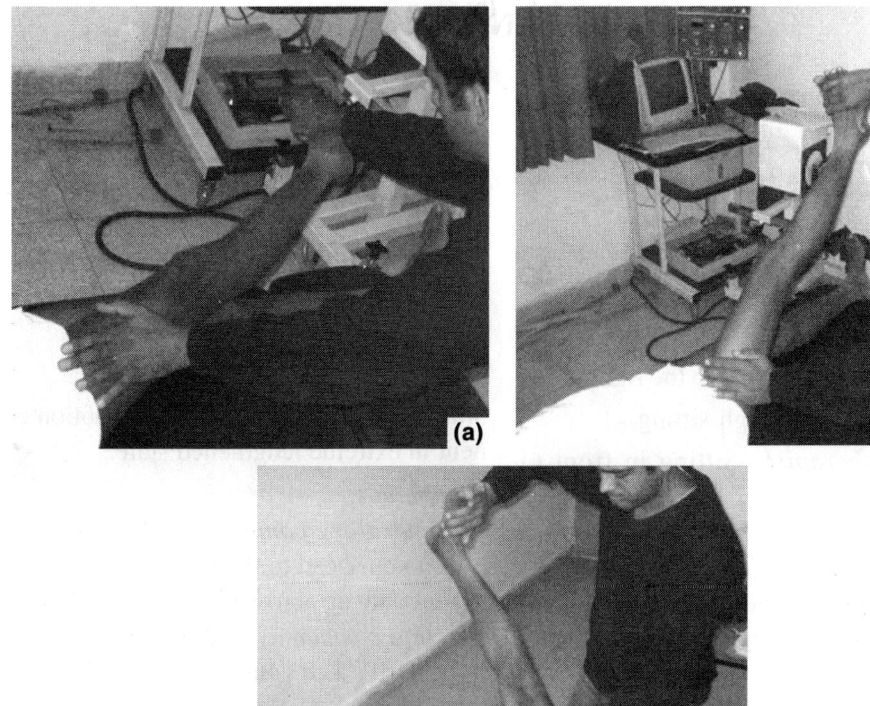

Figs 14.11a to c: D_2 flexion pattern

Commands are given as follows:

1. "Place the limb backward!", "Point your toes down!" (This position places all the flexion components in extreme lengthened state).
2. "Rotate the limb externally, pull the toes up and in! Turn your heel!"
3. "Take the foot up across the midline!"
4. "Now point the toes down, outward and turn the heel in!"
5. "Take the foot down away from the midline toward the initial position!"
6. Now perform the same and speak the commands as you perform.

Diagonal D_2 Flexion and extension pattern with knee straight

Motion components: Same as D_2 Flexion and Extension.

Position of the patient–Standing.

Position of the therapist–Standing in front of the patient.

Commands are given as follows:

1. Ready (Place your limb backward across the midline, point the toes down).
2. "Turn the heel out! Point the toes up and out!"
3. Take the foot up and away from midline.
4. Turn the heel in and point the toes down and in.
5. Take the foot down, across the midline.
   Repeat the same pattern and speak the commands as you perform.

HEAD AND NECK

FLEXION WITH ROTATION TO THE RIGHT

Free Active Motion

Motion components:
- Rotation of head (atlanto occipital joint) to the right.
- Rotation of cervical spine to right.
- Flexion of the cervical spine to the right.

Position of the patient—High sitting.

Position of the therapist—Sitting in front of patient.

Commands:
- *Preparatory commands* are given to make the patient understand as follows—You are going to turn your head to the right then you have to pull it down to touch the right chest with your chin.
- *Action commands*—"Turn your head!", "Pull your chin down!" and "Pull your head down!"

  Repeat the same pattern and speak the commands as you perform.

Facilitation and Reinforcement

Position the patient in supine lying take the head and neck out of plinth. Therapist stands at the head of patient, grasps the occiput by one hand and chin by other hand. Place all the components in extreme lengthened position.

Commands:
- *Preparatory command*—You are going to turn your head to the right then you have to pull it down to touch the right chest with your chin.
- *Action commands*—Now "Turn your head!", "Pull your chin down!" and "Pull your head down!"

  Therapist resists all the strong components while assists the weak components through their optimal range of motion in accordance with normal timing.

EXTENSION WITH ROTATION TO THE LEFT

Free Active Motion

Motion components:
- Rotation of the head to the left.
- Rotation of the neck to the left.
- Extension of the neck.

Starting position—Place all the motion component in extreme lengthened state.

Commands:
- *Preparatory commands*—You are going to turn your head to the left then you have to lift your chin up across the midline.
- *Action commands*—Now "Turn your head to the left!", "Lift your chin up!", "Push your head back".

  Repeat the same pattern and speak the commands as you perform.

Facilitation and Reinforcement

Position of patient is supine lying, therapist stands above the head at the edge of treatment table. Therapist grasps the occiput by left hand and chin by the right hand.

Place all the motion components in the extreme lengthened state.

Commands:
- *Preparatory command*—You are going to turn your head to the left then you have to lift your chin up across the midline.
- *Action commands*—Now "Turn your head to the left!", "Lift your chin up!" and "Push your head back!"

  Therapist resists the stronger components of neck extension but assists weaker component through their optimal range of motion in accordance with normal timing.

UPPER TRUNK

FLEXION WITH ROTATION TO THE RIGHT

Free Active Motion

Motion components:
- Rotation of the head to the right.
- Flexion with rotation of the cervical spine to the right.
- Flexion with rotation of the thoracic spine to the right.

Position of patient—Supine lying, the right upper extremity is placed at the initial position of D_1 Extension pattern, while left hand holds the right wrist.

Position of therapist—Standing at the right side of the patient.

Commands:
- *Preparatory command*—You are going to turn your head to the right and then you have to pull yourself up and over toward your right hip joint.
- *Action command*—Now "Pull yourself up!", "Turn toward right!", "Pull your chin down!", "Pull your head down!" and "Pull your arms toward your right hip!"

Repeat the same pattern and speak the commands as you perform.

Facilitation and Reinforcement

Position of patient and therapist remains same as free active motion.

Action command: "Pull yourself up!", "Turn toward right!", "Pull your chin down!", "Pull your head down!" and "Pull your arms toward your right hip joint!"

The therapist resists all the strong component but assists the weak distal components through their optimal range of motion in accordance with normal timing.

EXTENSION WITH ROTATION TO THE LEFT

Facilitation and Reinforcement

Motion components:
- Rotation of head to the left.
- Extension with rotation of cervical spine to the left.
- Extension with rotation of the thoracic spine to the left.

Position of patient—Supine. The left hand is placed at the right hip joint and right hand grasps it at the wrist joint.

Position of therapist—Stands at the left side of the patient, places right hand over the occiput while left hand is used to grasp the patient's left hand.

Commands:
- *Preparatory command*—You are going to turn your head up, then pull your arm up away from the midline toward the left shoulder.
- *Action command*—"Push my hands up!", "Turn toward left", "Pull your arm toward left across the away from the midline!" and "Straighten your back!"

The therapist resists all the strong components but assists the weak components through their optimal range of motion accordance with normal timing.

CHAPTER-15

Mat Activities

INTRODUCTION

A normal individual performs activities such as rolling, getting up from lying position etc. independently day to day life usually in the bed or floor. But a person with physical impairment finds difficult to do so. Therapist teaches methods and techniques to carry out such activities independently usually on mat as it provide large base of support (BOS) and low center of gravity (COG), hence known as mat activities. These activities are also prerequisite for independent ambulation.

An exercise mat is a good surface firmer than most beds, making it an easier surface to learn mat activities. At the same time, a mat should be soft enough to allow the inevitable tumbles without injury.

COMMON MAT ACTIVITIES

These activities are:
  i. Rolling
  ii. Prone on elbows
  iii. Prone on hands position
  iv. Hook lying.
  v. Bridging
  vi. Quadruped position.
  vii. Sitting: a. Long
                 b. Short
  viii. Kneeling
  ix. Half kneeling.

Rolling

It is roll over from supine to side lying/prone or from prone to side lying/supine.

Rolling generally progresses from log rolling to segmental rolling. Log rolling produces movement of the entire trunk as a unit around the longitudinal axis of the body. Segmental rolling is a progression from log rolling. In segmental rolling either the upper or the lower segment of the trunk moves independently while the other is stabilized.

Techniques to facilitate rolling are:
a. Flexion of the head and neck with rotation may used to assist movt. from supine to prone positions.
b. Extension of the head and neck with rotation may be used to assist movement from prone to supine positions.
c. Both the hands are clasped, elbow fully extended and shoulder flexed upto 100–110°. Patient creates momentum by swinging the extremities from side to side (Fig. 15.1).

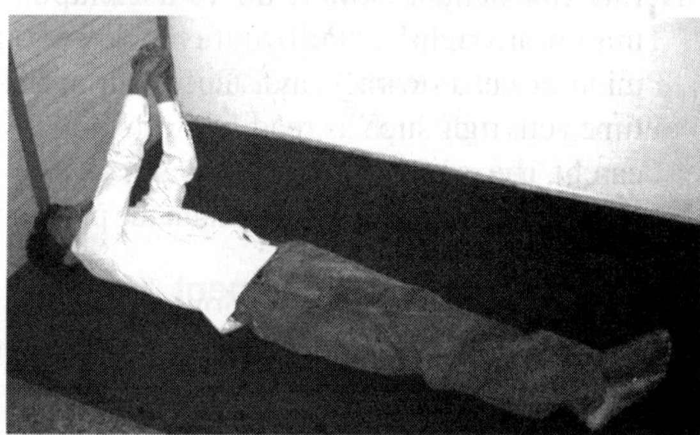

Fig. 15.1: Rolling

d. Crossing the legs one over the other also facilitates in rolling. The upper leg is towards the direction of rolling. For e.g., if a patient wants to roll towards the right side, the left leg should over the right one.
e. PNF patterns such as U/E – D_1 flexion and D_2 extension and L/E – D_1 flexion can also be used to facilitate rolling.

Prone–on–Elbows

This position provides weight bearing on elbows and forearm. The posture provides stability of glenohumeral joint co-contraction of scapular musculature, and improving head and neck control (Fig. 15.2).

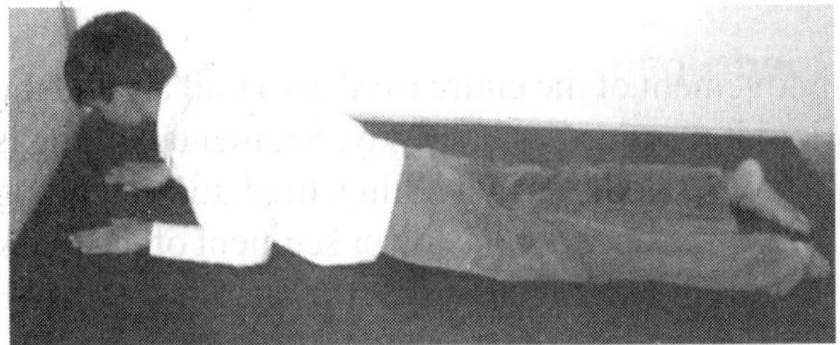

Fig. 15.2: Prone on elbows

Prone on elbows should cautiously be used in patients with:

- Cardiac or respirating problems.
- Shoulder or elbow pathology
- Marked hip flexor tightness and contracture
- Excessive lordosis of lumbar spine.

The position should progress in the following manner:

a. Initially patient should try to assume and maintain the position for few to several minutes with or without assistance. During this time activities such as reading, watching TV can be incorporated.
b. Patient should then try to maintain the position independently.
c. Weight shift in lateral directions should then be started which may progress to difficult anterior posterior directions also.
d. Activities such as peg lifting, writing, page turning (during reading), ball squeezing etc. can be used (contact guarding and verbal cues are given wherever necessary).

Prone on Hands

This is the intermediate position between the prone on elbows and quadruped positions. From prone on elbows position, patient fully extends his elbows. In this position BOS reduces and COG becomes more higher. The weight is born on hands, wrists, elbows and shoulders (Fig. 15.3).

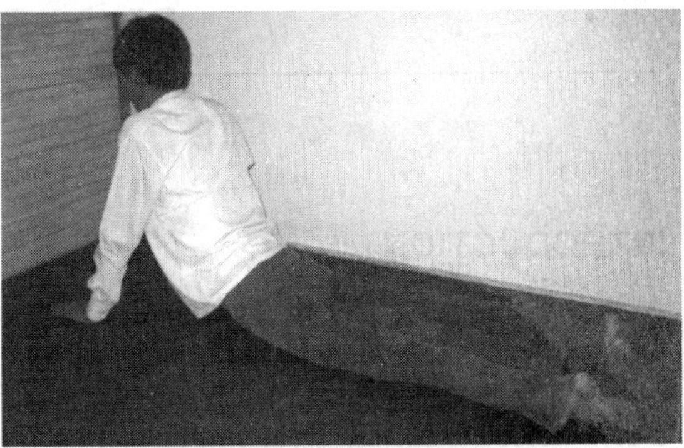

Fig. 15.3: Prone on hands

Precautions for this position is same as for prone on elbows.

Progression takes place in the following manner:

a. Initially patient should try to assume and maintain the position for few to several minutes with/without assistance.
b. Patient should then try to maintain the position independently.
c. Weight shift in lateral directions should then be incorporated.
d. Final step is performed in the form of push ups in prone position which is also helpful in increasing strength of triceps, brachii and pectoralis major.

Clinical implications of prone–on–elbows and prone–on–hands position: Both of these positions are carried over to do floor–to–stand transitions by paraplegic patients.

Hook Lying

The patient is in supine position with hips and knees flexed and feet flat on the floor or mat surface. In this position BOS is large and COG is lower than earlier two positions. Patient performs lower trunk rotation by swinging the lower extremity side to side (Fig. 15.4).

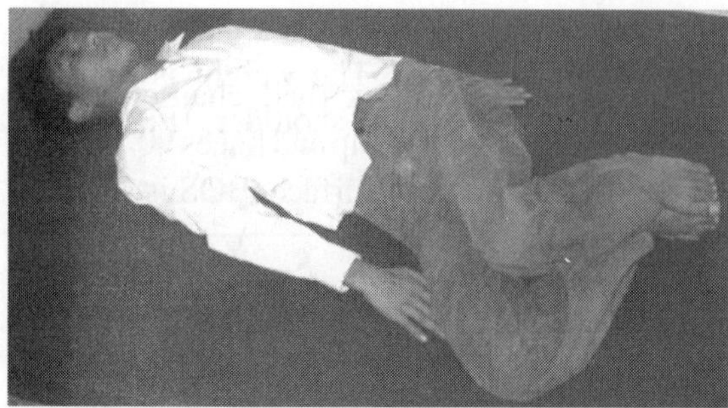

Fig. 15.4: Hook lying

Contanet guarding and verbal cues may be used and gradually weaned off as the progression takes place.

Gradual Resistance for lower extremity movement and decrease knee and hip flexion may also be used to increase the level of activity.

Bridging

The patient is in hook lying position, elevates his pelvis off the mat surface. In this position BOS reduces and COG becomes higher (Fig. 15.5).

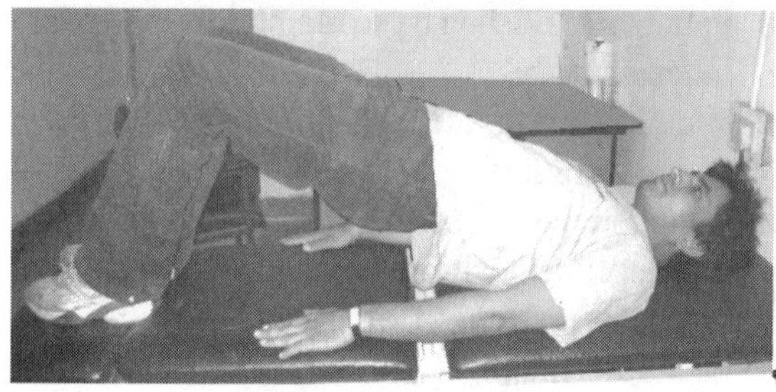

Fig. 15.5: Bridging

Progression of the activity takes place in following sequence:

a. Initially patient assumes and maintains position with or without assistance.
b. Independent maintenance of the position.
c. Elevation of the pelvis off the mat then again depressing it on the mat, is performed several times.
d. Resistance can be given on the anterior superior iliac spine.
e. Decrease the angle of hip and knee flexion.

Clinical implications of bridging:
• Improves pelvic mobility
• Strengthens low back and hip extensors.
• Helpful for using bed pan
• Relieves pressure
• Lower body dressing (Manual contact and verbal cues are provided as per need).

Quadruped

In this position the patient bears weight on all four limbs (Fig. 15.6).

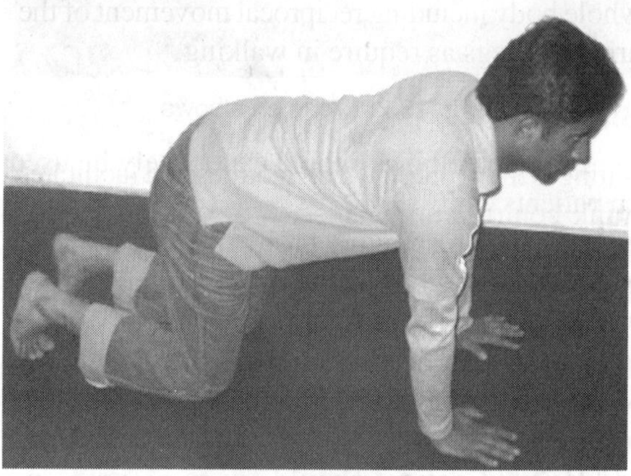

Fig. 15.6: Quadruped

The BOS is smaller the COG is higher than the bridging position.

Patient usually goes in quadruped position from prone– on–elbows or prone on hands position.

Progression of the activity takes place in the following sequence:

a. Initially patient assumes and maintains the position with assistance for few minutes.
b. Patient should then try to maintain the position independently for several minutes.
c. Weight shifts in forward, backward and side to side direction can be incorporated.
d. Raising of one of upper limb and bearing weight on rest of the 3 limbs.
e. Raising of one of upper limb and contralateral lower limb.

Increase the time gradually for d and e.

Clinical implications
- Patient weight bearing on lower extremity joints (step towards weight bearing in erect positions)
- Strength and mobility required for so many functional activities by upper extremities.

Functional activities such as cleaning floor, gardening (planting seeds and weeding) can be used to teach static and dynamic stability of quadruped position.

When balance and stability have been achieved in quadruped, crawling may be started. This activity facilitates the co-ordination of the whole body including reciprocal movement of the arms and legs as require in walking.

Sitting

Sitting is the position which requires and facilitates trunk control and balance. It also allows some amount of weight to be born by upper extremity. There are 2 forms of sitting needed to be practiced.
a. Long sitting.
b. Short sitting.

Long Sitting

Patient sits with knees fully extended; hips flexed hands may or may not support the upper body weight (hands may be positioned laterally, posteriorly or anteriorly with relation to pelvis) (Fig. 15.7).

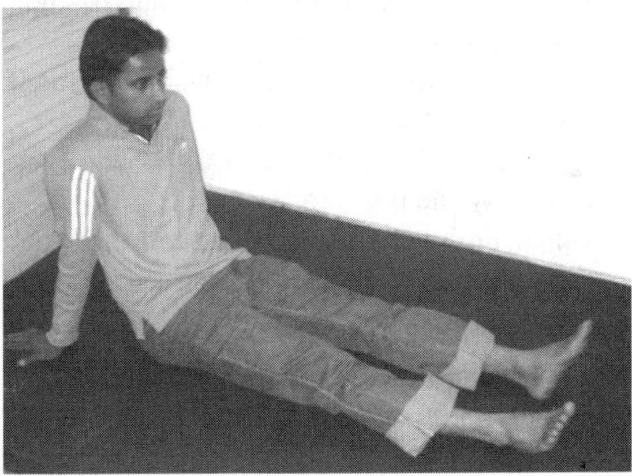

Fig. 15.7: Long sitting

Short Sitting

Patient sits on high surface (bed, chair etc) with knees at the edge making hip and knees 90° flexed and feet flat on the floor surface. BOS is smaller than long sitting.

Progression of the both positions may take place in following sequence—(patient usually progresses from long sitting to short sitting).
a. Initially patient assumes and maintains position with support.
b. Patient raises one hand placing the weight on other one. He repeats the movement with other hand.
c. Patient sits independently without any external or hand support.
d. Patient performs activities such as ball throwing (light to heavy weight), clapping overhead etc.
e. Push ups in both type of sittings should be performed with or without push up blocks. Increase the number of repetitions gradually.

Kneeling

Patient comes into kneeling position (hips extended and knees flexed at 90°) from quadruped position and bears weight on both the joint. This position also improves trunk pelvis control and upright balance. The BOS is smaller and COG is higher as compared to sitting (Fig. 15.8).

Progression may take place in following manner:
a. Initially patient assumes and maintains position with assistance for few seconds.
b. Patient assumes and maintains position independently for few minutes.
c. Patient shifts weight from one to other knee.
d. Ball throwing and other activities should be performed.
e. Kneel walking would be the final progression for the kneeling position (Fig. 15.9).

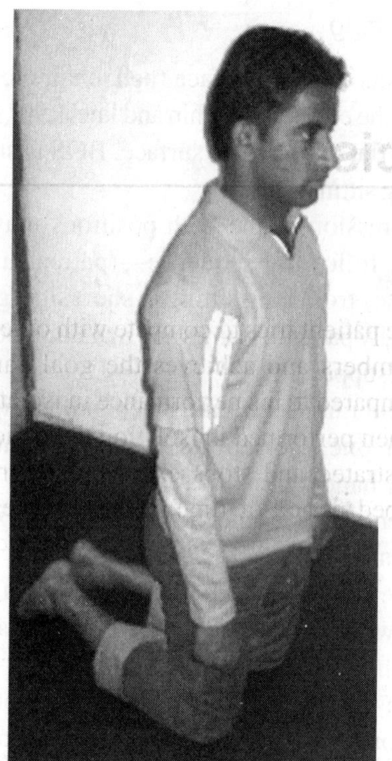

Fig. 15.8: Kneeling

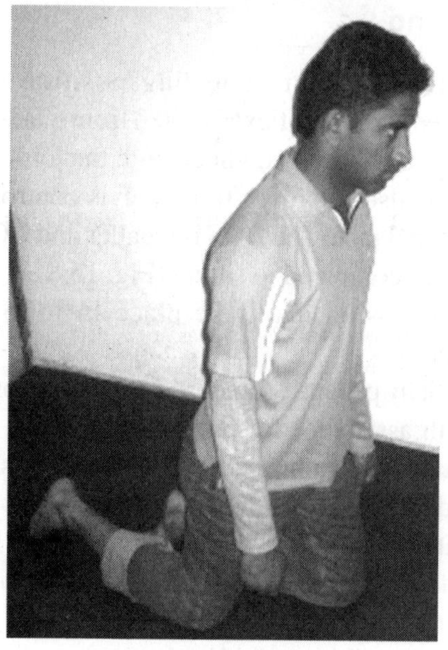

Fig. 15.9: Kneel walking

Half Kneeling

Patient assumes the position as shown in Figure 15.10. The BOS is larger than kneeling while COG is same. The limb which lies posteriorly bears more weight. This position improves pelvic control (lateral), hip extension and ankle and knee movement.

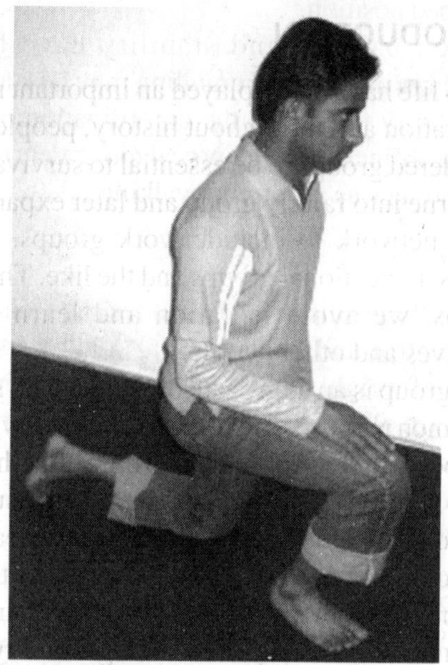

Fig. 15.10: Half kneeling

Progression takes place in the following manner:

a. Initially patient assumes and maintains position with support.
b. Patient then tries to maintain position without support and for longer period of time.
c. Weight shift from one limb to other and even anteriorly and posteriorly.
d. Upper limb activities such as ball throwing (light to heavy weight) peg lifting and clapping etc.

(**Note:** Contact guarding/manual support is given wherever necessary in all the positions or activities).

CHAPTER-16

Group Exercises

INTRODUCTION

Group life has always played an important role in civilization and throughout history, people have considered groups to be essential to survival. We are borne into family group and later expand our social network to include work groups, social groups, recreational groups and the like. Through groups, we avoid isolation and learn about ourselves and other people.

A group is an aggregate of people who shares a common purpose which can be attained by group members interacting and working together. In group exercise the patient gets a measure of individual attention and at the same time learns to take some responsibility for his own effort while working with others. A group for exercise usually comprises of 6–8 patients having same type of disability and would benefit from exercises which are similar in character. There is also consideration for modification of exercise in terms of repetition, range, speed etc. to suit the need of every member of the group.

All group members perform the exercises together and get supervised by the therapist for any change and modification in the performance.

Rationale for Doing Exercises in Group

1. The patient gets stimulation from other members of the group to perform the exercise in a more better way.
2. The patient does not feel isolated and depressed which is very common due to disability.
3. The patient tries to compete with other group members and achieves the goal earlier as compared to his performance in isolation.
4. When performed in isolation the patient gets frustrated and stops exercises before prescribed period of time as he observes no or little improvement but in group exercises he observes other's improvement and tries to achieve for himself.
5. The therapist saves time and many patients can be treated simultaneously. It is very practical for the setting where therapist to patient ratio is more.
6. The patient develops in himself a sense of responsibility which further helps in home exercise program.
7. The patient leaves to improve interpersonal relationship which is usually affected after disability.

Disadvantages of Group Exercises

Group exercises might not always be successful due to:
- Improper selection of patients.
- More or uncontrolled number of group members.
- Poor explanation of the instruction etc.

Formation of group:
- Space and other requirements.
- Selection of patients.
- Number of patients.
- Instruction to patients.
- Group types and levels.

- *Space and other requirements:* Big space is an essential prerequisite for group exercises so that multiple number of patients can perform the exercises together at one place. A big hall with 6–8 plinths or beds and space for mat activities for 6–8 persons is more practical.

  Equipment such as dumbells, sand bags, therabands etc. should also be in multiple numbers.

  Instrumental music or music of other type which suits the rhythm of exercise is always preferred. All the walls of exercise room or hall should be provided with big mirrors to give visual feedback of patient's performance.

- *Selection of patients:* Patients should be selected as per the similarities between their impairments and also the therapeutic needs.

  Clinically patient who has undergone number of individual sessions and expected to do home exercise program, can be selected as a candidate for group exercises.

  If patient does not fit to any of the group its better to continue with the individual treatment.

- *Number of patients:* As already discussed an ideal choice is between 6–8 patients per group, if this number exceeds then it would be difficult for the therapist to explain the instructions properly and to supervise their performance. And if the number of patients are less than 6 than it would not give the effect of group and all the benefits of group may not be obtained.

- *Instructions to the patients:* Therapist should discuss the importance of group exercises. He should give clear instructions to all the group members together in group exercise room or hall. It would be better if therapist demonstrates the exercises to be performed. In some set up video films of the group exercises prior to start the session is also preferred. Written instructions or hand outs can also be used to impart clear understanding of the group exercises.

- *Group types and levels:* Different types of groups are formed on the basis of age, sex, type of impairment, body part involved; patients are assigned to the respective type of group.

  Levels of groups are formed on the basis of intensity and nature of exercises. As the patient progresses, his level may be changed accordingly.

CHAPTER-17

Balance and Coordination Exercise

BALANCE

INTRODUCTION

The most traditional definition of balance is the ability to maintain one's center of gravity over a base of support. But recent researches have changed this definition, emphasizing on various factors affecting balance.

Balance is now defined as the state of physical equilibrium (maintenance of one's center of gravity) achieved when vestibular, visual and somatosensory information which is integrated in the central nervous system.

Constraint in maintenance of balance:
- Neuromuscular coordination deficits.
- Loss of sensory acquity.
- Musculoskeletal limitations.
- Sensory organization deficits.
- Fine motor control impairment.
- Inability to adapt motor responses.
- Feed forward or predictive deficits.
- Cognitive deficits.

Anatomical lesions leading to balance dysfunction:
- Lesions of the motor cortex.
- Lesions of corticospinal tract.
- Lesions of sensory pathways including cerebellum.
- Lesions of vestibular system.
- Loss of compensatory pathways such as vision.

Diagnostic conditions manifested by balance dysfunction:
- Stroke.
- Guillain Barré syndrome.
- Multiple scelerosis.
- Peripheral lesions—receptors in the ear, vestibular nerve.
- Ataxia.
- Head injury etc.

Maintaining balance is a complex interaction of the neuromuscular and musculoskeletal systems. Difficulty in maintaining balance may result in apprehension about movement or fear of falling.

Motor or Movement Strategies

These are normal movement patterns used to counteract balance perturbation or disturbances.

i. *Ankle strategy*—involves shifting the centre of gravity (CoG) forward and backward by activating muscles in a distal-to-proximal sequence. With forward sway, gastrocnemius is activated first, followed by hamstrings, then paraspinal muscles (Fig. 17.1). With backward sway, the anterior tibialis is activated first, followed by quadriceps, then abdominals.

This strategy is most commonly used when disturbances are small within the base of support.

ii. *Hip strategy*—involves shifts in the CoG by flexing or extending the hips. It has a proximal pattern of muscle activation. With forward sway, abdominals are activated first, followed by quadriceps (Fig. 17.2). With

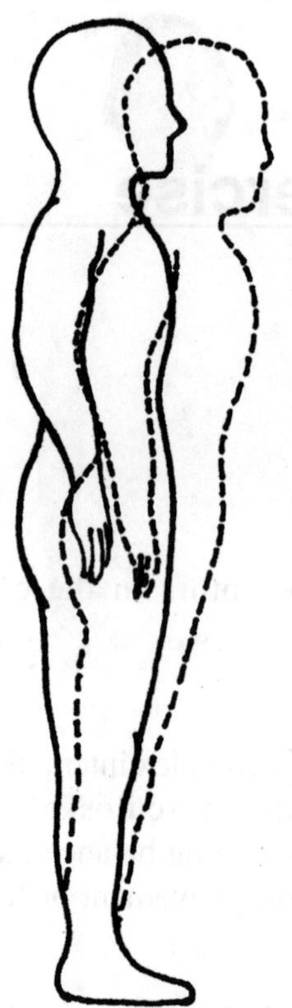

Fig. 17.1: Ankle strategy

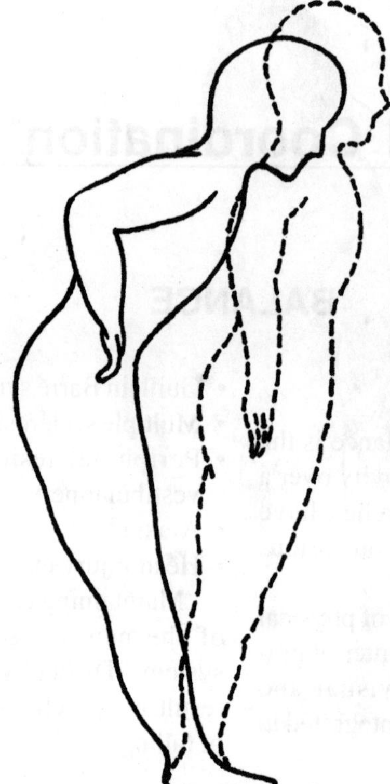

Fig. 17.2: Hip strategy

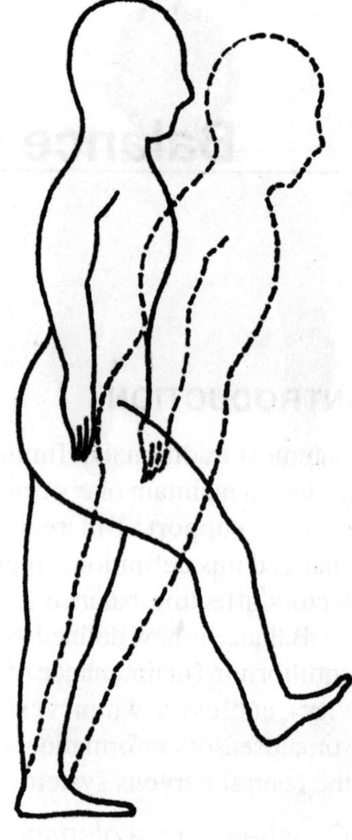

Fig. 17.3: Stepping strategy

backward sway, paraspinal muscles are activated first followed by hamstrings.

With sideward sway gluteus medius is primarily activated. This strategy is seen when a greater force challenges balance or when the support surface for the feet is small.

iii. *Stepping strategy*—realigning the base of support with a stepping movement. Stepping can be in forward backward or lateral direction (Fig. 17.3).

This strategy is used in response to fast and large balance disturbances.

iv. *Suspensory strategy*—lowering the center of gravity towards the base of support, i.e. flexion of the hip, knee and ankle (Fig. 17.4).

This strategy is used during standing or in ambulation to lower the body center of gravity closer to the base of support, which provide more stability. For e.g.: Cricketer uses this strategy while catching ball.

Evaluation for Balance Dysfunction

It is important to determine which component of balance is the cause of dysfunction. Evaluating the cause of balance dysfunction guides the therapist in development of treatment.

Points of Evaluation

- Patient's history.
- Association with head movement.
- Limitation of functional mobility.
- Falling tendency.
- Vertigo/nausea.
- Musculoskeletal system (ROM and Muscle strength).
- Sensory system:
  - vestibular

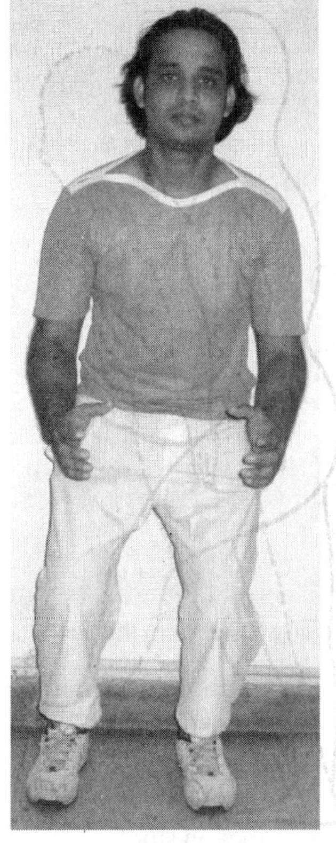

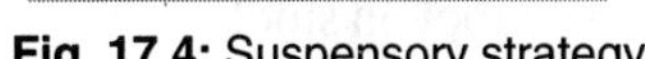

Fig. 17.4: Suspensory strategy

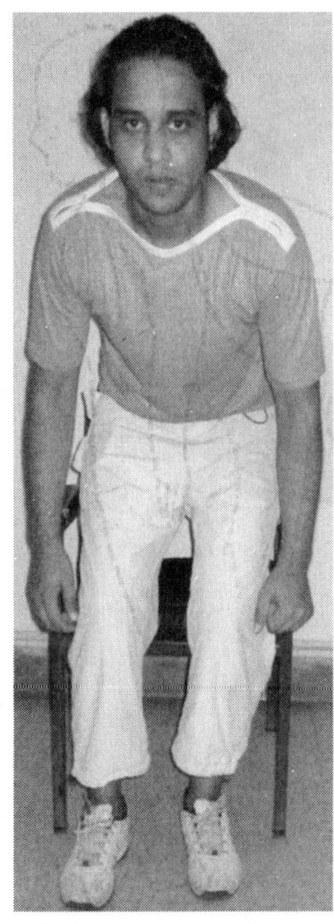

Fig. 17.5: Sit to stand

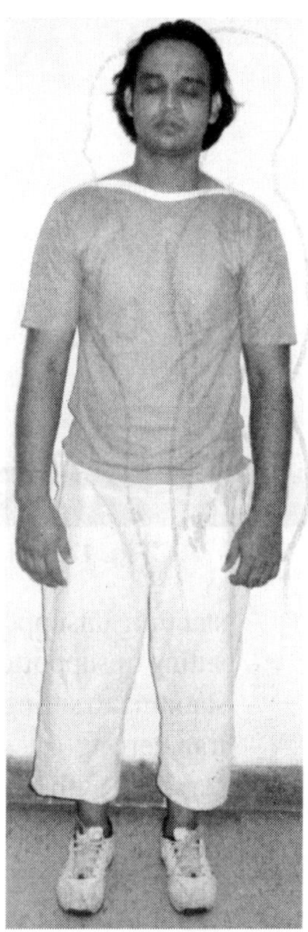

Fig. 17.6: Romberg's test

- visual and somatosensory (touch, proprioception, kinesthesia etc.)
- Motor/movement strategies
  - present or normal
  - present but limited or delayed
  - present but inappropriate for the particular context or situation
  - abnormal
  - absent.
- Function activity/position such as
  - rolling
  - supine-to-sitting
  - stable sitting
  - sit-to-stand (Fig. 17.5)
  - transfers
  - ambulation
  - climbing stairs.
    [*Romberg test (standing balance with eyes closed) suggests a somatosensory problem] (Fig. 17.6).

Hall pike test—The patient is in long sitting position on plinth and instructed to move into supine position. During this movement the therapist guides the head into extended and rotated (45°) off the end of the cervical spine. On reaching supine with the head extended and rotated, the therapist observes for the presence of nystagmus and asks how patient feels (Fig. 17.7).

Repeat the test again with other side of rotation. Complaints of vertigo, nausea and the presence of nystagmus are indication of vestibular dysfunction.

a. *Berg-balance scale*—This ordinal scale (0-4: 0—unable to perform, 4—able to perform the task safely and independently). Evaluates patient performance on 14 tasks commonly performed in day-to-day life.

Items of the scale are:
- sitting to standing

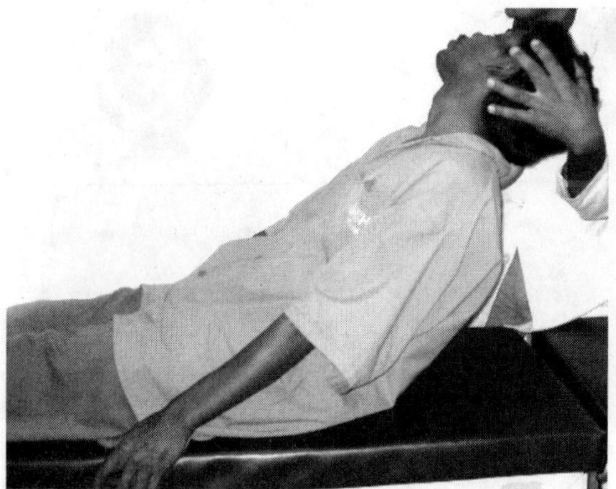

Fig. 17.7: Hall Pike test

– standing unsupported
– sitting unsupported
– standing to sitting
– transferring
– standing with eyes closed
– standing with feet together (Fig. 17.8)

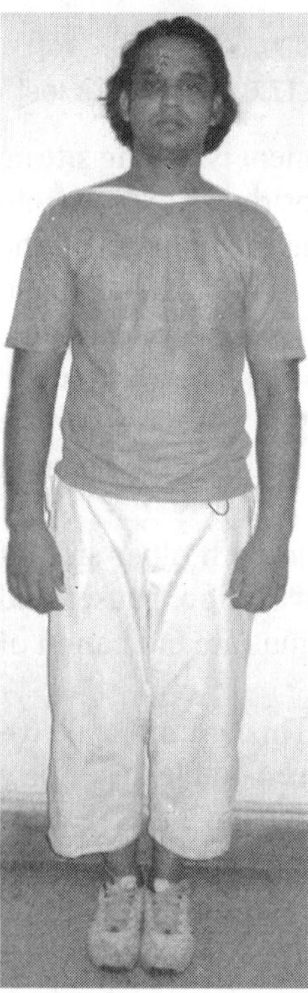

Fig. 17.8: Standing with feet together

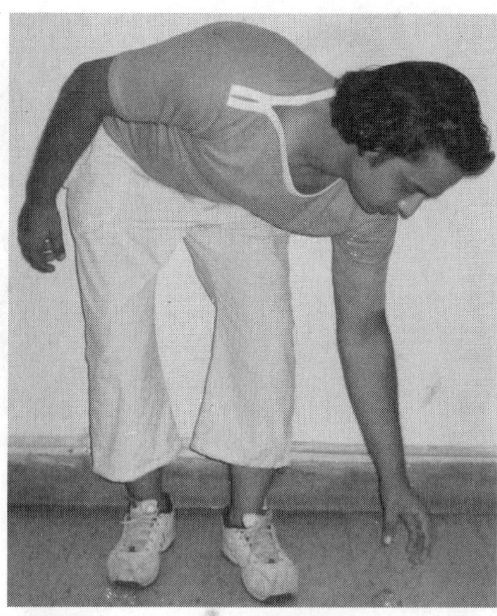

Fig. 17.9: Retrieving object from the floor

– reaching forward without stretched arm
– retrieving object from floor (Fig. 17.9)
– turning to look behind (Fig. 17.10)
– turning 360°
– placing alternate foot on stool
– standing with one foot in front (Fig. 17.11)
– standing on one foot (Fig. 17.12).

b. *Functional reach test*—This test uses a yardstick/marked scale, mounted onto a wall at the height of patient acromion process. The patient stands barefoot in a normal, relaxed stance on footmark, beside the wall (where yardstick is mounted).

The patient then extends one arm, with hand made into fist. Placement of the third metacarpal along the yardstick is recorded. The patient then reaches forward as far as possible without losing balance or take a step forward. Placement of the third metacarpal is again recorded (Figs 17.13a and b).

(The upper extremity is not allowed to touch the wall during the procedure).

Functional reach = Final measurement – Initial measurement

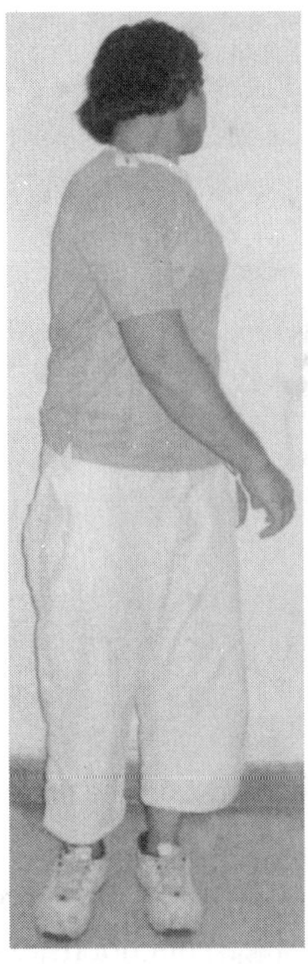

Fig. 17.10: Turning to look behind

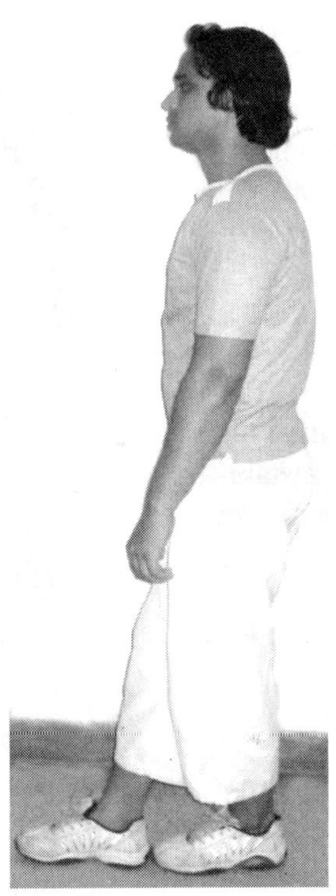

Fig. 17.11: Standing with one foot in front

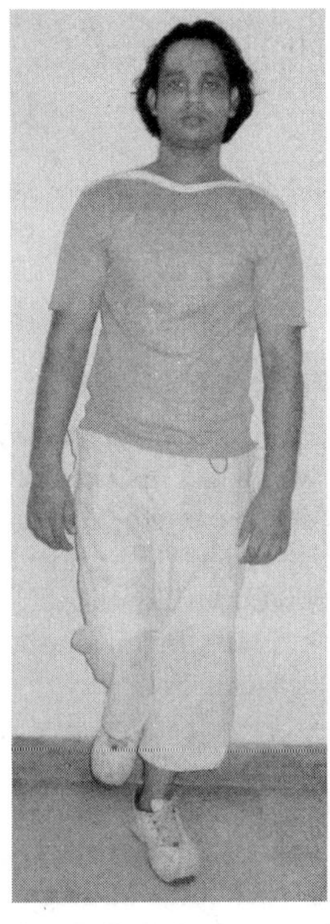

Fig. 17.12: Standing on one foot

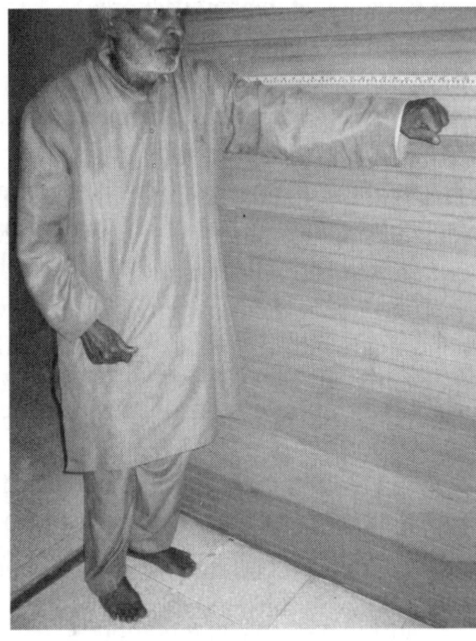

Fig. 17.13a: Functional reach test (initial position)

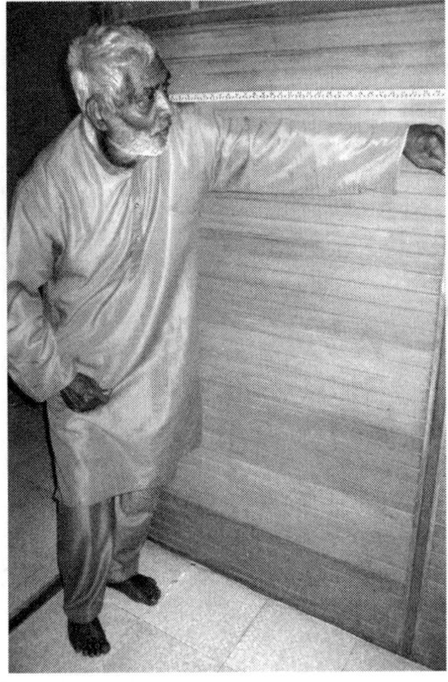

Fig. 17.13b: Functional reach test (final position)

Duncan *et al.* (1990) reported normal functional reach as per the age:

20-40 years old : 16.73 inches (men)
                   14.64 inches (women)
41-69 years old : 14.98 inches (men)
                   13.81 inches (women)
70-87 years old : 13.16 inches (men)
                   10.47 inches (women).

Balance Exercises

i. *Exercises for weakness*—The muscles which are responsible for postural instability, needs to be strong. This can be achieved by variety of therapeutic exercises. Such as:
   - Active exercises
   - PNF (Proprioceptive Neuromuscular facilitation.
   - PRE (Progressive resistive exercise)
   - Isokinetic etc.

ii. *Exercises for movement strategies*—If patient exhibits weakness or prior control in a particular strategy, he should practice positions which facilitate the activation of muscles require for that strategy.

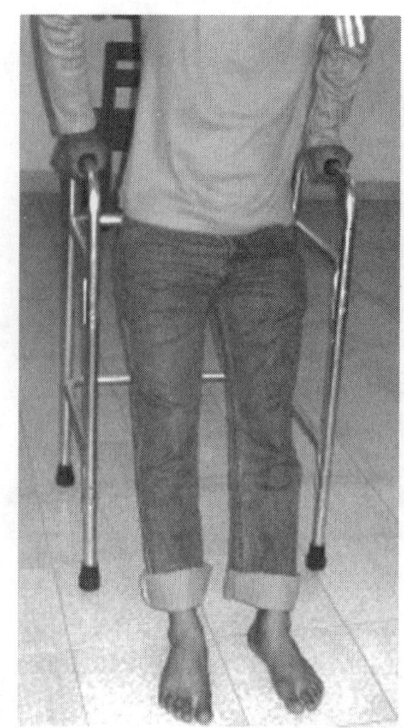

Fig. 17.15: Facilitation of ankle dorsiflexors with walker

For e.g. Patient having poor dorsiflexors finds difficulty in using ankle strategy for balance. He should practice following positions to facilitate the dorsiflexors.

a. Sitting on therapeutic ball with feet on the floor, ball is rolled posteriorly by the therapist, dorsiflexors get activated (equilibrium response) (Fig. 17.14).

b. Standing in parallel bar or walker, patient practices leaning posteriorly with small range in starting and then gradually increasing the range. Same facilitation is achieved (Fig. 17.15).

iii. *Static balance exercises*—These are performed to improve control in sitting and standing positions.

Patient follows the following sequence for developing sitting or standing control (he may skip any step in which he has good control).

a. *Sitting:*
   - sitting with two hands support
   - sitting with one hand support
   - sitting unsupported

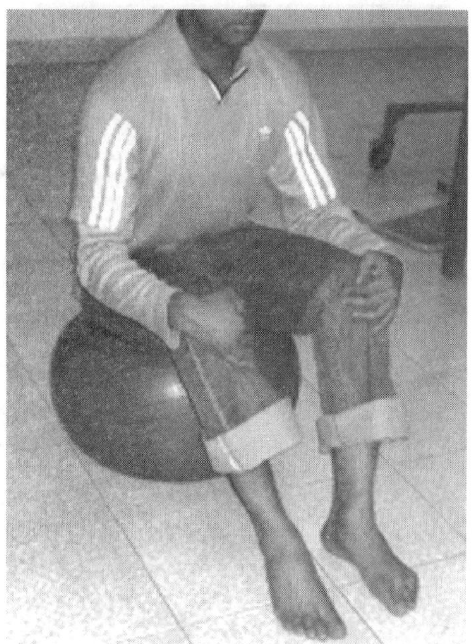

Fig. 17.14: Facilitation of ankle dorsiflexors on therapeutic ball

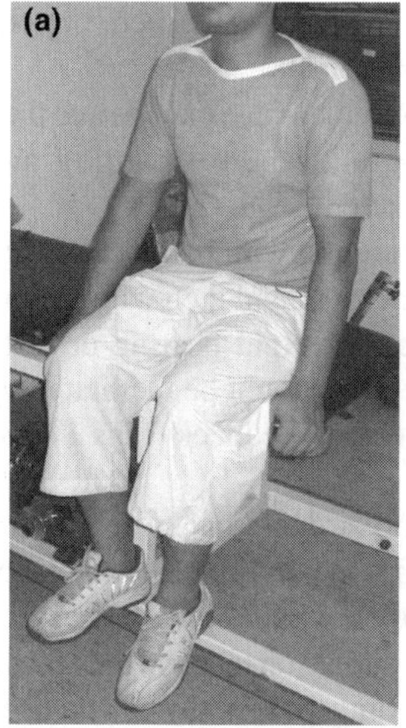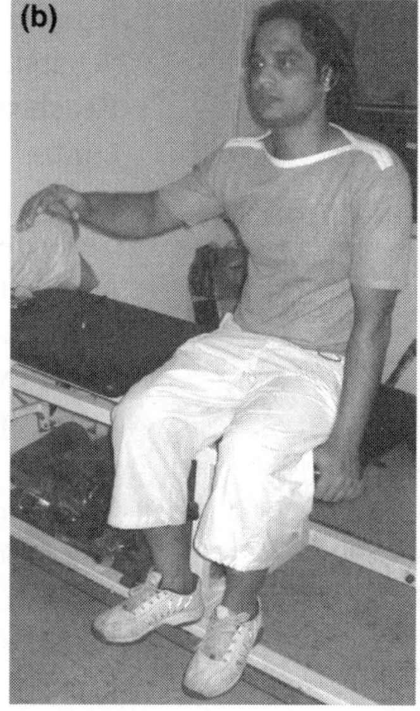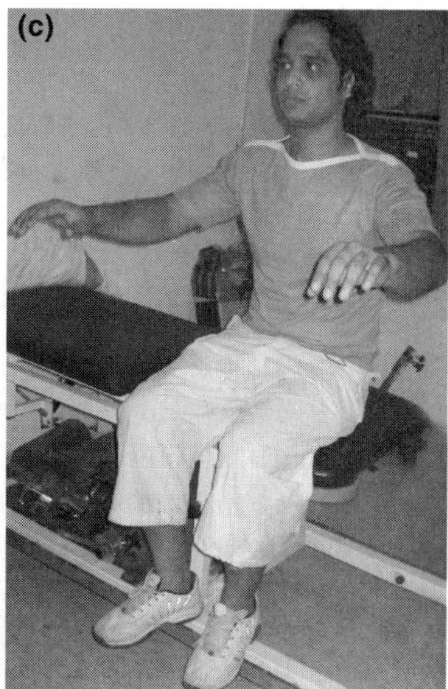

Figs 17.16a to c: (a) Sitting with both hand support, (b) Sitting with one hand support, and (c) Sitting without hand support

- change the sitting surface (hard to soft) (Figs 17.16a to c).
  b. *Standing:*
    - standing in parallel bar with two hands support (Fig. 17.17a)
    - standing with one hand support (Fig. 17.17b)
    - standing unsupported (Fig. 17.17c)
    - change the base of support (wider to narrower)
    - tandem standing (one foot in front of other) (Fig. 17.17d)
    - standing on one leg (Fig. 17.17e).

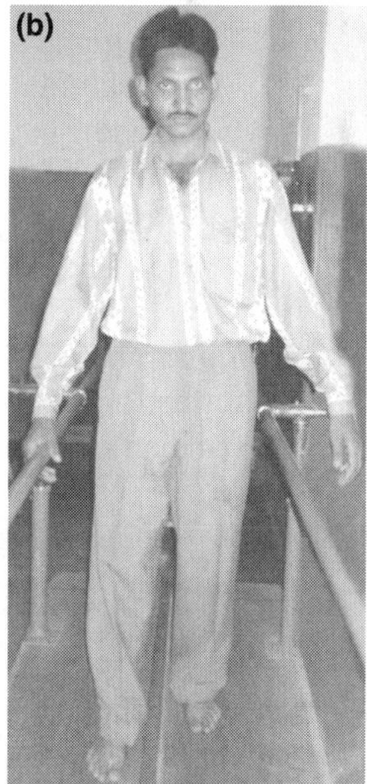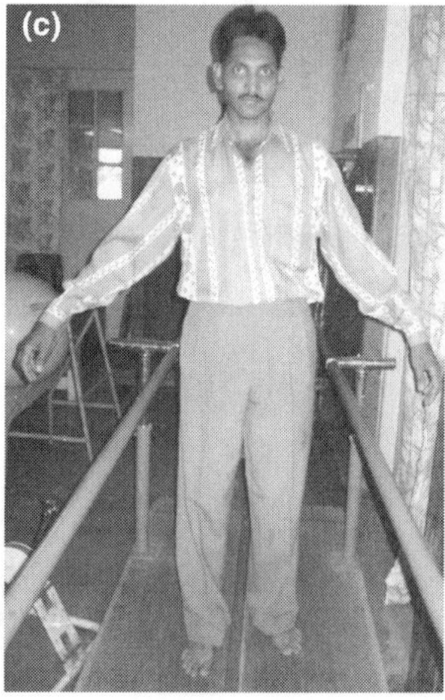

Figs 17.17a to c: (a) Standing with both hand support, (b) Standing with one hand support, and (c) Standing without hand support

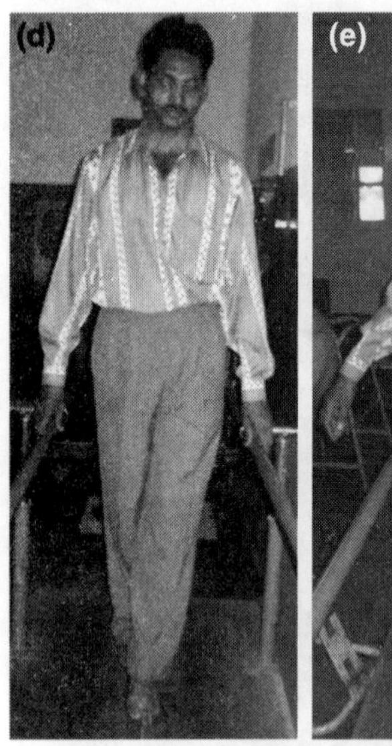
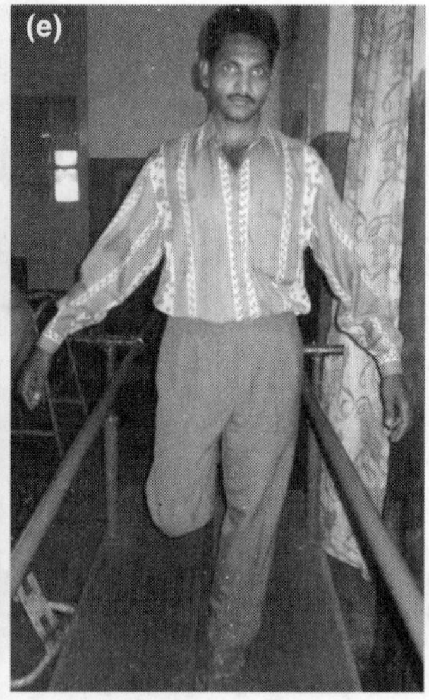

Figs 17.17d and e: (d) Tandem Standing and (e) Standing on one leg

iv. *Dynamic balance exercises*
  • After achieving unsupported sitting, patient is asked to look up and down, and from side to side, which activate the vestibular system.
  • Reaching activities on same side and then contralateral side both in sitting and standing position.
  • Sitting to standing with both hands support then one hand and then without any support. Equal weight bearing on both lower extremity should be facilitated by visual and verbal feedback (Figs 17.18a to c).
  • Stepping forward and backward can be practised first in parallel bar with one or two hands then without parallel bar.
  • Standing to supine on mat and then move back to standing. Same may be practised by going to prone position from standing. Each movement activates the vestibular system in addition to challenging the patient's dynamic balance (Figs 17.19a to f).

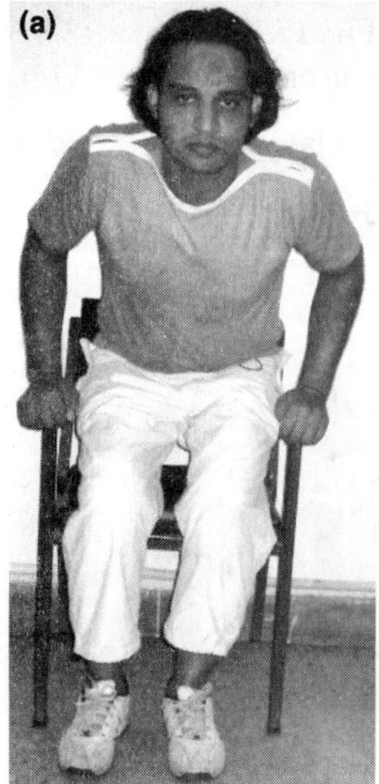
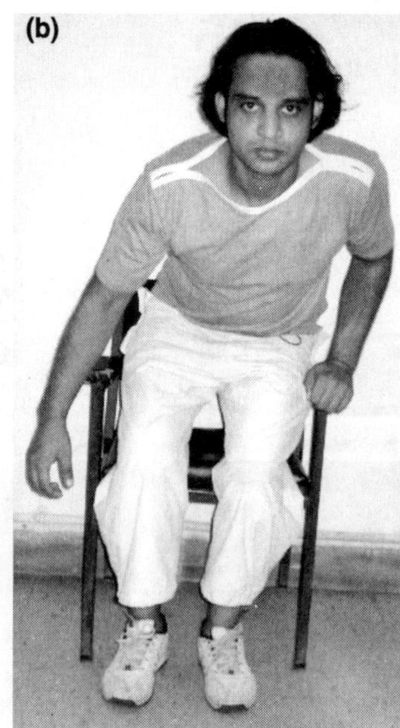
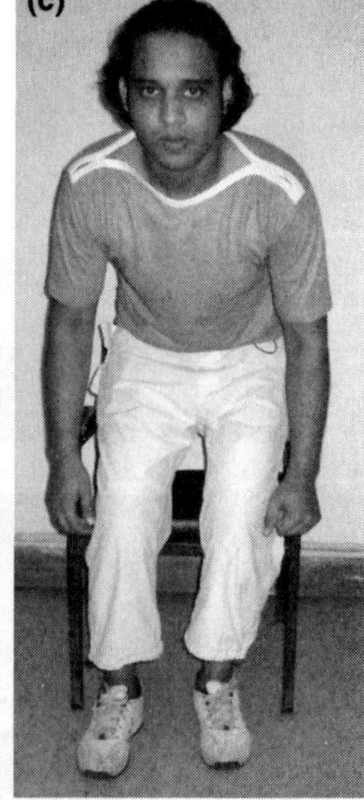

Figs 17.18a to c: (a) Sit to stand with both hand support, (b) Sit to stand with one hand support, and (c) Sit to stand without hand support

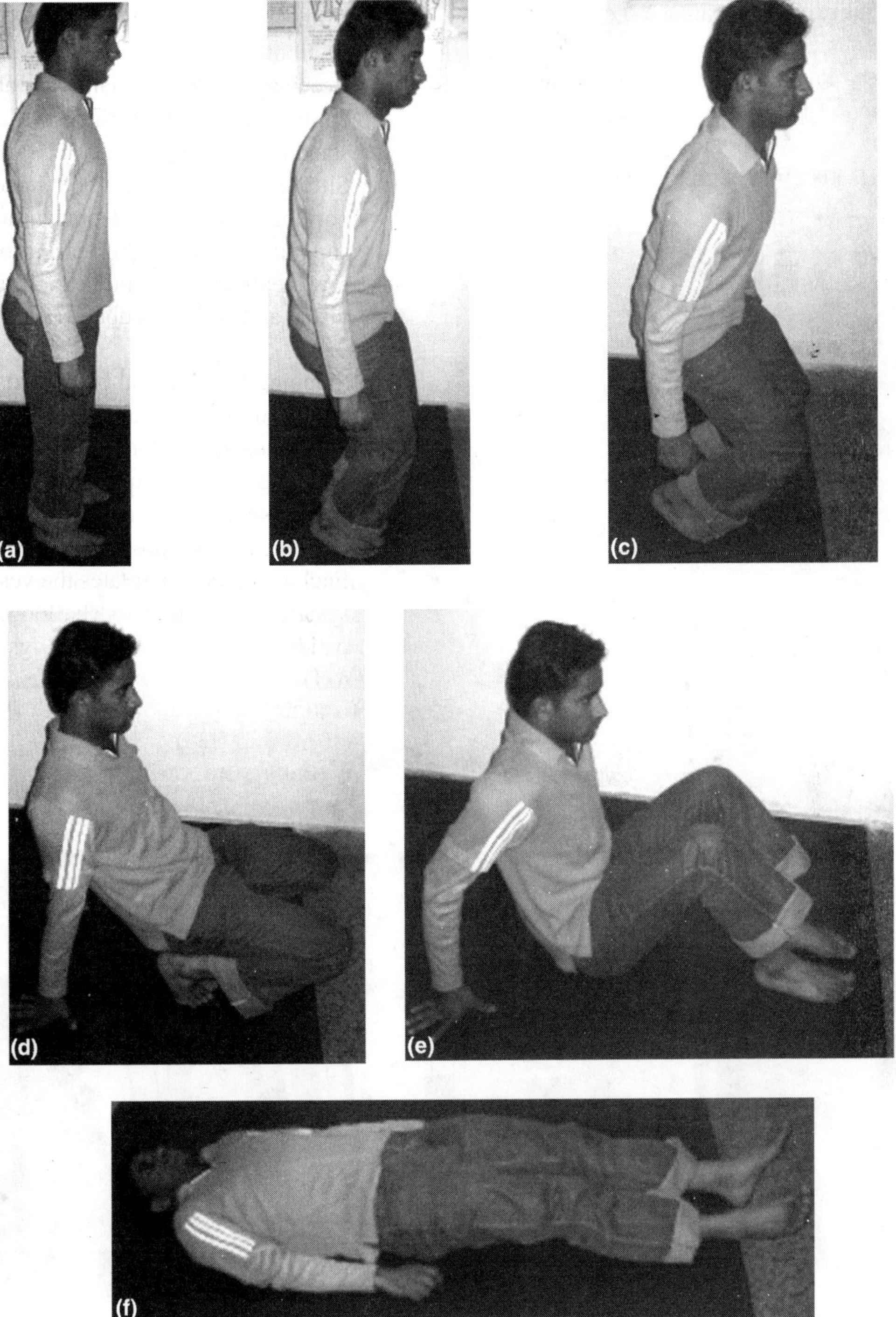

Figs 17.19a to f: Standing to supine

- Trunk dynamic balance and strength can be achieved by throwing and catching (at head level, overhead and either side) by therapy balls of various sizes and weights in a variety of positions such as kneeling, half-kneeling, sitting and standing (Fig. 17.20).

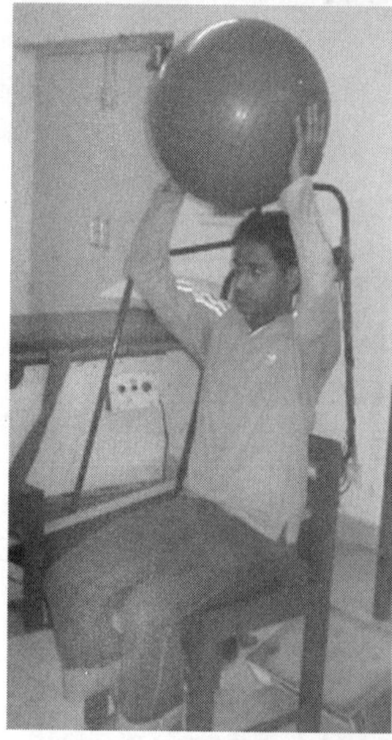

Fig. 17.20: Ball throwing in sitting position

- Gait activities should be practised in parallel bar then with assistive devices (walker → cane) and then without any device (Figs 17.21a to d).
  Patient should practice:
  - side stepping (Fig. 17.22a)
  - walking forward
  - crossing legs (Fig. 17.22b)
  - walking backward (Fig. 17.22c)
  - walking on heels (Fig. 17.22d)
  - walking on toes (Fig. 17.22e).
- Balancing on vestibular board or wobble board may be practised to facilitate weight-shift in backward/forward and side to side direction (Fig. 17.23) (In starting this activity may be performed between the parallel bars).
- Ball kicking activities should be incorporated to improve stability on one leg and dynamic movement with other leg (Fig. 17.24).
- Walking through obstacles (Fig. 17.25).
- Walking on different surfaces (hard to soft) (Fig. 17.26).
- Walking with various speed (slow to fast).

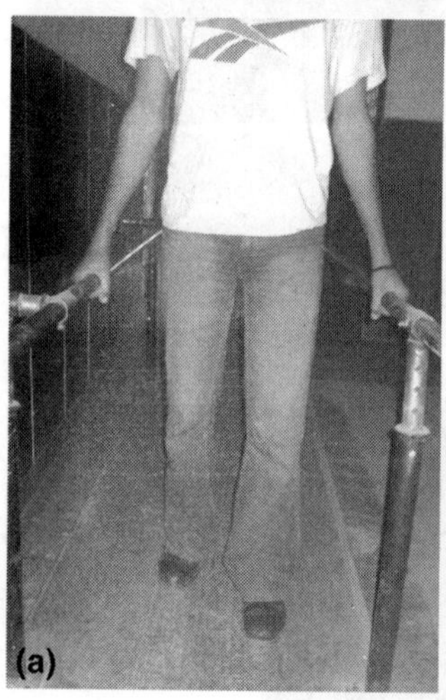
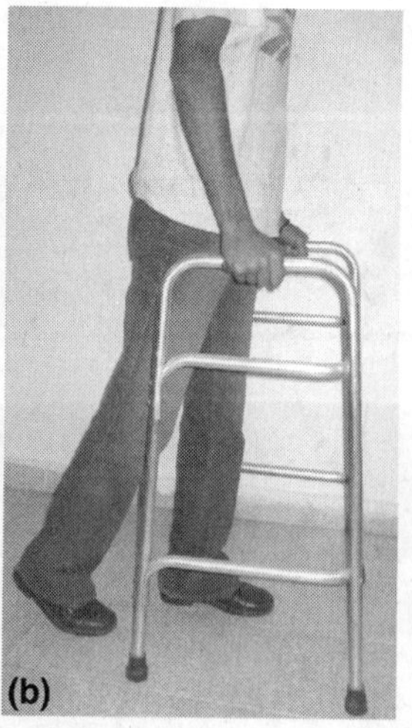
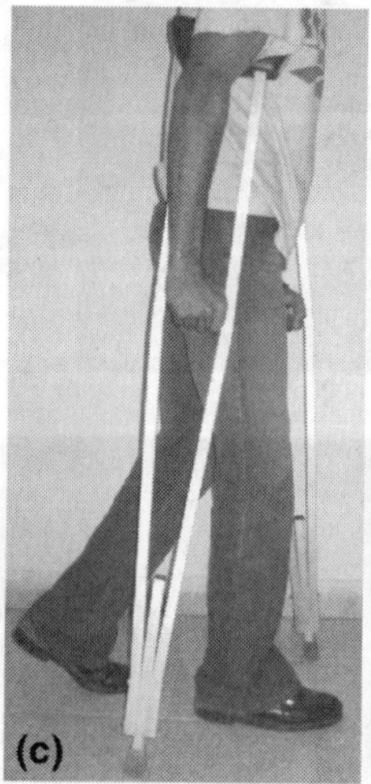
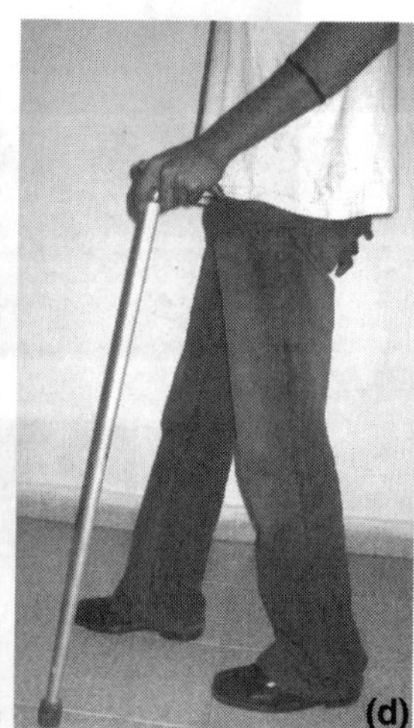

Figs 17.21a to d: (a) Walking with parallel bar, (b) Walking with walker, (c) Walking with crutches, and (d) Walking with stick

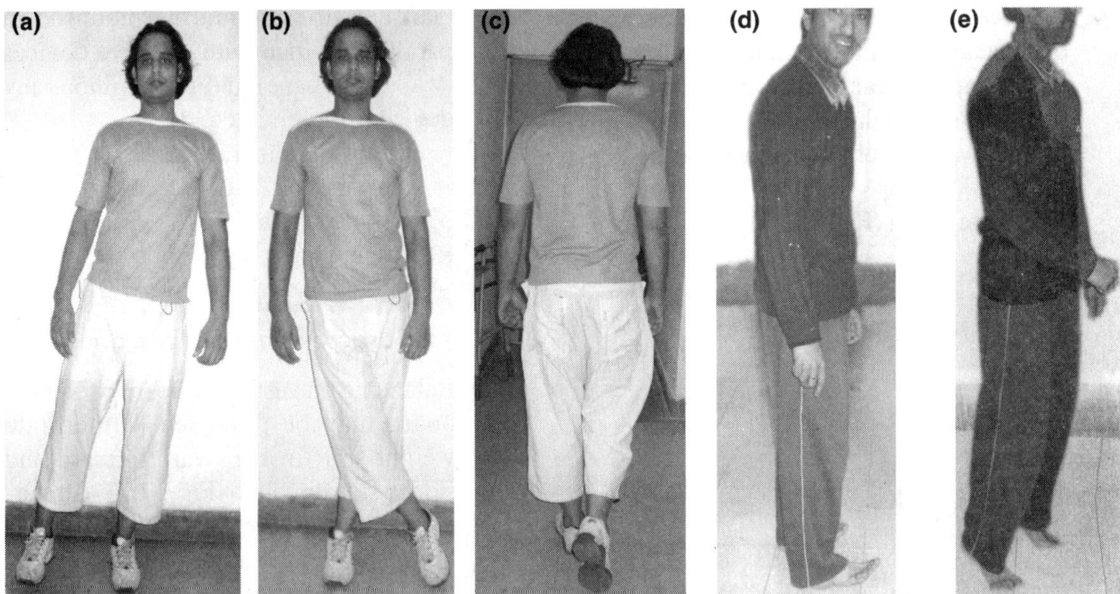

Figs 17.22a to e: (a) Side stepping, (b) Crossing legs, (c) Backward walking, (d) Walking on heels and (e) Walking on toes

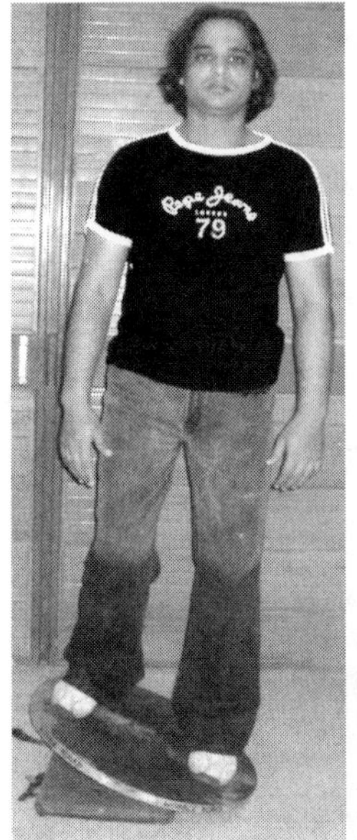

Fig. 17.23: Balancing on wobble board (side to side)

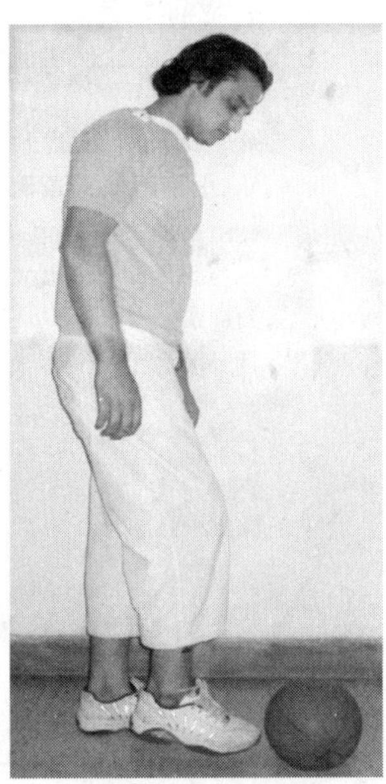

Fig. 17.24: Ball kicking

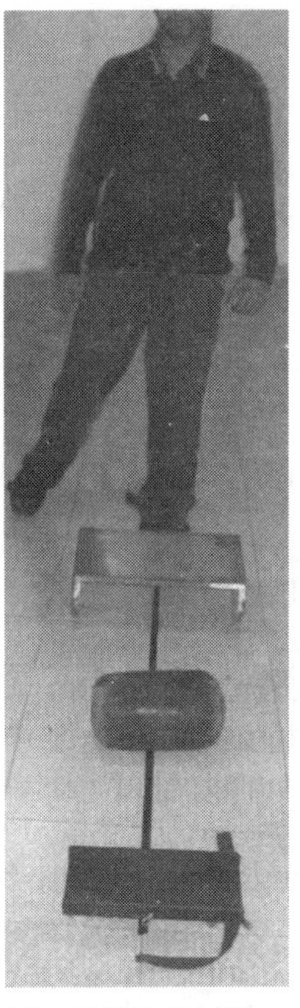

Fig. 17.25: Walking through obstacles

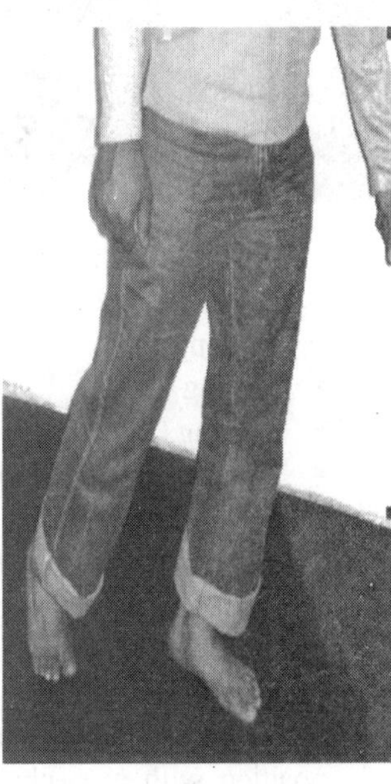

Fig. 17.26: Walking on soft surface

v. *Aerobic exercises*—Patient with balance dysfunction become deconditioned because of self imposed immobility arising from the fear of loosing balance.

Following aerobic exercise can be performed:

- Static cycling (Fig. 17.27)

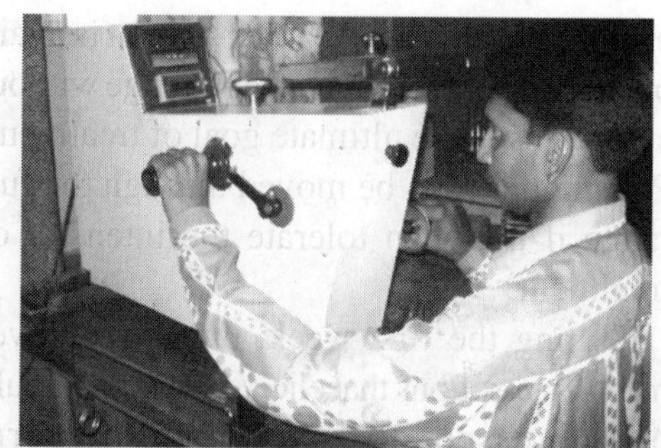
Fig. 17.28: Upper extremity bicycle ergometer

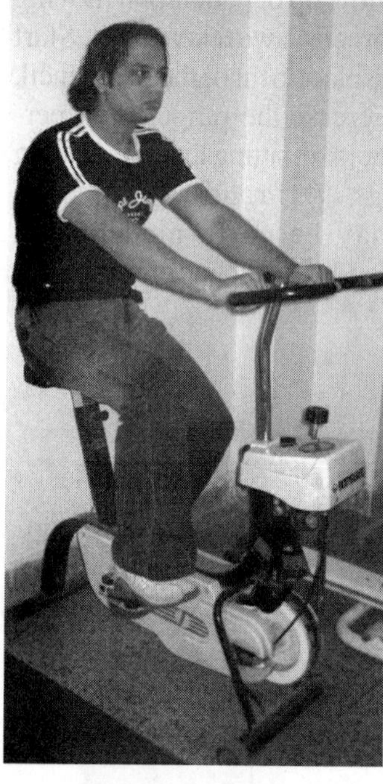
Fig. 17.27: Static cycle

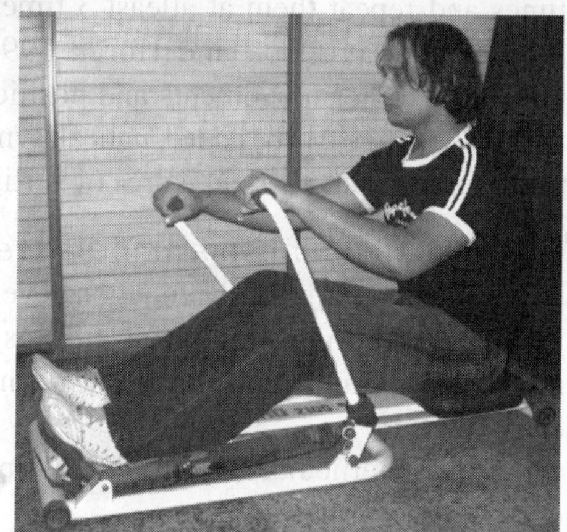
Fig. 17.29: Rowing

- Upper extremity bicycle ergometer (Fig. 17.28)
- Walking
- Jogging
- Rowing (Fig. 17.29)
- Trampoline etc. (Fig. 17.30).

vi. *Balance exercises for vestibular dysfunction habituation exercises*—are those which habituate the patient in positions of eliciting symptoms of vertigo and nystagmus.

Patient is gradually brought to the desired position, with every change in position symptoms might reappear. Positions are maintained at every change until the symptoms disappear. As the symptoms are gone, the

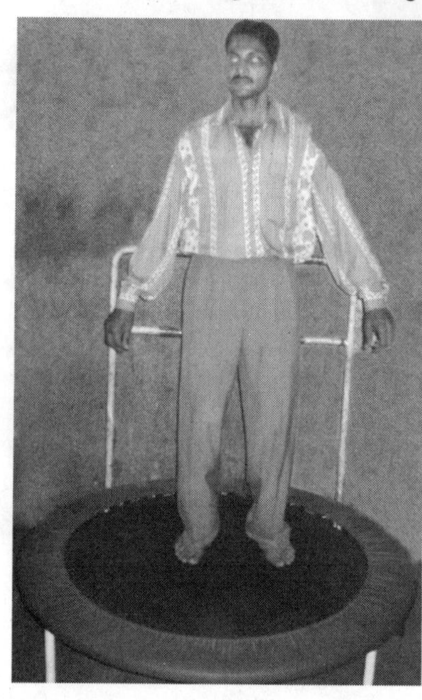
Fig. 17.30: Trampoline exercise

change towards the desired position is again made. Moving through the full range without symptoms is the ultimate goal of treatment. Patient may also be moved through the full range if they can tolerate the intensity of treatment.

During the first week, only two movements or positions that elicit symptoms should be addressed. Patient should perform movements and positioning activities 5 to 10 times and repeat them at atleast 3 times a day (Shumway-Cook and Horak 1990). Gradually, other movements and positions that elicit vertigo can be added, until all symptoms diminish and patient is free of vertigo.

Exercises for muscle imbalance—

Patients with vestibular dysfunction develop muscle imbalance due to strategies to minimize head and trunk movement that may cause vertigo.

For e.g. Sternocleidomastoid, latissimus dorsi might become tight.

Exercises for vestibular-ocular reflex—

The vestibular-ocular reflex may be impaired in patients with vestibular dysfunction. The following exercises may be used to increase vestibular-ocular reflex (Denham, 1996):

a. *Visual tracking exercise:* Instruct the patient to follow tip of pencil/pen moving in various direction with head still. Start with small displacement of the pen/pencil, gradually increase the range. First perform the exercise in sitting then in standing position (Figs 17.31a and b). Further the exercise may be performed during walking ascending/descending stairs.

b. *In sitting position:* Eyes are fixed while the head is moved passively by the therapist. First perform slowly, then with increasing speed, progressing to active movement of head.

Once patient can perform actively, exercise may be performed during standing, walking, and walking while reading a magazine (Fig. 17.32).

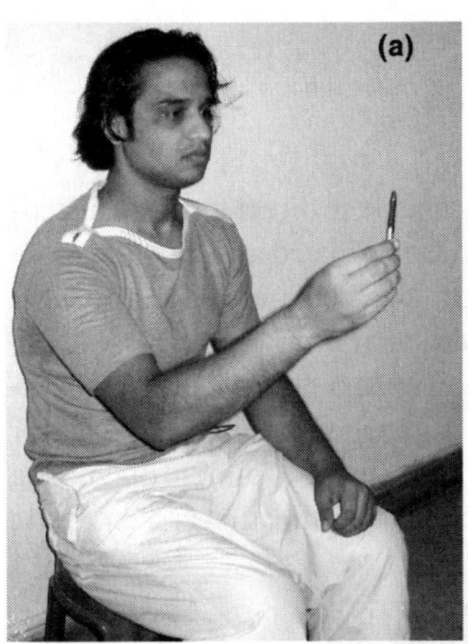
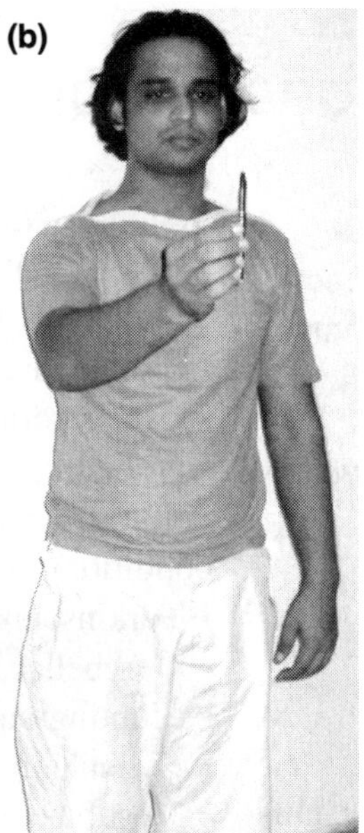

Figs 17.31a and b: Visual tracking exercise (a) While sitting, and (b) While standing

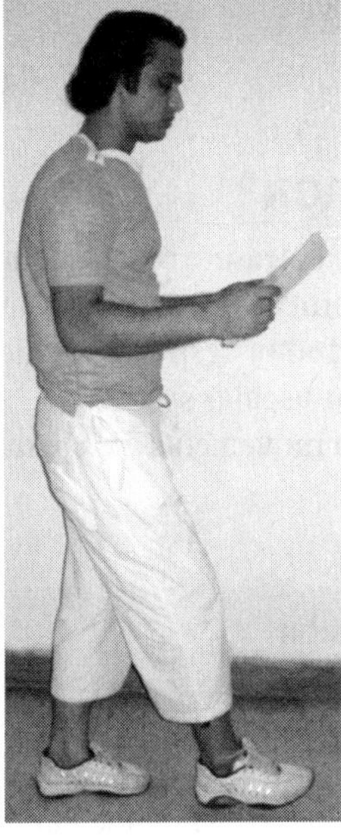

Fig. 17.32: Walking while reading magazine

vii. *Management for somatosensory loss*
- Modification of external environment.
- Compensation by visual feedback.
- Standing and walking barefoot on different textured surfaces.
- Use of weighted belts, and back support in chairs to improve trunk alignment which is impaired because of somatosensory loss.
- Walking with weight tied on knee and ankle joints (Fig. 17.33).
- Overuse of visual compensation should be discouraged.

Exercises for balance dysfunction may be modified as per the stage of condition, pathology, capability, interest and age of patient.

Precautions must be taken while giving balance exercises. Patient should be provided appropriate support/guidance/supervision as per the need. Environment should be safe enough to prevent any injury from fall during therapy session. Verbal and visual feedback should always be used whenever necessary.

Balance control learnt should be incorporated in real life functional activities.

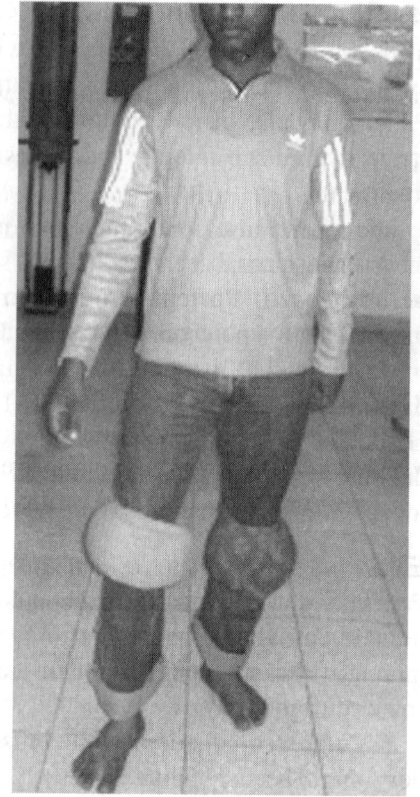

Fig. 17.33: Walking with weight tied on knee

COORDINATION

INTRODUCTION

Coordination is a measure of the quality of movement. It is the ability to carry out smooth, accurate and controlled motor responses which depends on intact neuromuscular system.

Coordinated movements are characterized by appropriate:
- Direction
- Distance
- Muscular tension
- Speed and
- Timing.

Coordination deficits occur when muscle fails to fire in sequence, or when the central nervous system (CNS) is unable to direct movement activities accurately. Coordinated movement require adequate strength and range of motion (ROM) to complete a particular task.

Incoordination occurs due to CNS lesions—Cerebellar, basal ganglia and dorsal (posterior column) lesion. The most common diagnostic conditions in which incoordination is seen are:
- Parkinsonism
- Cerebellar ataxia
- Huntington's disease
- Sydenham's chorea
- Vestibular dysfunction
- Cerebral palsy.

Signs of Incoordination

A. *Due to cerebellar dysfunction*
   i. *Asthenia*–Generalized muscle weakness.
   ii. *Hypotonia*–Decreased in muscle tone. (Decreased in resistance to passive movement and muscle may feel abnormally, soft and flaccid).
   iii. *Dysmetria*–is an impaired ability to judge the distance or range of a movement (Figs 17.34a and b):
      • Hypometria-underestimation.
      • Hypermetria-overestimation.
   iv. *Dysdiadochokinesia*–is an impaired ability to perform rapid alternating movements.
   v. *Tremor*–An involuntary oscillatory movement resulting from alternate contractions of opposing muscle groups.

   Kinetic or intentional tremor—occurs during voluntary movement of extremity tends to increase at the end of the desired movement or when the speed increases.

   Postural or static tremor—observed (back-and-forth oscillatory movements) when an individual tries to maintain standing posture.
   vi. *Dyssynergia*–is the movement decomposition describes a movement performed in a sequence of component part rather than as a single, smooth activity.
   vii. *Rebound phenomenon of Holmes*–Normally, when application of resistance to an isometric contraction is suddenly removed the limb will remain in approximately the same position. This ability gets impaired in patients with cerebellar dysfunction.
   viii. *Nystagmus*–Rhythmic oscillatory movements of the eyes.
   ix. *Dysarthria*–Disorder of the motor component of speech articulation, characterizcd by slow, slurred, hesistant, inappropriate pauses and prolonged syllables.
   x. *Gait disorder*–Wide base of support.

B. *Due to basal ganglia lesion*
   i. *Bradykinesia*–slowness of movement manifested by decreased arm swing, slow shuffling gait, lack of facial expressions,

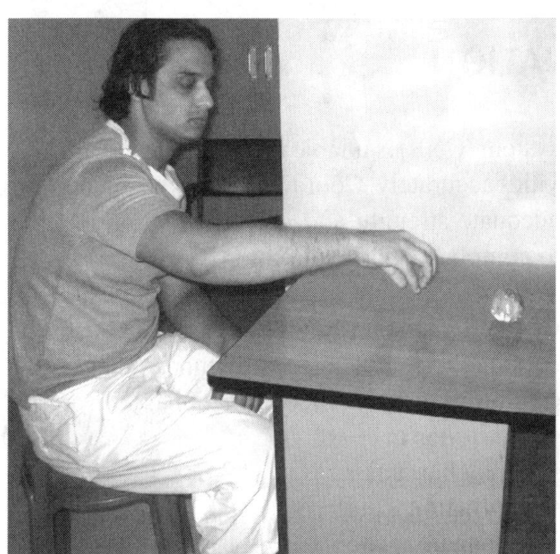

Fig. 17.34a: Dysmetria (hypometria)

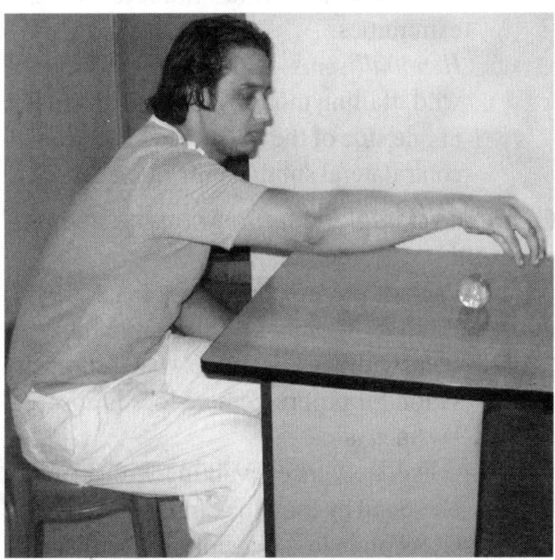

Fig. 17.34b: Dysmetria (hypermetria)

difficulty in initiating or changing direction of movement or in stopping a movement once begun.

ii. *Rigidity*–is an increase in muscle tone causing greater resistance to passive movement.

Lead pipe rigidity– is a uniform constant resistance throughout the range of movement.

Cogwheel rigidity–is characterized by 'give' and 'relaxation' and when the extremity is moved passively (combination of lead pipe tremor and tremor).

iii. *Resting tremor*–Tremors observed at rest especially in distal upper extremity in the form a 'pill-rolling' movement. These tremors disappear with movement.

iv. *Chorea*–involuntary, rapid, irregular and jerky movements.

v. *Athetosis*–Slow, involuntary, writhing, twisting, "worm like" movements usually seen in distal part of upper extremity.

vi. *Dystonia*–Twisting, bizarre movement caused by involuntary contraction of the axial and proximal muscles of the extremities.

vii. *Hemiballismus*–Sudden, jerky, forceful wild, flailing motions of the arm and leg of one side of the body (seen in lesion of contralateral subthalamic nucleus).

C. *Due to dorsal (posterior) column involvement*

i. Lack of proprioceptive feedback.

ii. Positive Rhomberg's sign—inability to stand with eyes closed (as visual compensation for proprioceptive loss is absent).

iii. Dysmetria.

iv. Gait disturbances-walking with an audible sound by foot (to compensate for proprioceptive loss by auditory feedback).

Tests for Coordination

Presence of incoordination can be tested in standing or during walking (equilibrium) and sitting position (Non-equilibrium). All these tests would make clearly observable one or other signs of incoordination (discussed earlier).

Tests in Standing or During Walking

I. *Standing:*
a. in normal posture
b. with feet together/narrow base of support (Fig. 17.35)
c. with one foot directly in front of the other (Fig. 17.36)
d. on one foot (Fig. 17.37)

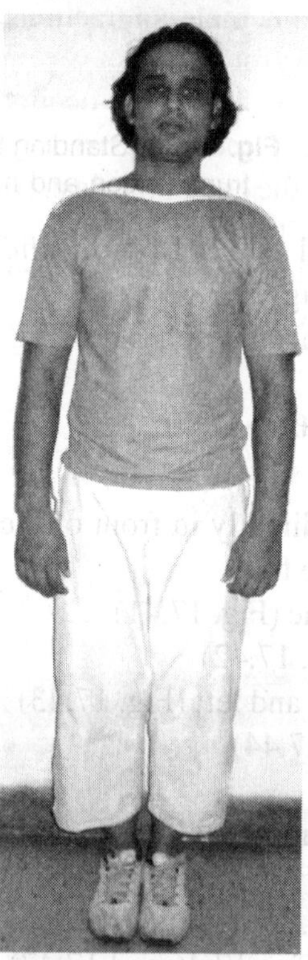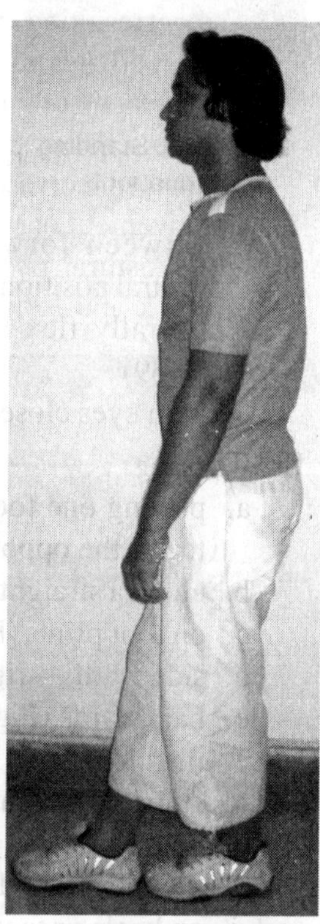

Fig. 17.35: Standing with feet together   **Fig. 17.36:** Standing with one foot in front

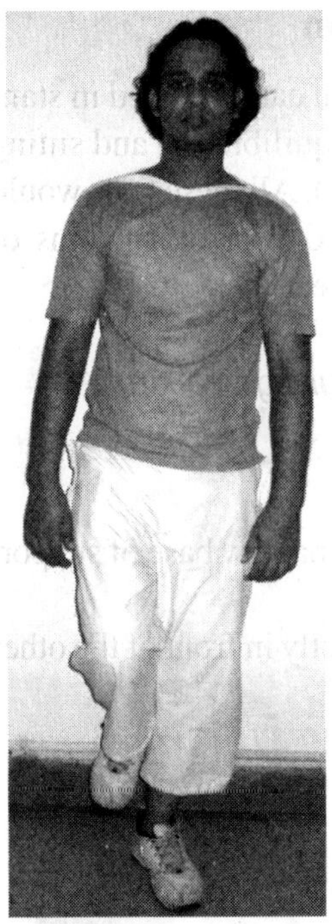

Fig. 17.37: Standing on one foot

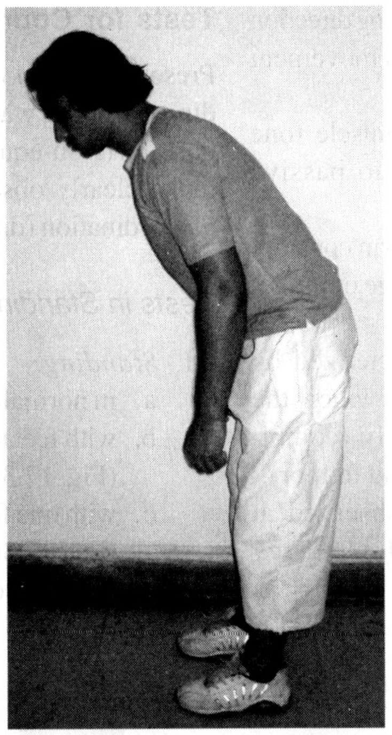

Fig. 17.38: Standing between forward trunk flexion and neutral position

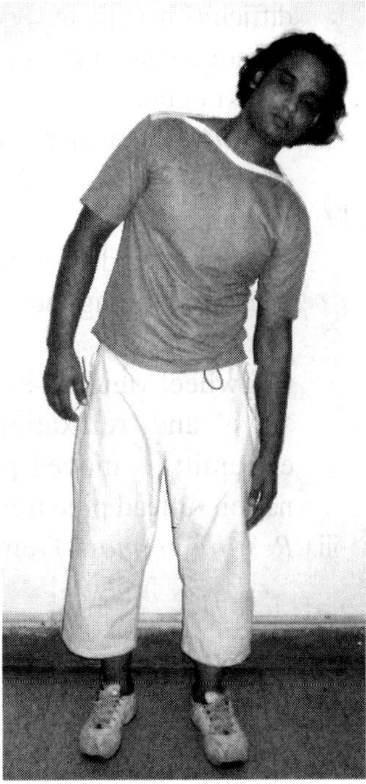

Fig. 17.39: Standing lateral flexion

e. between forward trunk flexion and neutral position (Fig. 17.38)
f. laterally flex trunk to each side (Fig. 17.39)
g. with eyes closed (Fig. 17.40).

II. *Walking:*
a. placing one foot directly in front of the toe of the opposite foot
b. along a straight line (Fig. 17.41)
c. on foot prints (Fig. 17.42)
d. side wards—right and left (Fig. 17.43)
e. backwards (Fig. 17.44)
f. march in place
g. stop and start abruptly
h. with turning at 90°, 180° and 360°
i. around circle (Fig. 17.45)
j. on heels or toes (Figs 17.46 and 17.47)
k. with step over or around obstacles (Fig. 17.48)
l. with different speeds.

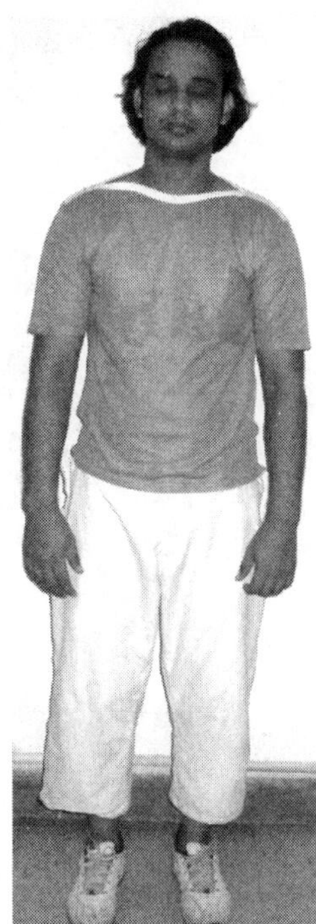

Fig. 17.40: Standing with eyes closed

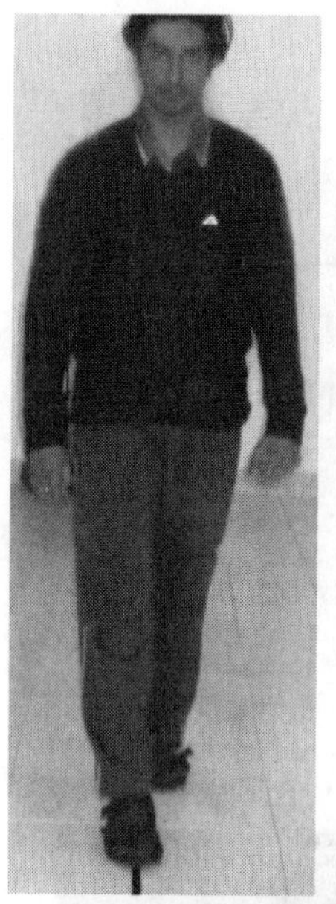

Fig. 17.41: Walking on a straight line

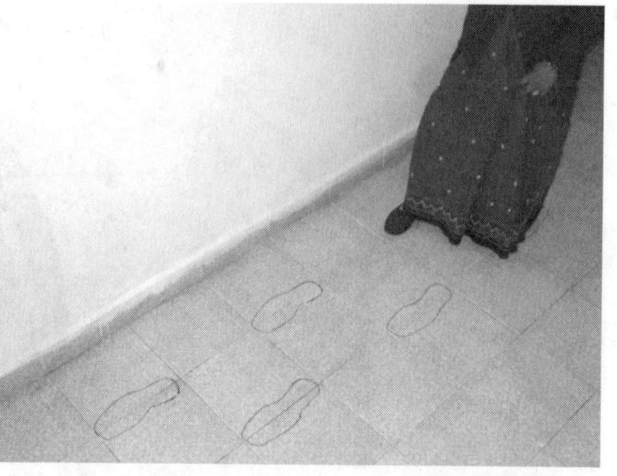

Fig. 17.42: Walking on foot prints

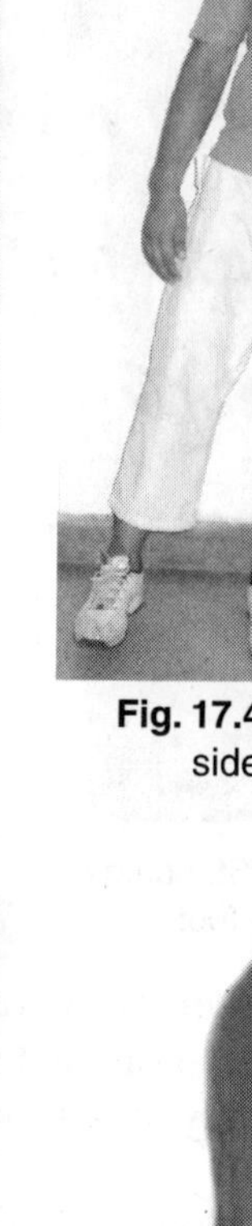

Fig. 17.43: Walking side ward

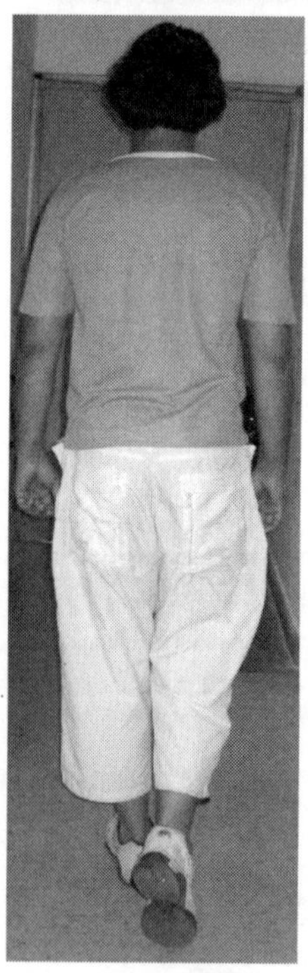

Fig. 17.44: Walking backward

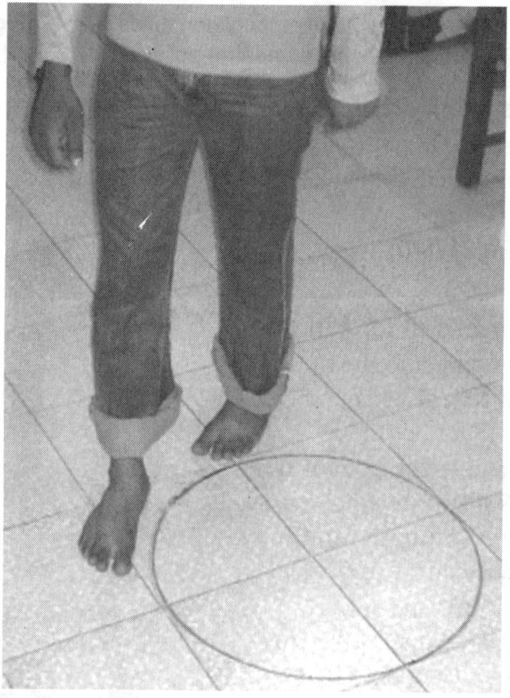

Fig. 17.45: Walking around circle

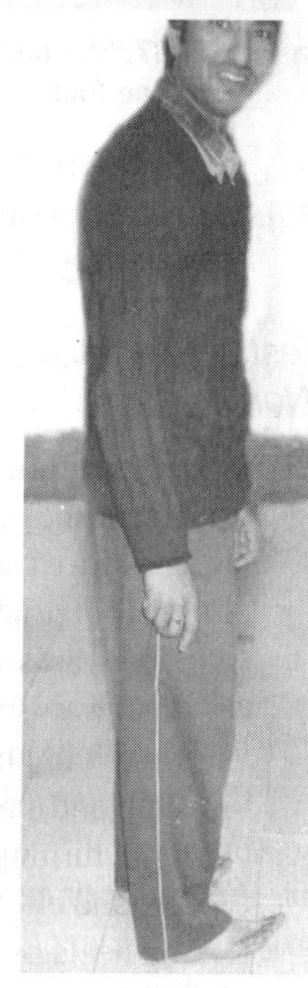

Fig. 17.46: Walking on heels

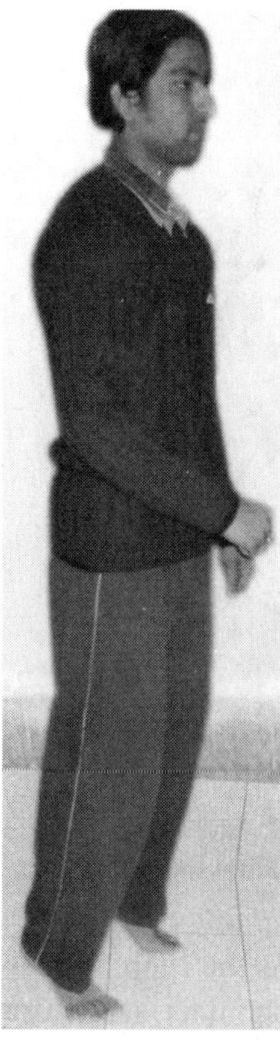

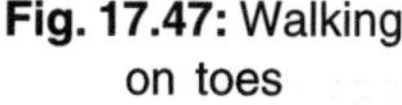

Fig. 17.47: Walking on toes

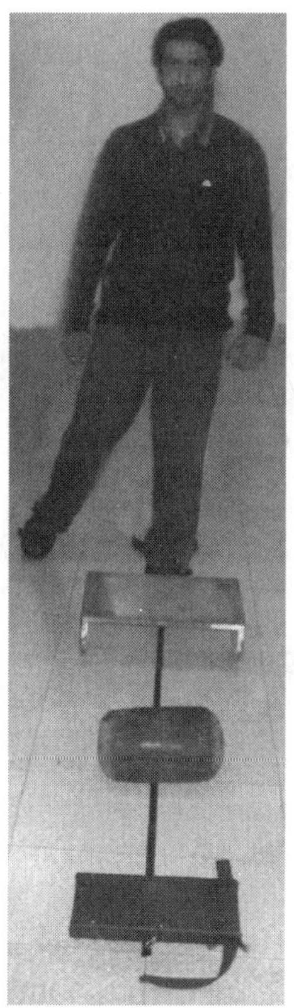

Fig. 17.48: Walking through obstacles

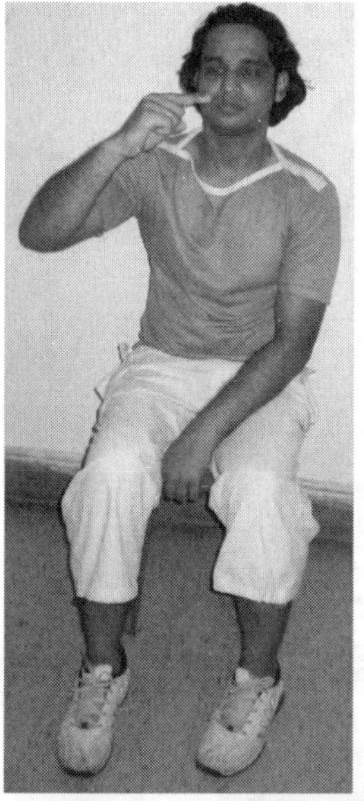

Fig. 17.49: Finger to nose test

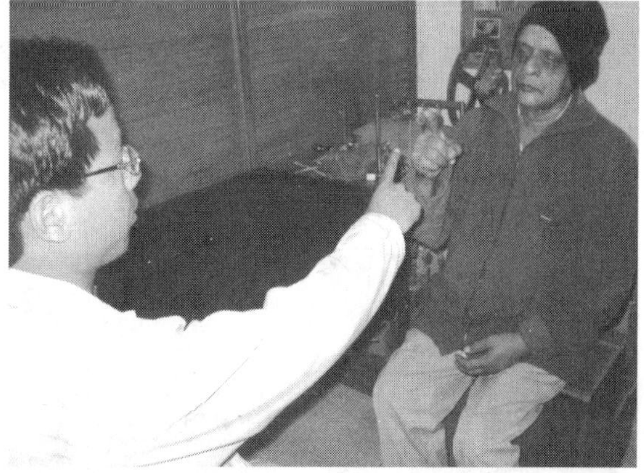

Fig. 17.50: Finger to therapist finger

Tests in Sitting or Supine Position (Non-equilibrium)

i. *Finger to nose*—The patient is asked to bring the tip of the index finger to the tip of the nose. Movement can be repeated number of times (Fig. 17.49).

ii. *Finger to therapist finger*—The patient is asked to touch therapist's finger held in various positions (therapist sitting in front of the patient). Movement can be repeated number of times (Fig. 17.50).

iii. *Finger to finger*—With shoulders abducted at 90°, patient is asked to bring both hands towards the midline and approximate the index fingers from opposing hand (Fig. 17.51).

iv. *Alternate nose to finger*—The patient alternately touches the tip of his nose and the tip of the therapist's finger (held in various positions) with index finger (Fig. 17.52).

v. *Finger opposition*—The patient touches the tip of the thumb to the tip of each finger in sequence.

vi. *Pronation/supination*—The patient is asked to do pronation/supination alternately with elbow flexed at 90°.

vii. *Alternate heel to knee (supine position)*—The patient is asked to touch the knee and

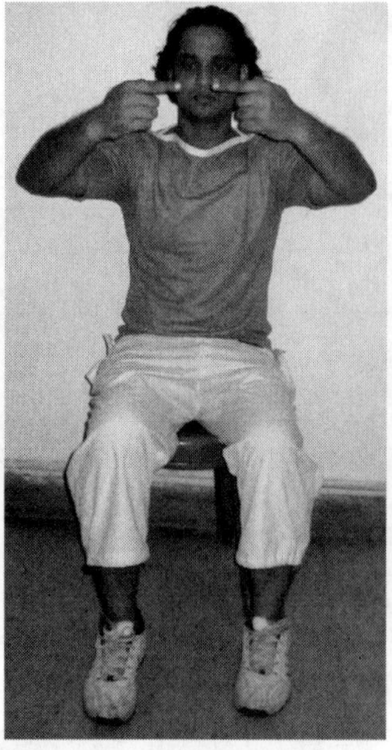

Fig. 17.51: Finger to finger test

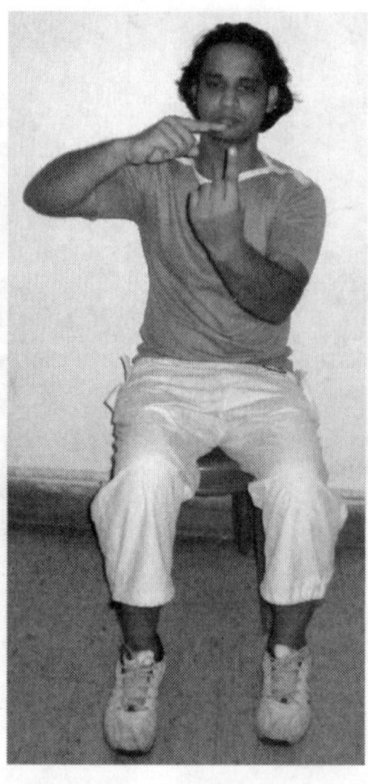

Fig. 17.52: Alternate nose to finger test

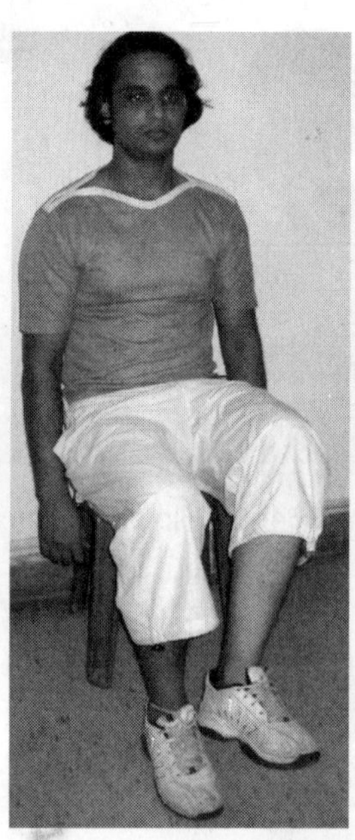

Fig. 17.53: Alternate heel to knee test

big toe alternately with the heel of the opposite extremity (Fig. 17.53).

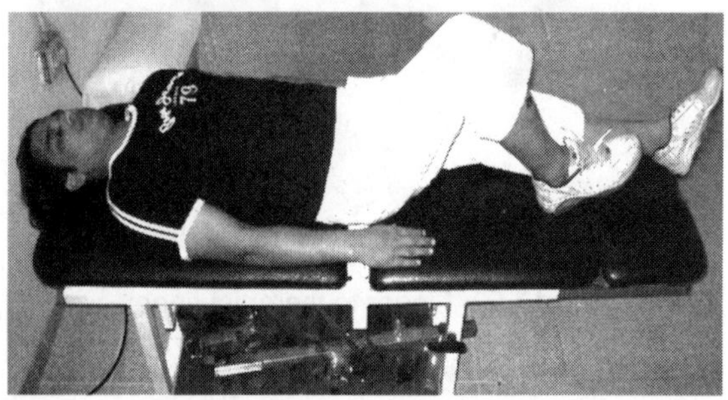

Fig. 17.53: Hip and knee flexion

viii. *Drawing an imaginary circle in the air with either upper or lower extremity.*

 ix. *Position holding*—Patient is asked to hold upper or lower extremity in any position.

  x. *Rebound test*—The patient is asked to do elbow extension, the therapist applies resistance to produce an isometric contraction of triceps. Resistance is suddenly released. Normally the opposing muscle group (biceps) will contract and controls the limb. (Other muscle groups such as shoulder abductors and flexors, elbow flexors can also be tested).

COORDINATION EXERCISES

Frenkel's exercises were designed to enable voluntary relearning of movement through repetition and retraining of functional patterns. Frenkel's exercises are performed while patients are supine, sitting or standing. Patients should perform each activity slowly with visual input to help control movement.

The exercises as described by Caliet, cited in Licht (1965) are:

I. *In supine, have the patient perform the following movements:*
  i. Flexion and extension of each leg at the knee and hip joints; abduction and adduction with knees flexed; later, abduction and adduction with knees extended (Figs 17.54a to c).

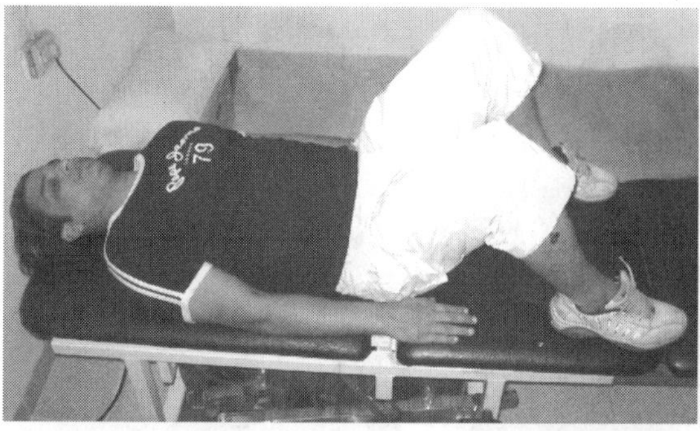

Fig. 17.54b(i): Hip abduction with knees flexed

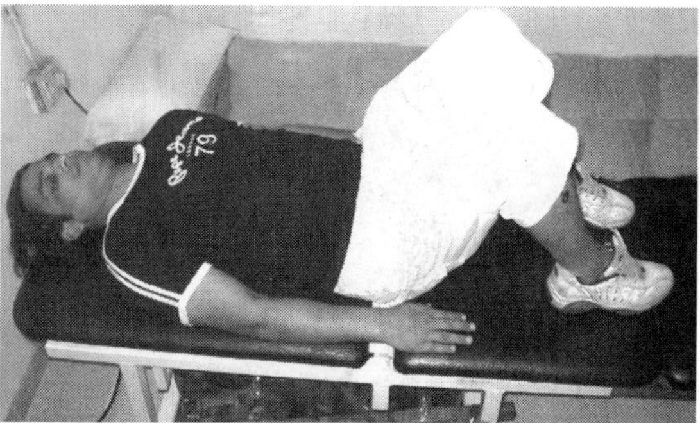

Fig. 17.54b(ii): Hip adduction with knees flexed

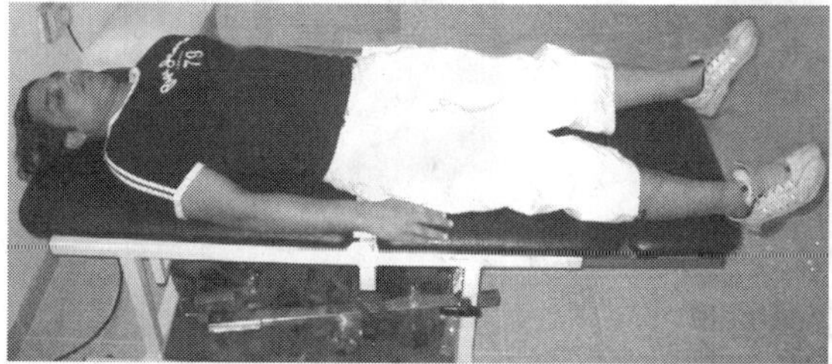

Fig. 17.54c(i): Hip abduction with knees extended

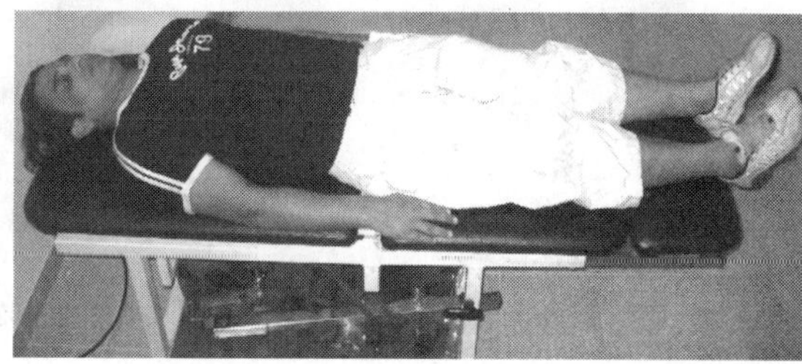

Fig. 17.54c(ii): Hip adduction with knees extended

ii. Flexion and extension of one knee at a time, with heel raised from the bed (Fig. 17.55).

iii. Knee flexion with and heel placed on some definite part of the opposite limb; for example, on the patella, or the middle of the leg, with the ankle and toe, then changing positions (Figs 17.56a and b).

iv. Knee flexion with, heel placed on the knee of the opposite leg, and is glided down the tibia to the ankle joint and back to the knee (Fig. 17.57).

v. Flexion and extension of both legs, together with knees and ankles held close together (Fig. 17.58).

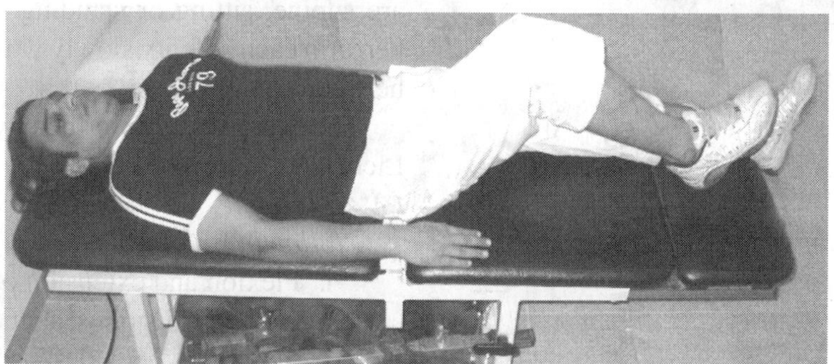

Fig. 17.55

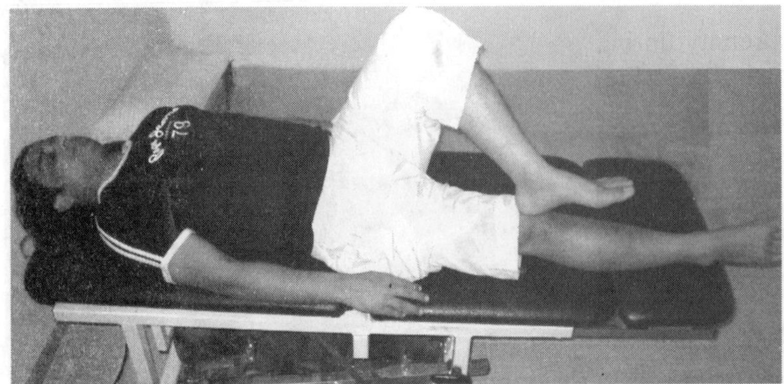

Fig. 17.56a

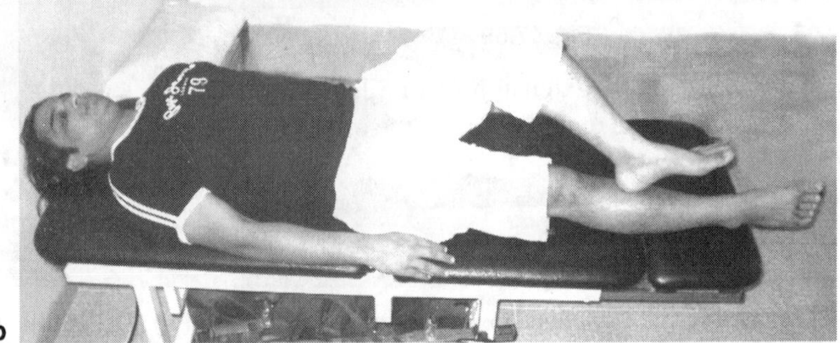

Fig . 17.56b

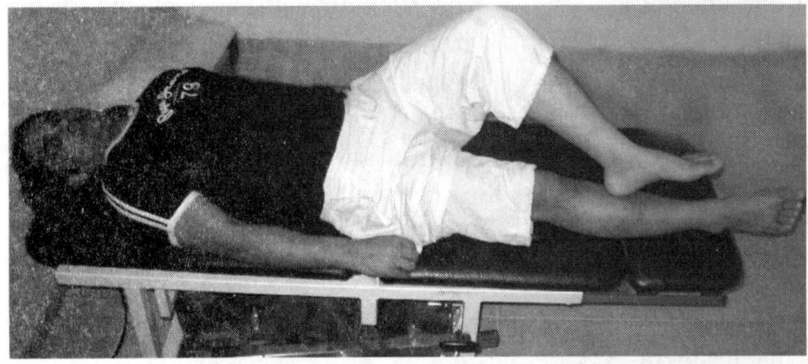

Fig. 17.57

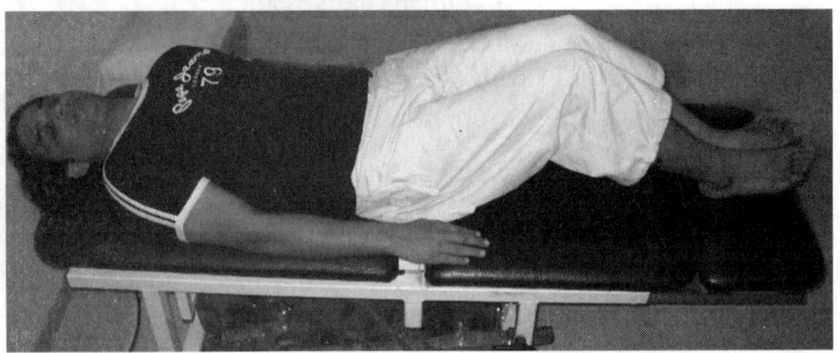

Fig. 17.58

vi. Flexion of one lower extremity during extension of the other (reciprocal) (Fig. 17.59).

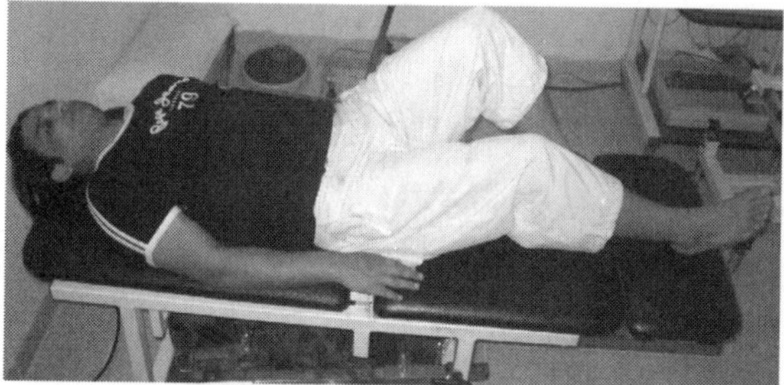

Fig. 17.59

vii. Flexion or extension of one leg during adduction or abduction of the other (Fig. 17.60).

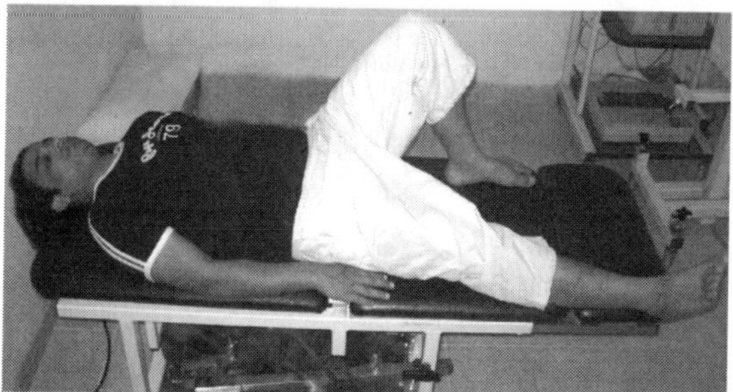

Fig. 17.60

II. *When patient can perform exercises (i) to (vii) of easily, he should perform them with their eyes closed.*

III. *In sitting:*

i. Try to place the heel of foot into the therapist's hand. The therapist changes the position of his or her hand after each attempt (Fig. 17.61).

ii. Maintain sitting unsupported for several minutes.

iii. Raise each knee alternately and place each foot firmly on the ground on traced footprint. This task may be performed in sitting or standing position (Fig. 17.62).

iv. Rise from a chair and then sit again holding knees together (Fig. 17.63).

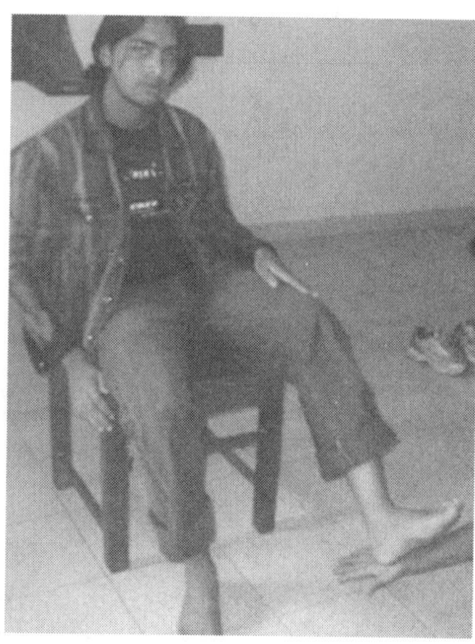

Fig. 17.61: Patient placing heel on therapist's palm

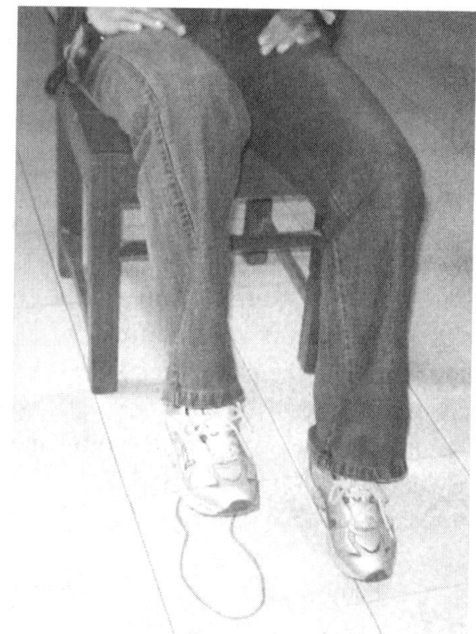

Fig. 17.62: Patient placing foot on marked foot print (in sitting position)

v. Place feet forward and backward on a straight line, then repeat on a zig-zagged line. These exercises may be performed in both sitting and standing position.

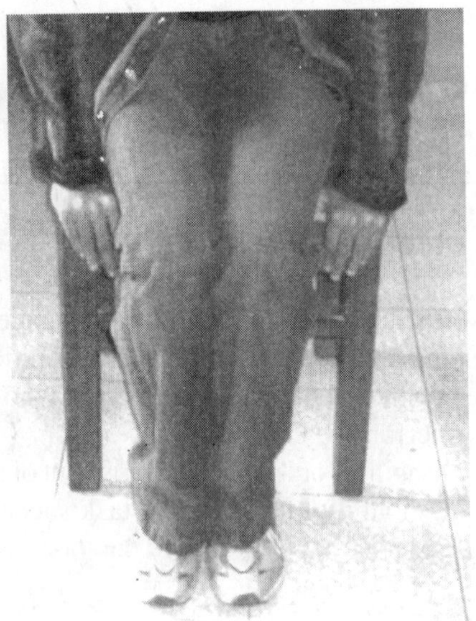

Fig. 17.63: Sit to stand with feet together

IV. *During walking:*
  i. Walk between two parallel lines (Fig. 17.64).
  ii. Walk on foot tracings placed on the floor.

OTHER ASPECTS OF MANAGEMENT FOR INCOORDINATION

1. *Functional activities*—To improve the coordinated movements of functional task, it is important that the patient repeat those tasks. The key to improving coordination is to vary the distance and speed of the movement to enable successful completion of the task and gradually retrain muscle activity.

   For e.g.:
   a. Draw numbers or alphabet on paper
   b. Practice writing
   c. Don and Doff shirts
   d. Brush teeth
   e. Comb hair
   f. Pick up small objects from floor/table.

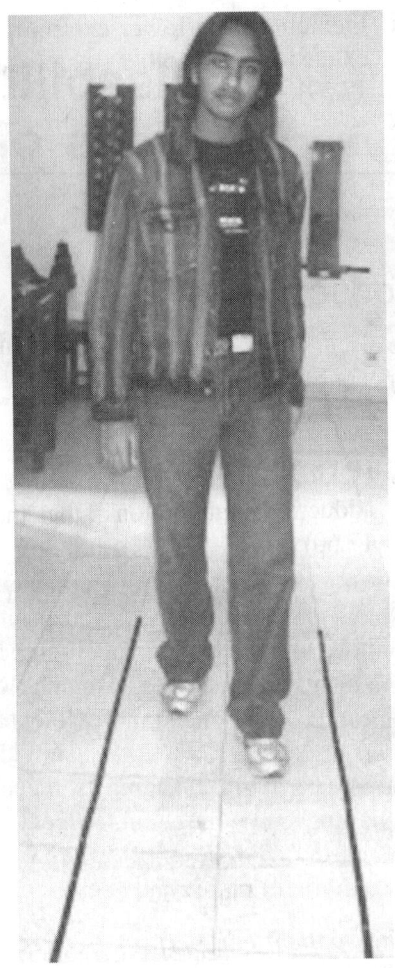

Fig. 17.64: Walking between parallel lines

2. *Proprioceptive neuromuscular facilitation (PNF)* discussed in Chapter 14.
3. *Weight bearing activities through proximal joints* (Standing, kneeling, sitting on mats and weight bearing through involved upper extremity).
4. *Sensory cues*—Use of sensory cues such as visual feedback, manual guidance, verbal cues etc. during exercises or practising functional task enhance the treatment outcome.

CHAPTER-18

Disability, Function and Activities of Daily Living (ADL)

INTRODUCTION

Before discussing more about function and ADL the concept of disability must be clearly understood.

CONCEPTS OF DISABILITY

As long as human kind has existed there has inevitably been impairment and disability. The life giving proccsscs of gestation and birth themselves can result in physical and mental incapacities that affect individuals activity of daily living. Natural disasters such as earthquakes, tsunami, flood and hurricanes, accidents of all kinds, violent aggression, wars also creat disability. Even without all this, the process of life and aging itself guarantees that if we live long enough impairment of some sort will occur.

The definitions of disability describe what the person cannot do. The phrases used are "lack of ability to perform an activity", "reduction of a person's activity", and "inability to engage in any substantial gainful activity." Such definitions are based on the belief that it is the person who cannot do or perform.

"Disability" or "nonability" arise out of an individual's inability to perform a task successfully because of an insufficiency in one or more areas of functional capability: Physical function, mental function, agility, dexterity, coordination, strength, endurance, knowledge, skill, intellectual ability or experience. "Disability" requires a conceptual definition; it is the gap between what a person can do and what the person needs or wants to do. Medically, disability is physical impairment and inability to perform physical functions normally.

Evolution of Models of Disability

Terminology in the field of disablement continues to breed confusion and controversy across and within discipline. Therefore, it is essential to discuss various models of disability (Fig. 18.1).

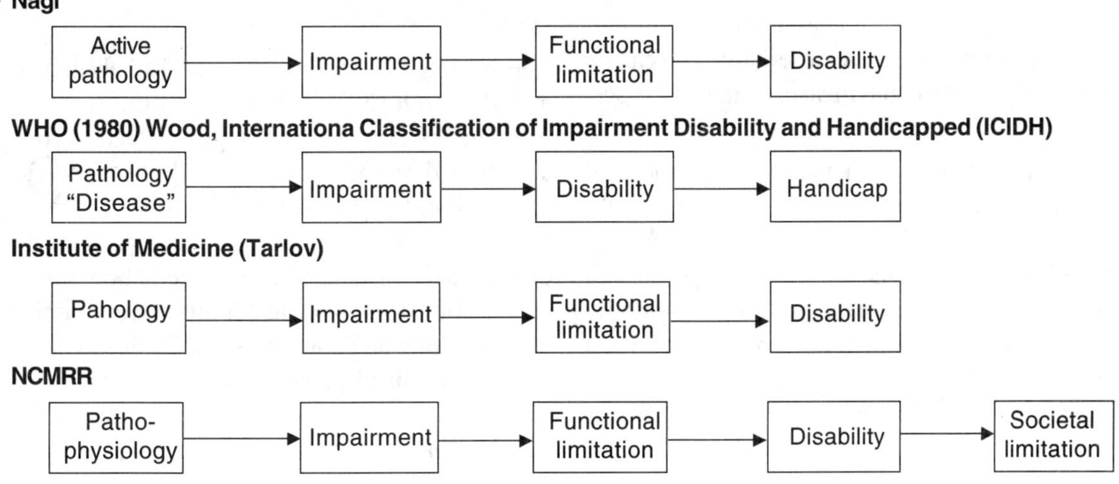

Fig. 18.1: Various models of disability

SAAD NAGI (1969)

Nagi, a sociologist was the first to provide a model of disability process. He suggested four stages in the disability process: active pathology, impairment, functional limitation and disability.

Active pathology: Interruption or interference with normal processes and efforts of the organism to regain normal state.

Impairment: Anatomical, physiological, mental or emotional abnormalities or loss.

Functional limitation: Limitation in performance at the level of the whole organism or person.

Disability: Limitation in performance of socially defined roles and tasks within a socio-cultural and physical environment.

WORLD HEALTH ORGANIZATION (1980) ICIDH

It is the most commonly used and internationally accepted conceptual model of disablement. It was proposed by Wood, he suggested four levels of disablement.

Pathology: is a disease or trauma that causes changes in the structure or function of the body or of a specific tissue or organ. Example: Arthritis.

Impairment: Occurs at the organ level and is defined as "any loss or abnormality of psychological, physiological or anatomical structure or function." Impairment are observable and can be objectively defined and measured in most cases.

Example: Loss of joint motion, amputation.

Disability: Occurs at personal level and is defined as "any restriction or lack (resulting from impairment) of ability to perform an activity in the manner or within the range considered normal for a human being." Disability is most commonly defined in terms of dependent functioning within one's personal sphere.

Example: Dependent Activities of Daily Living.

Handicap: Occurs at societal level is defined as "a disadvantage for a given individual that limits or prevents the fulfillment of a role that is normal (depending upon age, sex, social and cultural factors) for that individual." Handicaps may affect expected roles such as employee, family member, and community member. Example: lack of access to a pubic place because of wheelchair confinement.

The WHO model assumes unidirectional causality (impairments cause disability that cause handicap).

INSTITUTE OF MEDICINE (IOM)

For approximately 10 years, the ICIDH model remained unchallenged. Then two models were published concurrently; IOM and NCMRR. IOM was adapted directly from the Nagi model. The IOM model defines disability as "a function of the interaction of the person with the environment". The IOM model identified a subset of factors that could modify the relationships between impairments, functional limitations and disability. These factors include biology, environment (physical, social and psychological), life style and behavior. These factors are independent variables that can modify all levels of disablement process and affect quality of life.

NCMRR MODEL (1993)

The National Centre for Medical Rehabilitation and Research (NCMRR) changed the structure of model by creating five stages instead of four. The first three are defined similarly to Nagi's model. The term "pathophysiology" is substituted for "active pathology". The difference is in the definition of "disability" and "societal limitation".

Disability is defined as a limitation or inability in performing tasks, activities, and roles to levels expected within physical and social context. Societal limitation is a restriction attributable to social policy or barriers that limit fulfillment of roles.

RECONSIDERATION OF DISABLEMENT MODELS

The multiple models of disability have produced confusion. They limit our ability to define disability. Additionally, there are major criticisms of the existing models. First, they have overemphasized the medical model. A second major criticism is that the models have assumed causal relationships between the different levels. For example in some models disability is directly caused by the observed impairments; whereas in reality, impairments may explain 25% or less of the variance in disability or handicap. A third criticism of the existing models is that a unidirectional relationship exists between the levels. This unidirectional representation does not allow for reverse effects. For example, handicap (rolc limitation) may cause less mobility (disability), and less mobility causes declines in strength and endurance (impairment). Most importantly, the unidirectional representation implies that disability is not reversible. Lastly, the models are expressed in negative dimensions (handicap) rather than positive (enabling) terms (i.e., residual abilities).

Given these limitations, the two initiatives in 1997 put forth additional models to characterize disability.

MODIFIED IOM MODELS (1997)

The new IOM model clearly defines disability as the interaction of person with the environment and includes a bi-directional dimension (possibility of improvement). Disability has been moved from being a part of the process to being a product of interaction of the individual with the environment.

NEW WORLD HEALTH ORGANIZATION MODEL (1997-2001)

The WHO has recently modified the 1980 model of the disablement classification with its new name ICF-International Classification of Functioning in 2001.

ICF-defines component of health and some health related components of well being (such as education and labour). The ICF domain can, therefore, be seen as health domains and health related domains. These domains are described from body, individual and societal perspectives.

ICF has two parts each with two components (Tables 18.1 and 18.2).

Table 18.1: Definitions of the component of ICF

1. Functioning: Refers to all body functions, activities and participation as an umbralla term.
2. Disability: Serves as an umbrella term for impairment, activity limitation and participation.
3. Body functions: Are the physiological functions of body systems (including psychological functions).
4. Body structures: Are anatomical parts of the body such as organs, limbs and their components.
5. Impairments: Are problems in body function or structure such as organs, limbs and their components.
6. Activity: Is the execution of a task or action by an individual.
7. Participation: Is involvement in a life situation.
8. Activity limitations: Are difficulties an individual may have in executing activities (activity limitations replaces the term "disability" used in 1980 verson of ICIDH).
9. Participation restrictions: Are problems an individual may experience in involvement in life situations (replaces the term "handicap" used in 1980 version of ICIDH).
10. Contextual factors: Are the factors that together constitute the complete context of an individual's life and in particular the background against which the health states are classified in ICF.
11. Environmental factors: Constitute a component of ICF and refers to all aspects of the external or extrinsic world that form the context of an individuals life and as such, have an impact on that person's functioning. Environmental factors include physical world and its features, the human made physical world, other people in different relationships and roles, attitudes and values, social systems and services, and policies; rules and laws.
12. Personal factors: Are contextual factors relate to the individual such as an age, gender, social status, life experiences and so on (which are not currently classified in ICF).

Table. 18.2: An overview of ICF

	Part 1: Functioning and disability		**Part 2: Contextual factors**	
Components	Body functions and structures	Activities and participation	Environmental factors	Personal factors
Domains	Body functions Body structures	Life areas (tasks, actions)	External influences on functioning and disability	Internal influences on functioning and disability
Constructs	Change in body function (physiological)	Capacity Executing tasks in a standard environment	Facilitating or hindering impact of features of the physical, social and attitudinal world	Impact of attributes of the person
	Change in body structure (anatomical)	Performance Executing task in the current environment		
Positive aspect	Functional and structural integrity	Activities participation	Facilitators	Not applicable
	Functioning			
Negative aspect	Impairment	Activity limitation Participation restriction	Barriers/hindrances	Not applicable
	Disability			

Part I: Functioning and disability
a. Body functions and structures
b. Activities and participation

Part II: Contextual factors
a. Environmental factors
b. Personal factors

Each component can be expressed in both positive and negative terms.

DOMAINS FOR THE ACTIVITIES AND PARTICIPATION

In ICF the domains for the Activities and Participation components are given in a single list that covers the full range of life areas (from basic learning or watching to composite areas such as interpersonal interactions or employment). They are as follows:
1. Learning and applying knowledge
2. General tasks and demands
3. Communication
4. Mobility
5. Self care
6. Domestic life
7. Interpersonal interactions and relationships
8. Major life areas (education, work and employment and economic life)
9. Community, social and civic life.

INTERACTION BETWEEN THE COMPONENTS OF ICF (Fig. 18.2)

At this time, the new ICIDH-2 (ICF) classification appears to be the best model for conceptualizing impairment and disability. It acknowledges the complex and dynamic interactions between a given health condition, the environment, and personal factors. The relationships between impairment, activity limitations and participation restriction are not assumed to be unidirectional. For example one may have impairment without activity limitations (disability) or limitations in participation (handicap) or one could have activity limitations (disability) without limitations in participation (handicap). On the other hand one could have limitations in activities or participation

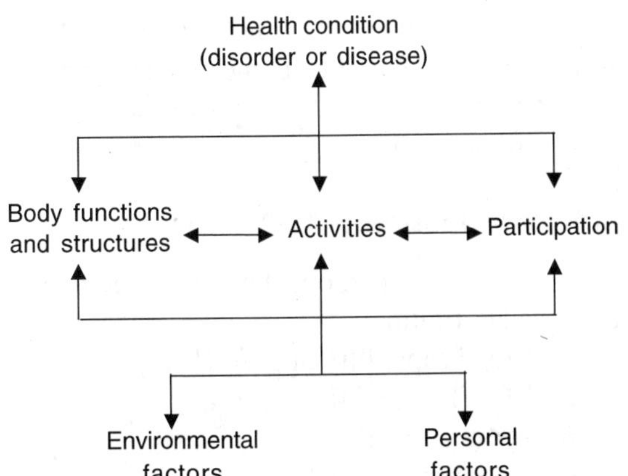

Fig. 18.2: Interatction between the component of ICF

without documented impairments (e.g. Pain). This model also recognizes that limitations in partici-pation may secondarily produce limitations in activities which may also produce impairments. For example, inability to participate in fitness programs may cause poor performance in daily activities which can produce impairments (decreased cardiovascular endurance and diminished muscle strength).

UNIVERSAL APPLICATION OF ICF

There is a widely held misunderstanding that ICF is only about people with disabilities; in fact it about all people. The health and health related states associated with all health conditions can be described using ICF. In other words, ICF has universal application.

FUNCTION

Function, in rehabilitation terms, is what humans do or how humans act. Functional activities encompass all those tasks, activities and roles that makes the individual independent. The ultimate aim of any rehabilitation program is to make the individual independent in all those functions which he used to perform before the trauma/disease.

Human functions can broadly be divided into:

i. Basic or personal activities of daily living (BADLs)
ii. Instrumental activities of daily living (IADLs)
iii. Work activities
iv. Sports/recreational activities.

Basic ADLs

Basic or personal ADL consists of the following activities:

a. Eating activities (using utensils, cup/glass, taking food/drink to the mouth, breaking bread etc.)
b. Hygiene activities (brushing teeth, bathing, toileting, combing hair, shaving etc.)
c. Bed activities (moving in bed, managing pillows and blankets, reaching for objects etc.)
d. Dressing activities (putting on/taking off shirts, trousers etc.)
e. Transfer activities (bed-to-chair, sit-to-stand from chair and toilet, into a car etc.)
f. Walking activities (walking on level surfaces and uneven surfaces, negotiating curbs, ascending and descending stairs).

Instrumental ADLs

To live independently in a community an individual should be able to perform following functional tasks known as IADLs.

a. Meal preparation (cutting vegetables, stirring etc.)
b. Household work (Dusting, mopping floors, washing dishes etc.)

c. Communication (writing, using telephone etc.)
d. Shopping
e. Driving
f. Gardening
g. Having sex.

Work Activities

These comprises of physical demands that a worker may need to perform a job:
a. Lifting
b. Carrying
c. Stooping
d. Pushing
e. Pulling
f. Reaching
g. Manipulating
h. Climbing
i. Sitting
j. Standing
k. Walking.

Sport and Recreational Activities

These skills are required to perform any sport or game:
a. Walking: Forward, retro and side ways.
b. Jogging: Forward, retro, on grass, on a track, on hills, in water etc.
c. Jumping: Vertical, forward, retro, side to side, on a level surface, from a height, etc.
d. Throwing: Underhand, overhand, two handed (with different size and weight of ball).
e. Catching: Two handed, one handed (with different size and weight of ball).
f. Batting: Cricket bat, tennis and badminton recquet, hockey stick etc.
g. Swimming: Back stroke, crawl stroke, breast stroke etc.
h. Sprinting: Forward, retro, on grass, on a track, on a basket ball court etc.

ADL Training is a method to make a particular activity possible for the client to perform with the help of a special device, splint, piece of equipment or specific technique.

Factors Influencing ADL Training

The following factors should be considered before starting ADL training:
i. Physical capability of the client:
   a. Muscle strength
   b. Joint range of motion
   c. Coordination
   d. Sensation
   e. Balance
   f. Cognitive and perceptual skills
   g. Cardiopulmonary endurance.
ii. Culture and values of the client
iii. Family support
iv. Environment (in which activity has to be performed)
v. Financial assistance.

Goal of ADL Training

The ultimate aim of any ADL training for the client is to achieve maximal level of independence is different for every client. For e.g. Walking independently may be the maximal level for a person with lower extremity amputation. But self care, feeding and communication with assistance or device may be the maximal level for quadriplegic.

Evaluation of ADL

Consists of evaluation of those activities which the client was performing before the disability or when he is expected to perform as per his socio-cultural context (In case of congenital or early life disability).

Parameters of ADL Evaluation

ADL is evaluated on basis of three parameters:
1. Level of independence—different levels are:
  • Independent

- Supervision
- Minimum assistance
- Moderate assistance
- Maximum assistance.

2. Time—Amount of time required to perform an activity.
3. Accuracy—How accurately the client perform the ADL.

Sequence of ADL Training

ADL training has to be given in the following sequence:

- BADL → IADL.
   For self care activities:

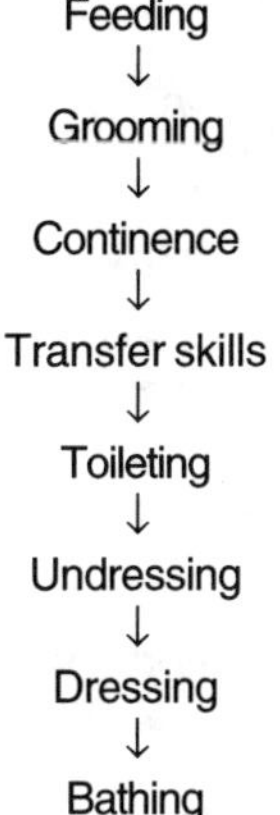

Basic Principles of ADL Training

i. Make out which ADLs are possible and which are impossible to achieve.
ii. Explore the alternate methods of performing the activities.
iii. Use any assitive devices that may be helpful.
iv. Determine the amount of assistance required (from no assistance to maximal assistance).
v. Progression of training:

a.
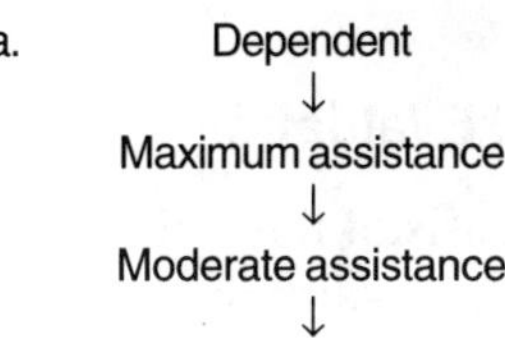

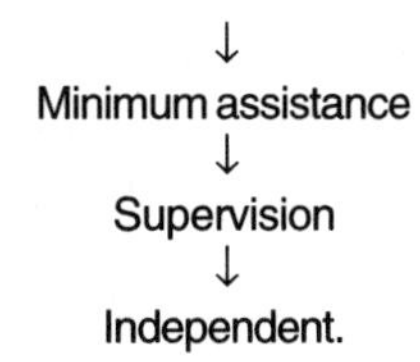

b. Few tasks → more tasks
   Simple tasks → complex tasks.

vi. Methods of teaching should suit the client's ability.
vii. Each activity should be broken into small tasks and then each task into several small steps. Then step by step teaching should be followed.
viii. Demonstration of each activity/task/step should be done by the therapist.
ix. Method of 'backward' or 'forward' chaining may be used while teaching ADL skills.

- Backward chaining: In this method therapist assists the client in all the steps of the task except the last step (which is independently performed by the client).

  When the last step is mastered, the therapist withdraws assistance from the second last step and the client performs the second last independently.

  The process is continued till the client achieves independence over all the steps.

- Forward chaining: The client practice and become independent in the first step of the task and rest steps is assisted by the therapist.

  Then therapist withdraws his assistance from the second step and the client performs the second steps.

  The process is continued till the client achieves independence over all the setps.

Guidelines for ADL training in the client with impaired muscle strength and/or limited range of motion:

1. Dressing activities
- Use one size larger garments.

- Use front opening garments.
- Use larger buttons or zippers.
- Use velcro if buttons/zippers are difficult to use.
- Use dressing stick
- Use reachers for picking up clothes.
- Use shoes without laces or with elastic or velcro types fasteners.
- Use button hooks.

2. Eating activities
   - Use adapted or built-up handles of utensils.
   - Use straws if it is difficult to drink with glass.
   - Use universal cuffs.
   - Use high table.
   - Use cups/glass with bilateral handles.

3. Bathing and grooming
   - Use hand held shower and flexible hose.
   - Use long-handled bath brush or sponge.
   - Use soap on a rope.
   - Use long or angulated handled comb/toothbrush.
   - Use reacher.
   - Use dressing stick
   - Use bathing stool with grab bar.
   - Safety issues:
     – use non skid tiles in bathroom/toilet
     – use grab bars.

4. Communication
   - Use holder for hand-piece of telephole.
   - Use dialing stick-hand, mouth or head held.
   - Use built up pen and pencils.
   - Use mouth stick or head stick from typewriter or computer.

5. Mobility and transfers
   - Use enlarged and padded grips on crutches, canes and walkers.
   - Use walker or crutch, bag or basket to carry objects.
   - Use raised chairs/toilet seats (easy to transfer from).

6. Home management:
   Use utility cart, reachers, adapted knifes, light weight utensils, etc.

Guidelines ADL training in the client with incoordination:

1. Weighted devices such as heavy plates or plates with weight attached, etc.
2. Suction bases, non skid mats or plate stabilized can also be used.
3. Weighted wrist cuffs can be used while performing ADLs.
4. Work height should be high enough to prevent bending, leaning or reaching.

Dressing activities for Hemiplegics
Figures 18.3a to i.

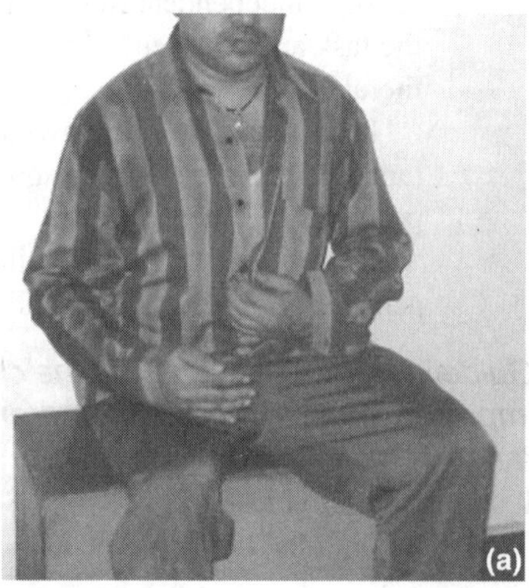
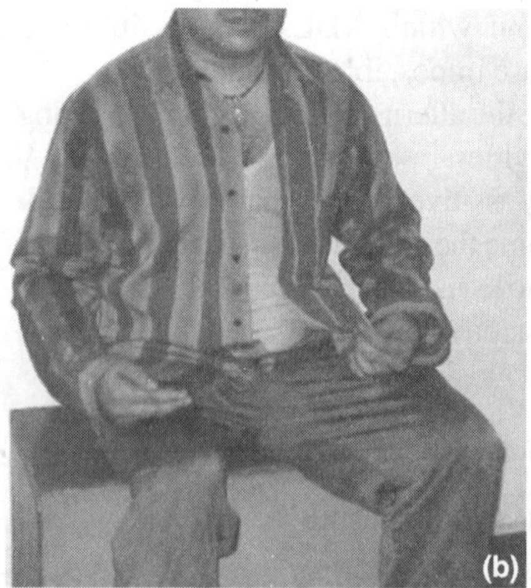

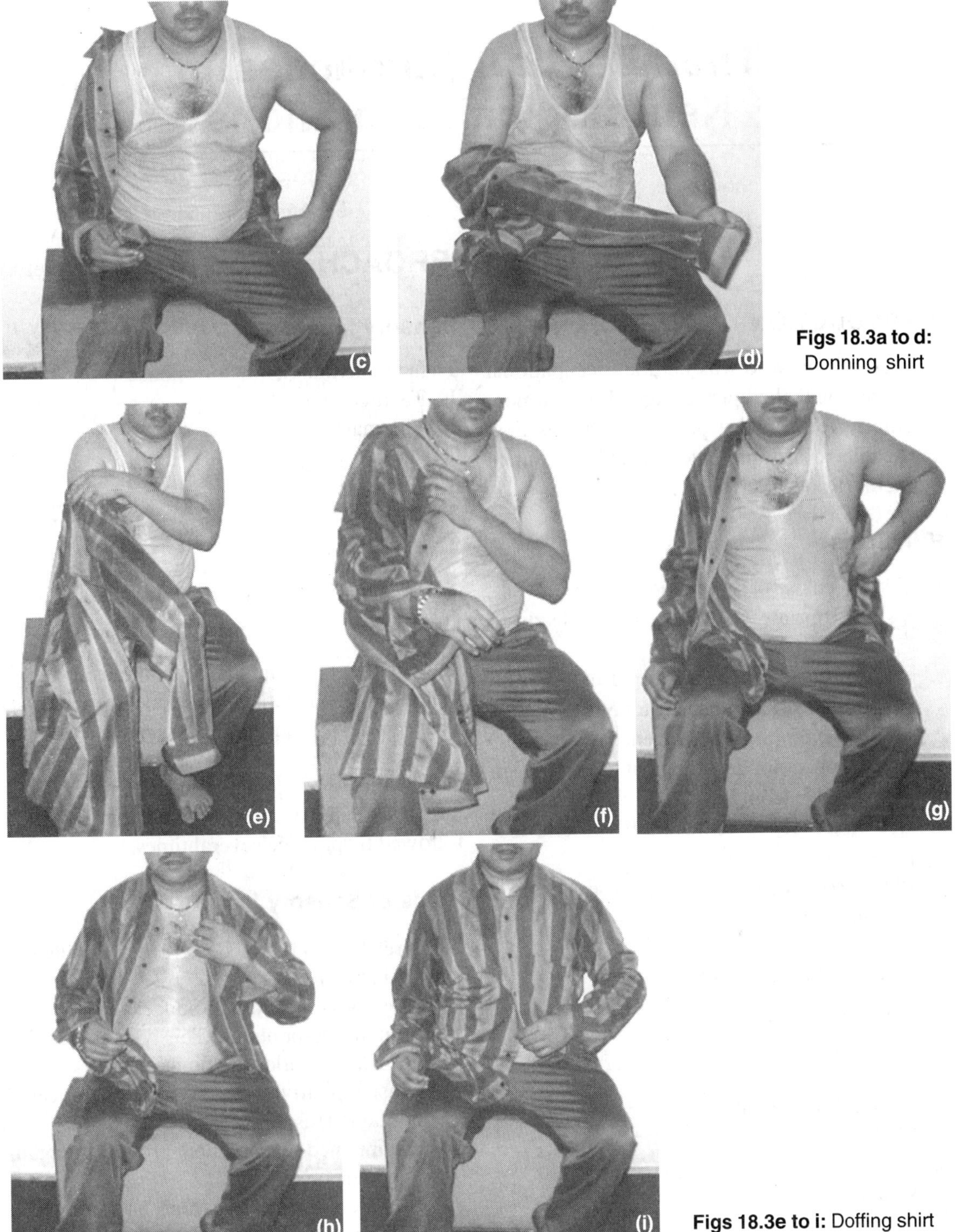

Figs 18.3a to d: Donning shirt

Figs 18.3e to i: Doffing shirt

CHAPTER-19

Therapeutic Approaches in Neurological Conditions

ROOD'S APPROACH

INTRODUCTION

Margaret Rood who was both an occupational and a physical therapist designed a treatment originally for cerebral palsy which was also applicable to any patient with motor control problems (Rood, 1976).

Principles

1. Controlled use of sensory stimulation
   - Appropriate sensory stimulus leads to specific motor response.
   - Appropriate sensory stimulus leads to normalization of muscle tone.
2. Use of developmental sequences
   - Sensorimotor development takes place in sequence from lower to higher level.
3. Use of activity to demand a purposeful response.
4. Practice of sensory motor responses is necessary for motor learning.

Levels of Motor Control

1. Supine withdrawal
2. Roll over
3. Pivot prone
4. Neck co-contraction
5. Prone on elbows
6. Quadruped
7. Standing
8. Walking.

Sensory Inputs

To facilitate/inhibit motor responses:
1. Tactile (cutaneous)
2. Thermal
3. Olfactory
4. Gustatory
5. Auditory
6. Visual
7. Proprioceptive (Stretch, resistance).

Method of Treatment

Sensory inputs are applied to facilitate or inhibit motor responses. Patients are made to go in developmental level sequentially starting from the level patient already has sensory inputs can be applied along with the developmental level. Finally use of purpose of activity should be incorporated followed by practice several times.

Rules of Sensory Input

Margaret Rood (1970), described four rules of sensory input:
1. A fast brief stimulus produces a large synchronous motor output. This type of stimulus confirms the reflex are functioning.
2. A fast repetitive sensory input produces a maintained response.
3. A maintained sensory input produces a maintained response.

   For e.g. Gravity—which has a constant effect on the sensory system. In all positions (standing, sitting or lying) the exteroceptors of the skin are in contact with a surface, thus discharging impulses into the nervous system.

4. Slow, rhythemical, repetitive sensory input deactivates body and mind.

For e.g. Slow rocking or soft music activates the parasympathetic system leads to generalized relaxation.

Sequence of Motor Development

Margaret Rood proposed four sequential phases of motor control:

1. *Reciprocal innervation/inhibition*—A phasic (quick) type of movement that requires contraction of the agonist muscles as the antagonist muscle relaxes. It is an early mobility pattern protective in nature.

2. *Co-contraction*—It is defined as simultaneous contraction of the agonist and antagonist muscles with the antagonist supreme.

It is a tonic (static) pattern which provides the ability to hold a position or an object for a longer duration.

3. *Heavy work*—It is described by stock Meyer (1967) as "mobility super imposed on stability." In heavy work the proximal muscles contract and move and the distal segment is fixed.

For e.g.—Creeping, in quadruped position the distal segments—wrist and ankles are in a fixed position. The neck and thorax (proximal joints) are stable whereas the shoulder and hip girdles are free to move.

4. *Skill*—It is the highest level of motor control and combines the effect of mobility and stability. In skilled pattern the proximal segment is stabilized while the distal segment moves freely.

For e.g.—Typing requires stability in proximal joints (shoulder, elbow) while skilled mobility in distal finger joints.

Outogenic Motor Patterns

1. *Supine withdrawal (flexion)*—Is a total flexion response towards the vertebral level of T_{10}. The flexion of the neck and the crossing of the arms and legs protect the anterior surface of the body.

It is useful in integration of the tonic labyrinthine reflex and for patients who do not have reciprocal flexion pattern and dominated by extensor tone.

2. *Roll over*—Rolling toward side causes:
   - Mobility pattern for the extremities and activates the lateral trunk musculature.
   - Stimulation of the semicircular canals, which in turn activate neck and extra ocular muscles.

   It is useful for patients who are dominated by tonic reflex patterns in the supine position.

3. *Pivot prone*—It is both a mobility pattern and a stability pattern. In this pattern there is full range of extension of the neck, shoulders, trunk and lower extremities. This position is difficult to assume and hold. It prepares the extensor muscles for upright positions and indicates integration of the symmetric tonic neck reflexes and the tonic labyrinthine reflexes.

4. *Neck co-contraction*—It activates both flexors and deep tonic extensors of the neck. It is the first real stability pattern. This pattern elicits the tonic labyrinthine righting reaction when the face is perpendicular to the floor and also promotes neck stability and extra-ocular control.

5. *Prone on elbows*—Weight bearing on elbows stretches the upper trunk musculature to influence the stability of the scapular and glenolumeral regions. In this position patient has better visibility of the environment and can do weight shift from side to side.

   The symmetric tonic neck reflex gets inhibited in this position.

6. *Quadruped position*—In this pattern lower trunk and lower extremities are in co-contraction. The patient can do weight shifts in forward/backward, side to side and diagonal directions. This provides mobility superimposed on the stability and prepares for equilibrium responses.

7. *Standing*—In this position weight is equally distributed on both legs after that weight shifting begins. The upper extremities are free to perform functions. Also standing brings in integration of righting reactions and equilibrium reacting.

8. *Walking*—Murray (1967) described gait as a normal locomotion that entails the ability to support the body weight, maintains balance and executes the stepping motion. Walking requires coordinated mobility and stability.

FACILITATION TECHNIQUES

1. **Tactile (Cutaneous) stimulation**—It causes stimulation of exteroceptors (end organs under the skin in subcutaneous tissues). These receptors respond to the external environment causes protective withdrawl responses and produces states of alertness and rapid movements of the limbs.

   a. *Light moving touch*—Touche is important for normal growth and development (Montague A, 1978).

   It has following effects:
   - Increases corticosteroid levels in the blood stream.
   - Increases resistance against disease.
   - Increases tissue repair.
   - Improves fluid and electrolyte balance.

   Margaret Rood used a light moving touch or stroking of the skin to activate the superficial mobilizing muscles.
   - *Application:* Finger tips, camel hair brush or cotton swab.
   - *Frequency:* 3-5 strokes, 30 seconds rest period between strokes.
   - *Area:* The first area is the area from the nose to chin, (after several stimulation infant may show response of flexion pattern of upper extremity and perhaps lower extremity.
   - Light stroking from the corner of the lip to the cheek. It activates neck muscles and the head tilts laterally toward the side of the stimulus.
   - Light moving touch to the navel or dermatome T_{10} in a midline to lateral direction-activates unilateral flexion pattern.
   - Light moving touch to the dorsal web spaces of the fingers and toes activates a withdrawl pattern of the extremities.
   - Light moving touch to the tips of the fingers or soles of feet facilitates a tickle withdrawl response of great magnitude.

   b. *Fast brushing*—Fast brushing by battery operated brush (introduced by Margaret Rood in 1964) is applied over the dermatomes of the same segment that supplies the muscle (myotome) to be facilitated.

   For e.g.—Stimulation of L_{3-4} dermatomes leads to the facilitation of quadriceps, tibialis anterior and detrusor urinae.

   The effect of fast brushing lasts for 30 minutes. The stimulus is applied for 3 to 5 seconds and repeated after 30 seconds.

   c. *Icing*—Ice is an extreme in thermal facilitation and has been used for facilitation of muscle activity and autonomic nervous system responses (Margaret Rood, 1954). Margaret Rood described three uses of ice:
   - Quick icing for patients having hypotonia (3 swipes, blott water after each swipe)

- Pressing ice cubes to the skin of a dermatome corresponding to myotome to be stimulated
- Ice to stimulate sympathetic nervous system and probably glandular output of the thyroid and adrenal glands.

  Ice should be used cautiously especially in patient having cardiac problems.
  Note: The exteroceptive stimulation can be unpredictable. In the 1970s M. Rood began to abandon the use of this stimuli and endorse the use of proprioceptive stimuli.

2. **Proprioceptive stimulation**—It refers to the facilitation of:
   - Muscle spindles
   - Golgi tendon organs
   - Joint receptors and the vestibular apparatus.

   Joint gives more control over the motor response. Proprioceptors adapt more slowly than exteroceptors and can produce sustained postural patterns (Buchwald J, 1967).

   a. **Heavy joint compression**—It is defined as joint compression greater than body weight applied through the longitudinal axis of the bone (Ager J, 1974).

   It causes co-contraction around joint under compression. This procedure can also be combined with ontogenetic patterns such as prone on elbows, quadruped, sitting and standing positions.

   The joint compression can be applied manually or by weighted cuffs or sandbags.

   b. **Stretch**—According to Rood stretch is a physiologic stimulus used to activate the proprioceptors in selected muscles of the body.
      - *Intrinsic stretch:* According to Rood it is the use of the intrinsic muscles to promote stability of the scapulohumeral rhythm.

        For e.g.—In prone on elbows, resistive grasp can enhance shoulder stability. Resistance is a form of stretching as it increases fusimotor activity of the muscle spindle.

   - *Resistance:* Rood emphasized the use of heavy resistance to stimulate both primary and secondary endings of the muscle spindle.

     When a muscle contracts against resistance it assumes a shortened length that cause the muscle spindles to contract so they readjust to the shorter length.

     According to Rood intermittent resistance graded to the desired motion is better than manual stretching for alleviating tight muscles.

   - *Stretch pressure:* It affects both the exteroceptors and the Ia afferent of the muscle spindle. The degree of stretch and pressure should be strong enough to cause defomation of skin and underlying superficial muscle:
     - lubricants can be used.
     - time of stimulus < 3 seconds.
     - can be applied directly over muscle or dermatomically.
     - use thumb, index and middle finger to stretch with pressure.

   - *Tapping:* It acts on the muscle spindle (afferent) and increases the tone of the underlying skeletal muscles.
     - it is done by tapping over the belly of muscles with finger tips
     - 3-5 times over the muscle to be facilitated.

   - *Vestibular stimulation:* According to De Quiros JB vestibular stimulation is a powerful proprioceptive input.

Therapeutic uses:
- to promote extensor patterns of the neck, trunk and extremities (Static labyrinthine system)
- to elicit subcortical responses, such as protective extension
- to activate antigravity muscles and their antagonist
- fast stimulation such as rocking stimulates while slow rhythmic rocking causes relaxation
- vestibular stimulation affects tone, balance, protective responses, bilateral integration and auditory language development.

- *Vibration:*
  - Frequency—High frequency—100 to 300 cycles/second.
    Low frequency—50 to 60 cycles/second.

  Uses:

  High frequency vibration is used to elicit tonic vibration reflex which stimulates contraction of muscle if applied directly over the belly. It also inhibits contraction of antagonist muscle and suppress stretch reflex.

  Low frequency vibration suppress pain perception, desensitize hypersensitive skin.

  Other factors:

  Vibration should be applied parallel to muscle fibers.

  Do not apply vibration over tendon, it may stimulate surrounding muscle through bone.

  Do not apply vibration with deep pressure as it is inhibitory.

Duration of application should not be more than 1 to 2 minutes (to avoid heat formation)

- *Osteopressure:* It is defined as pressure on bony prominences to facilitate or inhibit voluntary muscles.

  According to Margaret Rood, osteopressure produces a slower reaction and needs to be preceeded by a light moving touch. For e.g.—if light moving touch is applied to dermatome C_7 of the arm and pressure applied over the lateral epicondyle of the elbow, the arm extends.

  The underlying neurophysiology has not been understood properly.

- *Inhibition Techniques:* According to Rood following techniques may be used for inhibiting abnormal tone.
  - gentle shaking or rocking.
  - slow rolling
  - light joint compression
  - tendinous pressure
  - maintained stretch
  - rocking in developmental pattern.

- *Use of special senses for inhibition/ facilitation:* M. Rood used olfactory and gustatory stimuli to facilitate cranial nerves and to influence.

  Autonomic nervous system: Though she did not provide specific guidelines for their uses: Clinically following can be used:
  - pleasant orders for calming effect.
  - unpleasant order to produce primitive protective responses
  - noxious substances (such as vinegar) for activating muscles of mastication.

BRUNNSTROM'S APPROACH

INTRODUCTION

Brunnstrom approach or movement was given by sign Brunnstrom, a physical therapist in the year 1970.

This approach is exclusively for the patients with cerebrovascular accidents or stroke.

Principles

1. Reflexes and whole-limb movement patterns are normal stages of development. In stroke, development occurs in reverse pattern.
2. Reflexes and primitive movement patterns should be used to facilitate the recovery of voluntary movement after stroke.
3. Proprioceptive and other somato sensory stimuli can be used to facilitate movement or tonal changes.
4. Recovery in stroke patient takes place in following sequence:

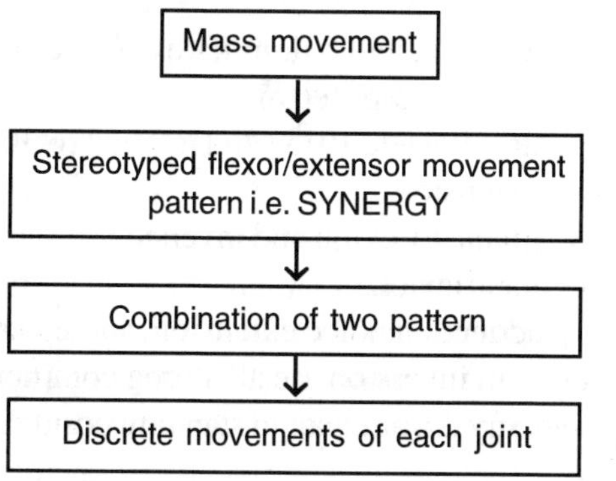

5. New correct movements achieved, must be practiced to be learned.
6. Treatment progresses in following sequence.

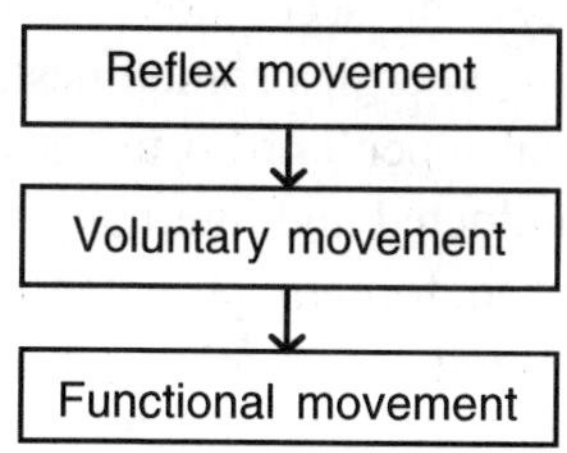

7. If voluntary effort leads to a response, the following sequence of contraction should be practiced:

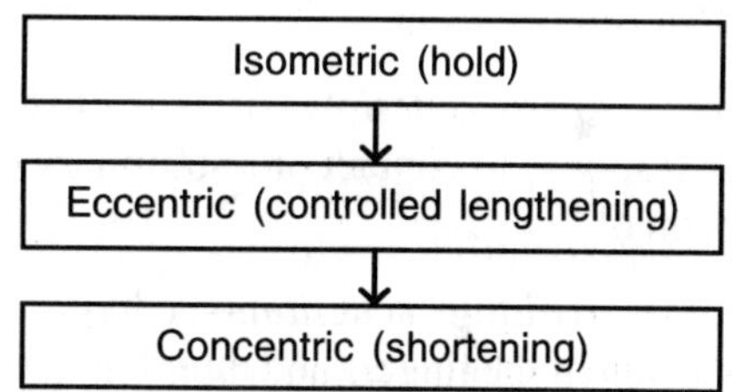

8. Reduce or wean off facilitation as soon as patient shows evidence of voluntary control.
9. Correct elicited movement, repeat to learn it.
10. Practice should include functional activities.

Definition of Terms

Synergy—is a movement pattern in which a group of muscles acting as a bound unit in a primitive and stereotypical manner.

The muscles are neurophysiologically linked and cannot act alone or perform all of their function. If one muscle in the synergy is activated, each muscle in the synergy responds partially or completely.

Associated reactions—are movements seen on the affected side in response to voluntary forceful movements in other parts of the body.

Homolateral limb synkinesis—is a mutual dependency between the synergies of the affected upper and lower limb. Similar type of movement occurs in affected upper and lower limb.

Limitation synkinesis—are associated reactions that facilitate the performance of difficult movement by performing the same movement on the opposite side.

Proximal traction response—is elicited by a stretch to the flexors muscles of one joint of upper limb which evokes contraction of all flexors of that limb including the fingers.

Grasp reflex—when deep pressure is applied to the palm and move distally over the hand and fingers, mostly on the radial side, adduction and flexion of fingers occur.

Instinctive grasp reaction—It is a closure of hand in response to contact of a stationary object with palm of the hand.

Instinctive avoiding reaction—A hyperextension reaction of the fingers and thumb in response to forward-upward elevation of the arm.

Souque's phenomenon—It is the automatic extension of the fingers when the shoulder is flexed.

It can be seen in only few patients though the position is helpful in facilitation of finger extension.

Ramiste's phenomenon—are associated reactions of hip abduction on a adduction. Resistance to hip abduction or adduction of the non involved extremity evokes the same movement of the involved extremity.

Components of Limb Synergies

Upper Extremity Flexor Synergy

It usually develops before the extensor synergy and composed of:
- Scapular retraction and/or elevation.
- Shoulder abduction and external rotation.
- Elbow flexion.
- Forearm supination.
- Wrist and finger—variable position elbow flexion is the strongest component movement to appear or to be facilitated. Shoulder abduction and external rotation are weak components.

Upper Extremity Extensor Synergy

Composed of:
- Scapular protraction.
- Shoulder horizontal adduction and internal rotation.
- Elbow extension.
- Forearm pronation.
- Wrist and finger—variable position.

Shoulder horizontal adduction and internal rotation are the strongest components of this synergy. They are the first movements to appear and to be facilitated. Elbow extension is a weak component.

Lower Extremity Flexor Synergy

Composed of:
- Hip flexion, abduction and external rotation.
- Knee flexion.
- Ankle dorsiflexion and inversion.

Hip flexion is the strongest component whereas hip abduction and external rotation are weak components.

Lower Extremity Extensor Synergy

This synergy usually dominates in the lower extremity and composed of:
- Hip extension adduction and internal rotation.
- Knee extension.
- Ankle plantar flexion and inversion.
- Toes dorsiflexion.

Hip adduction, knee extension, ankle plantar flexion with inversion are all strong component. This synergy is dominant in standing position.

Typical Arm Posture

When both synergies are developing and spasticity is marked, the strongest components of the flexion and extension synergies sometimes combine to produce typical upper limb posture in hemiplegia. The arm is adducted and internally rotated with the elbow flexed, forearm pronated and the wrist and fingers flexed.

Stages of Motor Recovery

Signe Brunnstrom observed that patient progresses through a series of recovery stages in a stereotypical fashion (Table 19.1).

Table 19.1: Stages of motor recovery in hemiplegia

Stage	Characteristics		
	Leg	**Arm**	**Hand**[*]
1.	Flaccidity.	Flaccidity; inability to perform any movements.	No hand function.
2.	Spasticity develops; minimal voluntary movements.	beginning development of spasticity; limb synergies or some of their components begin to appear as associated reactions.	Gross grasp beginning; minimal finger flexion possible.
3.	Spasticity peaks; flexion and extension synergy present; hip-knee-ankle flextion in sitting and standing.	Spasticity increasing; synergy patterns or some of their components can be performed voluntarily.	Gross grasp, hook grasp possible; no release.
4.	Knee flexion past 90° in sitting, with foot sliding backward on floor; dorsiflexion with heel on floor and knee flexed to 90°.	Spasticity declining; movement combinations deviating from synergies are now possible.	Gross grasp present; lateral prehension developing, small amount of finger ex-tension and some thumb movement possible.
5.	Knee flexion with hip extended in standing; ankle dorsiflexion with hip and knee extended.	Synergies no longer dominant; more movement combinations deviating from synergies performed with greater care.	Palmar prehension, spherical and cylindrical grasp and release possible.
6.	Hip abduction in sitting or standing; reciprocal internal and external rotation of hip combined with inversion and eversion of ankle in sitting.	Spasticity absent except when performing rapid movement; isolated joint movements performed with care.	All types of prehension, individual finger motion, and full range of voluntary extension possible.

From Brunnstrom S: Movement therapy in hemiplegia. New York, 1970, Harper & Row.

Evaluation

Evaluation for Brunnstorm approach includes following:
- Evaluation of sensory status of the patient.
- Level of recovery.
- Voluntary motor control.
- Influence of Reflexes and associated reactions.

S. Brunnstrom's gave *Hemiplegia classification and progress record,* but no data exists for its reliability support. Fugl Meyer *et al.* (1975) developed *The Fugl-Meyer Motor Test* whose reliability were determined to be strong and significant.

Goal of Brunnstrom's Approach

The main goal of this approach is to facilitate the patient's progress through the recovery stages that occur after the stroke.

The following techniques can be used to achieve this goal (Table 19.2).

Treatment

1. *Bed positioning:*
   - Proper positioning begins immediately after the onset of the stroke when the patient is in the flaccid stage.

Table 19.2: Techniques

- Postural and attitudinal reflexes (such as Tonic neck reflex, equilibrium and protective reactions etc.).
- Associated reaction.
- Homolateral limb synkinesis.
- Limitation synkinesis.
- Proximal traction response.
- Grasp reflex.
- Instanctive grasp reaction.
- Instinctive avoiding reaction
- Souque's phenomenon.
- Ramiste's phenomenon.
- Resistance
- Auditory stimuli (e.g. verbal cues)
- Sensory stimulus (e.g. rubbing/stroking skin over the muscle)
- Visual stimuli (e.g. use of mirror)

- Limbs should be placed in the most favorable position without interference from the hypertonic muscles.
- In absence of proper bed positioning the lower limb tends to assume a position of hip external rotation, abduction and knee flexion (due to weight of the limb, position is like flexor synergy of lower limb).
- In case, the extensor synergy dominates in lower limb, the recommended position is:
  - Supine.
  - Slight flexion of hip and knee (use towel or pillow).
  - Later support of leg by towel roll or pillow or sand bag to prevent external rotation and abduction.
  - Ankle supported for neutral position.
- In case, the flexor synergy dominates in lower limb, the recommended position is:
  - Supine.
  - Knee in extension.
  - Hip external rotation should be prevented as described earlier.

- The affected upper limb is supported on a pillow in a position that is comfortable for the patient. Abduction of humerus must be avoided. Patient is instructed to use the unaffected hand to support the affected arm when moving in bed.

2. *Bed mobility:*
   - Turning toward the affected side is easier than turning toward the unaffected side.
   - To turn toward the unaffected side, the affected upper limb is grasped by the unaffected hand, both the limbs are elevated upto 80°-90° of shoulder flexion with elbow extended. The affected lower limb is in slight flexion at hip and knee (supported by therapist). Patient turns an unaffected side by swinging the arms and the affected knee across the body towards the unaffected side. The momentum produced by upper limb helps in turning upper body and pelvis.

   As the patient develops control therapist support is withdrawn.

3. *Trunk control:*
   - To improve trunk control, the patient is gently pushed in forward, backward and side to side direction in sitting position.
   - First push towards the affected side to promote contraction on unaffected side then towards the unaffected side to facilitate contraction on affected side.
   - Improve control in all direction—trunk flexion, extension and rotation.
   - Patient crosses his arms with unaffected hand under the involved elbow and unaffected forearm supports the affected forearm. Therapist sitting in front of patient, supports the patient under the elbow and assists in trunk flexion (avoid any pull on the shoulders). This movement is also helpful in causing some amount of pain free movement of shoulder unconsciously.

- Trunk rotation is facilitated by using tonic neck and tonic lumbar reflexes.
4. Upper limb training
5. Hand training
6. Lower limb training.

Guide Lines for Treatment

Following are the guidelines given by signe Brunnstrom for treating Upper extremity, hand, trunk and Lower extremity during various stages.

Upper Extremity

a. *During stages 1 and 2:* The aim of treatment is to elicit muscle tone and the synergy patterns on a reflex basis.
   - To elicit flexor synergy, tap over the upper and middle trapezius, rhomboids and biceps.
   - To elicit extensory synergy tap over the triceps and stretch serratus anterior.
   - Passive movement through each of the synergy pattern.
   - Elicit flexor synergy first which should be followed by facilitation of the weak extension synergy.

b. *Stage 3:* The aim of treatment is to achieve:
   - Voluntary control for the synergy pattern.
   - Repeat alternate performance of synergy patterns.
   - Weight bearing.
   - Use bilateral rowing movements with therapist hold the patient's hands.

c. *Stages 4 and 5:* The aim of treatment is to break away from the synergies by mixing components from antagonistic synergies to perform new and complex patterns of movement:
   - Perform figure of 8 movement on table or board.
   - Following flexion movements can be performed to promote transition between stage 3 and 4.

- Hand to chin.
- Hand to ear (first affected then on the unaffected side).
- Hand to opposite elbow.
- Hand to opposite shoulder.
- Hand to forehead.
- Hand to top of head
- Hand to back of head.
- Other complex movements which re-presents stage 4, may also be practiced.
  For stage 4:
  - Arm to rear of body.
  - Arm raising forward to horizontal position.
  - Pronation—supination of forearms with elbows flexed.
  For stage 5:
  - Arm raising to side horizontal position.
  - Turning palms up and down, elbows extended.

d. *Stage 6:* Very few patients reached to this stage of upper limb. No specific training method is recommended.

Hand Training

Main objectives of hand training are:
- Achieve mass grasp by using proximal traction response and grasp reflex.
- Achieve wrist fixation for wrist. Facilitate wrist extension by tapping and fist closure simultaneously.
- Achieve active release of grasp:
  - This goal is difficult to achieve due to marked spasticity in finger flexors. Manipulation for active release of grasp—pull the thumb out of the palm, by gripping the thenar eminence while supinating the forearm passively.
  - Roll fingers into flexion to stretch extensors.
  - Pronate forearm while maintaining thumb extension.
  - Use Sougue's phenomenon.
  - Stroke over the inter phalangeal joints.

– Reinforce by individually stretching the finger extensors of each digit.

Trunk

- To elicit balance responses, patient is gently pushed in forward, backward and sideward directions.
- First push toward the affected side (to develop control on non affected side) then toward the non affected side (to develop control on involved side).
- Practice forward flexion of trunk by crossing arms with the non-affected hand under the affected elbow and the non-affected forearm supporting the affected forearm. Therapist may assist by supporting the patient under elbows. This also helps in achieving some pain free movement of shoulder.

- Return from trunk flexion position is actively performed by the patient (without therapist's support).
- Practice forward movement in oblique direction.
- Practice trunk rotation, first with therapist supporting the affected limb then without support.
  (Tonic neck and tonic lumbar reflexes can also be used to facilitate the response).

The basic principles for training of lower extremity follows the following sequence:

1. If voluntary control is absent in any movement or position, contraction of muscle is elicited reflexively.
2. Superimpose voluntary effort on the reflex contraction.
3. Use local facilitatory measures to reinforce the patient's voluntary effort.
4. Use the activated muscle in desired situation.

BOBATH APPROACH

INTRODUCTION

Berta Busse (physical therapist) and Karel Bobath (pediatric physician) born in Burlin, Germany, they practiced in London and developed Bobath concepts there.

Bobath has never conducted original research but hypothesized with the popular findings at the time and tried to explain the various theories.

Berta, during her practice, she observed and analyzed the normal movements and methods of relaxation of the muscles. The assessment of the muscle strength, activity of the muscles and their response to special relaxation methods formed the basis of her for abnormal motor coordination patients. She analyzed posture and movements, then practiced them variation until she learned how individuals perfected them. Her hands developed a great sensitivity to a muscle tone, its readiness to move and responsiveness to change.

Neural Development Technique (NDT) focuses on the analysis and treatment of sensori-motor impairments and functional limitations. This is a living concept, a problem solving approach that consists treatment and management of movements dysfunctions in individual with central nervous system pathophysiology.

Concepts

Following a cerebrovascular accident patient typically overuses the uninvolved side due to impaired sensory and motor function on the hemiplegic side. This also adds to posture, balance, strength, tone and coordination disturbances.

In Bobath approach the therapist develops a program to help the patient to avoid abnormal patterns of movement. This approach provides a foundation that promotes the highest level of functional recovery based on relearning normal movement rather than as compensation. One of the central principles of this approach is that alignment and symmetry of the trunk and pelvis are necessary for good alignment and symmetry of the extremities.

Patients with hemiplegia (stroke) exhibit abnormally high or low tone, which has to be inhibited or facilitated respectively.

Theories

Following are the various theories Bobath used for their clinical findings:
1. Reflex/Hierarchical Model.
2. System Theory.
3. Dynamic System Approach.
4. Neuronal Group Selection Theory.

Reflex/Hiererchical Model

It was developed by Jackson. Bobath used this to the maximum at the early stages. This theory states that a lesion in the higher centers would permit expression of normally suppressed patterns of movements which would then dominate the person's posture and movement. Bobath believed and thought that the CNS is organised as a hierarchy and divided into four functional levels of integration.
- Level 1 : Spinal level—Phasic, Primitive reflexes, stretch reflexes
- Level 2 : Pre pontine/Brainstem—Local, segmental, general tonic reflexes, mass synergies.
- Level 3 : Midbrain—Righting and protective reactions, excitatory and inhibitory control.
- Level 4 : Cortical level—Balance and equilibrium reactions or decrease voluntary control.

These four successive higher levels of neural integrative exert control over the preceding levels. Each level made use of the centrally controlled inhibition so that higher centres have the ability to suppress all but they require part of any intended movement.

The lower centres surrender their autonomy to the higher level during humenkind's development. This rigid model is generally being discarded today for in favor of more flexible models.

System Theory in NDT

Nicoli Bernstein a physiologist developed this theory. According to this motor behavior is an end product of a process of self organization of the body system which is not limited to the CNS alone. He has termed a "coordinative structure" because whenever two or more independent parts combine to perform as a functional unit or synergy they act as a unit.

Nicoli states that biological organisms, like other physical systems, are complex, multi dimensional, cooperative systems in which no one system has a priority for organizing the behavior of the system. In this frame work the task and the context of the behaviour becomes equally important parts of the system.

Dynamic System Approach

This is the extension of system theory, incorporating ideas of how complex system work together within physical world. It has emphasized more on the environment and body system as a strategies of intervention. This theory does not seem to support manual guiding and facilitating movement as a strategy for gaining the best movement possible for individual with motor dysfunction.

Neuronal Group Selection Theory

The dynamic theory is extended by Edelman (1987) and Sporns (1994) by offering a balance between maturation and interactive physical systems.

The theory explains that the recovery of the damaged brain can be fasten or achieved:
1. If the individual is engaged in activities that occur in functionally or developmentally appropriate environmental context and

2. If he or she is allowed to perform the movements which are required for specific tasks.

The Principles of NDT

- The individual should be seen as a whole person with a whole personality.
- A proper evaluation and assessment must be done based on observations and feeling the individual's responses.
- Treatment programmes are tailor made to meet the needs of the individual.
- Reassessment of the individual's responses to treatment is immediate and ongoing. Modifications are made immediately according to that.
- Key points of control are used during treatment to inhibit abnormal movement patterns and facilitate normal movement.
- The Physical Therapist, Occupational Therapist and Speech Therapist must work with the family and teach them how to manage the individual in functional activities, which is essential for effective treatment.
- The normal movements should not be superimposed on abnormal tone.
- All voluntary movements have automatic components.

Normalization of muscle tone may be accomplished by using one or more of the following techniques:

1. Weight-bearing over the affected side.
2. Trunk rotation.
3. Scapular protraction.
4. Anterior pelvic tilt.
5. Facilitation of slow, controlled movements.
6. Proper positioning.

Weight-bearing over the affected side: It is the most effective way of normalizing tone. With patients exhibiting low tone it is facilitative and with patients exhibiting high tone it can be inhibitory. It is helpful in normalization of tone, and providing sensory input to the hemiplegic side through proprioception.

Trunk rotation: It is another very effective way of normalization of tone and facilitating normal movement through the upper and lower extremity patients with hemiplegia usually move as a log or block without dissociation. Trunk rotation is helpful in breaking seen non-dissociated movement.

Scapular protraction: It is beneficial for patients exhibiting a flexion synergy of the upper extremity.

Anterior pelvic tilt: The posterior pelvic tilt is a position in which patients are usually seen. This position encourages abnormal posture resulting in increased hip extension, kyphosis of upper thoracic region and head and neck extension.

All these can be managed by position the pelvic forward.

Facilitation of slow, controlled movements: It is beneficial for high tone patients. It has been seen that quick movements increase the tone therefore it is recommended to use slower and more controlled movement.

Proper positioning: Abnormal postures promote compensatory movement and should be avoided. Proper positioning is very important during all the stages especially in the acute stage.

In sitting:
- Feet flat on the floor.
- Hips near 90° of flexion.
- Knees and ankles less than 90° of flexion
- Trunk extended.
- Head in midline and arm fully supported when working at the table.

In standing:
- Head should be in midline.
- Trunk symmetric.
- Weight equally distributed on both lower extremity.

MOTOR RELEARNING PROGRAM

INTRODUCTION

The Motor Relearning Program was developed by Australian physical therapists Roberta Carr and Janet Shepherd (1983) from their clinical experience and extensive review of contemporary movement science theory and research.

Characteristics of Motor Relearning Program (MRP)

1. Based on skill acquisition and motor development theories especially cognitive motor learning theory.
2. Considers factors other than central nervous system (CNS) damage that may be affecting performance.
3. Includes remediation of impairment and modification of environment.
4. Stresses on practice that fits the nature of the task.
5. Rejects assumptions of the reflex hierarchical model of motor control and of the traditional developmental theories.

Theoretical Basis of MRP

The Rood, Bobath, Brunstrom and Proprioceptive neuromuscular facilitation (PNF) approaches are based on a hierarchical model of motor control, which predicts that dysfunction in the motor cortex results in a release from inhibition of the more primitive brainstem and spinal networks. Treatment focuses on decreasing abnormal reflex activity and primitive movement patterns to facilitate normal movement.

Latest theories in movement science emphasize a distributed control, approach rather than a hierarchical model of motor control. According to this new model motor control depends upon number of structures in the central nervous system. Spinal level structures do not completely depend on higher centres for direct movement commands. Other hemispheric structures prepare the motor system to respond most efficiently to changing environment and task demands.

MRP is based on distributed control model and emphasize the interaction between the performer and the environment.

Interaction with environment for motor performance can better be understood by considering an example. Suppose a person wants to reach forward with one arm, reaching forward would depend upon many factors: the person's posture (sitting, standing, kneeling) and postural alignment, the shape and stability of the seat or supporting surface, how far away and in what direction the goal object is located and the presence of any obstacles between the individual and the goal object.

Motor performance skill of any task depends on the ability to perform the task in number of manners. Research has shown that simply practising movements in isolation of a goal or functional task will not lead to skill development. (Higgins and Spaeth 1972, Smyth 1984).

Carr and Shepherd emphasized on following issues which forms the foundation of Motor Relearning Program:

1. *Postural adjustments:* It is defined as automatic, anticipatory and ongoing muscle activation that enables an individual to maintain balance against gravity, optimal alignment between body parts and optimal orientation of the head, trunk and limbs in relation to the environment.

   It was advocated that postural adjustments can be learned only in the context of task performance. Furthermore, balance training in one position or for one task cannot be generalized to other position or for other task. That is postural adjustments has to be taught in various positions and number of tasks.

2. ***Compensator strategies:*** These are motor patterns or fixations which develop in response to obstructions to normal movement to enable an individual to achieve short-term success in movement or balance.

Effects of compensatory strategies may be reduced by:

a. *Prevention of abnormal muscle shortening:*
   - Postural education
   - Proper posture in lying, sitting and standing
   - Practice variety of motor tasks

   For e.g.: Standing up from sitting position with dorsiflexed ankle, several times a day would prevent shortening of gastro-cnemius.

b. *Prevention of fixation patterns:* Normally when we do tasks like skating or cycling for first time we contract maximum number of body muscles (especially flexors and extensors of trunk) to maintain our balance in posturally threatening situations. Similarly patients with neurological deficits use this pattern in normal day to day task. Most commonly fixation patterns used by such patients are pelvis-on-lumbar spine and scapula-on-thorax. The consequences of these patterns are difficulty in dissociating pelvis or scapula from their respective adjacent structures and lack of mobility of the limbs girdles limiting normal kinematics of upper and lower extremity.

   Motor relearning program stressed on prevention of such patterns by early introduction of training for balance and posture control.

c. *Prevention of muscle weakness:* Motor Relearning Program encourages therapists to "actively search for and detect small amounts of muscle activity as soon as they occur" (Carr and Shepherd 1987). MRP proposes following therapeutic interventions to counteract muscle weakness.

- Various positions of task performance to improve condition of muscle length and assisstive use of gravity.
- Educate patient about inefficient compensations and avoiding unnecessary muscle activity.
- Provide manual guidance to direct patient's performance of task.

3. ***Analysis of normal motor performance of functional tasks:*** One of the important assumption of MRP is that systematic research on how average people perform motor activities can provide a frame work from the treatment of physically impaired patients who must relearn what were once habitual, every day tasks. But research on analysis of normal human performance is limited.

   Tools like video cameras, force plate sensors, gait analyser and electromyographic polygraphs can be used to analyse such performance.

4. ***Motor learning:*** Motor learning has been defined as a set of processes associated practice or experience leading to relatively permanent changes in the capability for producing skilled action (Schimd tRA). This definition of motor learning reflects four concepts:

a. Learning is a process of acquiring the capability for skilled action.
b. Learning results from experience or practice.
c. Learning cannot be measured directly.
d. Learning produces relatively permanent changes in behaviour, thus short-term alterations are not thought of as learning.

The motor relearning program has a significant different approach to motor learning from the previous approaches designed to improve motor control.

It was assumed that practice of an exercise will generalize into improved performance of functional activity. But research does not approve this assumption. Therefore MRP proposes use of exercise with functional goal and varied context.

Approaches like PNF assumes that development takes place in a proper sequence (e.g. rolling → crawling → sitting → standing) as in infants. This forms the foundation for therapy in developing motor control for adult patients. To develop motor control one should follow the proper sequence by developing earlier pattern one would have good control over advanced pattern.

For e.g.: If patient develops good control over sitting it would aid him to develop good control in standing.

But MRP does not follow a developmental sequence. The MRP also disagree those who suggests that therapeutic intervention should proceed in a proximal to distal sequence.

For e.g.: While working on shoulder girdle, MRP encourages to work on hands, also through functional task.

In nutshell, previous therapeutic interventions for individuals with neurological deficits have focused on the patient as a recipient of facilitation and inhibition techniques provided by the therapist. In the MRP, the patient is an active participant in learning how to move functionally and to solve problem during performing functional task.

Therapeutic Intervention

The Motor Relearning Program provides guidelines for evaluating and improving motor control in seven functional daily activities:

1. Upper limb function
2. Orofacial function
3. Sitting up over the side of the bed
4. Balanced sitting
5. Standing up and sitting down
6. Balanced standing
7. Walking.

Carr and Shepherd do not propose any specific sequence for intervention among these seven functional categories. A four-step sequence may be followed to improve skill in a selected function:

Step 1 : Analysis of task
(Observation, comparison)

Step 2 : Practice of missing components
(Explanation of goal, visual and verbal feedback, manual guidance)

Step 3 : Practice of functional task
(Explanation of goal, visual and verbal feedback, manual guidance, Re-evaluation)

Step 4 : Transference of training
(Varied context, consistent practice, modification of environment, involvement of family members).

Guidelines for Evaluation

Detailed analysis of patient's performance of tasks within each of the seven categories of daily activities. The therapist observes the patient as he performs each task and then compares his performance with the normal performance associated with the task. Therapist should be keen observer and try to note the following:

1. Any missing components such as a lack of anterior pelvic tilt and hip flexion when rising to stand.
2. The absence of specific muscle activity.
3. The presence of any excessive or inappropriate muscle activity.
4. Compensatory motor behaviour such as hip-hiking during walking.
5. Incorrect timing of components within a movement pattern.

Guidelines for Treatment

The key to therapy is to adapt the task or the environment so that the person can achieve successful performance without compensation.

1. A functional task which is challenging yet attainable without any compensatory strategy, is selected and clearly explained to the patient.
2. Therapist modifies the patient's position and position of goal objects to match the level of motor as per the patient's capabilities.
3. The supporting surface on which the patient sits or stands is also carefully selected as per patient's postural control.
4. The MRP recommends five strategies for teaching the patient what he needs to learn:
    a. Verbal instruction.
    b. Visual demonstration:
        – by therapist.
        – with unaffected side/body parts of the patient.
    c. Manual guidance.
    d. Feedback:
        – about quality of performance of task.
        – should be timely and accurate.
        – should inform about movements to be repeated and movements to be avoided.
        – Positive feedback should be genuine.
    e. Consistent practice.
5. Movement component learned should be practised with complete functional task.

For e.g.: Component of bearing weight in elbow extended position should be incorporated in sitting to stand.

6. Once learned a task should be practised in varied context and different environmental and real life situation.

For e.g.: If a patient has learned to reach a glass on table, same task should be practised with cup in different position, at home, with friends etc.

Limitation of MRP

The MRP can't be applicable to patients with severe cognitive deficits which is not uncommon manifestation of stroke and other neurological conditions.

CONCLUSION

In conclusion the MRP is still relatively new and has some inconsistencies between its theoretical basis and actual clinical practice. Carr and Shepherd repeatedly emphasized on functional and goal oriented activities. They state and that they do not consider spasticity to be a significant problem of stroke and they give no recommendations for reducing abnormal tone.

CHAPTER-20

Therapeutic Approaches in Orthopaedic Conditions

PROGRESSIVE RESISTIVE EXERCISE (PRE)

Progressive resistance exercise was developed by De Lorme, which is based on 10 repetition maximum (RM). He first executed it on soldiers suffering from muscle weakness following second world war due to musculoskeletal injuries. A set of exercises was repeated 7 to 10 times per treatment session for five days a week. On the last day of the week (Friday) 10 RM was calculated and new exercise programme introduced for the next week. De Lorme called this method "Heavy Resistance Exercises".

The muscles strengthened by him were not disused but had lost strength from disuse. Later he implemented same exercises on poliomyelitis.

In 1948 De Lorme revised his original method and adopted the name progressive resistance exercise (PRE) because he believed the original name bore false implications since even muscles which could not contract against the force of gravity could be strengthened by this method.

Repetition Maximum (RM)

It is used in PRE to measure the strength of the given muscle, so that the muscle can be strengthened onward to its available strength. For example:

- 1 RM-is the maximum amount of resistance or load that can be lifted only once through available range of motion
- 2 RM-is the maximum amount of resistance or load that can be lifted twice through available range of motion.
- 10 RM-is the maximum amount of resistance or load that can be lifted ten times through available range of motion.

Assessment of RM (For example quadriceps muscles)

Appratus—Quadriceps table, De Lorme Boot and straps. Procedure—The patient is asked to sit in quadriceps table with proper back support, thigh is stabilized with straps. Hands should not be allowed to do any trick movements. De Lorme boot is attached with straps at just above ankle joint. Therapist manually assesses the strength of the quadriceps (which gives hypothesis that this patient can lift this much of weight). Then the weight is attached to the De Lorme boot and patient is asked to lift it in full range of motion. If patient lifts it easily then more weight is applied and patient lifts the weight. This involves a series of single repetition with progressively heavier weight until the 1 RM is achieved (Suppose 20 kg weight is lifted by the patient initially, then weight is increased to 20.5 kg and allowed to lift it through available range of motion, if it can also be lifted through full range of motion, weight is increased further to 21 kg and if this time patient is unable to extend it through available range of motion it means the 1 RM of this patient is 20.5 kg or this patient can extend the leg with 20.5 kg of weight once only in the prescribed or available range of motion.

The 10 RM is calculated by using the same method in which weight is applied to the De Lorme Boot and patient is allowed to extend the leg with the weight 10 times through available range of motion. The weight is increased progressively till the 10 RM is achieved (For example leg is extended with 10 kg for 10 times, if it can be lifted, weight is increased and leg is allowed to extend 10 times and is continued till 10 RM is obtained).

RM assessment is done following warm up exercises (cycling, jogging, push ups etc.) to prevent injuries to the muscles.

The following schemes are generally used in daily clinical practice by the therapist and trainers.

1. *De Lorme and Watkins*
   - 10 lifts with 1/2 10 RM
   - 10 lifts with 3/4 10 RM
   - 10 lifts with full 10 RM
        30 lifts for four times a week, progress 10 RM once weekly. Every 10 repetation.

2. *Mac Queen*
   - 10 lifts with 10 RM
   - 10 lifts with 10 RM
   - 10 lifts with 10 RM
   - 10 lifts with 10 RM
        Progress 10 RM every 1-2 Weeks.

3. *Zinovief (Oxford Technique)*
   - 10 lifts with 10 RM
   - 10 lifts with 10 RM minus 1 lb
   - 10 lifts with 10 RM minus 2 lb
   - 10 lifts with 10 RM minus 3 lb
   - 10 lifts with 10 RM minus 4 lb
   - 10 lifts with 10 RM minus 5 lb
   - 10 lifts with 10 RM minus 6 lb
   - 10 lifts with 10 RM minus 7 lb
   - 10 lifts with 10 RM minus 8 lb
   - 10 lifts with 10 RM minus 9 lb
        100 lifts for five time a week, progress 10 RM daily.
   - Every 10 lifts/repetitions are followed by brief period of rest.

HEAVY RESISTANCE EXERCISES

These exercises were first described by De Lorme in 1945 and used to restore the muscular power and volume after injuries. Athletes, sports persons and body builders use these exercises to increase the muscle girth and strength. Metal weights are generally used to apply resistance against the muscular effort after calculating the repetition maximum (RM). The resistance varies from individual to individual, age and the condition from which he or she is suffering.

PLYOMETRIC EXERCISES

It is the quick, powerful movement in which muscle or group of muscles contract eccentrically which is immediately followed by concentric contraction of the same muscle or group of muscles. For example during running or jumping when toes comes in the contact with the ground the gastrosoleus muscles contract first eccentrically than followed by concentric contraction (Fig. 20.1a to c).

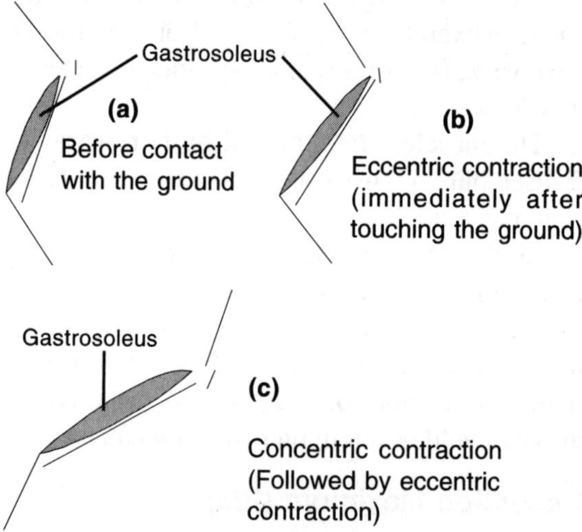

Figs 20.1a to c: Plyometric exercise

During the eccentric contraction (stretch phase), the work performance is enhanced by storing elastic energy in the muscles and during concentric contraction it is reused as mechanical work. This mechanical work is stored in the sarcomere cross bridges and can be reused during the following positive work if the muscles are contracted immediately after the stretch. The timing of the eccentric and concentric contractions, the velocity, and magnitude of stretch determines the ability of muscle to use the stored energy. A quick transition from eccentric to concentric contraction along with a high-velocity stretch of high magnitude produces the greatest benefits.

Bosco and colleagues found that the amount of elastic energy stored in a muscle during eccentric work determines the recoil of elastic energy during positive work.

Plyometric exercises are used to increase the reactivity of the nervous system and enhance the work performance. Before starting plyometric exercises an individual or athlete should undergo advanced exercise programme to build up muscle power, strength and endurance, because plyometric exercises are high level activities in which the muscle (mostly tendon part) is more susceptible to overuse injury.

Uses: Generally used for athletic training.

CLOSED AND OPEN KINETIC CHAIN EXERCISES OR TRAINING

Closed Kinetic Chain (CKC) Training

It is a method of exercise in which the distal segment is fixed and meets considerable external resistance, which prohibits or restrains its free motion. For example both feet (distal segment of the lower extremity) remain on the ground during partial squat to standing or *vice-versa*. The distal segment remains fixed while multiple proximal joints move in a functional manner with contraction of both agonist and antagonists for stabilization.

Examples of closed kinetic chain in upper extremity are-using the upper extremity to perform a wheel chair to bed transfer and push ups.

Closed kinetic chain exercises are more function-based and used for sport-specific muscle group. For example squating involves series of co-contraction of various muscles such as quadri-

ceps, hamstrings, gastrocnemius, and gluteus maximus, which require in many sports and general activities.

Although most of the scientific literatures concerning CKC activities is focussed on quadriceps rehabilitation after anterior cruciate ligament reconstruction, contrasting research by Hunger ford and Barry evaluated patellofemoral contact pressure areas during open kinetic chain exercises and closed kinetic chain exercises.

During closed kinetic chain exercises the cocontraction of the quadriceps and hamstrings decrease the anterior shear force in the knee joint and avoids any stress upon the maturing anterior cruciate ligament graft. These exercises (CKC) are safe to start in the first week of the ACL reconstruction because they generate low anterior tibial displacement and put the ACL graft at the lower risk for developing laxity. And this is the only reason why closed kinetic chain exercises favoured over open kinetic chain exercises after ACL reconstruction.

The cocontraction of quadriceps and hamstrings occurs in CKC exercises, with a progressive decrease in the hamstrings activity as the flexion angle of the knee increases, therefore CKC exercises should be limited to mini squat.

In lower extremities closed kinetic chain exercises appear to be more functional than open-kinetic chain exercises (OKC). During squating simultaneous extension occurs at the knee joint and hip joint. As a result of this movement, the rectus femoris muscle contracts concentrically (shortening) at the knee joint while at the same time it contracts eccentrically (lengthening) at the hip joint. Conversely, the hamstrings contract eccentrically (lengthening) at the knee joint and simultaneously contract concentrically across the hip joint. Therefore CKC causes concentric and eccentric contraction of the rectus femoris from half squat to standing and concentric and eccentric contraction of hamstring from standing to half squating. The concentric and same eccentric contractions at opposite ends of the muscle produce a pseudoisometric contraction. This type of contraction is used during functional activities such as walking, stair climbing, running and jumping and cannot be reproduced by isolated open kinetic chain (OKC) knee flexion and extension exercises.

Open Kinetic Chain Training

It is a method of exercise in which the distal segment of the extremity is free to move. For example—strengthening of quadriceps muscle on quadriceps table where the end segment of the extremity moves freely. In upper extremity such as throwing, strengthening of elbow flexors with dumbbell are the examples of open kinetic chain exercises. The open kinetic chain exercises are more useful in upper extremity as most of the functions are performed in open kinetic chain form.

Open kinetic chain exercises are recommended, especially in the intermediate phase of "bulking up" a severely atrophied muscle before more functional closed chain work is attempted (or along with low-weight closed chain work that emphasizes proper technique and mechanics).

For the upper extremities, open kinetic chain exercises are essential before return to sport because these exercises are similar to the limb movements used in most sports (e.g. the throwing motion).

MUSCLE ENERGY TECHNIQUES (METs)

The muscle energy techniques are derived from the osteopathy field and now being used most widely by clinician in the field of physiotherapy, orthopaedic and osteopathic medicine.

The variety of terms are used to describe the muscle energy techniques—According to:

- Liebenson, 1989 the muscle energy techniques are the "active muscular techniques of relaxation."
- Fred Mitcell Junior, 1958, son of Fred Mitchell Senior M (known for his incredible efforts into osteopathic field)—The patient uses his or her on request, from a precisely controlled position in a specific direction against a distinctly executed counter force.

Thus the muscle energy techniques are the muscle relaxation techniques in which manual resistance is applied against the active contraction of the muscle in the form of isometric or isotonic contraction which may be followed by gentle stretch.

Uses and Indications of METs

1. Severe pain because of severe muscle spasm followed by acute somatic dysfunction such as those with a whiplash injury.
2. Trigger points.
3. Fibrositic changes in the muscle.
4. Restriction of joint range of motion.

Effects of METs

- Muscle relaxation.
- Muscle strenthening.
- Decrease localized oedema/haematoma.
- Relieve passive congestion.
- Increase range of motion of the joint.
- Lengthening of muscles or soft tissues.

PRINCIPLES OF METs

Reciprocal Inhibition

As the name suggests it is the relaxation of antagonistic muscles. In this maneuver the agonist muscles which are shortened or tensed are not allowed to contract, because pain prevents the agonist muscle to contract, therefore opposite group of muscles (antagonist) are allowed to contract isometrically or isotonically against resistance which causes reciprocal inhibition or relaxation of the shortened muscles (antagonist).

Procedure

The shortened muscle is placed between a fully stretched or a fully relaxed state. The limb is held firmly but comfortably. The patient is instructed to contract the muscle (which is opposite to the shortened or tensed muscle,) isometrically or isotonically against manual resistance for 6-10 seconds. This technique allows agonist muscles to relax without contracting them (As the reciprocal inhibition is the component of both proprioceptive neuromuscular facilitation and muscle energy techniques, the some degree of rotational or diagonal movement may be incorporated during isotonic contraction).

Postisometric Relaxation (Lewit's PIR)—

As the name suggests "The physiological relaxation of muscle after isometric contraction." It is the type of hold relax exercise in which the contracted or tensed muscle is allowed to contract against the manual resistance. In this technique the patient is allowed to use the 10-20 percent of his available strength.

Procedure: The tensed or hypertonic (spasmed) muscle is lengthened into the restricted range of motion. Then the limb is held firmly but comfortably and patient is allowed to use 10-20 percent strength of his muscle against the manual resistance applied by therapist and also allows to take the deep breath during contraction. The contraction is allowed for 6 to 10 seconds.

In the next step of the techniques patient is instructed to relax the muscle and exhale then the muscle is again stretched into the restricted range of motion just short of pain and same step is followed again.

Janda's Postfacilitation stretch method—as the name suggest a stretch is given to the muscle just after the contraction. The method is generally used to elongate the muscle length, as well as relax the muscle.

Procedure—The tensed muscle is placed between a fully relaxed and fully stretched state. The limb is held firmly but comfortably and patient is instructed to contract the tensed or shortened muscle with full efforts for 6 to 10 seconds, then allowed to relax the muscle.

In the next step of manuever as the patient relaxes, a rapid stretch is given to the tensed or shortened muscle into restricted range of motion (new position) and held for 10 seconds which is followed by rest of 20 seconds.

The procedure is repeated 3-5 times per session

Isolytic technique—This is the type of resisted

isotonic eccentric contraction of muscle. The technique is used to elongate the muscle fibres by stretching them.

Suppose a patient is has shortened hamstrings. The hip joint is flexed at 30-45° (as it is convenient for therapist) with knee fully extended. The patient is then asked to contract the hamstrings, at the same time therapist maintains the knee extension and flexes the hip joint further which causes eccentric isotonic contraction of the hamstring muscles.

Initially patient offers 20 percent of available strength and the strength increases as the repetitions increase.

WILLIAMS FLEXION EXERCISES

In 1930 William proposed six lumbar flexion exercises. The aim of these exercises were to widen the intervertebral foramen and facet joints to reduce compression on nerve, strengthen the abdominals, stretch the back extensors, hip flexors, and reduce posterior fixation of the lumbosacral junction.

Six exercises are as follows:

1. Patient lies in supine with both knees flexed. While maintaining the position of legs, patient

bends the trunk forward with hip flexion and touches the toes.

2. The patient lies in supine with both knees flexed and contracts the abdominals.
3. Patient lies in supine with hip and knee flexion, holds the both knees with the hands and touches the chest with both knees.
4. In long sitting position repeatedly toes are touched with the hands.
5. In quadruped position one leg remains straightened and other is flexed at hip and knee joint.
6. Patient squats from standing to sitting with slight flexed trunk.

The first three flexion exercises increase the intradiscal pressure and further may increase the bulge of disc therefore should be contraindicated for acute disc herniation. Due to these contra indications William's exercises are rarely used in practice.

SPINAL STABILIZATION

It was first designed by Vollowitz and Morgan for the patients with lower back pain and is also called as functional spinal stabilization.

The stability to the spine is provided by static and dynamic stabilizers. Static stabilizers are—intervertebral disc, vertebral bodies, ligaments and facet joints, these stabilizers do not contract actively but they keep the spinal joints in proper alignment and are known as static stabilizers. Dynamic stabilizers are the structures which contract voluntarily during static and dynamic posture. Both static and dynamic stabilizers act on the spine and maintain the stability of the spinal segments.

Repetitive trauma or strain to the spine can weaken or decrease the ability of static and dynamic stabilizers to stabilize the spine and is the most common cause of pain.

Therapeutic exercises which train the patient to control posturally destabilizing forces during functional activities such as sittling, lifting, squatting and lunging etc. are known as *spinal stabilizing exercises.*

The prime function of these exercises is to increase the endurance and strength of the stabilizers of the spine so that the destabilizing forces can be controlled or eliminated, and this is the only instrument which can prevent chronic and recurrent pain. Learning to stabilize the back and self management skill is the key to prevent recurrence.

These exercise are progressed gradually from non weight bearing position (lying) to the weight bearing positions (sitting, standing) and include isometric contraction, which gradually progresses (as the condition of patient allows) to the functional activities such as—sitting, lifting, squating and lunging.

As the rule of these exercises, the exercise must start in pain free range. The lumbopelvic movement (anterior and posterior tilting) is the range of movement that is both safe and appropriate for the task at hand, and most of spinal stabilizing exercises are started with anterior and posterior tilts of the lumbopelvic joint. Sometimes it may be difficult to find the functional (painfree) range and therefore isometric exercises may only be initiated.

As the painfree range has been determined to be biomechanically safe or stable, it should be used in progressive exercise manner and if the condition of patient improves with the functional range, the exercise may progress form isometric to the isotonic.

In a comprehensive review, compelling evidence was presented that neuromuscular dysfunction is associated with lower back pain with changes in muscular strength and endurance of the trunk muscles and changes in activation amplitudes and synergistic muscle activation pattern reported for a variety of movement patterns.

• The dynamic stability approaches include building muscle strength and endurance and using neuromuscular control strategies required to maintain dynamic trunk stability. These strategies include (1) Selective recruitment of specific muscles and (2) Synergistic coactivation.

- McGill provides an excellent overview of the need for the trunk muscles to act in a synchronous manner to maintain stability, suggesting that even one muscle producing an inappropriate contraction (force) could result in the necessary force disrupt stability.

The present study focused on three exercises commonly prescribed in the management of LBP: the pelvic tilt, abdominal hollowing and trunk stability test level. The latter two emphasize the importance of a neutral spinal position and are claimed to recruit abdominals and trunk muscles in a manner consistent with dynamic stability training, lumbopelvic stability in particular. To date there are no measures other than EMG to substantiate that certain exercises elicit specific muscle activation patterns.

A recent EMG study of healthy subjects performing the three study exercises provided evidence that supported some and refused other previous claims associated with the pelvic-tilt and the abdominal hollowing exercises.

Concepts of Stabilization

1. The movement range (functional range) should be painfree.
2. The segment (Lumbar spine) should be moved in functional painfree range passively.
3. If functional range is not available, initially isometric exercise is recommended.
4. Gradually functional range is improved from isometric to isotonic, squating to sitting, walking and normal course of daily work. Thereafter advanced functional based exercises can be started.

McKENZIE

In 1981, RA McKenzie proposed a different method of treatment to back pain patients which is based on the patient's own normal spinal movements. The symptoms of patient can be reproduced and influenced by the movements and are observed during and after repeated movements or sustained movements.

The diagnosis and management in the McKenzie approach to mechanical disorders are based on the symptoms behaviour observed during and after repeated testing.

The aim of repeated movement testing is to influence the symptoms, and identify the movement which is painless and decrease the symptoms from distal part (peripheral) to the proximal part (central), which is known as centralization phenomenon. The painfree movement is only the treatment tool and is repeatedly performed to centralize the symptoms.

The movement which excerbates the symptoms from proximal to distal, or during repeated movement testing the movement which excerbates the symptoms from proximal to distal segment which is known as peripheralization, should not be administered as it may further increase the disease process.

The intensity and location of symptoms are identified while at rest, during repeated movements and sustained end range positions and are categorized into Postural, Dysfunction and Derangement syndromes.

Postural Syndrome

Pain is normally not present during repeated movements and end range movements but if the end range movements are sustained then only it can reproduce.

The syndrome can be treated by correction of posture. To achieve this the patient first achieves fully slouched position (in sitting, shoulders are drooped, trunk flexed, pelvis posterior tilted) and then fully straightened (chest is expanded, shoulder retracted and pelvis tilted anteriorly). The exercise is repeated for twenty times per session.

Dysfunction Syndrome

In this syndrome pain is reproduced at range of repeated movements, stops shortly on release of end range stress, and may radiate slightly. The symptoms remain unchanged after testing (no better or worse).

The symptoms are reproduced at end range of repeated movement as the shortened or tightened structures get stretched.

The dysfunction syndrome can be treated by stretching the shortened structures. Patient generated forces are sufficient in most of cases to stretch the shortened structures. The movement which causes pain at end range is ideally performed in a slow repeated movement fashion in sets of 10-15 every 2 hourly each day. The correction of posture is also the key factor.

Manual stretching procedures may also be introduced if the progress is slow.

Derangement Syndrome

Symptoms are altered during the movement or in the mid range or through the range and painful arc is present. During repeated movement testing symptoms may centralize or peripheralize.

The treatment is based on evaluation of movements that centralize the symptoms (the movement which reduce the symptoms from peripheral part to the proximal). Once the movement is identified that decreases peripheral symptoms is performed repeatedly in painfree range of motion. The movements which excerbate or peripheralize the symptoms should be discontinued.

MULLIGAN

Brian R Mulligan is a very familiar name in manipulative physical therapy practice. He has been involved in teaching of manual therapy in New Zealand and an abroad since early 1970s. He alongwith RA McKenzie and JC Cameron established the New Zealand Manipulative Therapists Association in 1968 and was made a life member of this body in 1988.

Mobilization with Movement

He has developed the new term "Mobilization with movement" (MWM), which was first implemented on spine to treat the musculoskeletal disorders of spine with SNAGS (sustained natural apophyseal glides) and then to the extremities. Today movement with mobilization covers all the joints of the body.

Similar to the maitland, Mulligan has also paid attention to the movement plane of the joint (Facet joints), which was described by Freddy M Kaltenborn, as lying across the concave articular surface.

Unlike other mobilization techniques, Mulligan has explained all the spinal mobilization techniques in weight bearing positions of the patient (standing or sitting). He considers this to be extremely important as so often with non weight bearing techniques, improvements gained are lost when the patient resumes in an erect posture (weight bearing position).

With the exception of PRP's (Pain relief phenomenon) all techniques are painless Which are quite different from the often quoted phases "No pain no gain".

Common techniques described by the Mulligan are as follows:

1. NAGS (Natural Apophyseal Glides)
2. Reverse NAGS
3. SNAGS (Sustained Natural Apophyseal Glides)
4. Self SNAGS
5. Spinal mobilization with limb movement.

CYRIAX

The Deep Transverse Friction Massage was given by James Cyriax. A London based orthopaedic practitioner. The cyriax massage is recommended to treat most of the musculoskeletal ailments. James Cyriax is also famous for his intraarticular injections.

According to cyriax to treat the musculo-skeletal ailments, it is very important for the practitioner to know where exactly is the problem or source or root of the symptoms. Once practitioner finds the location of lesion, the treatment must be directed directly on the lesion. The symptoms can not be improved if the treatment is being directed elsewhere of the lesion. For example, lateral epicondylitis patient may complaint symptoms over the dorsum of the forearm or down the elbow joint. If treatment is given over the dorsum of forearm, the lateral epicondylitis can not be treated. It is therefore find out the exact location of lesion (i.e. musculotendinous junction/part of the common extensors) and administer the treatment over the location of lesion.

To find out the location of lesion the practitioner must take proper history of patient and perform following maneuvers.

1. Examine the tender area.
2. Observe active range of movements—pain during active movement suggests that lesion/problem may be in the contractile structures, such as muscles.
3. Perform active resistive movements—pain on active resistive movements confirms the lesion may be in the contractile structures.
4. Perform passive movements—if above maneuvers do not reproduce symptoms, it may be said that contractile structures are intact and lesion could be elsewhere. If passive movements reproduce the symptoms of the patient the site of tension may be in the innert or non-contractile structures such as-ligaments joint capsule, cartilage, bursae or bones.

Deep transverse friction massage—The technique varies slightly from condition to condition but the principles remain constant.

1. *Lesion must be brought within reach of the therapist's finger:* For instance, in supraspinatus tendinitis the patients arm must be placed behind the back. This brings the tendon out of the acromion which would otherwise shield the entire structure.
2. *The tissue to receive the massage should be in appropriate tension (except muscle belly):* For instance in lateral epicondylitis if the technique is performed on tendon, the wrist and fingers should be flexed, forearm pronated and elbow is extended to put the tendon under tension. If the technique is being performed on the musculotendinous junction or muscle belly then common extensors of wrist should be relaxed, so the massage can penetrate deeply to tease the fibres apart.
3. *The treatment is applied by the therapist's finger tip.*

Procedure:

- The tip of finger (index) is placed on the skin, the finger tip moves with the skin over the underlying structures. The technique is to move the whole hand with the patient's skin and the therapist's finger moving as one, otherwise a friction burn of the skin may occur. Some practitioners put a piece of tissue paper between fingertip and the skin: this avoids the burn and absorbs sweat which might otherwise cause slippage. The index finger can also be reinforced by middle finger if more pressure is required.
- The friction must be across the fibres of the affected structures with sufficient amplitude of sweep to ensure that the frictional element (and not the pressure) is paramount.
- *Intensity:* The strength (pressure) of massage depends on the stage of this lesion. In acute cases it is given extremely gently and in chronic cases with greater rigour.
- *Duration of treatment:* Varies from condition to condition ranging from 5 min to 20 min.

Some discomfort may be caused during first few minutes which can be minimised by a gentle start. **If there is continuous discomfort, massage should be stopped immediately.**

- The treatment is directed on alternate days for 6 to 12 sessions although it depends on severity of symptoms.

Deep transverse friction massage on following:

1. *Muscular lesions*—The massage breaks down the adhesions formed by the scar tissue between individual muscle fibres.
2. *Muscle tendon*—The scar is eroded by the abrasive action.
3. *Ligamentous lesions*—The formation of adhesions during the period of healing is prevented by moving the ligament over bone in limitation of its normal behaviour.
4. *Tenosynovitis*—It appears that the manual rolling of the tendon sheath to and fro against the tendon serve to smooth off the roughened surfaces.

MYOFASCIAL RELEASE TECHNIQUE

Myofascial release (MFR) technique is given to release restrictions that are secondary to tonal dysfunction in children and adults. The long thening of superficial and deep soft tissue is accomplished by changing the viscosity of the fascia ground substance and by gentle and sustained stretch of the muscular elastic components of fascia.

This technique is usually given in conditions: such as cerebral palsy, stroke, head injury etc.

MUSCLE BENDING: It is also one of the myofascial lengthening technique like MFR which is performed on tendinous part of the muscles such as hamstrings, biceps brachii, hip adductors and pectoralis major.

Procedure: The muscle is placed in a relaxed position, then its tendinous part is grasped

---

Contd.

Contd.

---

between the thumb and fingers of both hands. In the next step the tendinous part is bent by giving pressure with the thumb and fingers of both hands moving away from each other.

The procedure of MFR on superficial and deep soft tissues is as follows:

Pectoralis—Patient is placed in supine position, therapist places three fingertips on the upper sternal end and moves the fingertips along the length of the muscle to the humeral end upto insertion.

Biceps Brachii—Any comfortable position of the patient is choosed. Therapist places three finger tips on the anterior aspect of the upper arm, over the origin of long or short head of biceps and then moves down vertically along the length of muscle to its insertion.

Forearm Muscles (Wrist flexors)—Thumbs of both hands are placed on origin of flexors (below the cubital fossa) then move in a lateral direction upto the wrist.

Palm—The both thumbs are placed on the palmer aspect of the wrist and move in a lateral direction upto the base of the metacarpophalangeal joints.

Rectus Abdominalis—The patient is placed in supine lying. Therapist places upper hand close to the xiphisternum and the lower hand close to the pubic symphysis. A pressure is applied with the upper hand in cephal direction and with the lower hand in caudal direction.

Posterior Neck Muscles—The patient (child) is placed in prone position on medicinal ball and therapist sits behind the child. Therapist places one hand on the base of occiput and the other is placed between the occiput and shoulder. The upper hand (occipital hand) stabilises the head and neck while lower hand is used to give a pressure in caudal direction towards the pelvis or towards the shoulder girdle in case of an asymmetry.

Lower Extremity

Hip Flexors—The patient is placed in supine lying, therapist stands at the side of patient. One hand is placed one inch lateral below the umblicus and other hand is placed on anterior aspect of the upper thigh (affected side). A pressure is applied in cephal direction with the upper hand and in caudal direction with the lower hand.

Adductors—The patient is placed in supine lying, therapist stands at the affected side of the patient. The knee is kept straight. Three fingertips are placed on the groin or origin of the adductors and run along the muscle belly of adductors (medial aspect of thigh) upto the insertion of the adductors. The pelvis is stabilized during maneuver to avoid hiking or lateral flexion. After every stroke from groin to knee the hip joint is abducted.

Hamstrings—The patient is placed in prone lying and therapist stands at the side of the patient. Three fingertips are placed on the ischial tuberosity and moved along the muscle fibres upto insertion of hamstrings.

Gastrocnemius—Patient is placed in prone lying, therapist stands at the side of the patient. Three fingertips are placed on the origin of the muscle and move down in a vertical direction upto the heel.

Plantar Fascia—The patient is placed in prone lying with knee flexion at 90°. Therapist stands at the side of the patient and grasps the patients leg at the ankle joint. The thumb of other hand is placed on little below the heel and move in a lateral direction up to the base of toes.

FUNCTIONAL REHABILITATION IN ORTHOPAEDICS

On past, functional rehabilitation was the ultimate goal only for the neurologically impaired patients. Although the patient with neurological deficit may have obvious motor control, motor performance, cognitive and perceptual problem. The orthopaedic patient may have subtle but similar problems to overcome.

Most of us have experienced that the patient who regained normal strength and motion could not perform his function. Orthopaedic injury may result in abnormal sensory feed back and altered neuromuscular control which may lead to decreased or abnormal movements. Functional training maximizes the use of sensory information mediated by the ligaments, capsule and/or musculotendinous unit.

Many studies have been done on this issue and it has been suggested to therapists to work on functional restoration along with strength and range of motion.

There are three approaches which can be used to achieve this goal:

1. A Total-Body approach
2. An Activity-Oriented approach
3. A Realistic approach.

A Total-Body Approach

The functional ability of a person depends on the proper interaction of all the body parts and brain. Hence functional restoration requires treatment of the whole body, not just the affected body part. The emphasis of therapy should not only be on strength, ROM, and gait but should also include balance, proprioception, coordination and agility.

An Activity Oriented Approach

The patient should demonstrate the ability to safely perform all the functional tasks necessary to return to his previous life style.

This tasks can be incorporated into standard strengthening and flexibility programs.

A Realistic Approach

Each patient has different needs and functions. The therapist alongwith patient must define the risks and rewards of desired functional goals and should work together to restore important functional activities as safely as possible.

For e.g.: In some conditions running, jogging may not be safe for the patient. To walk safely should be the goal.

Functional Exercise Equipment

The following equipments can be used during functional rehabilitation program for orthopaedic conditions.

1. Steps.
2. Balls–Basket ball, Football, Beach ball, Tennis ball, Medicinal ball etc.
3. Bicycles (upper and lower body).
4. Games.
5. Hand equipment—such as Baltimore thera-peutic equipment (BTE).
6. Stair climbing machine.
7. Surgical tubing.
8. Therabands.
9. Wobble boards.
10. Trampoline.
11. Work hardening equipment.
12. Tread mills.
13. Rowing machine.
14. Gym equipment–Weights, dumbells, barbells etc.
15. Chairs/Stool with different heights.
16. ADL Boards.
17. Self help devices–Reachers, adapted utensils, adapted writing tool, dressing stick etc.
18. Assitive devices–Walker, crutches and sticks.
19. Mobility devices–Wheel chair.

CHAPTER-21

Yoga and Asanas

INTRODUCTION

Yoga is a very old Indian practice that goes back to over 5000 years. The term 'yoga' comes from a Sanskrit word 'yuj', it means to yoke, to unite. In the most ordinary sense yoga means uniting the body and the mind with the soul. In a dualistic sense it also means uniting the soul with the supreme self. In yoga, through a step by step process we try to dissolve the ego consciousness in the soul consciousness. We practice yoga by withdrawing the mind and the senses from the myriad distractions of the world in order to obliterate the boundaries of identity and form we create for ourselves. This actually means to bring oneself to a disciplined way of life.

It is believed by ancient yogics that for human being to harmonize with the environment and themselves, they have to unite the spirit, mind and body, and for all of it to be united, there must be a balance in the physical, emotional and spiritual aspect of life. The way to maintain and achieve this balance is through meditation, breathing, and yoga postures. Thus, both the body and the mind are used when practising yoga exercises, as it requires perseverance and will power to be able to perform each of the yoga asanas. Yoga in the eastern countries believed to be a spiritual self-mastery meditation skill to keep the mind, body and soul together, whereas, in the western countries yoga is practised as physical exercise or alternative medicine rather than the spiritual self-mastery meditation.

CONCEPTS

In the history of the vast literature on yoga and in the present times, there have been several different conceptions of yoga. In terms of concepts one yoga may differ from another yoga because of the origin of that particular yoga was for a particular function. For example Hatha yoga and Ashtanga yoga (Raja yoga). The ashtanga yoga emphasizes on the ease and spontaneity in one's bodily postures or asanas while meditating, whereas, the hatha yoga employs hatha or violence and force and requires of hatha yogin , for example to stand on one leg, or hold the arms, or inhale smoke with the head inverted when meditating. Similarly, a kind of yogic samadhi or some sort of sidhi or perfection could be achieved by taking drugs or by reciting some mantras. In view of above, it may be learnt that one should not confuse with the other conception and that one should not speak of yoga without specifying the sense in which one is using the word and kind of yoga one is talking about. Now-a-days in the modern world the people have a concept towards yoga as identical with the practice of yogic asanas with the explicit aim not at spiritual upliftment, but better bodily health and reduction of and maximum possible freedom from psychological tension.

Yoga is neither a philosophy nor a religion but it is art which is value neutral such that it can be adopted as necessary part of the conceptual scheme or the training programme of any religion or philosophy.

Therapeutic Effects

The physical aspect of what is called yoga in recent years, the asanas, has been much popularized in the West. Physically, the practice of asanas is considered to:

- Improve flexibility.
- Improve strength.
- Improve balance.
- Reduce stress and anxiety.
- Reduce symptoms of lower back pain.
- Improve symptoms of asthma and chronic obstructive pulmonary disease (COPD).
- Increase energy and decrease fatigue.
- Shorten labor and improve birth outcomes.
- Improve physical health and quality of life measures in the elderly.
- Improve diabetes management.
- Reduce sleep disturbances.
- Reduce hypertension.

Conditions Required Before Yoga

Warm Up: It is important to perform warm up exercises to prepare the muscles for the yoga. Warm up exercises may be a brisk walk or jogging or simply some form of stretching of the muscles like movements of the neck, trunk, shoulder, hip and knee. These warm up exercises not only relaxes the muscles but also prepares the muscles for the extreme stretches require during the yoga asanas.

Empty Stomach: The stomach should be empty. The best suited time to practice the yoga is morning. Yoga may also be performed in the afternoon, but it should be with empty stomach or after 3-4 hours of the meal. Force or pressure should not be used, and body should not tremble.

Environment: The place where yoga is practised should be cleaned, spacious, fully ventilated and free of noises and pollution. Morning yoga in the park is considered to be the suitable conditions for the yoga practitioners.

Clothes: The yoga practitioners should prefer undergarments with loose and comfortable clothes.

TYPES OF YOGA AND ASANAS

A. YOGA

The Yoga Upanishads identify four types of yoga—Mantra yoga, Laya yoga, Raja yoga and Hatha yoga. In the Bhagavadgita we find karma yoga and bhakti yoga. Karma yoga means performing desire less actions as an offering to God.

Mantra Yoga: Involves continuous mental repetition of a mantra or some sacred syllable till the mind become completely absorbed in it.

Laya Yoga: Involves the dissolution of the lower self and the mental activity and the rising of the kundalini (energy from the base of the spine) to the tip of the head. Its more extreme version is Hatha yoga practised by some schools of Saivism such as the Nath yogis and the Kalamukhas. It involves the practice of some extremely difficult bodily postures, breathing practices and use of certain chemicals to gain complete mastery over the body and the mind.

Raja yoga or the king of the yogas is the most standard form of yoga, described by Patanjali in his Yogasutra it involves the practice of eight fold yoga, hence, it is also known as *Ashtanga Yoga*. Ashtanga means eight limbs (steps), which purify the practitioners' mind, reduce stress and anxiety by performing eight steps. Ashtanga is believed to derive its origin from ancient text yoga *Korunta*. It is aimed at channelling hyperactive young minds and restive bodies with the infinite energy of teenage boys. The concepts of each step (limb) is learned and practised carefully before progressing to the next. The following are the eight steps:

1. **Yama (Control):** It is the practice of restraints or precepts. The five restraints suggested by Patanjali are: not to be violent,

not to lie, not to steal, not to indulge in sex and not to be greedy.

2. **Niyama (Rules of Conduct):** It is the practice of five observance or discipline. Patanjali suggested five rules or observances: practice of purity, happiness, austerities or asceticism, study of the scriptures, and surrender to God.

3. **Asanas (Poses):** Asanas are the movements, postures of the body to make the body supple and fit.

4. **Pranayama (Breath Control):** It is the practice of regulating of the inspiration and expiration (breathing) for certain period of time to calm the mind and relax the body to experience higher states of consciousness.

5. **Pratyahara (Withdrawal of Sensory Perceptions):** It is the practice of withdrawal of the senses and mind from the sense objects. This is usually done by closing eyes, looking inwards and by focusing the attention on the area between the eyebrows or on the thoughts and feelings that arise in the consciousness.

6. **Dharana (Concentration):** It is the overcome of the sense of duality to which we are usually subject by concentrating the mind on a single point or object such as the image of deity.

7. **Dhyana (Uninterrupted Meditation):** Dhyana is the meditation, which can either be passive or active. Uninterrupted meditation can bring equanimity, tranquillity and inner happiness.

8. **Samadhi (Complete Equilibrium):** **Samadhi** is a state of self-absorption in which the movements of the senses and the mind cease and all distinctions between the knower and the known disappear. It is a state of unity and subjectivity in which mind comes to a complete rest while the practitioner remains conscious but absorbed in himself.

B. BASIC YOGA–ASANAS

Asanas are the physical movements or posture of the yoga practice and in combination with yoga it constitutes a style of yoga. In the yoga sutra, Patanjali describes asana as a "firm, comfortable posture" that refers specifically to the seating posture, most basic of all the asanas. Asanas are widely known as "yoga postures" or yoga positions. Raja yoga also known as king of all the yoga, has eight limbs (steps), the third step or limb of raja yoga describes the asanas. The Yogasutras is the most authoritative ancient scripture on yoga.

Asana later became a term for various postures useful for restoring and maintaining a practitioner's well-being and improving the body's flexibility and vitality, with the goal of cultivating the ability to remain in seated meditation for extended periods.

There are number of postures and movements in yoga, and although all of them are beneficial, some are more challenging than others. Initially basic yoga are taught to the clients/patients and as soon as the concepts of basic yoga are learned the therapist may progress to the advanced yoga. Progressing to the advanced yoga is one of the crucial steps and the therapist needs to screen the patients/clients as the advanced yoga require more flexibility and movements. The older population should be progressed carefully to the advanced yoga as they have osteoporotic bones, degenerative changes and limited flexibility of the joints. The following yoga asanas are explained as below:

(a) Sun Salutation or Surya Namaskar

Surya Namaskar or the Sun Salutation, which is very commonly practised in most forms of yoga, originally evolved as a type of worship of Surya, the Vedic solar deity. Surya the Hindu solar deity by concentrating on the Sun, for vitalization. It consists of yogasana and Pranayama. It is useful in all the age groups of people. A full round of surya namaskar is considered to be two sets of the twelve poses with the change in the second set where opposite leg is moved first. The twelve poses are mentioned as under (Fig. 21.1(i-xii)); the practitioner:

i. Stands straight with no lordosis in the lumbar and cervical spine, both the feet together and places both hands on the chest to join them. Inhales and recites some mantras (bija mantras).

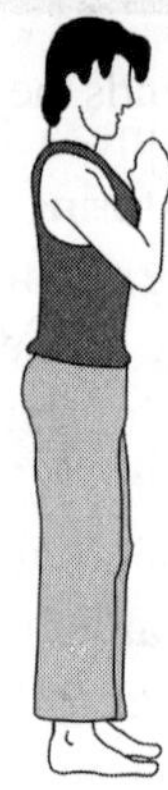

ii. Inhales and raises both the arms overhead, keeping the palms together.

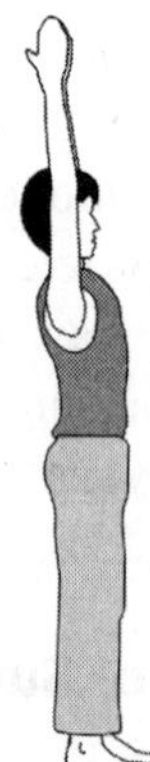

iii. Exhales and bends the trunk forward as much as possible without bending the knees. Patients with PIVD should avoid this asana.

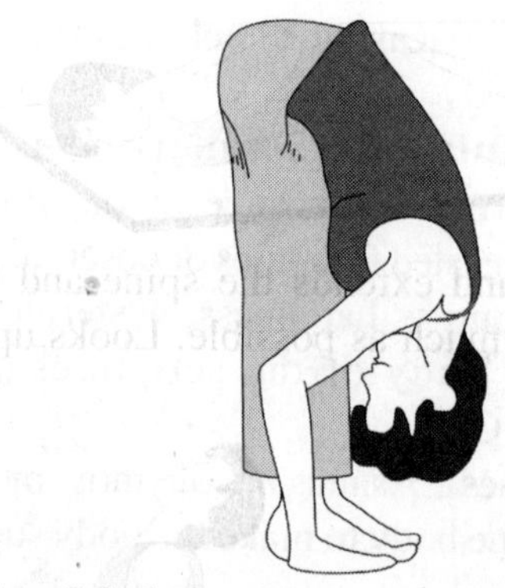

iv. Inhales and steps the right leg backwards, extends the neck, trunk and right hip joint. The left hip and knee is flexed fully.

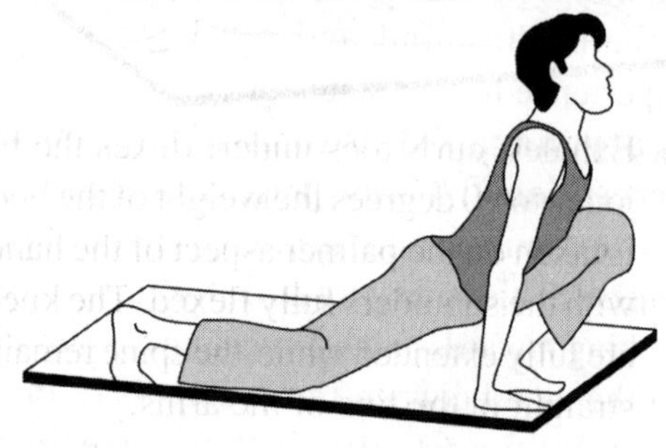

v. Exhales and takes the left leg back into plank position. The body is supported on the hand (palmer aspects). The neck, trunk, hips and ankles remain in the neutral position.

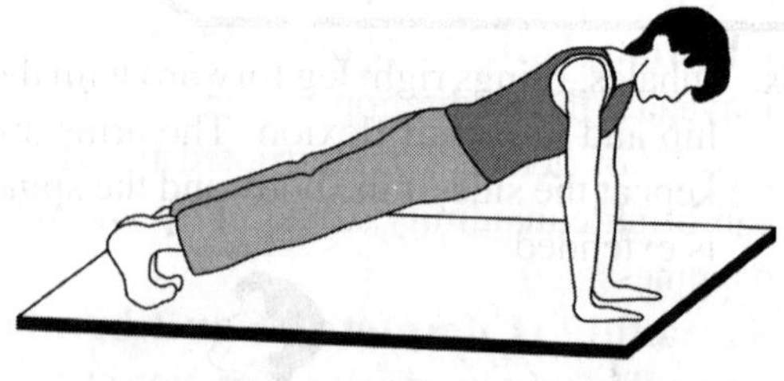

vi. Retaining the breadth, the forehead, chest, and knees are lowered to the floor by extending the shoulders and flexing the elbows. There is strong contraction of the shoulder flexors and elbow extensors, this strengthens the upper corset muscles too.

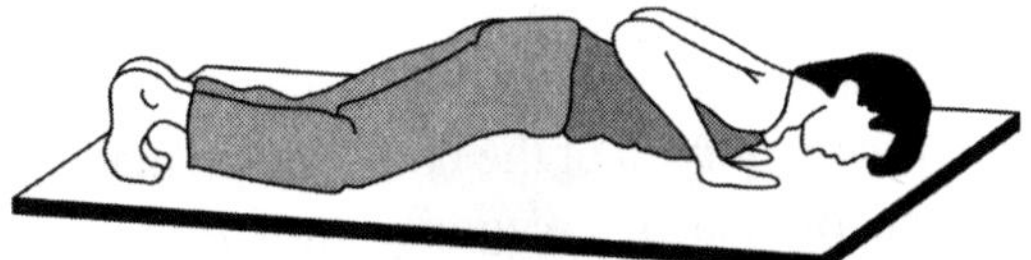

vii. Inhales and extends the spine and hip joints as much as possible. Looks up to the sky.

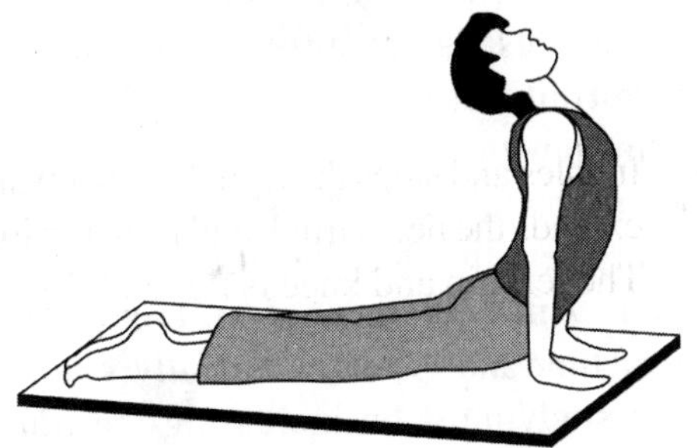

viii. Exhales, curls toes under, flexes the hip joints to 90 degrees the weight of the body is taken on the palmer aspect of the hands with the shoulders fully flexed. The knees are fully extended while the spine remains straight in the line of the arms.

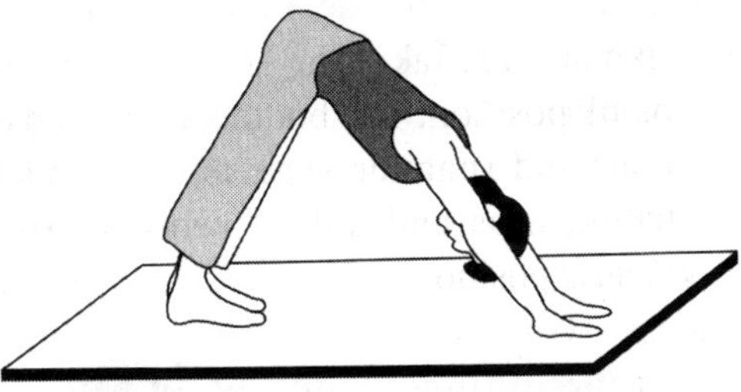

ix. Inhales, brings right leg forward with the hip and knee full flexion. The arms are kept at the side of the body and the spine is extended.

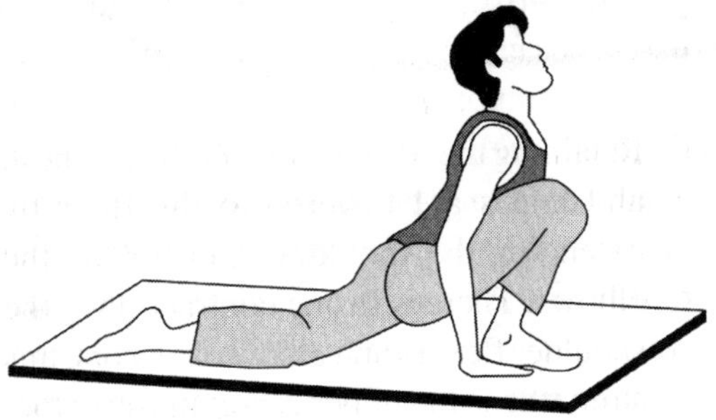

x. Exhales and flexes the spine as much as possible by touching the toes with the hands.

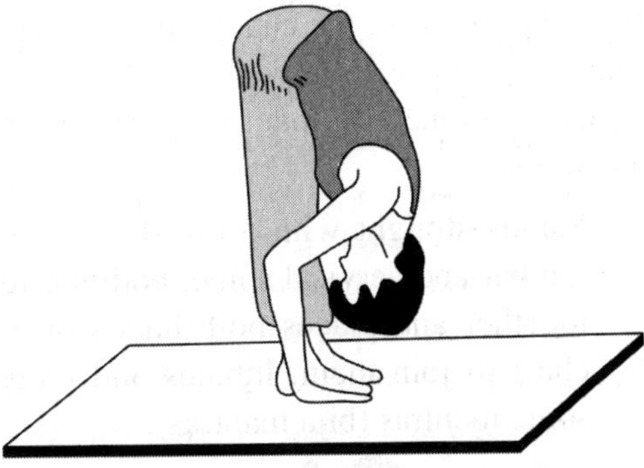

xi. Inhales and extends the knees, hips, spine and sholders.

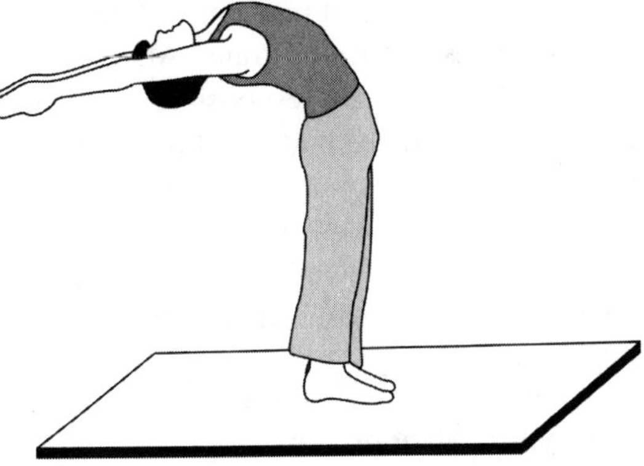

xii. Exhales and comes back to the pose of tadasana.

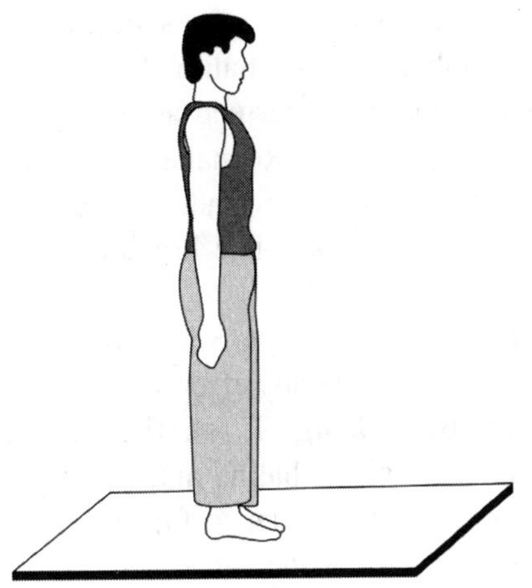

(b) Pranayama

Pranayama is the fourth limb or step of ashtanga yoga, as set out by Patanjali in the yoga sutra. Pranayama is made up of two words prana means breath or bio energy in the body and yama means control, hence, pranayama is the control of breath or bio (pranic) energy. It is done by regulating the breathing and holding the breath in between for certain periods of time to calm the mind and relax the body to experience higher states of consciousness. The practice is an integral part of both hatha yoga and ashtanga vinayasa yoga in the execution of asanas. Patanjali in yoga sutras mentioned pranayama as means of attaining higher states of awareness, holding of breath is an important practice of reaching samadhi.

Five Types of Prana: Prana, Apana, Vyan, Udana and Samana are responsible for various pranic activities in the body. Out of these Prana and Apana are most important. Prana is upward flowing and Apana is downward flowing. Practice of Pranayama achieves the balance in the activities of these pranas, which results in healthy body and mind.

Pranayama Procedure

The breathing procedure of the pranayama should be taught to the practitioner to avoid any harmful effects. Pranayama involves mainly of two activities inhaling and exhaling. In Yogasutras of Patanjali, inhaling is termed as Puraka and the exhaling is termed as Rechaka. The state when these two activities are made to halt has been termed as Kumbhaka. The breathing rate may be:

i. **Quiet Breathing:** Smooth continous naturally without any efforts.

ii. **Deep Breathing:** First, the movements concerned with inhaling and exhaling are to be controlled in order to further slow down the breathing, at the same time the need of oxygen for the body is to be lessened, so that the speed of breathing can further, slow down. The constitution of the body is such that if the need or use of oxygen is not reduced, it becomes difficult or rather impossible to control the process of breathing. The easy way to reduce the need of oxygen is to stop the movements of the body and try to relax all the muscles. After some time the practitioner finds it difficult to do the deep breathing further, at this juncture he or she should return to the neutral breathing and rest for a while. After taking rest the deep breathing should start again. After practising deep breathing with equal time and speed successfully, one should start studying it by increasing the time for exhaling. If inhaling (Puraka) is in four seconds, then exhaling (Rechaka) shall take 5 to 6 seconds instead of four. This needs special efforts. When a person succeeds in doing inhaling and exhaling at the ratio of 1: 1 for 10 to 15 minutes, he should double the time for exhalation. The ideal ratio for inhaling-exhaling is 1: 2.

iii. **Fast Breathing:** When the speed of the inhaling and exhaling is more than the deep breathing is termed as fast breathing. In the fast breathing the practitioner should increase the speed of inhaling and exhaling, however short breathing is not practised. The practitioner has to practice continue the cycle of quick breathing with constant practice. This sort of breathing is easy to understand and to practice also. The fast breathing clears the nasal passage and exercises the parts involved in the respiratory system. During fast breathing there is a feeling of whirling sensation in the head which may be considered to be normal, but as soon as it occurs the practitioners should return to the quiet breathing and then after some time comes back to the fast breathing. Making habit of the fast breathing can remove

Pranava Mudra for Pranayama–Body Gesture and Mental Attitudes

It may be performed in six different steps.

Type-1 Keep both the nostrils open and then inhale and exhale with both the nasal passages. This type is nothing but quick breathing with both the nasal cavities. One should inhale and exhale with as much speed as possible and for as much time as feasible. **Type-2** Take up Pranava Mudra and close the right nostril with the help of the thumb of the right hand, and inhale with left nostril and also exhale through the same nasal passage. In brief this type can be described as quick breathing with the left nostril. **Type-3** In this type left nostril is to be closed and the quick breathing is done with the right nostril. **Type-4** In this type close the right nostril and inhale with the left nostril, and then immediately close left nostril and exhale with the right nostril. In this way try quick breathing by changing the nostrils. **Type-5** This type of breathing is just opposite the previous one, that is, the left nostril is closed and inhaling is done with the right nostril, then immediately closing the right nostril, exhaling is done with the left nostril. **Type-6** This type of breathing is designed by combining previous two types, i.e., Type-4 and Type-5. First inhale with left nostril and exhale with right one, then inhale with right nostril and exhale with left nostril. Later continue the same process, i.e., inhaling and exhaling with left and right nostrils alternately. Further switch to fast breathing by increasing the speed of breathing. After sufficient practice the speed of breathing can be increased immensely.

such kind of sensation. To practice the fast breathing the practitioner sits in one of the following asasna: Padmasana, Vajrasana or Swastikasana. The eyes are closed and the practitioner concentrates in the breathing to achieve maximum results.

(c) Dandasana

Dandasana is derived from two words of Sanskrit danda mean stick and asana means posture. The practitioner sits on the floor with both the hip joints flexed to 90 degrees and knees extended fully. The arms should be rested on either side of the body the whole spine (lumbar, thoracic and cervical) is kept straightened the whole posture will look like an English alphabet "L". The legs will be parallel, whereas the body will be perpendicular to the floor. The practitioner remains in the dandasana pose for at least 2-3 minutes. The dandasana helps in strengthening core muscles, shoulder girdle and upper back extensors. The pose also helps in hamstrings and neck extensors stretching (Fig. 21.2).

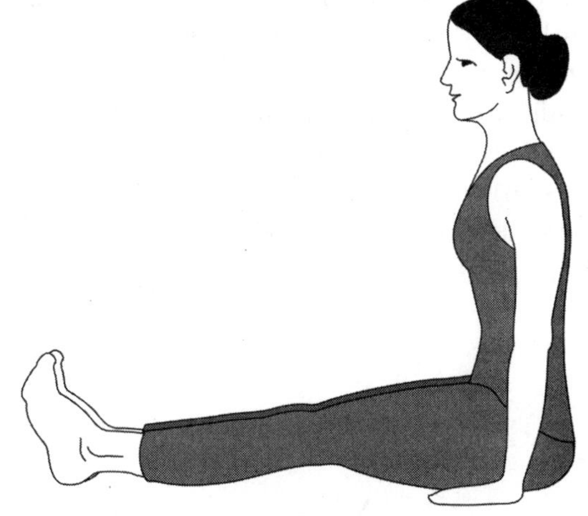

Fig. 21.2

Modifications

(i) The practitioner sits on the floor with the legs extended and spine straight. This pose helps in stretching of the hamstrings and strengthening of the core group muscles.

(ii) Gradually, practitioner expands the chest, drops the shoulder blades down and backward, inhales slowly throughout this entire pose and keeps the chin slightly lowered position. This pose is maintained for a minute or two.

(iii) The neck is flexed forward and then extended backward this helps in stretching of neck extensors.

(iv) The arms are flexed to 90 degrees with thumb in downward direction. Patient inhales and then flexes the shoulders further to the full range. This helps in improving the chest expansion and pectoralis stretching.

(v) The practitioner presses the thigh with the floor. The hip joints are rotated medially and laterally. The ankle joints are flexed and extended.

(d) Vajrasana

Vajra is derived from Sanskrit mean thunderbolt. Vajrasana makes the body exceptionally strong and healthy. The practitioner sits on the ankle and toes with both the knees flexion. The spine should be extended and both the hands placed on the knees. The practitioner sits on the ankle (dorsum) and toes with both the knees flexion. The spine should be extended and both the hands placed on the knees. The practitioner inhales and exhales slowly. While drawing the abdominal region inward (inhale) and expanding the chest, the practitioner should concentrate on breathing. Vajrasana helps in lowering blood pressure and strengthening of the core stabilizers (Fig. 21.3).

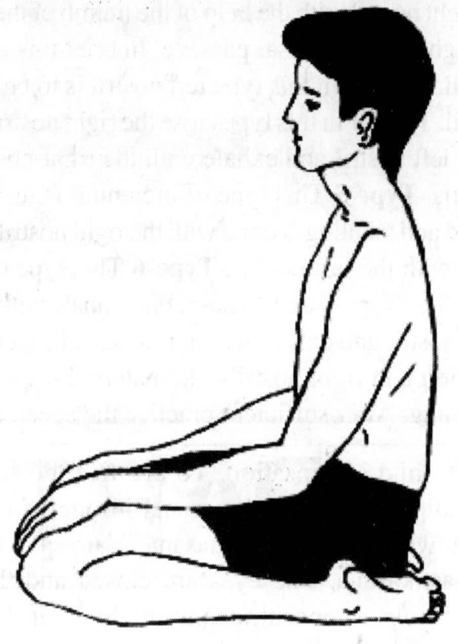

Fig. 21.3

PART - TWO

CHAPTER-22

Orthopedic Assessment

Assessment is the systematic approach of making a diagnosis to know how to approach treatment and to design an appropriate scheme of management. In order to make a diagnosis, and to design an appropriate scheme of management, it is essential for the examiner to understand each patient as fully as possible, irrespective of their social class and economical or cultural background. Interpretation of the clinical findings obtained during the subjective and objective examination enables the clinician to make a provisional diagnosis and scheme of management. Therefore, assessment is the cornerstone of effective clinical practice. The assessment includes following components:

A. Examination
B. Evaluation
C. Diagnosis
D. Prognosis
E. Intervention

A EXAMINATION

Examination is the process in which clinical data or findings are gathered by obtaining a history, performing a relevant system review, selecting and administrating special tests and measures. Examination has two parts subjective and objective. Moving step by step of the assessment from subjective examination to objective examination the clinician can reproduce the patient's symptoms and determine the level of the dysfunction or injury.

a. Subjective Examination

During subjective examination the examiner gathers information from the patient by asking the questions. such as: "Yes gentleman what is your problem"? When it started? How it started etc? The information collected during the subjective examinations depends on to a large extent on the quality of communication between the examiner and patient. Therefore, the examiner should establish a pleasant relationship with the patient to get an accurate information. Attempts are made to gather accurate information from the patient so that these may give clues in making the diagnosis and designing scheme of management. The examiner should ask the relevant questions. Not every question will need to be asked otherwise patient will get irritated and may distort the information. The subjective examination involves following:

i. *General Information:* During the general information the clinician obtains the following information from the patient: Age, Sex, Occupation, Height: Weight ratio, Reaction to stress and pain. *Consideration of Age:* The prevalence of the certain conditions are at the certain ages. The disc degen-eration starts at around age of 40 years, while onset of ankylosing spondylitis is before the age of 40 years. The patient over the age of 50 years presents with low back pain may be considered for the malignant disease, while, the patient below the age of 25-30 years with low back pain is considered for the mechanical or traumatic such as dysfunction at the intervertebral disc, appophyseal joints, ligaments, postural problems and malalignment and ruled out for the degenerative disease, hence, examiner must consider the age before progressing to the next element of the assessment. *Sex:* While obtaining general information, clinician should also consider the sex of the patient. The prevalence of some conditions or disease such as ankylosing spondylitis is higher in the males than females, hence, a female patient presents with the low back pain may be ruled out for the AS and may be considered for the mechanical or other conditions of back pain such as dysmenorrhoea, urinary tract and pelvic infection etc. *Occupation:* The people involved in the overhead activities are more prone to the shoulder impingement and anterior instability as overuse of the rotator cuff muscles fail to rotate and depress the head of humerus downward during the elevation. Activities such as lifting and carrying heavy objects with forward flexion of the spine may weaken the annulus fibrosus and end plate, and this may allow nucleus pulposus to bulge towards the annuls fibrosus. Therefore, in order to understand and reach to the exact cause of the problem the examiner should not skip the occupation of the patient taking into account.

ii. *Chief Complaint:* Why has the patient sought for treatment or referred to the physiotherapy department or clinic? The patient may come to the physiotherapist with following complaints: Stiffeners, giving way, instability, weakness, loss of function, for differential diagnosis, after trauma, surgery, manipulation under anesthesia, plaster removal following dislocation, injury or trauma. The complaint is always written in the patient's language. The therapist should establish a pleasant relationship with the patient and take him into

fully confidence and ask the questions such as:

a. **What was the Onset of Symptoms:** The pain and other symptoms may start with gradual or sudden onset. Symptoms start with gradual onset indicate an active pathology such as infection or inflammation if they do not subside with the rest. The mechanical back pain such as disc degeneration and faulty posture has the gradual onset but they respond to the rest and heat modalities. The symptoms start with sudden onset speaks about traumatic lesion, and there is probability of the injury to the ligaments, tendons, joint capsule, menisci, intervertebral disc, appophyseal joints or muscle tear/rupture etc.

b. **What was the Mechanism of Injury:** The patient explains how the injury took place. If patient is able to reveal the exact mechanism of injury, the clinician or examiner can reach to the exact site or structure. For an example below mentioned mechanisms are related to the particular structures. *Forward bending with lifting of heavy weight:* During forward flexion the line of gravity falls anterior to the midline which increases the extension moment arm, and requires more muscle work to stabilize the spine and lift the object. Initially the individual tries but fails to generate that much force in the midway, resulting rupture of the annulus fibrosus, end plate or posterior longitudinal ligaments and strain in the muscles that enables the intervertebral disc (nucleus pulposus) to prolapse posterior, and causes dysfunction at the facet joints and nerve roots. *Patient falls on outstretched hand:* During this mechanism there is excessive load on the distal radius and results in radial styloid fracture. Patient falls on the outstretched shoulder with abduction and external rotation produces large loads on the anterior stabilizers of the shoulder resulting in anterior shoulder subluxation or dislocation. *Twisting of the ankle joint with inversion and planter flexion:* The anterior wider part of the talus fits snugly in the mortise (space between two malleoli). In plantar flexion and inversion the anterior wider part of the talus comes out of the mortise and leaves the joint unstable, the anterior talofibular ligament fails to control the plantar flexion and inversion, eventually the ligament sprains.

c. **Area of Symptoms:** It is useful to record the area of the pain by using a body chart, because this helps in a quick visual reference. Sometimes the area where symptoms are originated remains silent or less symptomatic, for an example in an acute cervical disc herniation patient complaints more pain in the arm and forearm. Therefore, the examiner should correlate the distal symptoms with the cervical. The examiner should also understand the quality of the pain which helps in determining the area of lesion. The patient may complain on more than one area of symptoms.

d. **Severity or Intensity of Pain:** The patient is asked to indicate the description or number which best describes the intensity of their pain at its least and at its worst.
   i. Mild.
   ii. Moderate.
   iii. Distressing.
   iv. Horrible.
   v. Excruciating.

Visual Analogue Scale (VAS): It is a ten point scale starts from 0 to 10. Zero is no pain and ten is the unbearable pain. The patient is asked to indicate the point where his pain falls. This not only helps in understanding the intensity of the pain of the patient but also helps in the prognosis. For example in the first visit patient marks at five and after five treatment sessions he or she says that the pain is decreased in the intensity and now it is at point 2.

e. **Depth of Pain:** Pain situated deep down may be originated from bone and muscles whereas superficial pain is originated from the joints. The depth of pain may give some indication as to the structure at fault but, like quality, this can also be misleading.

f. **Irritability:** This is the length of time for which the person has to perform the activity to increase the pain, and conversely how long it takes before the pain settles to its former intensity. The purpose of assessing irritability of the disorder is to try to discern just how much movement the patient's disorder can be subjected to without causing an exacerbation. It can be measured as high, moderate or low. *High irritability:* The aggravating factor causes the pain to increase very quickly or instantly and then the pain takes a long time to settle back. *Moderate irritability:* The aggravating factors take longer to increase the symptoms. *Low irritability:* The aggravating factor can be performed for a long time before exacerbating the patient's symptoms and then as stopping the activity the symptoms subside rapidly.

g. **Behavior of Symptoms:** The pain and symptoms of the patient may be constant, intermittent or fluctuating. The examiner should ask when the constant, intermittent or fluctuating symptoms are present? or when they fluctuate? Does the patient has sleep disturbance? If yes, does it because of mechanical or inflammatory reason?

h. Aggravating and Relieving: What aggravates and eases the symptoms? The movement or posture that produces or increases the symptoms should be noted carefully. Patents with acute mechanical disorder usually find relief in the symptoms during rest but in chronic stage symptoms may also be present in the rest. These patients respond to the heat therapy treatment. Whereas, patients with inflammatory pain always complaint more pain in the rest and the symptoms decrease in activities probably due to engagement in the activities, however, as the disease progresses symptoms will be present in rest as well as in activities. There is no relief in symptoms with the heat therapy (infection).

i. Positional Factors: Most musculoskeletal pain is mechanical in origin and is therefore, made better or worse by adopting particular positions or postures that either stretch or compress the structure that are giving rise to pain.

j. Time Factors: Certain pathologies tend to be more painful at characteristic times of the day, for example, chronic changes are characteristically painful and stiff initially and arising from sleep.

k. Duration of the Symptoms: How long the symptoms are present? Is there any improvement in the symptoms since they have started? Mechanical pain usually improves with the time whereas, infective or inflammatory pain persists and increases in intensity with the time. **Intermediate:** Any relief in the symptoms even for a few minutes is considered intermediate, *example:* Mechanical pain. The patients

---

System Review
a. General Well-being: Weight, appetites, fever, appearance, sleep mood.
b. Cardiovascular and Respiratory: Exercise balance for simple, everyday things laid a flight of stain or moving the lawns .Chest pain, palpitations, swelling, caught and sputters.
c. Alimentary: Belly pain, nausea, vomiting bowel habits and nature of stools.
d. Genitourinary: Frequency of micturition by day and by night, incontinence, pain, frequency and duration of periods, sexual activity, and bladder function.
e. Nervous System: Headache, vision and hearing, weakness or disturbed sensation.
f. Locomotors: Joint pain, stiffness, range of motion, swelling, crepitus, contracture, tightness and deformity.

complaint less severe or no pain while resting in a particular position which releases the stress or load on the faulty structure.

iii. History: *Previous Treatments:* Has the patient received any treatment for this condition in the past, if yes what treatment has been taken? Was it effective or was the improvement partial? **Past Medical History:** Has the patient suffered any major operations or illness? This might affect the tissues and be a contraindication to particular treatments.

Examples:
i. Respiratory disease
ii. Cardiac disease
iii. Diabetes
iv. Rheumatoid arthritis
v. Epilepsy

Is the patient receiving or received oral steroid medications? Patients having chronic respiratory diseases, inflammatory bowel diseases or R.A., may receive oral steroid therapy. This treatment affects bone and produces tendency towards bruising. Medication used in the past or using for the present condition should also be noted carefully.

iv. *Observation:* After taking history, the next element of subjective assessment is careful physical observation of the **swelling, redness, muscle atrophy, posture, active movements and gait.** During an observation the patient should be undressed. The posture is reviewed (observed) from anterior, lateral and posterior. The examiner notes down the abnormalities in the posture and restriction in the active range of motion, if any, and the patterns of movements (such as compensatory movements and muscle substitutes to show the maximum results). The best way to find the abnormality in the posture and movements, is compared the clinical findings with the normal subjects (practice to observe the posture and movements on normal subjects). This is known as system review. For an instance the examiner finds the pulse rate of the patient 99 per second and when it is compared with normal it is termed as tachycardia but if the examiner does not know normal value it cannot be said that it is very high.

b. Objective Assessment

On the basis of data received from the patient or caregivers during the history and observation, the therapist establishes a kind of disorder in his mind and progresses to the objective examination for further confirmation of the disorder. It is worth to note before any movement tested, the therapist should have a clear appreciation of the disorder to know whether to limit test movements and so avoid exacerbation. Patients with acute injuries are required to provide history and the mechanism of injury. It is far wiser to delay the objective examination (less important of examination) for such patients over two to three days. Objective examination consists passive movements and some special tests, performed on the patient to produce a degree or kind of pain that is not the normal kind of discomfort that could be considered as an acceptable normal.

i. *Palpation:* The suspected site of symptoms is palpated for tenderness, temperature, sensation, crepitus and end feel. To elicit the tenderness, a palmer aspect of the thumb is placed directly on the site of symptoms and pressed gently. Pisiform aspect of the wrist may also be used to elicit the pain and symptoms. To feel the temperature, the dorsal aspect of the hand is placed on the suspected area. Increased temperature of the suspect area indicates an active inflammation or infection. To test the sensation, a test tube, cotton or tip of the finger is placed on the suspected area and patient is asked how he or she perceives it. To test the crepitus the examiner places hand on the suspected area of lesion and asks the patient to move the joint actively. Feeling of grinding or jerk during an active movements indicates crepitus. For an example to test the crepitus in the shoulder, the examiner places hand on the shoulder and the patient is asked to elevate the arm actively. The end feel is experienced with passive movements of the joints. The end range may be limited by the pain, swelling, spasm of the muscles, abnormal bony contacts and loose bodies which may give the feeling of empty, soft, firm and hard.

ii. *Special Tests:* The special tests and measures are performed to generate data by reproducing the symptoms of the patients impairments and functional limitations. These special tests and measures are based on medical safety, patient comfort, emotional, functional, social, vocational needs and financial resources. The following relevant examination may be performed by a therapist: aerobic capacity, joint integrity, and mobility, motor function, range of motion, muscle strength, cardiopulmonary functions (ventilation, respiration and circulation) posture and gait balance.

B. EVALUATION

Interpretation of the examination findings is the evaluation; it is one of the most critical stages in a clinical decision making. Evaluation is the dynamic process in which the therapist makes judgment based on data gathered during the subjective and objective examination. The therapist interprets the subjective and objective examination and clinical findings to understand the source or cause of the patient's impairments, disorder, functional limitations and disabilities. The clinical data may also be analyzed to determine the progression and stage of the sign and symptom, and stability of the condition.

C. DIAGNOSIS

Diagnosis is the dynamic condition of analyzing the clinical data gathered during the subjective and objective examination and evaluation; and organizing them into clusters, syndromes, or categories to help in determining the appropriate intervention and strategy for each patient. American Physical Therapy Association (APTA) has described the diagnosis as a label encompassing a cluster of sign and symptoms commonly associated with a disorder, syndrome or category of impairment, functional limitation or disability. Cluster is set of observations or data that frequently occur as a group for a single patient. Syndrome is an aggregate of sign and symptoms that characterize a given disease or condition.

Impairments

It is the loss or abnormality of physiologic, psychological, or anatomical structure or function. **Physiologic Impairment:** It can be defined as an alteration in any physiologic function such as reduced force or torque production, reduced endurance, reduced mobility, reduced balance and coordination, and altered posture and movement patterns. **Anatomic Impairment:** It can be defined as an abnormality or loss of structure, such as hip anteversion, structural genu varum, congenital or traumatic loss of an extremity. **Psychological Impairment:** It is an abnormality related to the psychological system. It is usual with the physiologic and anatomical patient to have some degree of psychological impairment. Physiotherapy treatment is more effective in improving physiologic impairment in terms of increasing functional strength, range of motion, improving balance and coordination and posture. Physiotherapy treatment has less role in improving the anatomical and psychological impairments.

D. PROGNOSIS

Prognosis is the determination of minimal improvement to maximal improvement expected at various intervals during the course of physical therapy intervention. The prognosis depends upon the health, underlying condition and age of the patient. A healthy patient shows faster improvement in the sign and symptoms than the patient who is having the history of underlying pathological condition such as diabetes of the same age. For an example a 65-year healthy patient with fracture of neck of femur managed with total hip replacement can walk with the toe touch weight bearing with the help of walker in

<table>
<tr><td colspan="2" align="center">Examination</td></tr>
<tr><td>Subjective</td><td>Objective</td></tr>
<tr><td valign="top">

- General information
- Chief complaint/History
  - Onset of symptoms
  - Mechanism of injury
  - Duration of symptoms
  - Area of symptoms
  - Nature and quality of symptoms
  - Intensity of symptoms
  - Aggravating factors
  - Behavior of symptoms
  - Irritability
- History
- Observation of:
  - Posture
  - Active movements
  - Swelling
  - Joint contour
  - Muscle atrophy and
  - Gait

</td><td valign="top">

- Palpation
  - Tenderness
  - Temperature
  - Sensation
  - Swelling
  - End feel
  - Crepitus
- Special Tests
  - Functional tests
  - Isometric tests
  - Joint play tests
  - Neural movement tests

- Radiological Examination

</td></tr>
</table>

the first week, this is the short term expected improvement of the patient. The long-term expected improvement of this patient is jogging without any pain and gait deviations after three months of the operation. On the other hand an ankylosing patient will be having poor prognosis as the disease is progressive which causes loss of movements of the spine and peripheral joints with the due course of time. The prognosis also depends upon the risk factors and response to previous interventions.

E. INTERVENTION

Intervention is the purposeful and skilled physiotherapeutic treatment of various methods, techniques, modalities and education administered towards the patient in order to improve pain, symptoms and functional impairments. An effective physiotherapeutic treatment requires thorough subjective and objective examination.

Clinical Decision Making

Clinical decision making is the dynamic process which involves vertical thinking and lateral thinking. *Vertical Thinking:* It is characterized by logical sequential predictable thinking. It is also known as conventional thinking or process of gathering data or information from the patient. It stays within a problem space. *Lateral Thinking:* It is concerned with the generation of new idea, and with looking things in a different way. It tends to restructure the problem space. The lateral thinking focuses not only on the problem space but also on the proximal and distal parts of the problem space. The therapist's assessment is more inclined to the clinical decision making.

Differential Diagnosis of General Conditions

1. **Infective Conditions:** Severe unremitting pain at rest with no history of injury, persistent pain at night, loss of weight, loss of appetite, unusual growth or lumps, no relief with medication or position or heat therapy.

2. **Inflammatory Conditions:** Pain at rest, morning stiffness, swelling (effusion or thickening), warmth, erythema, diffuse type of tenderness, loss of motion.

3. **Vascular:** Throbbing, diffuse type of pain.

4. **Neurological Conditions: Nerve involvement**—sharp, bright, lightning like. **Nerve root**—sharp, shooting. **Sympathetic nerve**—burning, pressure like, stinging, aching etc. **Upper motor neuron lesion**—spasticity, exaggerated tone, exaggerated reflexes, extensor planter reflex, spastic gait. **Lower motor neuron lesion**—flaccidity, decrease tone, diminish reflexes muscle wasting.

5. **Systemic diseases**.

Differential diagnosis of orthopedic conditions

Muscle	Nerve roots	Bone	Fracture	Mechanical
Cramping, dull, aching. **Tendinitis:** Localized tenderness, ecchymosis, palpable defect in the muscle, weakness, resisted movement painful. Pain may be in the mid range also. **Strain:** Ecchymosis, palpable defect in the muscle, weakness, pain at extreme ranges on passive stretching.	Sharp, shooting, bright, lightning-like.	Deep situated, dull, nagging.	Sharp, severe in intensity, intolerable.	Pain during activities, tenderness, crepitus, aggravates in particular position/posture which put the pressure on the damaged structure, relieves at rest and night. Mechanical pain may be degenerative, disc herniation, muscle strain, ligaments sprain, and may arise from acute or chronic repetitive injuries. Patients with chronic mechanical pain may have morning stiffness and pain at rest but these respond to the heat therapy and stretching exercise.

Assessment Proforma

Subjective Assessment

- **General Information**
  - Name   :
  - Age   :
  - Sex   :
  - Address   :
  - E-mail ID/contact no.   :

- **Chief Complaint**
  - Pain   :
  - Stiffness   :
  - Weakness   :
  - Instability   :
  - Giving way   :
  - Post fracture stiffness/swelling   :
  - Referred for differential diagnosis   :

- **History of Symptoms**
  - Onset of symptoms: Gradual/sudden   :
  - Mechanism of injury   :
  - Duration of symptoms   :
  - Area of symptoms   :
  - Nature and quality of symptoms   :
  - Intensity of symptoms (VAS)   :
  - Aggravating/relieving factors   :
  - Behavior of symptoms   :
  - Irritability   :

- **Medical History**
  - Hormonal disease
    - Hypo/hyperthyroidism   :
    - Diabetes   :
    - Parkinson's disease   :

- – Hypertension/seizures
- – Medications, NASAIDs/steroids :
- – Previous surgeries/implants :
- – Drugs interaction/allergy :
- **Observation of:**
  - – Posture from
    - ❑ Anterior view :
    - ❑ Posterior view :
    - ❑ Lateral view :
  - – Active movements
    - ❑ Flexion/Extension :
    - ❑ Abduction/Adduction :
    - ❑ Medial/Lateral rotation :
  - – Swelling: effusion/thickening :
  - – Joint contour :
  - – Muscle atrophy :
  - – Gait :

Objective Assessment

- **Palpation**
  - – Tenderness :
  - – Temperature :
  - – Sensation :
  - – End feel :
  - – Crepitus :
- **Special Tests**
  - – Functional tests

    i.

    ii.

    iii.

  - – Isometric tests :
  - – Joint play tests :
  - – Neural movement tests :

- **Radiological Examination**
- ....
- ....
- ....

Evaluation

- ....
- ....
- ....
- ....
- ....

Diagnosis

- Possible
- Classical
- Definite

Intervention

- ....
- ....
- ....
- ....
- ....
- ....
- ....

Re-Examination/Evaluation/Intervention

....
....
....
....
....
....
....
....
....

CHAPTER-23

Soft Tissue Injuries

MUSCLE STRAIN

When the muscle is loaded with an external force, the load is resisted primarily by the collagen fibrils. Initially tissues respond to the load by straightening from their resting crimped state, which may be upto 4% elongation in a linear fashion. The muscle fibers return to its normal resting length as the load is removed. If the load is high and causes elongation of the muscle fibers beyond 4% of its normal length, deformation occurs and muscle fibers never return to the normal length. The muscle is said to be strained.

Elastic Range

Due to external force there is elongation of the muscle fibers upto 4% which return to its normal length as soon as the load is removed.

Plastic Range

Due to extreme load there is elongation of the fiber beyond 4% of its length. The muscle fibers do not return to the normal length after removing the load. Elongation of the fibers beyond 4% of their normal length causes deformation and rupture of the muscle fibers, in turn the load on the remaining fibers increases.

Types of Muscle Strain

Muscle strain may either be an acute or chronic.

Acute Strain: Muscle strain occurs along a continuum from an acute micro traumatic injury to chronic micro traumatic overuse injuries. The acute traumatic injuries can cause muscle strain if a muscle is rapidly overloaded or overstretched and the tension generated in the muscle fibers exceeds the tensile capability of the musculotendinous junction unit. These strains occur near the musculotendinous junction and at random areas within the muscle belly.

Chronic Strain: The chronic traumatic injuries produce muscle strain if the muscles are involved in continuous repetitive activities. During the continuous repetitive activities the proximal muscles of the joint get fatigue, resulting in substitution with distal muscles. The distal muscles will be strained. For example when the shoulder muscles get fatigue during continuous repetitive activities or work, substitution with distal musculature occurs. In lower extremity, following fatigue of the gluteus medius and ilio-psoas muscles, the tensor fascia lata dominates over these muscles and is at risk for an overuse strain. [This situation is very similar to the chairperson of any party sitting on desk along with two members on each side, for press conference. In reply of a particular question, the chairperson apprehended and fails to answer as a lack of knowledge, that allows one of members to dominate over the chairperson and seeks attention of the media. The member has done a good job but he has to pay the price of dominating over the chairperson]. Improving the strength and recruitment patterns of the iliopsoas and gluteus medius can reduce the load on the tensor fascia lata and allow it to recover.

A thorough evaluation can determine the source of the overuse strain which may due to continuous repetitive activities. Work site assessment is necessary to prevent a recurrence of the muscle performance impairment. If left untreated, this impairment can quickly lead to disability. It should be treated with postural or motor program re-education and resistive exercises. The proximal muscles should be strengthened first followed by distal by using the progressive resistive exercise. The progressive resisted exercise should be directed to the proximal muscles, followed by distal muscles. Two to three sets (each set of ten repetitions) per day to form fatigue is generally recommended, but if not fatigue by 30-40 repetitions, then the resistance should be increased to form fatigue. The exercises will increase muscle performance. These may be progressed to a higher speed to challenge stability. In aforesaid example, to strength the hip abductors, the patient stands with one foot. A resistive theraband around each of the ankle is wrapped. The patient may hold the chair with the one hand for support and then the three sets of PRE are done.

Subtle Strain

This type of muscle strain is common when a muscle is continuously placed in a relatively lengthened, tension producing position. It is a gradual process. In upper crossed syndrome, there is a forward head posture. The head shifts anterior to the midline. This places lower trapezius muscles in a lengthened position. The trapezius lower fibers are at greater risk of overstretch strain. Such patients are need to be educated about the work station ergonomics. Correction of working style can improve the posture and reduce the muscles strain.

A. Hamstrings Strain

Hamstrings strain is frequently reported in clinics, and its diagnosis is one of the challenges for the clinicians. Most common cause of hamstrings strain is overuse of the muscles particularly, biceps femoris. Hamstrings participate in force couples around the lumbopelvic hip complex, contributing to posterior pelvic rotation, hip extension and indirectly hip medial and lateral rotation. However the hamstrings are the prime movers of the knee flexion.

During mid swing to initial contact the hamstrings decelerate the hip joint, while at initial contact and loading response, the biceps femoris is thought to decelerate tibial medial rotation that occurs with foot pronation. Weakness of the gluteus maximums and deep hip external rotators may lead to excess demand on the hamstrings to decelerate hip flexion during late mid swing and hip medial rotation at initial contact. The biceps femoris load is exaggerated (over used) because of force couple it contributes. The condition is aggravated if the weakness of gluteus maximus and deep hip lateral rotators are associated with fore foot varus. Underuse of the oblique abdominal muscles increase anterior tilting of the pelvis which may lead to overuse of the hamstrings because they must exert a posterior rotational force on the lumbopelvic region.

Overuse: Hamstrings strains are managed by strengthening of the gluteus maximus, deep hip external rotators and biomechanical correction of the foot. Sometimes clinicians focus on the symptoms and under estimate the cause of strain. This may improve the symptoms, but there are more chances of recurrence of hamstrings strain, which contributes to the poor performance. Hence, to treat the strains therapist must focus on the cause, not on the symptoms.

The exercises such as stomach-lying hip extension may be taught to the patient. This will not only strengthen gluteus maximum but also strengthens deep external rotators of the hip joint. These two commonly underused synergists (gluteus maximus and deep external rotators) of

> ### Stomach-lying Hip Extension
>
> The patient lies on the stomach on a firm surface, and an adequate thickness of pillow is placed under torso. The patient is instructed to pull the belly toward the spine (belly tuck in), in the next hip is extended barely off the floor, and is held for at least six seconds. Three sets of 30 repetition may be performed. As the force generating capability and kinesthetic awareness improves sufficiently, stomach-lying hip extension exercise is progressed to the functional activities such as walk stance, step up and step down.

hamstrings contribute to the hamstrings overuse strain. The aim of stomach lying hip extension exercise is to improve force generating capability and kinesthetic awareness of the muscle to the extent that is adequate to allow it to fully participate in a function of task. (The patient with overuse hamstrings strain usually give inadequate force generating capability to participate in a functional task).

B. Gluteus Medius Muscle Strain

Gluteus medius strain is not very common, but may strain functioning in a chronic gradual, continuous stretching. Patients with leg length discrepancy (functional or structural) often present with stretched gluteus medius of the normal side, due to adduction of the normal side hip joint. The gluteus medius strains are treated with leg length correction in case of structural LLD. If LLD is functional then the treatment should be focused on the strengthening of the muscles contributing to the functional leg length discrepancy in conjunction with stretching. The exercise may progress to the functional activities such as walk stance, step up and step down.

C. Lumbo-Pelvic Musculature Strain

Similar to the hamstrings, the lumbo-pelvic muscles may be strained of trauma, overuse and gradual continuous stretch. Traumatic injuries such as road traffic accident usually cause strain to the spinal extensors and multifidus muscles. Overuse strains are usually occur in population whose job involves repetitive flexion and rotation of the lumbo-pelvic region. It often involves the oblique abdominal strain on a crew team.

D. Anterior Scalene Muscle Strain

The anterior scalene muscle is usually strained if it is overused. Patient complaints pain in the upper thoracic spine and the area of first rib. The function of the muscles is cervical flexion, ipsilateral side flexion and contralateral cervical rotation. Weakness or underuse of the deep neck flexors, contralateral rotators, ipsilateral side flexors of neck and diaphragmatic can force anterior scalene muscle to work more; resulting in shortening of the anterior scalene muscle.

Treatment of overuse of the anterior scalene muscle should be focused on strengthening of the underused muscles such as deep neck flexors, ipsilateral side flexors, contralateral rotators and diaphragmatic muscles (anterior scalene muscle also acts as an accessory respiratory muscle). The second part of the treatment should be focused on the stretching of the anterior scalene muscle. To stretch the muscle the first rib is stabilized and patient is instructed to bend the neck to the contralateral side and rotate to the same side. While maintaining the side flexion and rotation the neck is extended for further stretching of the muscle.

E. Middle and Lower Trapezius Strain

The patient with forward head posture (protracted shoulders and head) can place the middle and lower trapezius in an overstretched position. Functioning in overstretched position can cause strain to the middle and lower trapezius muscles.

Patients often complaint pain in the middle border of the scapula. Treatment is focused on the correction of the forward head posture (correction of the protracted head and shoulders and upper thoracic kyphosis). This includes strengthening of deep neck flexors, rhomboids, middle and lower trapezius; and stretching of pectoralis major, upper cervical extensors, trapezius upper fibers and anterior scalene muscles.

F. Posterior Deltoid Strain

In patients with anterior instability, the head of humerus translates (excessively) anteriorly as the anterior capsule is lax. Therefore, posterior deltoid muscles contract eccentrically to control anterior excessive translation of the head of humerus. The posterior deltoid fibers are strained as they are overused in order to prevent anterior excessive translation of the head of humerus. These patients complaint pain in the posterior aspect of the shoulder girdle (posterior deltoid).

LIGAMENTOUS SPRAIN

The end range of the joint is mostly resisted by the inert structures such as ligaments and joint capsule. For an example, when the joint is moved beyond its normal limit it is resisted by the joint capsule and ligaments, but if the force is high and beyond the capacity of these structures, there is stretching or disruption in the continuity of the ligaments or joint capsule. Sprains may also be associated with muscle strain injuries. Patients with ligament sprain usually presents with pain, swelling, ecchymosis and joint instability. However, mild sprain does not cause swelling and instability.

The severity of the sprain depends upon the degree of mechanism of injury. Patients usually complaints pain in the extreme ranges when the disrupted or stretched portion of ligament or joint capsule is stretched. Sometimes patients complaints pain in the end range during the functional activities but the passive movements do not produce these symptoms, this is common in mild injuries, whereas in severe injuries the pain may be present throughout the range of motion. Instability and apprehension tests provoke the symptoms.

Classification

The sprains are graded as mild, moderate and severe, which involve microscopic tearing or stretching of the ligament or joint capsule fibers to complete disruption of the ligament.

- **Grade I or Mild Sprain:** It is a microscopic tearing or stretch of the ligament with little swelling and tenderness. There is no functional impairment and instability of the joint.
- **Grade II or Moderate Sprain:** It involves macroscopic partial tear of ligament with moderate swelling and tenderness. There is loss of functional status of the joint. Joint instability or ligamentous laxity is present.
- **Grade III or Severe Sprain:** Complete or nearly complete tear of the ligament with severe swelling, tenderness and ecchymosis. There is gross functional impairment. Mechanical joint instability is present.

Management

The management depends upon the severity of the sprain. PRICE is administered to improve sign and symptoms. Grade I and Grade II sprains are managed with PRICE, controlled activities and exercises, whereas, grade III sprains may require surgical intervention.

i. **Protection (P):** The activities which put load in the sprained ligament should be avoided. The supportive or assistive devices such as sling, splint, cane, crutches and walker should be used in order to avoid the weight on the joint and ligament.

ii. **Rest (R):** The ligament which is sprained should not be allowed to stretch, hence end range movements should be avoided.

iii. Ice (I): Ice towel or ice pack over the area should be applied for ten minutes to reduce swelling and accelerate healing of the tissues. The application of ice should not be more than ten minutes as it may cause dilatation of the vessels that can increase the swelling in the joint. However, it can be repeated every hour.

iv. Compression (C): Grade I sprains are usually treated with short term immobilization in the form of elastic crepe bandage to prevent swelling and movements. Grade II sprained joints are immobilized in the elastic crepe bandage or brace with limited weight bearing. Grade III sprained ligaments need to be immobilized in the plaster of paris.

v. Elevation (E): Swelling is very usual after ligamentous sprain. The leg should be elevated above the level of heart. To do this two or three pillows may be placed under the ankle joint at night. The leg may also be placed on the stool when the patient is sitting at the work station.

ANTERIOR TALOFIBULAR LIGAMENT (ATFL) SPRAIN

It is estimated that one inversion injury of the ankle occurs for every 10000 people each day. Ankle sprain constitutes 7-10 percent of all admission to the hospital emergency departments. 50 percent of such injuries occur during sport activities.

The stability of the ankle is provided by the ligaments, muscles and bony configuration. The peroneous longus and bravis on the posterolateral side and tibialis posterior, flexor digitorum longus, and flexor halluces longus on the medial side contribute to the dynamic stability. The passive stability is provided by the medial, lateral, posterior ligaments and the syndesmosis. The lateral ligaments complex such as anterior talofibular ligament (ATFL), calcaneofibular ligament (CFL) and the posterior talofibular ligament is most commonly affected in the ankle injuries (Fig. 23.1).

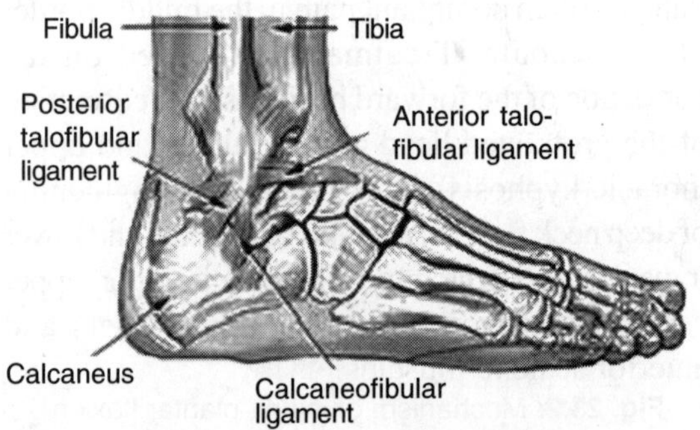

Fig. 23.1: Lateral ligaments complex

The ankle joint remains more stable (closed packed) at the neutral position because the wider anterior portion of the talus fits snugly into the ankle mortise. Plantar flexion of the ankle rotates the posterior narrowed talus into the mortise, resulting in a much loose fit (loose packed), with a particular tendency towards inversion. The anterior talofibular ligament is relaxed at the neutral position and taut in a plantar flexion with inversion. It is the primary restraint against inversion during plantar flexion.

When the ankle is plantar flexed the anterior talofibular ligament becomes taut in order to prevent excessive plantar flexion as the anterior wider portion of the talus is replaced with the narrowed posterior portion of the talus to the mortise and the ankle joint becomes unstable (loose packed). The growth plate in the children is particularly vulnerable to fracture because it is weaker than the surrounding ligaments, bone and the periosteum. Usually anterior talofibular ligament sprain occurs in isolation but if the injury is severe it may be combined with the calcaneofibular ligament sprain. The lateral collateral ligament sprain is classified as grade I, II and III (Fig. 23.2).

- **Grade I or Mild Sprain:** It is a microscopic tearing or stretch of the anterior talofibular ligament with little swelling and tenderness. There is no functional impairment and instability of the joint.

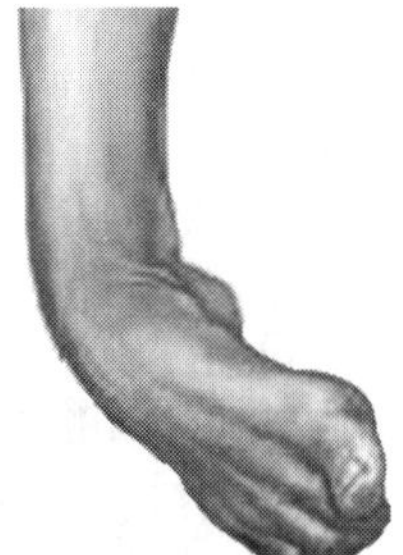

Fig. 23.2: Mechanism of injury, plantar flexion with inversion

- **Grade II or Moderate Sprain:** It involves macroscopic partial tear of the anterior talofibular ligament with moderate swelling and tenderness. There is loss of functional status of the joint. Joint instability or ligamentous laxity is present.

- **Grade III or Severe Sprain:** Complete or nearly complete tear of the ligament with severe swelling, tenderness and ecchymosis. There is gross functional impairment. Mechanical joint instability is present. Grade III sprains are further classified on the basis of degrees of injury. First degree sprains: There is complete rupture of the anterior talofibular ligament. Second degree sprain: There is complete rupture of the anterior talofibular and calcaneofibular ligament. Third degree sprain: There is a dislocation of the joint with ATFL, CFL and posterior talofibular ligament (PTFL) sprains (Fig. 23.3).

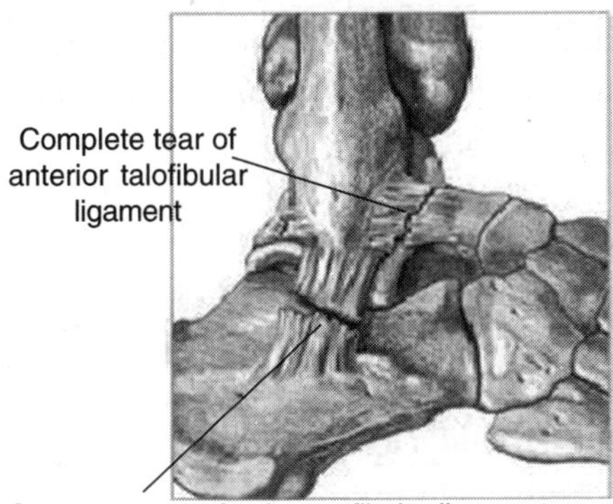

Fig. 23.3: Type III sprain

Clinical Features

The patient usually recalls the mechanism of injury and presents with tenderness on anterior edge and at the tip of the fibula with swelling around the joint, in case of calcaneofibular ligament sprain. Haemorrhage continuous 6 to 12 hours. Patient complaints that pain aggravates when the foot goes into the plantar flexion and inversion, however no pain occurs in the dorsiflexion. Ecchymosis may occur, indicating injury to blood vessels in the area (Fig. 23.4).

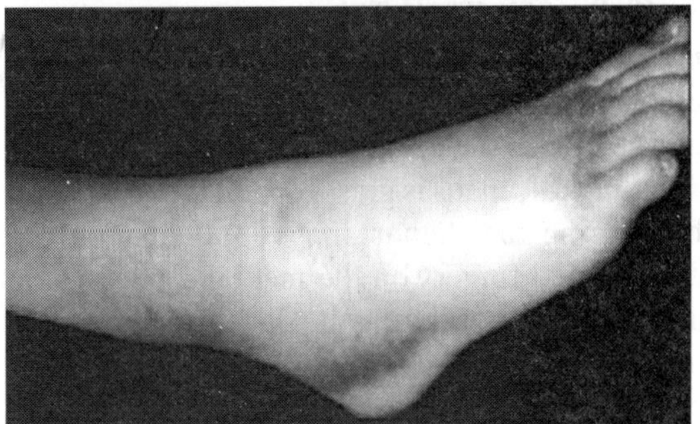

Fig. 23.4: Swelling around the ankle joint

Physical Examination

A comprehensive history and evaluation helps in diagnosing the severity and type of ankle sprain. Radiographic imaging techniques may need to be used to rule out fractures, complete ligament tears, or instability of the ankle mortise. The anterior drawer test and the talar tilt test are usually reproduce the symptoms and identify the ligaments sprain.

Anterior Drawer Test: The patient lies supine, ankle joint is taken out of the plinth. The therapist stands at the side of ankle joint, stabilizes distal tibia with one hand and holds the heel in slight plantar flexion with the other hand. While stabilizing the tibia, the heel is drawn anteriorly with respect to the tibia. Translation greater than 5 mm or difference in the anterior translation from the asymptomatic ankle suggests a tear of the ATFL. The test may also be performed in the sitting position (Fig. 23.5).

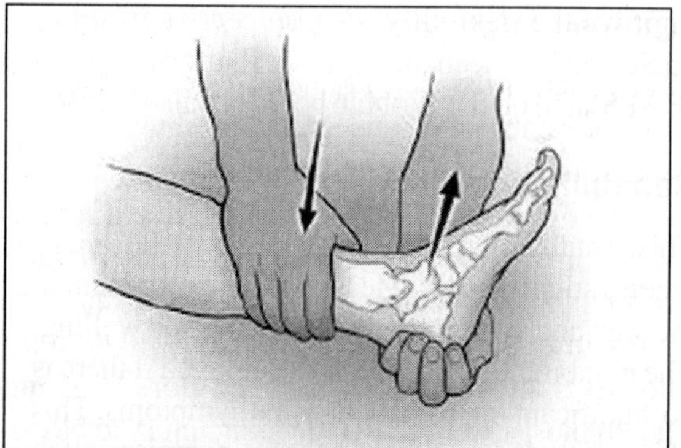

Fig. 23.5: Anterior drawer test

Talar Tilt Test: This tests the integrity of the calcaneofibular ligament. The patient sits comfortably and the therapist stands at the side and stabilizes the distal tibia with one hand. The talus and calcaneus is grasped with the other hand by placing the thenar and hypothenar on the dorsum and fingers on the medial aspect of the ankle. While stabilizing the distal tibia the talus and the calcaneus is inverted as a unit with respect to the tibia. A positive finding of more than 5 mm with a soft endpoint indicates a combined injury to the ATFL and CFL.

Management

Based on the diagnosis and an understanding of ligament healing properties, a progressive treatment regimen can be developed. The initial emphasis is made on accelerating healing, controlling inflammation and associated pain and swelling. Healing of a ligament sprain as in most of soft tissue injuries follows a process of inflammation, repair and remodelling. During the reparative and remodelling phase, the goal is to progress the rehabilitation appropriately to facilitate healing and restore the strength and proprioception.The controlled stress helps in promoting healing and results in a stronger repair.

Grade I and II Sprains Treatment

Immediately after injury, PRICE principle is followed to reduce haemorrhage, swelling,

inflammation and pain. Most of ankle sprains can be managed successfully with a non-surgical approach.

1. **Protection:** The ankle joint is immobilized (protected) in a functional brace or removable cast boot (for grade II), at the neutral position. Early weight bearing is allowed with the help of axillary crutches (Fig. 23.6).

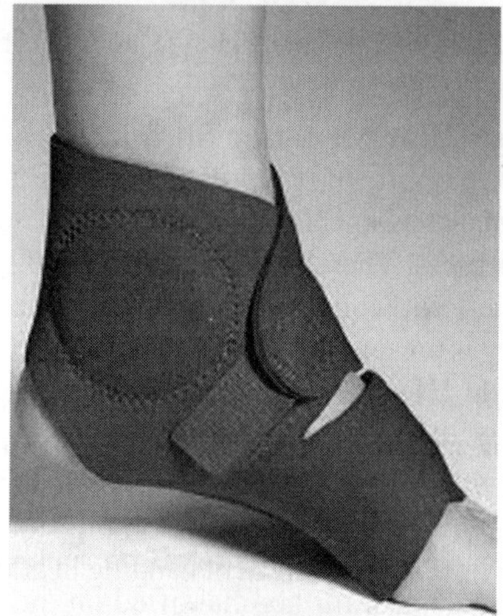

Fig. 23.6: Brace

2. **Rest:** Plantar flexion and inversion must be avoided in order to avoid the stress on ATFL.
3. **Ice:** Ice bag or cryocuff are applied for 10 minutes gently on the ankle joint to prevent hemorrhage and swelling. During ice application, the vasoconstriction occurs in the first ten minutes which is followed by vasodilatation. The therapist must not allow vasodilatation to occur especially in the acute stage (Fig. 23.7).

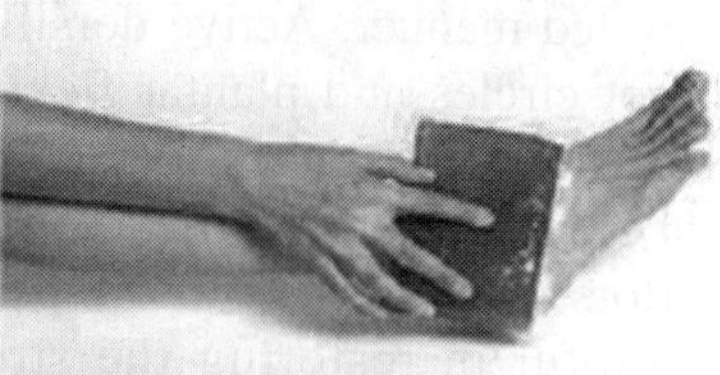

Fig. 23.7: Ice pack over the ATFL

4. **Compression:** Compression with an elastic bandage is beneficial in preventing the swelling especially when the foot is in dependent position such as in sitting and walking. Vasopneumatic compressions are also helpful in controlling pain and swelling (Fig. 23.8).

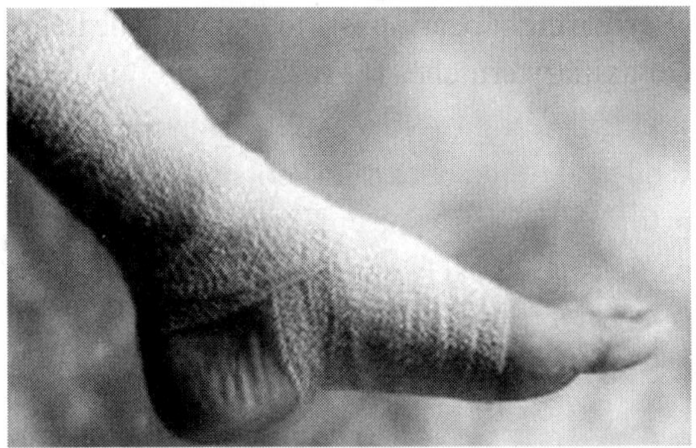

Fig. 23.8

5. **Elevation:** The leg is raised above the heart level in order to increase venous return from distal to the proximal part. The patients are also advised to keep the foot on the stool or chair while sitting instead of hanging in gravity dependent position.

Initial Phase

The ankle joint is immobilized (protected) in a functional brace or removable cast boot (for grade II), at the neutral position. Early weight bearing is allowed with the help of axillary crutches. The functional brace or cast boot must be accompanied with the rest, ice, compression and elevation till the end of this phase to achieve optimal results. After 3-4 days of injury, exercises are initiated as the patient shows improvement in the pain and swelling. *The exercises must not interrupt the repair process*; hence, these should be in a controlled manner. Active dorsiflexion, inversion, foot circles and plantar flexion are initiated in the pain free range. *Strengthening:* Submaximal isometric of dorsiflexors, plantar flexors, evertors and invertors in the pain free range are helpful in restoring the strength. *Stretching*: Calf stretching should be initiated to improve the flexibility. *Proprioceptive training* on Seated Biomechanical Ankle Platform System (BAPS) and on the Wobble board are also helpful.

Rehabilitation Phase

This usually starts after one week of the injury when patient reports at least 90% improvement in the sign and symptoms such as pain and swelling. The rehabilitation phase may be delayed if there is no significant improvement in the symptoms. This phase introduces weight bearing exercises such as heel raise, toe raise (initially bilateral followed by unilateral heel raise), stair and mini squatting (30 degrees bilateral knee flexion). The isometric exercises are progressed to the theraband and weight cuff resisted exercises.

Functional Phase

The patient may return to the normal activities. This phase usually starts after second week of the injury. The aim of treatment is to regain full strength, proprioception training, stability of the joint and return to the sport. The theraband and weight cuff resisted exercises remain same but more resistance. Incorporation of multidirectional agility drills can begin at this stage. Start with controlled exercises that are on both legs.

- Brisk walk followed by figure of eight, zig zag cutting and jogging. Begin jumping forward and backward over a line.
- Progress to jumping laterally over a line.
- Progress to box drills: Draw on the floor with tape and number the boxes starting in the upper left corner and progressing clockwise.
- The athlete may return to the sport if he/she gains full confidence, and muscle strength equivalent to the contralateral leg.
- The plyometric and proprioceptive training exercises and running is also started at this phase before return to the sport. On level ground, begin single leg standing exercises incorporating sport specific exercises such as kicking a ball, catching and throwing a ball, or

Syndesmosis Sprains

The syndesmosis sprains are usually occur in combined with other ankle joint sprains. It is the disruption of the distal tibiofibular and interosseous membrane. The distal tibiofibular ligament attaches at the distal end of the tibia and fibula which plays important role in maintaining the mortise space. The anterior wider portion of the talus remains in the mortise at the neutral position.Disruption of tibiofibular ligaments resulting in diastasis, or widening of the mortise at the talocrural joint.

Mechanism of Injury: The tibiofibular ligament disrupts if there is pronation and eversion combined with internal rotation of the leg when the foot is fixed on the ground or extreme dorsiflexion of the ankle joint. The *external rotation* and dorsiflexion forces the talus into the mortise, resulting widening of the talocrural joint which eventually disrupts the tibiofibular ligament and the interosseous membrane. The patients with syndesmosis sprains complaint pain in the anterior and posterior ankle joint particularly when trying to push off of the affected ankle. The patient does not bear the weight on the affected ankle joint.

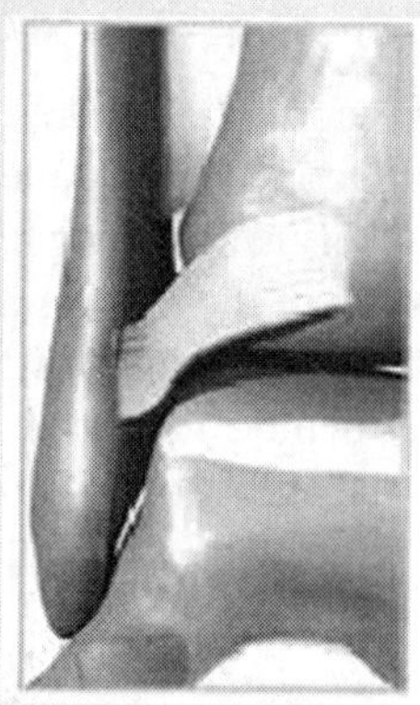
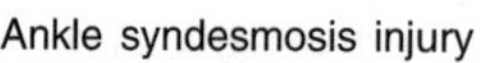
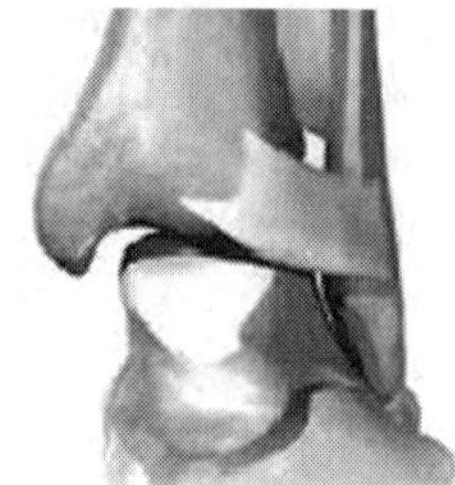

Physical Evaluation: Pain, swelling and tenderness around the ankle joint with inability to bear the weight on the joint are the common clinical findings of the syndesmosis sprain. The following physical tests may further confirm the sprain. *Squeeze Test* – Patient sits comfortably on the plinth.Therapist stands at the side, stabilizes the knee joint with one hand and grasps the anterior proximal leg with other hand and squeezes gently. If the test elicits pain in the tibiofibular ligament and interosseous membrane or syndesmosis area, it suggests syndesmosis sprain.**External Rotation Stress Test:** The patient sits comfortably on a treatment plinth with knee flexion to 90 degrees. The therapist sits comfortably at the side and stabilizes the distal tibiofibular joint with one hand and grasps the ankle at neutral position with other hand. While stabilizing the joint the foot is rotated externally. In case of positive test, the patient will complaint pain in the syndesmosis area. **Tibiotalar Shuck Test:** The examiner stabilises the leg with one hand and grasps the talus with other hand. While stabilizing the leg the medial and lateral force is applied to the talus alternatively. Pain in the syndesmosis region or feeling of the looseness may indicate syndesmosis sprain.

Management: The syndesmosis sprains are treated conservatively with cast immobilisa-tion for 4-6 weeks followed by rehabilitation program similar to the Grade I and Grade II ATFL sprains. The syndesmosis sprain with unstable and widened mortise is often managed with surgical fixation.

swinging a bat. Progress to standing on an air filled or foam cushion. Begin by keeping the exercise, such as catching a ball, close to the body. Progress to throwing the ball farther from the body to force the athlete to shift his center of gravity.

Prevention of Recurrence of ATFL Sprain

Poor compliance with therapy may predispose to functional instability of the ankle joint, therefore, to prevent reinjury, proprioceptive rehabilitation should continue until the athlete demonstrates improved functional skills particular to the individual's sport. Upon initial return to sport, the athlete should continue to support the ankle with tapping or a brace. The patient should be encouraged to continue home exercises program to ensure full restoration. Technique training (on jumping and landing), proprioceptive training, and orthosis have all shown to decrease risk of reinjury.

Grade III Sprain Treatment

The grade III first degree sprains are successfully treated with non-operative conservative treatment. Immediately after injury, the PRICE principle is followed to reduce haemorrhage, swelling, inflammation and pain. There has been much debate over the treatment of Grade III sprains whether these should be managed with immobilization or surgical repair. One school of thought recommends surgical repair followed by immobilization and rehabilitation. Others suggest immobilization followed by rehabilitation. It is concluded that the surgery should be recommended if there is involvement of other ligaments sprains such as calcaneofibular and tibiofibular ligament. The rehabilitative management including exercises remain almost same as Grade II and II sprains.

Surgical Management

The surgery should be reserved for the patients with chronic ankle instability. Most surgeons prefer surgical reconstruction of the ATFL especially second and third degree of grade III sprains where other structure such as CFL and syndesmosis sprains are also involved.

A graft is taken from gracillus or semitendinosus tendon. A tunnel is made on the talar neck on the insertion of the ATFL. A transfibular tunnel directed anterior to posterior through the fibula tip to a blind ending tunnel in the calcaneus at the insertion site of the CFL is also made. An ATFL graft is inserted in the tunnel through talus to the fibula. The CFL graft is also inserted in the tunnel through calcaneum to the fibula.

ANTERIOR CRUCIATE LIGAMENT SPRAIN

Introduction

Anterior cruciate ligament is a primary restraint to the anterior translation of the proximal tibia throughout the range of motion, however, it has more restraining power in the last 30 degrees of the extension. Although functioning independently, an ACL and PCL guide the instant centre of rotation of the knee, thereby controlling the joint arthrokinematics.

An ACL sprains most commonly causes knee joint instability than does sprains to other knee ligaments. In the past, an ACL tear could end the career of the athletes or result in the need for surgery and a year or more of rehabilitation. In the 1970s, ACL reconstruction were done through large arthrotomies, using extraarticular reconstruction followed by immobilization of the knee joint. To get rid of prolong immobilization and arthrotomies new approach of reconstruction "arthroscopy" was introduced in the 1980s. In the 1990s, the concept of "accelerated" rehabilitation evolved in an effort to return to the field quicker than ever.

Anatomy

The anterior cruciate ligament arises from the posteromedial corner of medial aspect of lateral femoral condyle in the intercondylar notch. It inserts in a fossa in front of and lateral to anterior tibial spine. It is made up of multiple collagen fascicles surrounded by an endotendinium and enveloped in a synovial membrane. The anterior cruciate ligament is innervated by the tibial nerve. The blood supply is received from the middle genicular artery. The bony attachments of the ligament at distal and proximal do not receive a significant blood supply from the artery. It is the reason of poor healing of the ligament after the injury (Fig. 23.9).

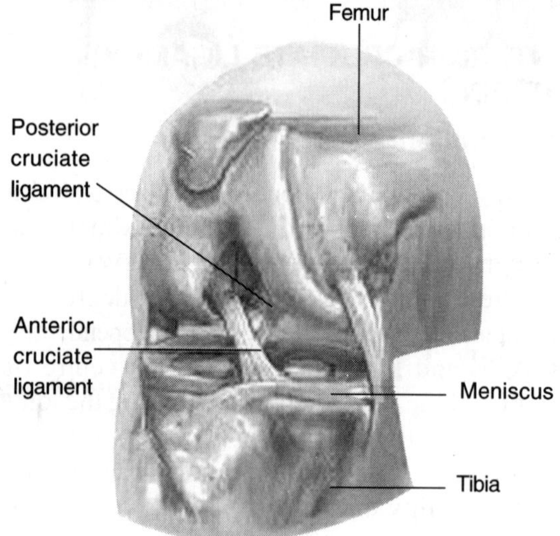

Fig. 23.9: Anterior and posterior cruciate ligaments

The anterior cruciate ligament is composed of two principal parts: small anteromedial band and a larger bulky posterolateral portion. The small anteromedial bundle becomes tight in flexion. The large posterolateral band moves anteriorly and becomes loose in flexion, on the other hand in extension it becomes tight. The posterolateral bulky portion of the ligament limits anterior translation, hyperextension and rotation of the knee joint whereas anteromedial bundle provides more rotational control which is in an axial position.

Epidemiology

Female soccer and basket athletes have the rates of ACL injuries more than the male soccer and basket athletes. Male and female basket athletes have similar rates of contact and non-contact ACL injuries whereas female soccer athletes have more non contact ACL injuries than male soccer athletes. Women have wider pelvis, shorter femurs, and less developed thigh muscles than males, these differences form a more lateral proximal reference point and increase lateral pull of the quadriceps on the patella and put medial stress on the knee joint.

A notable finding on gender difference in an ACL tears in relationship with physical abilities by researchers (Mountcastle *et al.*) is that women are three times more likely to have an ACL injury than men due to variations of hormone levels and greater ligament strength in men than in women. Most importantly, there is substantial differences in neuromuscular coordination and control in landing. Women also have less hip and knee flexion range of motions. The higher Q angle combined with their weakened hip muscles strength also makes them more prone to an ACL sprain as the greater Q angle increases force on the patella and in turn there is more anterior translation of the proximal tibia on the femur. Some authors have concluded that there is slight difference in gender ACL tear. On the other hand, there were significant gender differences in ACL injury rates when particular specific sports and physical activities were compared.

Etiology

The etiology of an ACL injuries has multifactorial theories. Two of them are extrinsic and intrinsic. *Extrinsic:* The athletes who improve their extrinsic elements are not prone to the ACL injuries. The extrinsic elements are improved through attending the different training sessions prior to the play. These training sessions help in improving the body movements in sport, muscle strength and coordination, shoe surface interface, and level of skill and conditioning. *Intrinsic:* The intrinsic elements are the anatomical structures such as joint laxity, limb alignment (valgus or varus), notch dimension, and the size of the ligament. These intrinsic elements contribute to the ACL injuries.

Mechanism of Injury

An ACL injuries usually occur during soccer and basketball play in young athletes and most often from skiing in the older people. The strong contraction of the quadriceps muscles places a significant stress (anterior tibial shear force on the ACL), especially when the knee is between 0 degree and 30 degrees. An ACL tear often occurs as the result of quick deceleration, hyperextension, or marked internal rotation of the tibia on femur, and does not involve the contact with other individual or athlete. This usually occurs when the athlete lands on the leg and quickly pivots in the opposite direction (valgus twisting injury). In this mechanism the posterolateral large bulky portion of the ACL gets sprained. This possibly disrupts the ACL with minimal injury to other structures such as medial and lateral meniscus and medial collateral ligaments (Figs. 23.10 a-b).

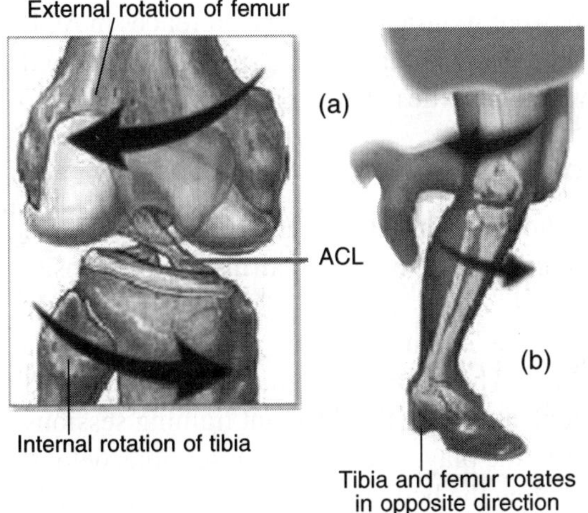

Figs. 23.10a-b: Mechanism of injury

The significant stress on an ACL, causes plastic deformation (sprain) with loss of collagen cross linkage. Rupture of the ACL usually occurs as a single fibre mass failure rather than sequential fibre failure; this possibly explains why, partial ACL injury is less common than the complete tear (Fig. 23.11).

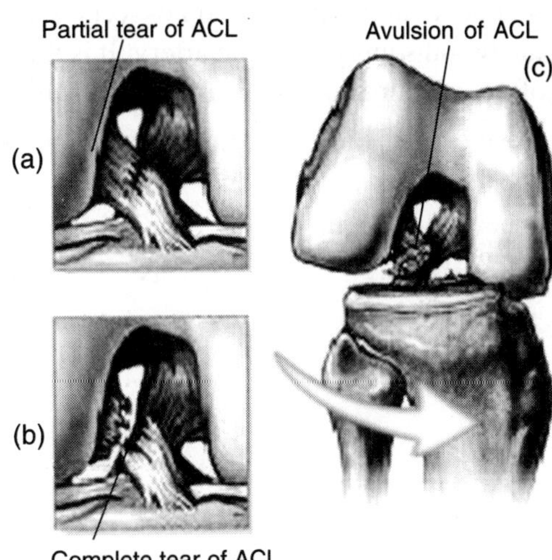

Fig. 23.11a-c: a. Partial tear, b. complete tear, c. avulsion of anterior cruciate ligament

Clinical Features

The acute ACL rupture is characterized by hemarthrosis, pain and instability. Athletes may experience a popping sound after impact, swelling and instability usually a "wobbly" feeling. Pain may also be a concerned factor and may range from moderate to severe. However, some patients continue their routine work by neglecting the instability and pain, which can have devastating consequences, resulting in a massive cartilage damage, and increase risk of secondary osteoarthosis.

Physical Examination

The therapist can make a provisional diagnosis of the ACL tear by performing some physical test because some of physical tests have very good sensitivity to the ACL tear. However, the patient needs to get an MRI done to determine the integrity of the ligament especially before arthroscopic treatment.

1. **Anterior Drawer Test:** The patient lies supine with the knee flexion to 90 degrees. Examiner sits on the forefoot of the patient of side which is being examined and holds the proximal tibia with both the hands. The examiner pulls the proximal tibia anteriorly on the femur. A test is positive if there is an excessive displacement of the proximal tibia on the femur without firm end feel compared with normal knee joint (Figs. 23.12a-b).

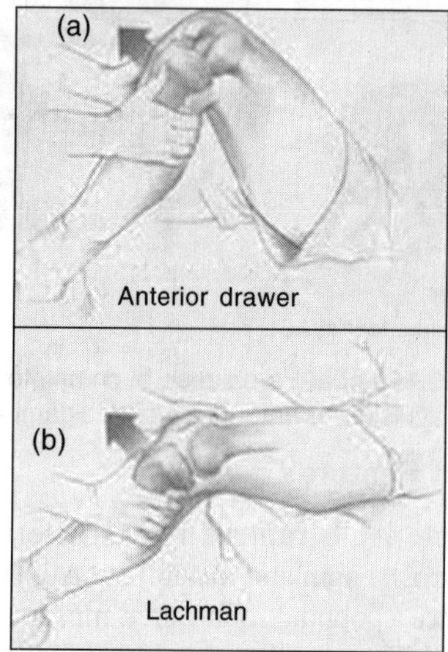

Figs. 23.12: a. Anterior drawer and b. Lachman test

2. **Lachman Test:** This test is named after orthopedic surgeon John Lachman. The test is recognized by most of clinicians as the most reliable and sensitive clinical test for the determination of anterior cruciate ligament integrity, superior to the anterior drawer test commonly used in the past for an ACL evaluation. The patient lies supine with the knee flexion at 20 to 30 degrees with external rotation of the leg (as per Bate's guide to physical examination). The examiner stabilizes

the distal femur with one hand and holds the proximal tibia with the other hand. While stabilizing the distal femur the proximal tibia is translated anteriorly on the femur. Anterior translation of tibia more than 12 mm, associated with a soft end-feel indicated a positive test for an ACL sprain or tear.

3. **Pivot Shift Test:** The patient lies supine, therapist stands at the side which is being examined, grasps the heel with the one hand and places other hand on the lateral aspect of the knee to apply valgus stress on it. The leg which is being examined is taken slightly out of the couch edge to flex it upto 30 degrees. At the flexion of 30 degrees a valgus stress is applied to the knee joint and then it is extended gently. A click or pop sound is felt while extending the knee joint with the valgus stress because there is anterior displacement of the lateral tibial plateau on the lateral femoral condyle.This test assess the ACL insuffi ciency (Fig. 23.13).

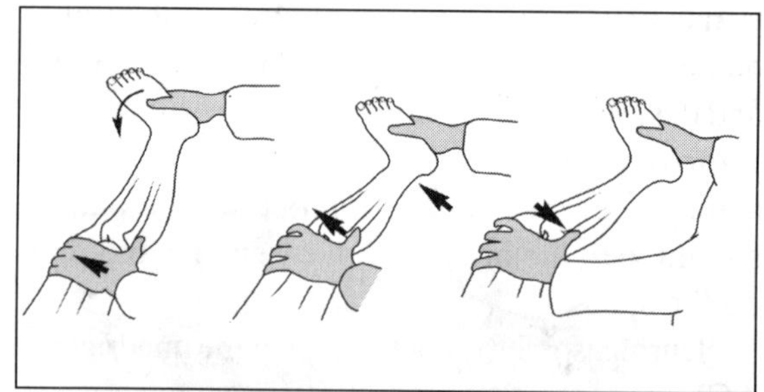

Fig. 23.13: Pivot shift test

Patients who have evaluated for an ACL injury should also be evaluated for other injuries such as meniscus and collateral ligaments, that often occur in combination with an ACL tear.

Management

There is much debate over the management of the ACL sprains, which patient requires reconstruction and which not is not clear. Athletes with ACL tear, who require high demand sports activities cannot return to the sport without reconstruction of the ligament. However, patients with low demand activities may continue with the torn ACL, but this may lead to secondary osteoarthrosis and meniscal tears especially posterior horn of the medial meniscus.

Partial ACL Tear Management

Partial tears are managed with the conservative treatment especially if the patients are of low demand activities. Immediately after injury, the PRICE principle is followed to reduce haemorrhage, swelling, inflammation and pain. The leg is elevated above the level of the heart and ice is applied for 10 minutes three to four times daily. Elastic crepe bandage is applied over the knee joint to prevent further hemarthrosis. The torn ligament is less likely to restrict the anterior translation of the tibia over the femur, therefore, knee brace or orthosis with the extension lock is advised to prevent the anterior translation of the tibia as it may cause further damage to the torn ligament. The stair climbing and descending is not allowed till the satisfactory improvement in the sign and symptoms is achieved, however, if it is required, the patient should lock the brace in full extension and then do the stairs.

During isometric contraction of the quadriceps, ACL is stressed more at 30 degrees, whereas at 90 degrees ACL remains unstrained. Active knee extension between 50 and 110 degrees does not strain the anterior cruciate ligament. At 90 degrees of flexion, an ACL accounts for approximately 85 percent of resistance to anterior drawer test.

The hyperextension of the knee joint develops much higher forces on ACL than PCL. At 5 degrees of hyperextension, the force on the anterior cruciate ligament is ranged between 50 and 240 newton. In normal ACL, in neutral rotation, application of 100 newtons of anterior force produces: 2-5 mm of anterior translation at full extension, 5-8 mm of anterior translation at 30 degrees of flexion and after 30 degrees as the flexion increases, an anterior translation of the tibia decreases. This biomechanical behaviour of the anterior cruciate ligament has an important clinical significance in administering the exercises especially in the acute stage.

Open Kinetic Chain Exercises

Open kinetic activities generate more isolated muscle contraction and thus allow for more specific muscle strengthening. The stabilizing effect of the muscle may be lost as soon as the fatigue of that particular muscle occurs and can put the ACL at great risk. These exercises place a significant force on the ligament between 0 and 30 degrees, therefore should not be used in the acute phase, particularly between 0 and 30 degrees. The open kinetic strengthening of the quadriceps in the form of isometric can safely be used between 60 and 100 degrees of flexion as the ligament in this range remains unstrained, however the resistance should be mild to moderate. The open kinetic strengthening of the hamstrings muscles is safe and often advised in the treatment of ACL injuries as these exercises do not cause any anterior translation of the tibia.

Closed Kinetic Chain Exercises

Closed kinetic chain exercises cause co-contraction of both the agonist and antagonist group of the muscles with progressive decrease in hamstrings activity as the flexion angle of the knee increases. Closed kinetic exercises by allowing agonist muscle activity, may not provide focused strengthening, but may provide a safer environment for an ACL in the setting of fatigue. Closed kinetic chain exercises in the first 30 degrees of the flexion produce less anterior translation of the tibia than the open kinetic chain exercises, this is because contraction of the hamstrings does not allow excessive anterior translation of the tibia. But further increase in flexion angle of the knee decreases the contraction of the hamstrings and increases anterior tibial translation. Therefore, mini squatting (between 0 and 30 degrees) exercise with the brace may be advised to an ACL injury patients.

Arthroscopic Reconstruction of the Anterior Cruciate Ligament

Reconstruction of the ligament is the choice of treatment as an anterior cruciate ligament does not heal independently because of inadequate blood supply to the ligament. Athletes with ACL tear usually require reconstruction in order to perform sharp movements safely with stability. The surgery is advised after swelling and inflammation subsides. This procedure does not repair the ligament, instead, it reconstructs an ACL by using other ligaments or tendons of the body. There are two options for the ACL graft selection; allograft and autograft. Autograft are the patients own tissues, which may be from hamstrings tendon or patellar tendon. Allografts are cadaveric tissue sourced from a tissue bank. Patella tendon bone autograft and hamstrings tendon autograft are the most common and preferred and tend to produce the best results.

Patellar Tendon Bone Autograft

The central 1/3 of the patellar tendon is removed along with a piece of bone from patella and tibia. The advantage of this graft is that the patella tendon and ACL are relatively having same length and it uses a bone to bone attachment that helps in accelerating early healing process. The central 1/3 bone patellar tendon bone graft has an initial failure strength of upto 2977N, which is higher than the intact ACL. The current trend is that the initial strength must exceeds that of the normal ACL to maintain sufficient strength as the strength of graft is decreased during the healing stage. PTB graft has disadvantage of common knee pain due to the removal of the bone from the patella. **Hamstrings Graft:** Two tendons are taken from the hamstring muscles, and wrapped together to form a graft (new ACL ligament). This has an advantage of not having pain in the anterior joint and also requires small size incision. The disadvantage of this graft is that it takes longer time to heel because there is no bone to bone healing and tendon to bone connection takes relatively long to become rigid. After implantation, an ACL graft undergo sequential phases of avascular necrosis, revascularisation, and remodelling. Ultimate load to failure and graft stiffness in a patellar tendon autograft can drop as low as 11% and 13% respectively of the normal ACL.

Femoral and Tibial Tunnel

The appropriate landmarks for femoral and tibial tunnel is one of the key points to be considered before starting the procedure. Most common error is non-isometric tunnel placement within intercondylar notch rather than its normal posterior position. Anterior placement of the graft (femoral) relative to normal anatomical insertion of ACL results in high strain on graft in flexion. Posterior placement of the graft results in excessive tightening of the graft in knee extension. Posterior tibial tunnel placement may be preferred to avoid anterior cruciate ligament graft impingement with the intercondylar roof. More medial starting point for tibial tunnel, may allow for better alignment of femoral tunnel.

Post-Operative Management of the ACL Reconstruction

Post operative treatment of an ACL reconstruction include: Immobilization in a brace, early motion, strengthening, assisted weight bearing, light sports at 6 months, and competitive at 8 months or later.

- **Bracing:** The knee joint is immobilized in a brace following ACL reconstruction to protect the donor graft. The brace is worn in the first 4-6 weeks all the day and night in a full extension; however, it may be removed or unlocked during the exercises. After six weeks it is replaced with a functional brace, which is advised till the athlete return to the competitive sport. The brace is unlocked while sleeping (after 4-6 weeks). Biomechanical studies of healing ACL graft performend in animals have shown that the graft requires a long time to revascularization and that the biomechanical behaviour of the graft never returns to normal. Functional knee braces provide a protective strain-sheilding effect on the ACL graft when anterior shear loads and internal torque are applied to the knee in the non weight bearing condition. However the strain shielding effect of functional braces decreases as the magnitude of anterior shear and internal torque applied to the knee increase.

- **Weight Bearing:** Toe touch weight bearing with crutches is allowed for 4-6 weeks to prevent anterior translation and any strain on the newly fitted graft. The toe touch weight bearing status of the patient, how long it is recommended, greatly depends upon the surgeon, therefore, further progression of the weight should be done with the consultation of the operating surgeon. Usually after 4-6 weeks weight bearing as tolerance may be initiated with the assistance of crutches followed by full weight bearing.

- **Exercises: Initial Phase: 0-4/6 weeks,** Initially active assisted quadriceps sets, gluteus maximus sets, hamstrings sets, ankle pump exercises are started in a brace to prevent the graft. Straight leg raising, and side leg raising initiated with brace in full extension (locking). Assisted active knee flexion and extension in a brace in high sitting position also

helps in improving flexion. These exercises are administered for 4-6 weeks. At the end of four weeks patient should achieve full extension and 90 degree flexion and 100 degree flexion by the end of six weeks. Extension lag is one of the complications of the ACL reconstruction, and if not corrected initially, it can cause anterior knee pain, quadriceps weakness, and early patella-femoral osteoarthritic changes. Any sign of loss of terminal extension should be observed carefully from the beginning of the exercises, and if, present, it should be managed with locking the brace in full extension especially in the first four to six weeks. Loss of flexion is not a major problem as it does not hamper the functional activities and can be gained easily by using the contract relax exercises, however, anteriorly placed graft may limit the terminal flexion permanently. *Strengthening Exercises:* Isometric resistance exercises of the quadriceps should be started with the angles which do not strain the graft. After four weeks isometric exercises at 80, 90 and 100 degrees can safely be initiated as at these angles the graft remain unstrained. Isometric strengthening of the hamstrings can be started at any angles. *Closed kinetic chain exercise* may also be started after 4-6 weeks. Mini squatting is the choice of close kinetic chain exercise in the first thirty degrees of the flexion as it allows co-contraction of the quadriceps and hamstrings and does not produce much anterior tibial translation, but as the flexion increases the action of the hamstrings decreases on the tibia and anterior tibial translation increases, therefore beyond thirty degree flexion squatting is not advised. *Eccentric Strengthening Exercises:* A muscle force producing capacity is most optimal when an external force exceeds that of the muscle while the muscle lengthens.

Hence, the potential to improve muscle strength by overloading the tissue is greater with eccentric strengthening than with concentric strengthening. Recent evidence suggests that the application of progressive, high force eccentric resistance exercises to the involved limb can be used safely to increase muscle volume and strength in ACL reconstructed individual.

CONTUSION

Contusion is the disruption of blood vessels below the skin, anywhere in the body. A direct blow to the skin is the main cause of the contusion; however, there is no break in the skin occurs. The blood comes out of the vessels, accumulates in the deeper tissues and forms a clot, known as hematoma. Ecchymosis is seen in the area. It may be absent if the deep tissue hematoma is formed.

Patients complaint pain and swelling in the area with painful movements. If the injury is superficial, ecchymosis is seen on the skin over the contusion. Tenderness is also the dominant feature of the contusion. Patients usually reveal the mechanism of the injury. The severity of this type of injury can be deceptive.

The contusions are managed with PRICE. Contusion of quadriceps and biceps brachii should be treated with caution as these muscles are at risk of ectopic bone formation (myositis ossification).

MUSCLE CRAMP

Muscle cramp is an involuntarily and forcibly contraction of the muscle or group of muscles, that lasts few seconds to minutes or occasionally longer. It is not uncommon for a muscle to recur multiple times until it finally resolves. Typically, cramps cause an abrupt, intense pain in the involved muscle which may be experienced as mild twitches to excruciatingly painful. The cramp may involve few fibers of the muscle or whole muscle or several muscles of same action (agonist or antagonist). Every individual experiences cramp at some time in their life, usually in the third decade of life and become increasingly as the age progresses, however, children may also experience cramps of muscles. Cramp may occur to any skeletal (voluntary) and organ (involuntary) muscles (rarely), however, it is more commoner in the skeletal muscles such as calves ("charley horse"), quadriceps, hamstrings and intrinsic muscles of the foot.

Etiology

The cause of the cramp is unknown, however, it is believed that inadequate stretching before exercises, muscle fatigue, exercising in the heat, and imbalance in the levels of electrolyte such as sodium, potassium, chloride, calcium and phosphate in the blood may contribute to the muscle cramps.

Pathology

The voluntary contraction of the agonistic muscles require relaxation of the antagonistic muscles. Cramps can occur when antagonistic muscles fail to relax properly due to myosin fibers not fully detaching from actin filaments. In skeletal muscle, ATP must attach to the myosin heads for them to disassociate from the actin and allow relaxation. The absence of ATP in sufficient quantities means that the myosin heads remains attached to actin. An attempt to force a muscle cramped in this way to extend (by contracting the opposing muscle) can tear muscle tissue and worsen the pain. The muscle must be allowed to recover (resynthesize ATP), before the myosin fibers can detach and allow the muscle to relax.

Prevention

Adequate conditioning of the muscles and stretching prior to any exercises or sports activities, adequate nutrition and hydration, attention to safety when exercising, and attention to ergonomic factors may help in prevention of the cramps.

Management

Stretching of the muscle may help in relieving the cramps. With exertional heat cramps due to electrolyte abnormalities (primarily sodium loss and not calcium, magnesium and potassium) appropriate fluids and sufficient salt improves symptoms.

BURSITIS

Bursitis is an infection or inflammation of the fluid-filled sac (bursa) that lies between a tendon and skin, or between a tendon and bone. The condition may be acute or chronic. Activities that involve excessive and repetitive forces on the inter-tissue junctions frequently lead to an inflammation to the bursa.

Bursa is a small fluid filled sac lined or water bag similar to synovium; they usually are located at inter-tissue junctions that encounter high friction during movements. The inter-tissue junctions involve skin, tendons, or muscles, ligaments over bony prominence. Bursa may or may not communicate with a joint.

Origin

Bursa is very much similar to tendon sheath and the synovial membrane. Some bursae are simply extension of the synovium membrane others are formed by external to the capsule. Occasionally the cavity of the bursa communicates with the cavity of the synovial joint (suprapatellar bursa and subscapularis bursa communicates with knee joint and shoulder joint respectively).

There are two types of the bursa:

a. **Anatomical:** Those anatomically or normally present (over the patella and olecranon); and

b. **Adventitious:** Such type of bursa develop over a bunion, an osteochondroma, or on spine due to kyphosis. The adventitious bursa are produced by repeated trauma or constant/prolonged friction or pressure. These bursae have a lack of true endothelial or synovial lining. The adventitious bursa which develops in response to an abnormal and excessive friction (such as subcutaneous bursa) develops over the tendocalcaneous in response to badly fitted shoes should not be confused with anatomic bursa.

Functions

Muscles are the drivers of the joint, their contraction produces movement on the joints (bones move in opposite direction) this encounters high friction in the inter-tissue junctions. The functions of the bursae are to reduce friction, protect delicate structure from pressure, help the joint to move with ease, lubricate and cushion pressure points and provide a slippery surface that has no friction.

[**Example:** When a zip lock small water bag is placed between the hands and then hands are rubbed on each other. The movements would be smooth and effortless this is exactly how a bursa functions as a smooth, slippery surface between two moving inter-tissue surfaces].

Causes

Acute or chronic trauma such as overuse, and sustain repetitive stresses can cause excessive load on the bursa. Acute or chronic pyogenic infection, low grade inflammatory conditions such as gout, syphilis, tuberculosis or rheumatoid arthritis may also cause bursitis. Trauma or injury can cause inflammation in the tendon which is termed as tendonitis that may put some degree of stress on the bursa and causes bursitis. However, it is not clear whether tendonitis causes bursitis or bursitis causes tendonitis, but most of time both conditions occur combined (follow each other).

Mechanism

Chronic repeated trauma allows gradual accumulation of synovial fluid in the bursa, in turn the bursa becomes swollen, inflamed and rough. The smooth gliding bursa now acts as gritty and rough within an already confined space that leads to friction in the inter-tissue surfaces. The movements become irritating and painful which further contribute to the bursitis and tendonitis.

Clinical Symptoms

A dull ache, stiffness in the area around the bursa or joint line may be experienced. Symptoms aggravate with movements and pressure. Redness and swelling may be observed occasionally in the area of inflamed bursa in case of superficial (subcutaneous) bursitis. The extreme movements can put the stress/pressure on the bursa and cause pain. The resistance against the contraction at extreme ranges can also aggravate the symptoms.

Hip Joint Bursitis

Bursitis associated with gluteus maximus muscle may be of three types:
- Trochanteric bursitis.
- Subgluteal bursitis.
- Iliopsoas or iliopectineal bursitis.

Trochanteric Bursitis

Trochanteric bursa lies between the insertion of the tendon of the gluteus maximus and the vastus lateralis. Trochanteric bursitis may either be infectious or non-infectious. Infectious trochanteric bursitis may be caused by an acute pyogenic infection or a tuberculosis (Fig. 23.14).

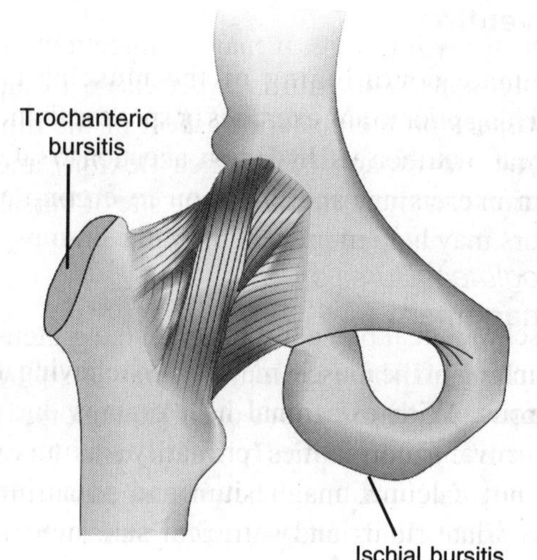

Fig. 23.14: Trochanteric bursitis

a. Tuberculosis is rarely seen now except of in some developing countries was fairly common in this bursa in the past. To make a diagnosis, cultures from fluid of bursa should be taken for pyogenic organism and acid fast bacteria. Patients present with localized pain with or without previous history of tuberculosis. Pain aggravates in the night or during rest.

b. Non-infectious or traumatic trochanteric bursitis pain will be around the lateral aspect of the hip. It is common in middle aged older people engaged in sports activities such as running, tennis, gardening etc. Patients typically complain of lateral hip pain over the outer thigh or difficulty in walking. The hip pain is usually aggravated by direct pressure; depending upon the degree of inflammation and swelling, pressure sensitivity ranges from mild morning pain and stiffness to intolerance to sleeping on the affected side. Patients may rub the thigh when describing the pain.

Subgluteal Bursitis

Subgluteal bursa is usually a large and multi locular, separates the deep surface of the gluteus maximus from the greater trochanter and the short rotator of the hip joint. It may be infectious or non-infectious. The pain is experienced in the deep tissues on the posterior aspect of the hip. Extreme hip flexion (with knee flexion) and adduction can elicit the pain in the site of bursa.

Ischiogluteal Bursitis

The ischiogluteal bursa lies between the gluteus maximus and the ischium. It may also be infectious or non-infectious or inflammatory, is more commoner in individuals who have secondary occupations. The prolonged sitting causes constant irritation in the bursa which becomes swollen and inflamed.

Iliopsoas Bursitis

It is also known as iliopectineal bursitis, the largest bursa around the hip joint, which covers anterior hip joint capsule and extends proximally into the pelvis posterior to the iliopsoas. Iliopsoas bursitis can cause pain in the anterior aspect of hip joint with an ilioinguinal mass. Hip flexion and resistance to the extension of the hip joint may produce pain (Fig. 23.15).

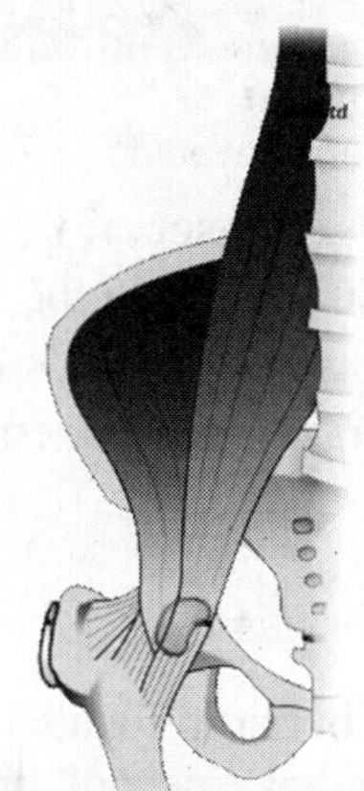

Fig. 23.15: Iliopsoas bursitis

Knee Joint Bursitis

The knee joint has as many as fourteen bursa. They are situated wherever skin, muscle, or tendon rubs against bones. Some important bursae, are discussed as below: (Fig. 23.16)

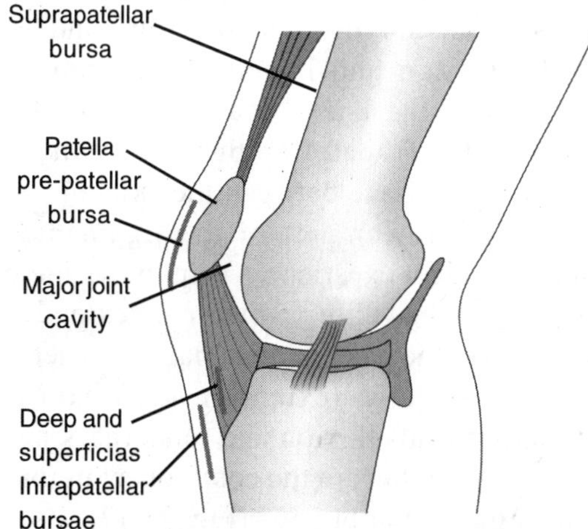

Fig. 23.16: Knee joint bursitis—suprapatellar, infrapatellar and pre-patellar

Suprapatellar Bursitis

In the front of the patellofemoral joint there is no capsule. Quadriceps over the suprapatellar region produces enormous friction during the knee joint movements. To reduce the friction between quadriceps and suprapatellar region an adventitious bursa is formed which is known as suprapatellar bursa. The bursa communicates with the joint. Pain in the superior aspect of the knee joint is usually caused by the suprapatellar bursitis which is more common in runners and jumpers. Suprapatellar bursitis is usually the result of direct trauma to the bursa from either acute injury or repeated microtrauma.

Physical examination may elicit tenderness in the anterior knee just above the patella. Passive flexion as well as active resisted extension of the knee will reproduce the pain. Sudden release of resistance during this maneuver will markedly increase the pain. There may be swelling in the suprapatellar region with boggy feeling on palpation. Occasionally the suprapatellar bursa may become infected which produces systemic symptoms, such as fever and malaise, as well as local symptoms, including rubor, color and dolor.

Infrapatellar Bursitis

Infrapatellar bursa is a small deep situated bursa between the tuberosity of the tibia and the patellar tendon and is separated from the synovium of the knee by a pad of fat. The superficial infrapatellar bursa lies in the subcutaneous tissue between the skin and the front of the lower part of the ligamentum patellae. Patient experiences pain in the site of the bursa, and swelling which may extend on either side of the patellar tendon. Loss of active terminal extension (extension lag), pain on resistance to full flexion and tenderness near the patellar tendon are the common symptoms of the infrapatellar bursitis (Fig. 23.17).

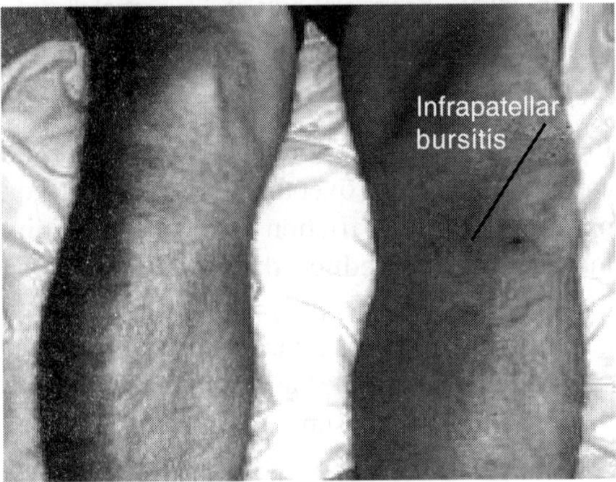

Fig. 23.17: Infrapatellar bursitis with marked swelling

Prepatellar Bursitis

The prepatellar bursa lies in the subcutaneous tissue between the skin and front of the lower half of the patella and the upper part of the ligamentum patellae. The direct trauma such as a fall on the patella, or by recurrent minor injuries (housemaid's and namaaz position) are the common causes of traumatic prepatellar bursitis. Pyogenic prepatellar bursitis especially in children is also common (Figs. 23.18a-b).

Prepatellar bursitis is very common in those whose occupation demands prolonged kneeling,

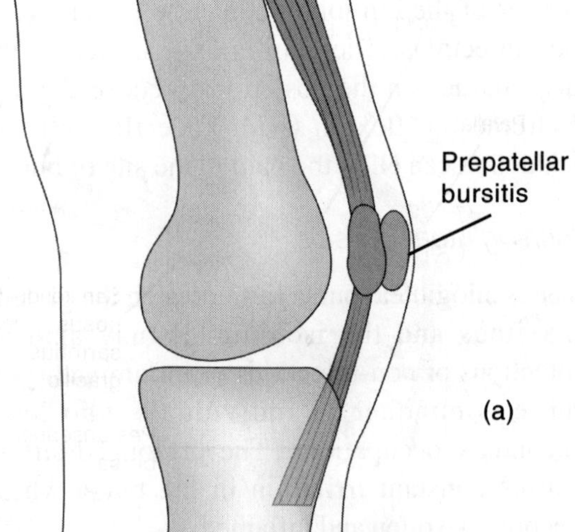

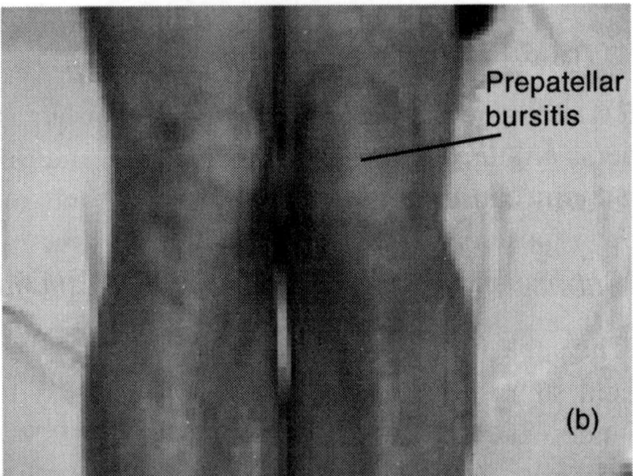

Figs. 23.18a-b: Prepatellar bursitis with redness and swelling

e.g., carpet layers, housemaid's and namaaz prayers. Indeed, effusion into the bursa sac are popularly known as housemaid's knee because in kneeling, the bursa comes into contact with the ground.

Pes Anserine Bursitis or Voshell's Bursitis

The pes anserine bursa is located between the proximal anteromedial aspect of the tibia and the undersurface of the pes anserinus muscle tendons (gracilis, semitendinosus and sartorius). Pes anserine bursitis also known as Voshell's bursitis is a commonly missed causes of medial knee joint pain (Fig. 23.19).

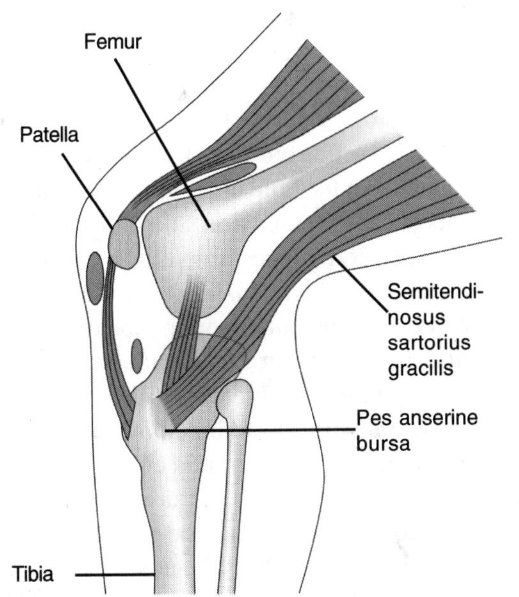

Fig. 23.19: Pes anserinus bursitis

Shoulder Joint Bursitis

Subacromial Bursitis or Sub Deltoid Bursitis

The subacromial bursa lies between the deltoid and supraspinatus muscle. It extends upwards underneath the acromion process and the coraco acromial ligament. The subacromial bursa reduces the friction and permits the greater tuberosity of the humerus to rotate inwards under the acromian process during the abduction and rotation of the shoulder. Although the subacromial bursa becomes inflamed more often than any other bursa, the inflammation is rarely primary in the bursa: rather it results from tendonitis of the rotator cuff of the shoulder with or without calcification. Codman (1934) described bursitis as an entity. The tendon of the supraspinatus lies just below the subacromial bursa. Injury to the supraspinatus tendon produces some inflammatory changes, but it may be painless until the adjacent brusa (subacromial) is involved which, being abundantly supplied with vessels and nerves produces the symptoms of which the patient complains. Pain in the shoulder which may radiate down the lateral arm and aggravates while overhead activities (flexion with internal rotation) is the common symptom of the subacromial bursitis (Figs. 23.20a-b).

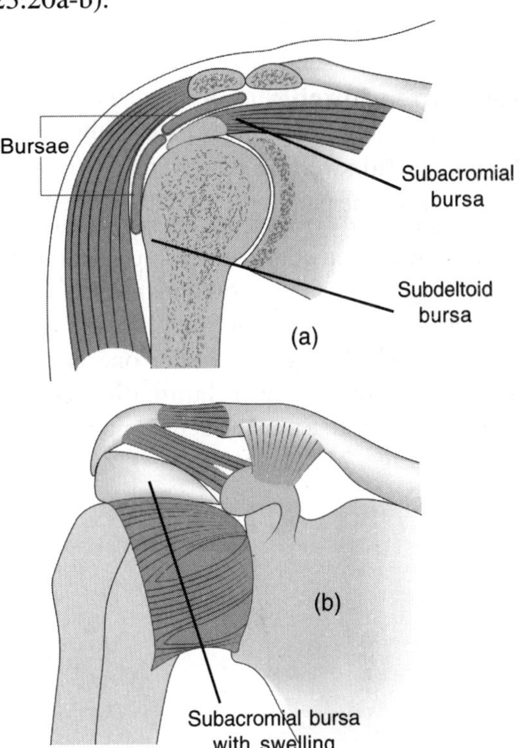

Figs. 23.20a-b: a. Subacromial bursa, b. Subacromial bursa with swelling

Neer has described the maneuver to test the subacromial bursitis as passive shoulder flexion and internal rotation. Patient should complain pain at the end range. The test is not so sensitive to the bursitis as other conditions may also produce the same symptoms. Hawkins and Kennedy described the test which has more sensitivity than Neer. It involves forward flexion at 90 with internal rotation which brings the greater tuberosity under the acromian arch and reduces subacromial space, contributes to further impingement in the bursa.

Subscapularis Bursitis

The subscapularis bursa lies on the anteromedial surface of the humeral head between the tendon of the subscapularis muscle and the capsule of the shoulder and communicates with the joint. Traumatic subscapularis bursitis is not very common.

Elbow Joint Bursitis

Olecranon Bursitis

Clinically there are two olecranon bursa; one lies between the tendon of the triceps muscle and the posterior ligament of the elbow and the olecranon; the other lies between the attachment of the olecranon and the skin. The later one is more prone to inflammation.Inflammation in the subcutanenous bursa may be acute or chronic or infectious (Figs. 23.21a-b).

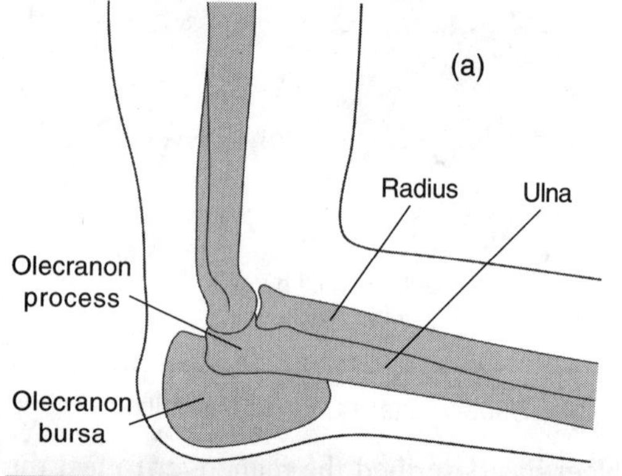

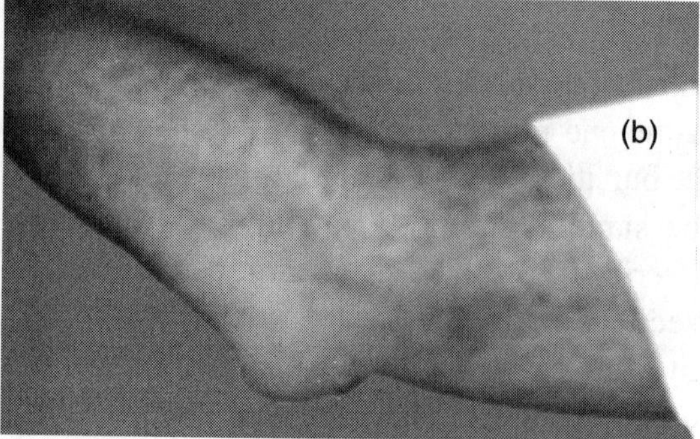

Fig. 23.21a-b: Olecranon bursitis with marked swelling

Olecranon bursitis is not common in children below seven years because the bursa does not develop at this age. Traumatic bursitis may be caused by a direct blow, fall on playing surface or chronic repeated trauma with gradual accumulation of the fluid in the bursa. For example students during examination study for long hours at a stretch and place their elbow (posterior aspect) on the table. This is the most common cause of olecranon bursitis with repeated trauma and direct pressure on the olecranon. It is also known as minor's or student's elbow.

Pain on pressure, posterior elbow swelling and pain in flexion are the common clinical findings. In case of septic brusitis the area is warm and erythematous and pain may be in the night and rest also. For differential diagnosis the bursa is aspirated and the fluid is examined for white cells crystals and bacteria and cultured for micro organisms (stain and cultural studies).

Retrocalcaneal Bursitis: Pain in the posterior aspect of the heel at the insertion of tendo-achilis may be arisen from retrocalcaneal bursitis. There are two bursae retrocalcaneal and subcutaneous calcaneal bursa. Retrocalcaneal bursa is a deep bursa, situated anterior to the Achilles tendon between calcaneus and Achilles tendon, whereas, subcutaneous calcaneal bursa is a superficial bursa situated posterior to the Achilles tendon between skin and Achilles tendon. Retrocalcaneal bursitis may be caused by bursal impingement between the Achilles tendon and an excessively prominent posterosuperior Aspect of the calcaneus (Haglund deformity) during dorsiflexion of the ankle. Retrocalcaneal bursitis may be unilateral or bilateral and may be associated with gout, rheumatoid arthritis, and seronegative spondyloarthropathies. Recent studies suggest that a misaligned subtalar joint axis in relation to the Achilles tendon (measured in terms of joint inclination and deviation) can result in an asymmetrical force load on the tendon disrupting normal biomechanics. Tight or poorly fitted shoes that produce excessive pressure on the posterior heel is also one of the cause of the retrocalcaneal bursitis (Fig. 23.22). This altered joint axis is associated with an increased risk for Achilles pathologies, including bursitis. Swelling and redness with warmth and pain on pressure may clearly be apparent.

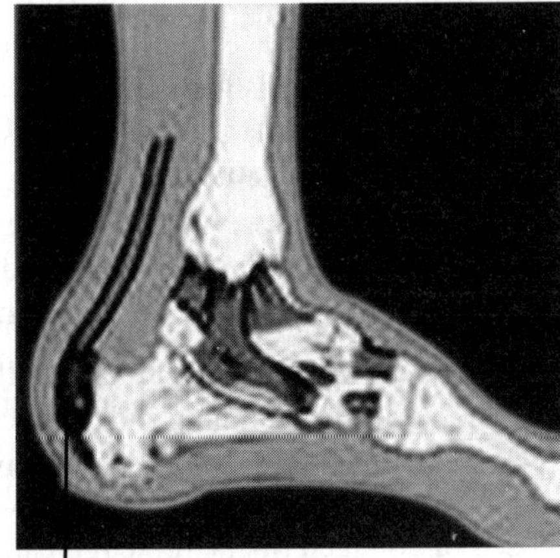

Fig. 23.22: Retrocalcaneal bursitis

Treatment

- Cryotherapy.
- Contrast bath.
- Continuous ultransound with the intensity of .9w/cm^2.
- Gradual progressive stretching of tendo-Achilles.
- Shoe modification.
- Corticosteroid injections–After fair trial of above treatment.

Management

The treatment of bursitis is determined by its cause and secondarily by pathological changes in the bursa. In most of the cases surgery is not needed. Modification in the activities–correction of posture–should be given priority. Traumatic bursitis often responds favorably to conserative treatment and aspiration and injection of an appropriate steroid preparation, but infectious bursitis may require surgical intervention.

- Aspiration and injections of an appropriate drugs.
- Incision and drainage when an acute supportive bursitis fails to respond to non-surgical methods.
- Excision of chronically infected and thickened bursa and removal of an underlying bony prominences.

The infected bursa should be examined for organism and also treated with an appropriate antibiotics. Aspiration and injection of antibiotics may be the second step. Dressing should be applied after aspiration, surgical drainage is occasionally needed.

The surgical excision of the bursa is required for repeated bouts of bursitis that interfere with functional activities and for chronically damaged and infected bursa, particularly if calcaneal osteomyelitis is present.

Management of Traumatic Bursitis

Prevention: Any activity which makes the inflammation of the bursa worse, should be avoided.

- Avoid repetitive activities that put excessive load or stress.
- Lose weight if it is needed.
- Modification in the shoe.
- Maintain strength and flexibility of the muscles.

Cryotherapy: Application of ice packs twice or thrice daily with minimum of fifteen minutes can reduce the inflammation. Ice packs are readily available in the market should be recommended.

Pulsed Ultrasound Therapy: 3 MHz ultrasound for subcutaneous bursitis and 1 MHz ultrasound with high intensity and low duty cycle for deep situated bursa can be recommended, so that ultrasound energy may reach to the deep situated bursa.

Contrast Bath: Moist heat therapy is an effective in relieving the muscle spasm. Contrast bath may also be recommended for retrocalcaneal bursitis.

CHAPTER-24

Arthritis

Arthritis is derived from two Latin words arth and itis. Arth means joint and itis means inflammation, hence, arthritis is defined as inflammation in the joint. As far as osteoarthritis is concerned, it is an essentially non-inflammatory disease, the disease does not commence with the inflammation, hence, it should not be called as arthritis. Therefore, the latest definition of the arthritis is given as: any process by which a joint is damaged is known as arthritis. There are two processes which involves joint destruction: inflammatory and degenerative.

OSTEOARTHRITIS

Osteoarthritis is essentially a non-inflammatory degenerative disease of the atricular cartilage which is characterized by thinning and destruction of the joint surface, new bone (osteophyte)

The Articular Cartilage: The articular cartilage is composed of collagen fibers, proteoglycans and water. These substances contribute to the shape, size and elastic properties of the cartilage which make cartilage more resistant to the repeated mechanical stresses.

- Collagen fibers and proteoglycans (keratin sulphate and condroitin sulphate) contribute upto 20 percent.
- Water contribute upto 80 percent (Figs. 24.1a-b).

In terms of biphasic material, the articular cartilage is composed of a porous permeable collagen proteoglycan solid matrix filled by the freely movable interstitial fluid (approximately 25% by wet weight). In addition to solid and fluid there exists an additional ion phase when considering articular cartilage as a triphasic medium. Therefore biomechanically articular cartilage should be viewed as a triphasic material.

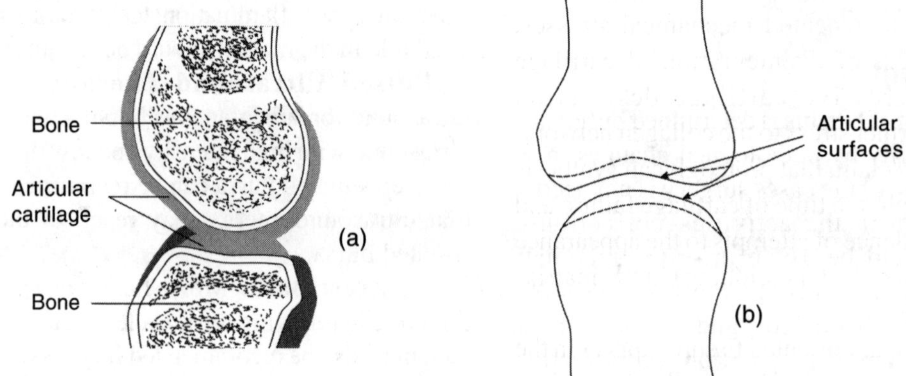

Figs. 24.1a-b: Normal hyaline articular cartilage

formation and capsular fibrosis. As the disease is an essentially non-inflammatory it should be termed as osteoarthrosis instead of osteoarthritis, however, both osteoarthritis and osteoarthrosis terms are used interchageably and has same meaning.

It affects commonly weight bearing joints such as the knee, hip and spine, moreover the individual joints are affected with differing frequency in men and women.

Pathogenesis

It is thought that early failure of the collagen fibers network (loosening of the collagen network) enables the proteoglycans to attract more water molecules. The increased water contents in the cartilage allows abnormal expansion of the proteoglycans and thus tissue swelling. *Associated with this change is a decreased in a cartilage stiffness and increase in cartilage permeability.*

In the next stage of degeneration, the proteoglycans of cartilage contain lower concentration of keratin sulphate than the normal while the concentration of condroitin sulphate increases. *Associated with this change the proteoglycan concentration in the cartilage falls.* At this stage there is decreased in a cartilage stiffness and increased in cartilage permeability. The cartilage losses its elasticity and becomes less resistant to repeated mechanical stresses, and the process of disintegration of cartilage begins. Progressive cartilage destruction contributes further stress to the collagen network. (Some authors claim that proteoglycan synthesis is increased upto the time of cartilage failure and there is an evidence of attempts to the appearance of chondrocyter clusters (cloning) in the matrix-depleted cartilage).

Perpendicularly oriented fissures appear in the superficial zone and they gradually extend into the deeper. Due to these fissures there is detachment of the small articular cartilage fragments into the joint space where they are eventually degraded. The progressive loss of thickness of the articular cartilage may lead to surface abrasion and complete exposure of bone in areas of peak overload. Eventually there is loss of full thickness of the articular cartilage, where the articular cartilage is composed of a bony articular plate polished from the grinding interaction of bone articulating with bone. Revascularization of the remaining articular cartilage produces osteophytes which may project to the periarticular structures (peripheral unshared areas) (Figs. 24.2a-b and 24.3).

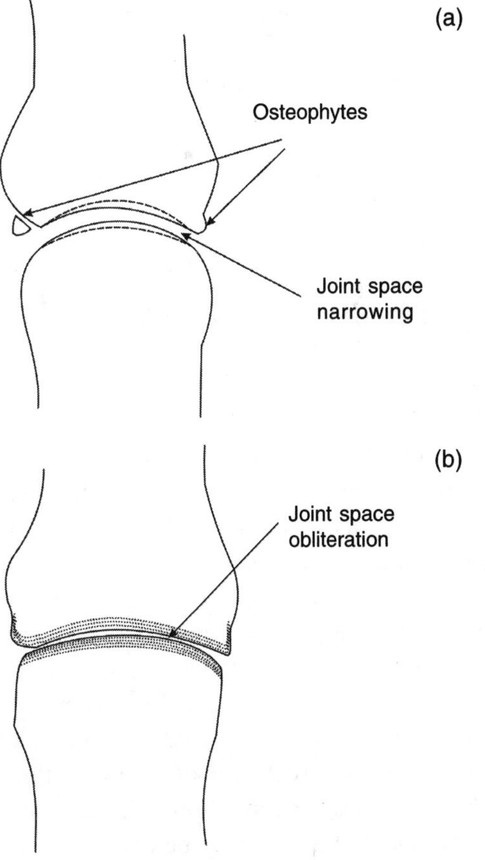

Fig. 24.2a-b: Degenerated articular cartilage, loss of joint space and osteophytes

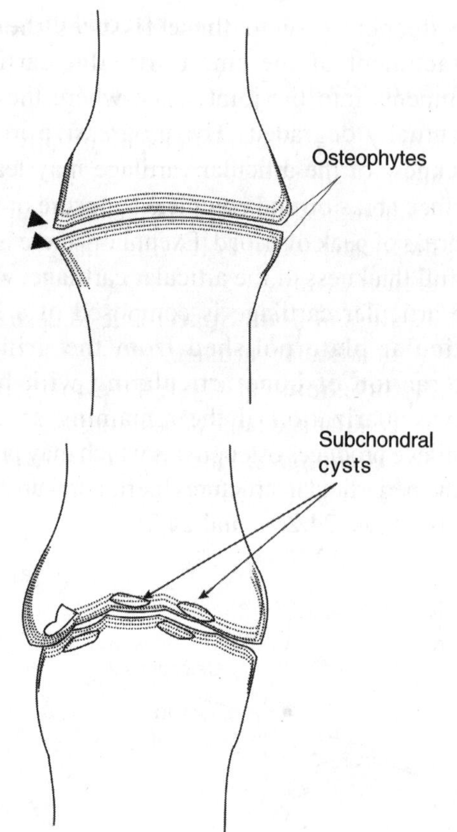

Fig. 24.3: Degenerated articular cartilage with joint space obliteration, osteophytes and subchondral cyst

The osteophytes deposit onto the synovium and then penetrate to the sub synovial layers and the resultant fibrosis may extend to the capsule. The capsule loses its elastic properties, becomes thickened, and its volume is decreased. Finally there is limitation in the range of motion. Loss of full thickness of cartilage allows exposure of the subchondral bone. 'Cracks' in the subchondral bone plate permit pressure transmission to the cancellous bone resulting in cyst formation.

The advanced changes include some type of subluxation such as widening of the joint of one side, horizontal translation, angular deviation etc. Small pieces of cartilage may be dislodged and develop loose bodies which can result in locking of the joint and episodic severe pain.

The Wear Mechanism of the Cartilage May Commence or Begin in Three Ways

1. **Interfacial Wear:** There is direct contact of the weight bearing surfaces (articular cartilages) with no lubrication film separating them. This is the commoner problem in the obese and the individuals whose job is long standing such as nurses, hair dressers. The interaction of the weight bearing joint surfaces causes adhesions—the fragment adhere to each other and abrasion—the tissue is scrapped by harder one.
2. **Fatigue Wear:** The deformation of the underlying weight bearing joint surface may occur if there is repeated micro trauma to the surfaces.
3. **High Impact Wear:** High impact activities such as jumping and running may increase the stress and load on the cartilage with insufficient time for internal fluid distribution.

These wear mechanisms put excessive load and alter the normal load bearing mechanism of the cartilage. This whole phenomenon disrupts the collagen fiber proteoglycan matrix and predisposes cartilage to early degeneration.

Clinical Sign and Symptoms

- Pain.
- Muscles guarding (spasm).
- Stiffness.
- Swelling.
- Tenderness.
- Crepitus.
- Decrease range of motion, flexion contracture, extension lag.
- Angular and rotatory deformities.

Pain is the dominant clinical feature which is aggravated by the activities those put more stress on the affected cartilage. Usually pain is more common in the form of discomfort and stiffness. Initially it is worsen on rising from bed, and again at the end of a day's activities and relieved by the rest. As the disease progresses there is involvement of the synovium and the capsule, which limits the range of motion of the joint and produces swelling (synovial and capsular thickening) and the joint becomes deformed. The muscles guard the joint by preventing the painful movements, resulting in shortening of the muscles which further decreases range of motion. Initially pain is poorly localized and is dull aching nature. It is relieved by rest but when the other structures such articular, periarticular, and capsule are involved, pain may also be experienced during rest and at night.

Types of Osteoarthrosis

- Primary osteoarthrosis.
- Secondary osteoarthrosis.

Primary Osteoarthrosis: The exact cause is not known but the following factors are believed to contribute to the causation of primary osteoarthrosis. Obesity, genetic, heredity, multiple endocrine disorders and multiple metabolic disorders. However no cause is barrier.

Secondary Osteoarthritis (Demonstrable Abnormalization): The secondary osteoarthrosis occurs ten years earlier then the primary osteoarthrosis and is more severe. Anything which alter the line of force or put excessive load on the articular cartilage can contribute to the secondary osteoarthritis. The predisposing factors to secondary osteoarthrosis are as under:

- *Obesity.*
- Fracture, trauma, Perthes disease.
- Infection, tuberculosis.
- Metabolic disorders–Diabetes and parathyroidism.
- Inflammatory arthritis–Rheumatoid arthritis.
- Hemophilia, syringomyelia.
- Coxa-vara, coxa-valga, ante-version of femur.
- Joint instability–subluxation, excessive translation.

- Overuse of intraarticular steroid therapy.

Investigations

- Laboratory investigations are usually within normal limits.
- Radiological findings are the most important diagnostic tools. Following changes can be seen on X-rays:
  1. **Loss of Joint Space:** Due to destruction of articular cartilage.
  2. **Subchondral Cyst:** Due to increased cellular and bone deposition.
  3. **Osteophytes:** Due to revascularization of the remaining cartilage and capsular traction.
  4. **Loose Bodies:** Due to fragmentation of osteoclondral surface.
  5. **Deformity and Malalignment:** Due to destruction of capsular ligament and ligamentous laxity.

Radiographic evaluation should always be considered in a standing or weight bearing position of anteroposterior view. For patellofemoral joint a lateral view is required as it is a skyline view of the patella. For lateral compartment of the tibiofemoral joint posteroanterior view should be taken in a standing with the knees in 30 degrees of flexion this is because the medial compartment involves degeneration of distal femur and central tibia, and lateral compartment involves degeneration in the posterior femur and posterior tibia.

TIBIOFEMORAL JOINT OSTEOARTHROSIS

Introduction: The human knee joint, the largest and perhaps most complex joint in the body, is a two joint structure composed of the tibiofemoral and patellofemoral joints. The knee joint transmits loads, participates in motion, aids in conservation of momentum and provides force couple for activities involving the leg.

- 80% of patients develop medial compartment resulting in varus or bow legged deformity.
- 05–10% of patients develop lateral compartment resulting in a valgus or kneed deformity.
- A small percentage of patients develop rotatory deformity of tibia that causes significant patellar maltracking or sublaxation. It is common in an arthritic knee but is surprisingly seldom a source of symptoms.
- **Panarticular Arthritis:** The involvement of both tibiofemoral compartments (medial and lateral) and patellofemoral joint.

Degenerated Articular Cartilage: In the degenerative process the concentration of proteoglycans in the cartilage falls. The proteoglycans organize the collagen fibers in the articular cartilage. As the concentration of the proteoglycans falls the collagen fibers becomes disorganized. At this stage the cartilage looses its elasticity and becomes less resistant to the repeated mechanical stresses and the process of disintegration begins. Perpendicular oriented fissures appear in the superficial zone and gradually extend into deeper zone. These fissures promote detachment of small articular cartilage fragments into the joint space where they are eventually degraded. There is progressive loss of thickness of the articular cartilage. The cartilage looses its full thickness (bone articulating with the bone (Figs. 24.4a-d).

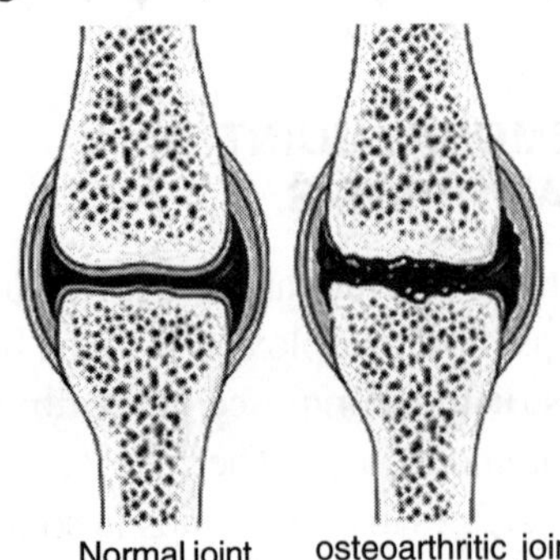

Fig. 24.4a: Knee joint osteoarthritis normal and degenerated cartilage

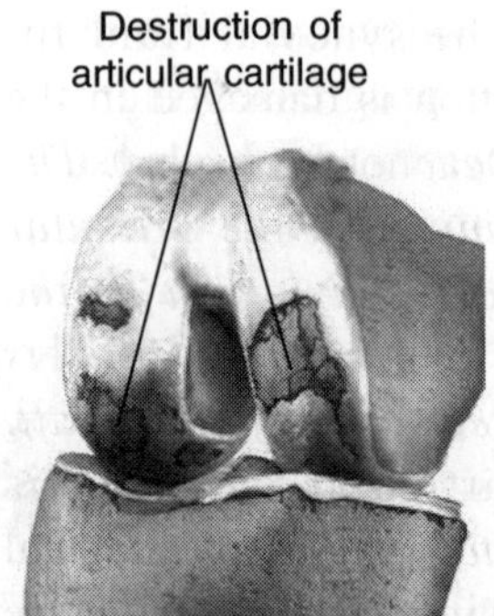

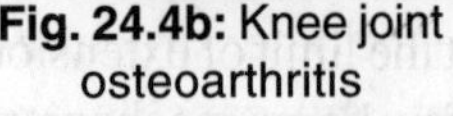

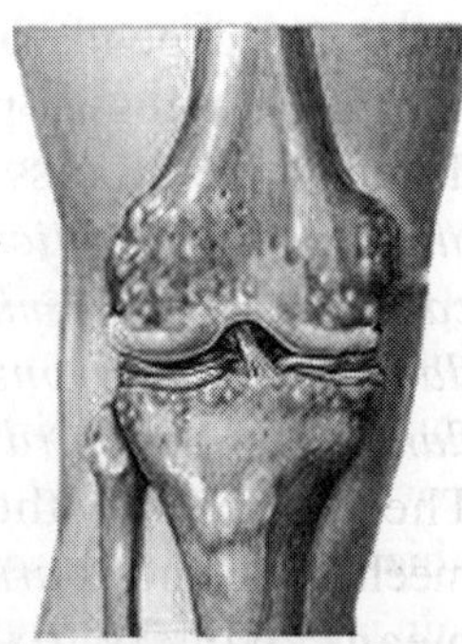

Fig. 24.4b: Knee joint osteoarthritis

Fig. 24.4c

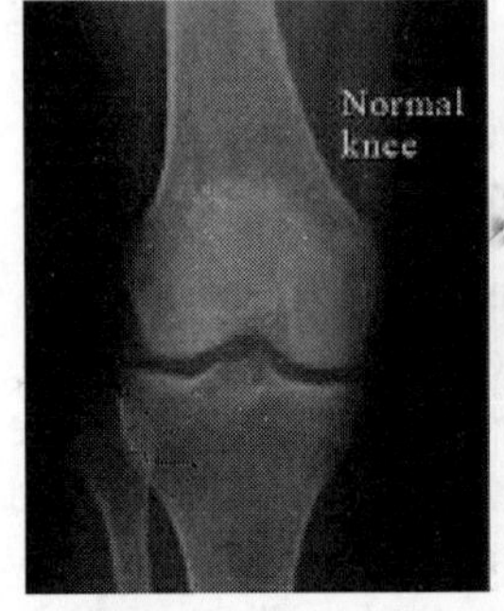

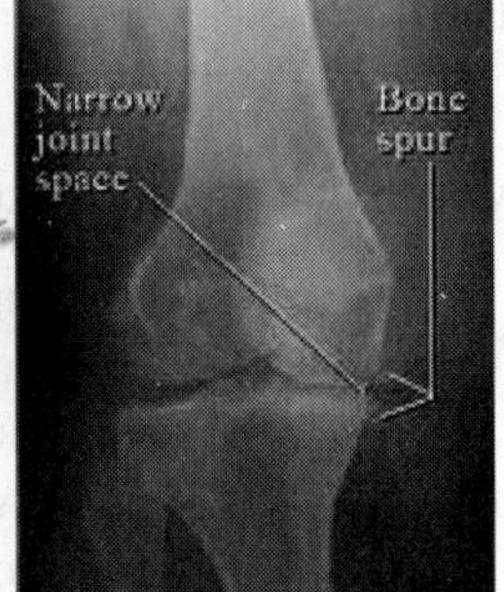

Fig. 24.4d: Knee joint osteoarthritis X-rays

Radiological Grading of the Knee Osteoarthritis

0 – Normal.

1 – Doubtful narrowing of joint space and possible osteophytic lipping.

2 – Definite osteophytes, definite narrowing of joint space.

3 – Moderate multiple osteophytes, definite narrowing of joint space, some sclerosis, and possible deformity of bone ends.

4 – Large osteophytes marked narrowing of joint space, severe sclerosis, and definite deformity of bone ends, subchondral cyst may also be present.

Involvement of the Medial Meniscus in Degenerative Disease: The lesion in the meniscus may be of two types: The complete longitudinal tear and horizontal cleavage in the medial meniscus. The fibrocartilage of medial meniscus depends on the synovial fluid for nutrition. Once this portion is damaged in the degenerative process it cannot be healed. *The meniscus then inflicts injury to the articular cartilage of the femoral condyle just as the damaged soft bronze of a bearing inflicts damage to the hard steel of the crankshaft.* The damage to the articular cartilage is mechanical and is *arrested only* by mechanical means, namely, excision of the structure interfering with movement at the limit of extension and in particular with the screw home mechanism (Fig. 24.5).

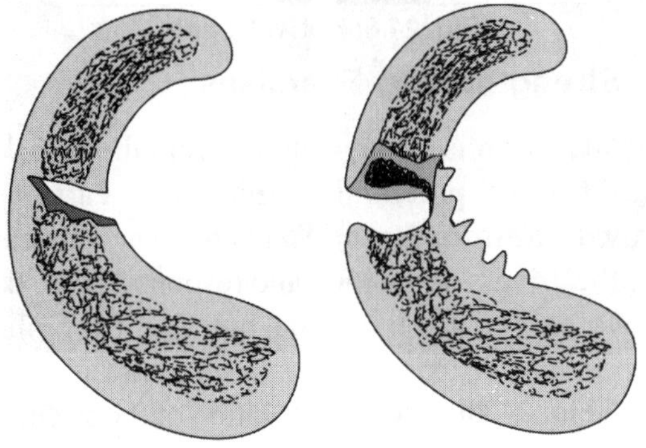

Fig. 24.5: Medial meniscus degeneration with longitudinal tear and horizontal cleavage

Internal Torsion of Tibia: The medial rotation may be associated with varus deformity, however, it is not necessary. The varus deformity and internal rotation of the tibia varies in degrees. If the medial rotation is associated with varus deformity the rotational component takes more responsibility for the degenerative changes. When the tibia a medially rotated in order to produce a gait in which the feet look directly forward instead of crossing over one another in the act of walking the tibia must be rotated laterally by the action of biceps.

In mid stance, tibia rotates laterally on the femur to achieve full extension and closed packed position of the knee joint. This is the most stable position of the tibiofemoral joint. Lateral rotation of the tibia on the femur from flexion to full extension (in mid stance) is termed as "screw home mechanism". The patients with tibiofemoral osteoarthrosis finds difficulty in rotating the tibia laterally on the femur. This would compromise the screw home mechanism, and contribute to the further destruction of the medial compartment of the tibiofemoral joint.

Tibial Torsion in Patients with Medial-Type Osteoarthritic Knees

The normal lateral tibial torsion rotation is considered as approximately 23 degree. As the osteoarthrosis progresses the lateral tibial torsion decreases. The rate of decrease in lateral tibial torsion in patients with osteoarthrosis is more in the proximal tibia than in the distal. There is a correlation between reduction of lateral torsion with the radiographic stage of osteoarthrosis of the knee and general osteoporosity.

Measurement of Tibial Torsion

A simple clinical method to measure the tibial torsion is to have the patient sit with the legs hanging over the edge of the examination table. The angle formed by the second metatarsal ray and the tibial tuberosity is measured. The tibial torsion is approximately equal to the mean of the two angles. In another similar method of tibial torsion measurement, an angle formed by the transmalleolar axis and the edge of the table is measured. The tibial torsion is approximately equal to the mean of the two angles.

Clinical Features of Tibiofemoral Joint

Pain and stiffness in the knee joint which aggravates in weight bearing are the dominant features of osteoarthritic knee joint. There is pain on pressure (tenderness) on the medial joint line. The knee joint space is decreased on X-rays. As the disease progresses the patient finds difficulty in walking and stair climbing. The terminal ranges may be limited. In an advanced stage an angulatory and translatory deformities can be seen in the knee joint which predispose to the deformities such as bow leg and internal torsion of the tibia.

MANAGEMENT

1. Pain and Stiffness

Pain and spasm in the joint is actually a protective type or muscle guarding. Due to degenerative changes the thickness of the cartilage is decreased and joint space is reduced resulting in laxity of the ligaments. This whole procedure is responsible for instability of the joint. Therefore, during weight bearing or movements there are unwanted movements of articular surfaces. *If patient avoids the movements, pain can be reduced, but limiting the movements can have an adverse effect on the muscles.* The muscles become tight, which further contributes to the pain and stiffness, and limits the range of motion. This whole cycle makes the patient disabled and the activities of the daily living are compromised.

Pain and muscle spasm can be relieved by using some heating modalities such as paraffin wax bath, hot water bag and hot pack. The hot water bag is easily accessible in the market, and can be used by filling the hot water in the bag. The bag covers the painful area. Initially a towel can be placed between the bag and the painful area but it can be removed as the temperature of the water falls. The total time should be at least 15-20 minutes and it can be repeated twice or thrice a day. The hot water bags are preferred over electric pads for their moist heating effects. Short wave diathermy and interferential therapy may also be advised for their deep heating and analgesic effects respectively. Patient may also be advised pocket TENS for its effectiveness in relieving pain and spasm by acting on the pain gait (Fig. 24.6).

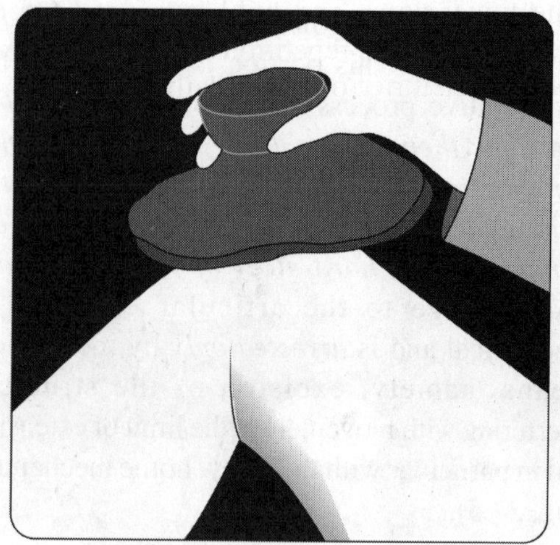

Fig. 24.6: Hot water bag

2. Strengthening Exercises

Regular exercises may help in strengthening the muscles and potentially stimulating cartilage growth. ***Restoration of Strength:*** The muscles are the drivers of the joint and responsible for the movements. Not only that but also they play important role in providing the dynamic stability to the joint. Therefore, restoration of the strength of the muscles is one of the goals of the treatment.

Ten Muscle Strengthening Exercises:

i. **Quadriceps Sets:** In lying with the knee straight a towel roll is placed under the knee joint. While pressing the towel down, knee is extended fully. The position is held for at least 6 seconds. After 6 seconds of contraction muscles is relaxed. Several repetitions of 15-20 may be performed thrice daily (Fig. 24.7).

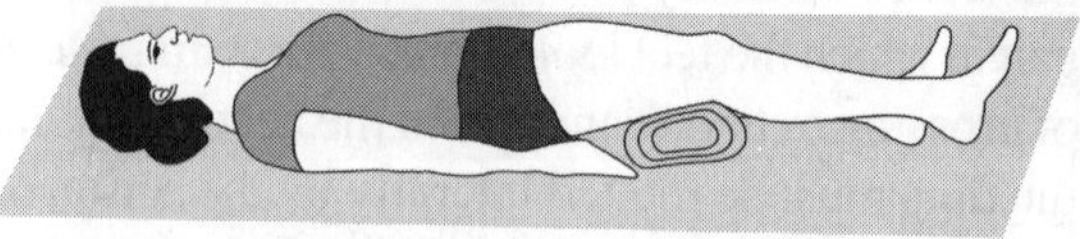

Fig. 24.7: Quadriceps sets

ii. **Gluteus Maximus Set:** In lying with the knee straight a towel roll is placed under the knee joint. The patient is instructed to press the towel down and hold it for at least 6 seconds. Several repetitions of 15-20 may be performed thrice or twice daily (Fig. 24.8).

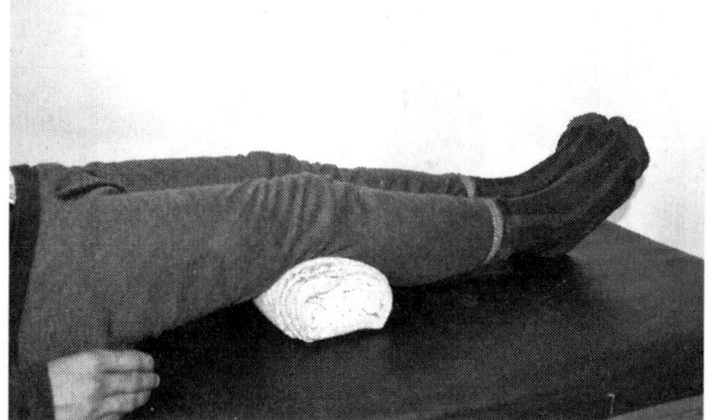

Fig. 24.8: Gluteus maximus set

iii. Ankle Pump Exercise: While keeping towel roll under the knee the ankle joint is moved up and down (Figs. 24.9a-b).

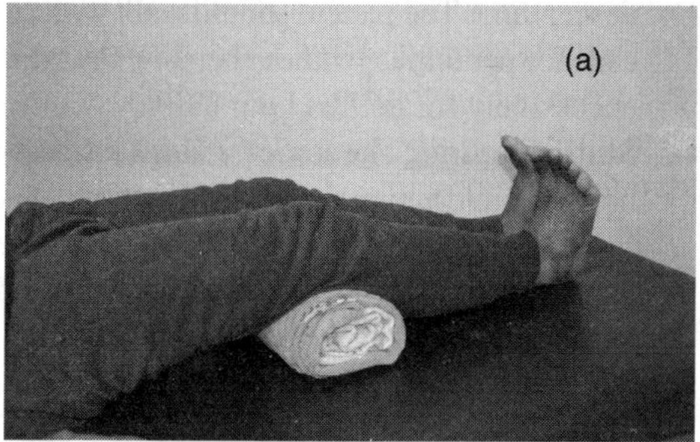

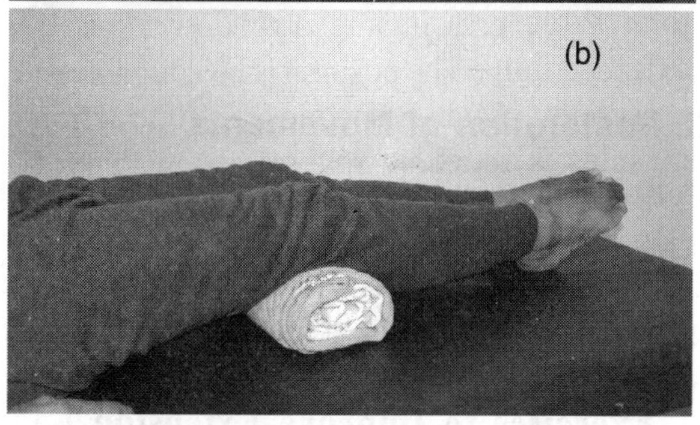

Figs. 24.9a-b: Ankle pump exercise

iv. Straight Leg Raising: While keeping the leg straight the patient is asked to raise it above around 60-70 degrees at the hip joint (Fig. 24.10).

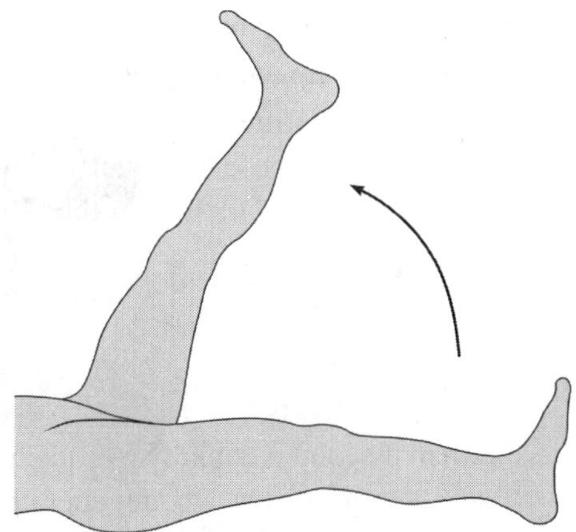

Fig. 24.10: Straight leg raising

v. Side Leg Raising: The lower leg is flexed out of the bed at around 20 degrees of the hip and knee joint (supine). In the next the affected leg is raised upto 70 degrees in side lying. Several repetitions of 15-20, two to thrice daily may be performed (Fig. 24.11).

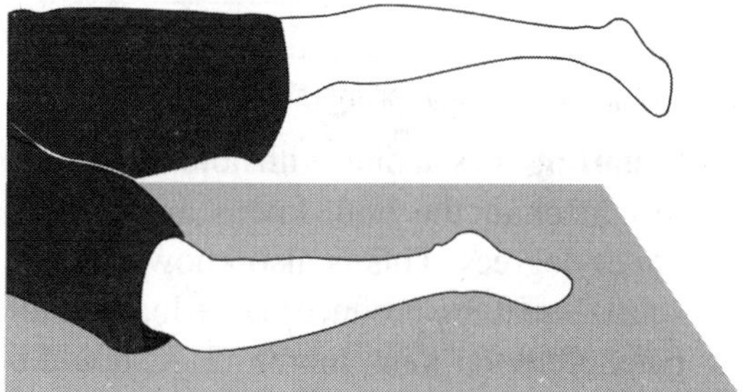

Fig. 24.11: Side straight leg raising

vi. High Sitting/Sitting on Table: The weight cuff of 1/2 kg, 1 kg, or 2 kg, as per tolerance of the patient is tied at the ankle joint. The knee joint is flexed and extended for 10 times. After 10 repetitions patient should take brief period of rest to allow the muscles relaxed. This completes one set (10 repetitions). The total 3 sets may be performed with brief period of relaxation between the sets. The weight can be increased after one or two weeks as the strength of the muscles (quadriceps) increases. In case exercise increases pain and symptoms, weight cuff may be taken off and knee is straighten up and bent down without weight (Fig. 24.12).

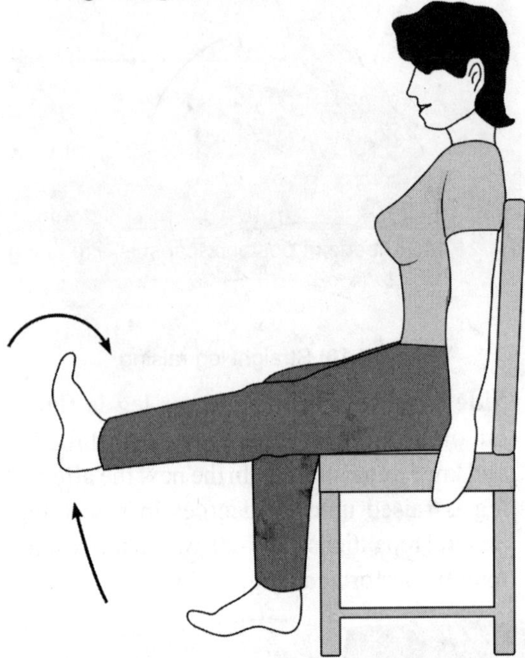

Fig. 24.12: High sitting/sitting on table

vii. **Squatting:** In standing with holding the back rest of chair the both knees are bent for 15-20 degrees. This is also known as mini squat. Squatting produces large loads on the patellofemoral joint, therefore, it should be avoided or limited to the 15-20 degrees (mini squat) (Fig. 24.13).

viii. **Swimming:** Swimming is the best exercise for the patient with osteoarthrosis of the knee and hip joint. The movements are performed against the resistance (water) without placing the excessive load on the joint. The exercise also increases the overall cardiovascular endurance. It reduces weight of the body too.

ix. **Walking:** If the arthritis changes are chronic, patient should walk with the stick or cane on the opposite hand. Walking is the safe and it produces minimal stresses on the knee joints

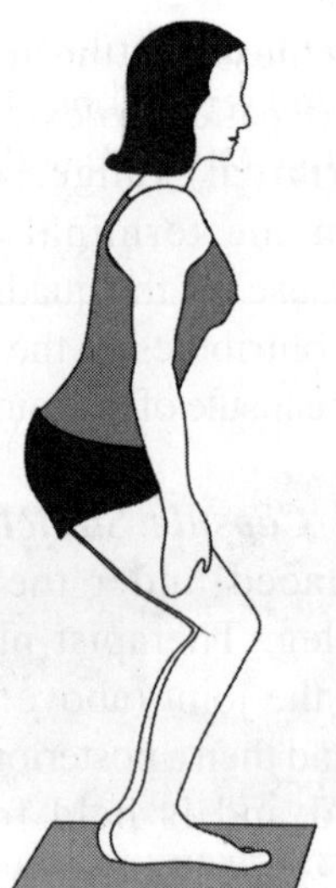

Fig. 24.13: Squatting

comparing with the stair climbing and descending. The patient should walk with 90 cadence per minute without bending the trunk excessively for half an hour daily.

x. **Static Cycling:** The static cycling can easily be accessible and patient can do cycling with resistance as per tolerances. Initially the exercise on the bicycle should be started without resistance for a short period of time. After one week as the muscles conditioned, both resistance and the time can be increased as per tolerance.

3. Restoration of Movements

Following reduction of muscle spasm, pain, and restoration of strength the third priority of the therapist should be given in obtaining full range of movements. It can be achieved by performing some exercises.

i. **Exercises to Improve Extension Lag:** Extension lag is an active loss of terminal extension. Once the active and passive extension is lost the joint becomes deformed and is known as extension lag. Loss of terminal extension is very common in osteoarthrosis.

Pain and stiffness are the main factors in preventing the patient to extend the knee to the end (terminal) range. Avoidance of extension in the terminal range causes weakness (disuse) of the quadriceps muscles that further contributes to the extension lag. The posterior capsule of the joint also becomes light.

a. *Posterior Capsule Stretching:* A towel roll is placed under the ankle of the affected leg. Therapist places both the hands on the joint (above and below the patella), and then a posterior directed force is applied and is held for at least 10 seconds. This will increase the flexibility of the posterior capsule. The pressure should be so gentle that it should not aggravate the symptoms. The exercise must be followed by the active extension. Patient should be taught to do the exercise at home (Figs. 24.14 and 24.15).

b. *Quadriceps Strengthening:* The towel roll is placed under the knee, and patient is instructed to extend the knee joint as much as possible. At the end range the therapist can assist the active movement. This recruits the quadriceps muscles fibers responsible for terminal extension.

c. *Surge Faradic Current:* Surge faradic current may also be beneficial in improving the extension lag by stimulating and recruiting the quadriceps muscles fibers. The patient is instructed to contract the muscle simultaneously with the current as much as possible.

ii. **Exercises to Improve Flexion:** The patient lies prone and therapist stands at the side of the patient. The knee joint is flexed upto the range where limitation starts. This position is held firmly and the patient is instructed to extend the knee joint. The therapist applies resistance against the concentric contraction of the muscles. Several repetitions are

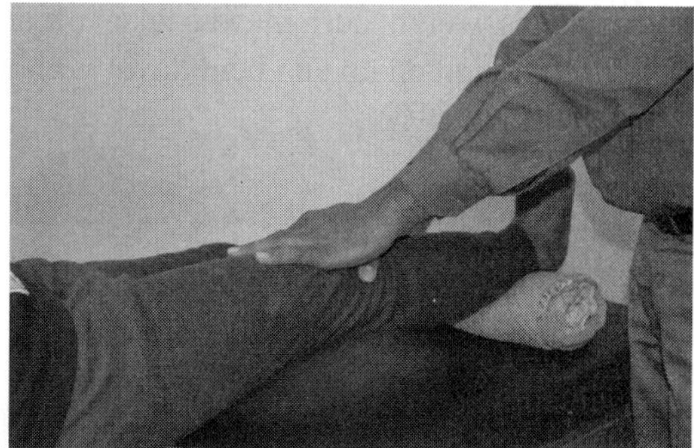

Fig. 24.14: Knee joint posterior capsule stretching

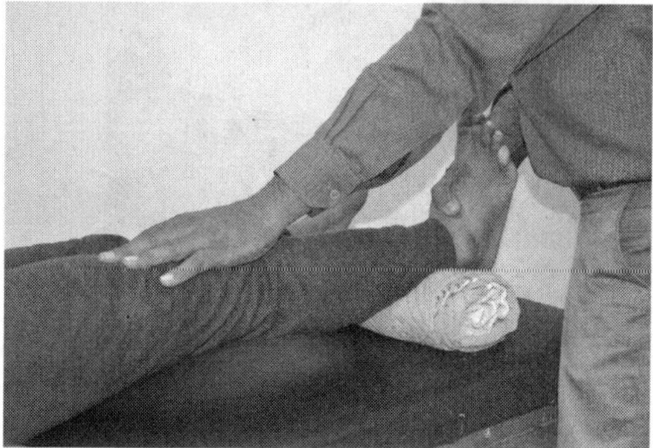

Fig. 24.15: Posterior knee joint capsule stretching with distraction of the joint

performed till a significant improvement in the flexion is achieved. Hot pack along the length of the quadriceps may prove more significant results (Fig. 24.16).

4. Weight Loss

The osteoarthrosis is a degenerative disease which is more common in weight bearing joints. The articular cartilage of the obese patients transfer more weight, hence, these patients have more chances of disruption of the proteoglycans and collagen fibers. The cartilage looses its physical properties and eventually there is loss of full thickness of the cartilage. The patients who attend the swimming pool, and do the regular walking can reduce the weight of the body. Avoiding oil content in the diet may also help in reducing the fat. Successful weight loss dramatically relieves pain and symptoms in the arthritic knee joint.

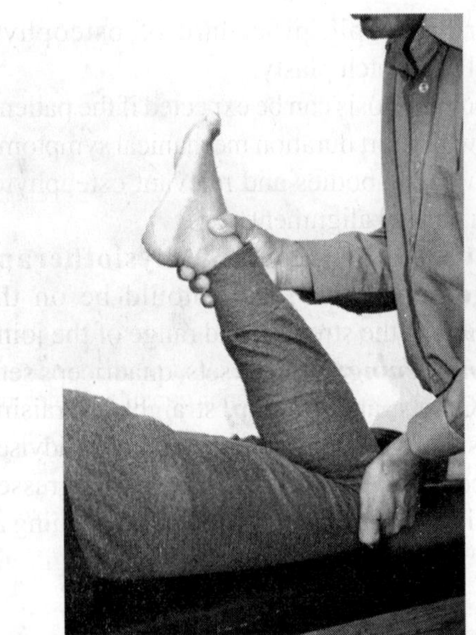

Fig. 24.16: Exercise to improve flexion

5. Activity Modification

Any activities which place more stress on the cartilage should be avoided.

i.   Discontinue high impact activities, change to low impact.
ii. Avoid stair climbing, kneeling and squatting.
iii. Do not use low chair.
iv. Use western toilets.

6. Orthotic Management, Aids and Appliances

The assistive devices and orthotic aids such as knee braces, are used to improve functions of moveable parts of the body or to support, align, prevent, or correct deformities. Splints or braces help in correcting joint alignment and weight redistribution.

i.   **Shoe Modification:** It has been observed that the patient with flat foot (loss of medial arch of the foot) complain pain in the medial or anterior aspect of knee joint. The flat foot changes the direction of weight distribution in the joint and also alters the quadriceps angle as it produces internal rotation of the tibia. The flat foot is possible if the intrinsic muscles of the foot are weak. The problem can be solved out by raising the medial arch of the shoe. In young population medial arch can be developed by some form of exercises and electric stimulation. These patients may do the exercise such as pulling the towel with the toes and walking on sand. But it is difficult to develop the arch in the middle aged population, therefore raising medial arch of the shoe can correct the alignment of the tibia and reduce the pain and symptoms.

ii. **Cane on Opposite Hand:** By holding the cane with opposite hand, the arthritic leg is progressed forward to the body with the cane. The weight of the body is taken on the cane and arthritic knee simultaneously, hence the load of the arthric knee is transferred to the stick or cane.

iii. **Knee Cap:** It provides passive stability to the knee joint and may be worn while walking and climbing stairs. It should not be made habit as it may decrease the strength of the muscles.

iv. **Braces:** Some custom made braces are beneficial in unloading the joint especially when unilateral compartment is affected. The unilateral joint space can be increased significantly by using a mechanical device "screw" and transferring the weight on the brace instead of joint. The disadvantages of braces are: they are very expensive, and most of the patients quit wearing quickly secondary to bulkness, and inconvenience. Some patients may also be benefited from a light neoprene knee sleeve, which may improve proprioceptive feedback.

7. Hyaluronic Acid Injections

Hyaluronic acid injections are having limited value in relieving pain and symptoms. They appear to work best before there is bone-on-bone crepitus. Studies have shown that these injections are of equal benefit of non-steroidal anti-inflammatory drugs. However, other studies show that hyaluronic sodium to be no better than placebo.

8. Supplements

It is believed that the supplements such as glucosomine, and chondroitin sulphate (cartigen, free flex fort) helps in regenerating the cartilage, however no studies claim such results. The supplements are moderately expensive with no side effects. These supplements are initially advised for three months, and if found no improvement may be discontinued or if patients wish to try and derive great benefit they may use for more than three months.

Surgical Intervention

The patients who do not get benefited with the conservative treatments and present constant pain and symptoms may be elected for surgical intervention.

Arthroscopy

The patients with normal mechanical alignment who fail to respond to a conservative management (administered at least for 3-6 months) and mild to moderate arthritis (grade 2 and 3 on radiographs) may be considered for arthroscopic debridement. The arthroscopic procedure should be considered palliative, temporary for patients with arthritic knee joint.

As the degenerative disease progresses, the degenerated articular cartilage and synovial tissue release pro-inflammatory cytokinase that induces chondrocytes to release lytic enzymes leading to degradation of type-2 collagen and proteoglycans. The arthroscopic procedure (lavaging) may "dilute" or "wash out" these inflammatory mediators, although the effect is temporary. Grade 2 and 3 osteoarthrosis with osteophytes, tibial spine pain and extension lag may be benefited

from arthroscopic procedure of osteophyte removal and notch plasty.

Good prognosis can be expected if the patients present with short duration mechanical symptoms, effusion, loose bodies and relevant osteophytes but with normal alignment.

Post Arthroscopic Physiotherapy Management: The focus should be on the restoration of the strength and range of the joint.

a. ***Strengthening:*** Gluteus sets, quadriceps sets, VMO sets, ankle pump, straight leg raising and side leg raising exercises should be advised thrice daily. Exercises should be progressed to mini squat, cycling, jogging and running as patient shows improvement in the sign and symptoms.

b. ***Stretching:*** Iliotibial band, lateral patellar retanaculam, quadriceps, gastrocnemius, iliopsoas and posterior capsule of the knee joint should be stretched.

Osteotomy

The involvement of medial compartment of the knee joint produces varus deformity as the full thickness of the articular cartilage is lost. These patients may be advised for a valgus producing, high tibial osteotomy. Patients with greater than 10 degrees of varus may undergo supracondylar osteotomy which do not interfere with subsequent total knee replacement. However, eventually, a total knee replacement requires in the due course of time, for this reason osteotomies are performed rarely.

Total Knee Replacement (TKR)

The replacement of both the articular surfaces with the foreign material (implant) has become choice of treatments now-a-days. Patients with incapacitating pain, functional impairment, flexion deformity or contracture, valgus, varus deformities and those who failed to respond to the fair trial of conservative treatment require total knee joint replacement.

Implants: Cemented, cementless or hybrid prosthesis may be selected for the surgery. The selection of prosthesis depends upon the age, health and integrity of the bones. Semi-constrained prosthesis are used for most of the patient as these may correct flexion contracture upto 45 degrees and angular deformities upto 25 degrees. The total expected life span of the prosthesis is considered of 15-20 years, however, it may be decreased if the patient is young and dynamic. On the other hand the life span of the prosthesis is increased if the patient is sedentary (Figs. 24.17 and 24.18).

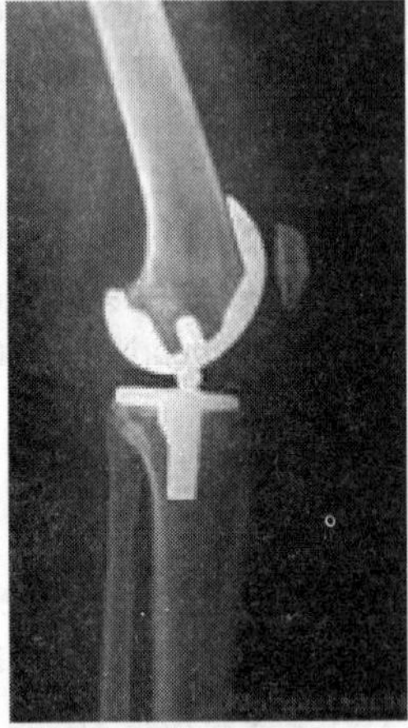

Fig. 24.17: X-ray—Total knee joint replacement

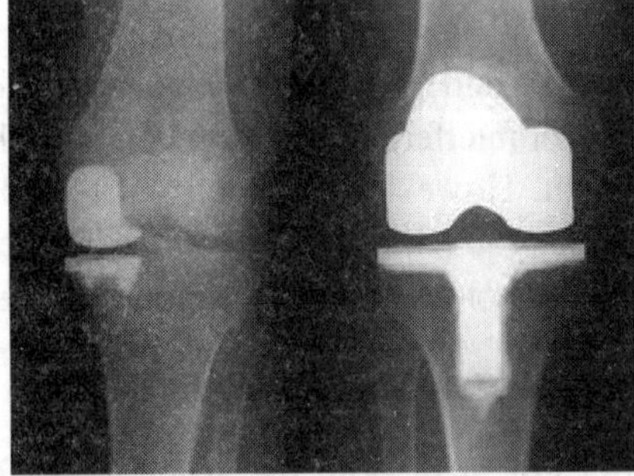

Fig. 24.18: X-ray—a. uni-compartment replacement, b. total knee replacement

Pre Operative Physiotherapy Treatment

a. **Restoration of Range of Motion:** The muscle energy and PNF techniques such as hold relax, contract relax and reciprocal inhibition help in relaxing the muscle and improving range of motion. Anterior and posterior glides with distraction and stabilization (proximal part of the joint) helps in stretching of the joint capsule and regaining range of motion.

b. **Restoration of Muscle Strength:** To restore the strength the exercises such as quadriceps sets, gluteus sets, ankle pump, SLR, side SLR, and mini squat should be administered and taught to the to do at home.

c. **Breathing Exercises:** Deep breathing and spirometer exercises are taught well before the operation to improve cardiovascular endurance.

Post-Operative Physiotherapy Management

As soon as patient comes out of the operation theatre he or she is allowed to walk as per tolerance or as advised by the surgeon. The exercises such as quads sets, gluteus maximus sets, ankle pump, SLR, side SLR and hamstring sets are started from the day one, two to three times daily. The patients should achieve 90° of flexion at the end of 14th day of operation. Following should be the goals of therapist:

1. **Reduction in Pain:** Ice pack, cryotherapy on mediolateral joint or along the length of quadriceps. It should not be placed directly on the stitch line.

2. **Restoration of Strength:** Initially isometric quads sets, hamstrings sets, gluteus maximus sets, ankle pumps, SLR and side SLR should be started from the day one twice daily. The closed kinetic chain exercises such as mini squat may also be initiated following discharge of the patient. The strengthening exercises in high sitting (isotonic) with resistance may produce pain and symptoms, hence, should be initiated without the resistance and progressed to the resistance as the sign and symptoms improve.

3. **Restoration of Range of Motion:** Patient should achieve at least 90° of flexion in the

14 days of operation. To improve flexion the patient is placed in supine lying position, therapist stands at the side of the leg which is being treated. Therapist holds the ankle with one hand and grasps the knee joint with other hand. The patient is encouraged to flex the knee joint as much as possible. Therapist should make efforts in increasing range of motion actively by commanding him such as yes very good, you are doing very well. In case, if patient finds difficulty in achieving flexion upto 90° at the end of second week, the therapist may go for reciprocal inhibition of the quadriceps. In high sitting position, the knee joint is flexed as much as possible, at the point where limitation starts the knee joint is stabilized and ankle joint is held firmly with the other hand. Now the patient is instructed to flex the knee joint against the resistance. The strong contraction of the hamstrings will allow quadriceps muscles to relax and helps in improving flexion range of motion. After removal of the stitches (usually after two weeks), hold relax, and contract relax of the quadriceps may be initiated to improve flexion range. The reciprocal inhibition technique is only indicated if there is severe muscle spasm and pain which does not allow the patient to contract quadriceps (contract relax, hold relax), hence, hamstrings are contracted to relax the quadriceps muscles.

Passive movements may increase post-operative pain, spasm and symptoms; hence, these should be avoided at initial stage to increase range.

Extension Lag: Following total knee replacement pain and spasm is the common complaints of patient. Patient keeps the leg in flexed position by placing pillow under the knee joint as it relieves pain. To correct extension lag a pillow is placed under the ankle joint and a posterior directed force is applied to the knee joint with distraction. Several repetitions of posterior directed force help in regaining full extension of the knee joint. Quadriceps strengthening also helps in achieving full extension.

PATELLOFEMORAL JOINT OSTEOARTHRITIS

The degenerative process may also involve the underlying surfaces of the patellofemoral joint. Pain and stiffness in the anterior part of knee which aggravate with the activities such as squatting, stair climbing, descending, running and jumping are the common features of the patello-femoral arthrosis. If the tibiofemoral joint is intact and only patellofemoral joint is involved the patient will not complain pain while level walking as the patellofemoral ground reaction forces almost negligible in level walking. On the other hand patient with tibiofemoral and patellofemoral will complain pain in both stair climbing and level walking. Extension lag may also present as the disease progresses (Figs. 24.19 and 24.20).

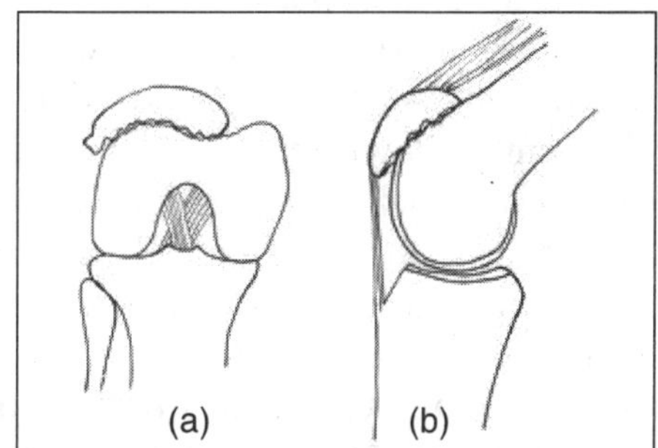

Fig. 24.19: Patellofemoral osteoarthritis a. anterior posterior view, b. lateral view

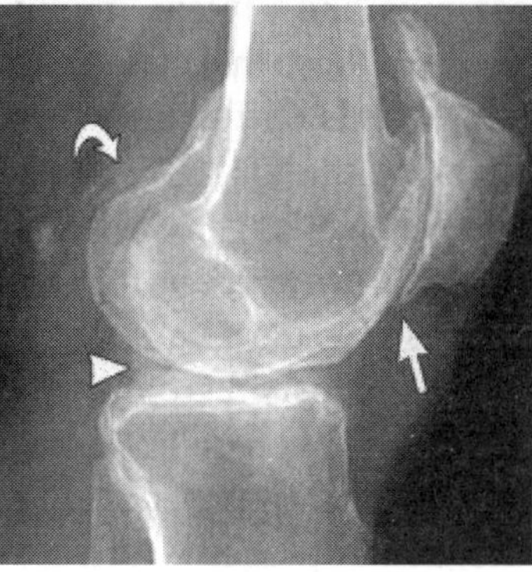

Fig. 24.20: X-ray–lateral view, patellofemoral osteoarthritis

Patellar Mal Tracking

Normally patella moves on the trochlear groove of the femur. Lengthening or shortening of the muscles displaces the patella from trochlear groove to one of the epicondyles of the femur. Therefore ground reaction forces of the patello-femoral joint shifts to either of epicondyles, which leads to disruption of cartilage of one of the epicondyles of femur. The most widely accepted theory regarding the cause of patellofemoral pain suggests that the symptoms are the result of excessive patellofemoral joint stresses owing to abnormal patellar tracking. The patellar mal tracking is thought to generate excessive stress on the medial or lateral epicondyle of femur resultant the patellofemoral joint reaction forces alter and the contact area between the patellofemoral joint surface decreases. This causes pain, irritation and degeneration in the articular cartilage. The following factors contribute to the patellar mal tracking:

i. **Weakness of Hip External Rotators:** Insufficient contraction of hip external rotators may allow internal rotators to rotate the femur internally (ante version). This will increase the Q angle and allow the patella to move on the lateral epicondyle of the femur during knee flexion.

ii. **Weakness of Gluteus Medius and Maximus:** One of the most common causes of the patellar mal tracking is weakness of the gluteus maximus and gluteus medius muscles. Weakness of these muscles causes the femur to fall inwards during the stance phase, thus increasing the Q angle, and so the lateral pull on the patella.

iii. **Weakness of the Quadriceps:** Weak quadriceps unable to keep the patella deeply into trochlear groove of the femur and resultant contact area of the patellofemoral joint is decreased, which leads to increase in stress on another area of the joint surface.

iv. **Pes Planus or Flat Foot: Foot Pronation or Flat Foot:** The tibia rotates laterally in mid stance to achieve full extension of the knee joint. This is known as screw home mechanism. Flat foot rotates the tibia medially which would actually decrease the 'Q' angle, and the lateral forces acting on the patella. Eventually the screw home mechanism is altered. To compensate for the lack of tibial external rotation caused by the failure of the foot to resupinate, the femur would have to internally rotate on the tibia such that the tibia was in a relative external rotation. Theoretically compensatory internal rotation of the femur would permit the screw home mechanism to allow for knee extension. In turn excessive internal rotation of the femur would move the patella medially with respect to the ASIS and tibial tuberosity, thereby increasing the 'Q' angle and the lateral component of the quadriceps muscle vector.

v. **Pes Cavus (High Arched Foot Supination):** It provides less cushioning during the stance phase, which can place more stress on the patellofemoral mechanism particularly in running.

vi. **Tightness of Tensor Fascia Lata (TFL):** The vastus medialis oblique works as a medial dynamic stabilizer for the patella. Weakness of a VMO allows lateral stabilizers to pull the patella on the lateral epicondyle of the femur. The patella tracks on the lateral epicondyle of femur instead of on the trochlear groove which predisposes the patellofemoral joint to osteoarthrosis. Iliotibial band is one of the lateral dynamic stabilizers of the patella. The short iliotibial band tilts and pulls the patella laterally as one of slip of the iliotibial band called the lateral retinaculum fibers attach into the lateral border of the patella.

vii. **Good Leg Arthropathy:** This is common in the patients whose one leg is short. Because of shortening of leg patient walks with the normal leg flexion. Normally during stance phase the knee remains extended which reduces ground reaction forces on the patellofemoral joint. Flexion during stance phase increases ground reaction forces on the patellofemoral joint and predisposes the joint to osteoarthrosis.

Patellar Mal Tracking Tests

The test should be done in full extension. In this position patella typically rests just lateral to the midline. As soon as the knee joint moves into flexion at around 10 to 20 degrees, the patella centers into the trochlear groove and proceeds to track in a relatively smooth and straight path with progressive knee flexion. In patients with patellar mal tracking the patella remains on the lateral epicondyle upto 30 degree of knee flexion and then suddenly jumps into the trochlear groove with a jerk and click sound.

This follows a J path and also knows as *J sign*. Patellar mal tracking may be associated with patellar tilt. Tightness of lateral structures, such as lateral retinaculum, vastus lateralis, or iliotibial band may cause lateral tilt of the patella. Normally the lateral border of the patellar can easily be elevated 0-20 degrees above the medial border. Less than 0 degree elevation of the lateral border of the patella suggests patellar tilt. In full extension the patella is observed carefully and patient is asked to contract the quadriceps. The test is considered positive for lateral tilt if the patella shifts (displacement) laterally.

Clark Sign: Patient lies supine with both the knees extended, therapist stands at the side, places one hand on the supracondylar aspect (patella) of the knee joint. The patella is pressed hard against the condyles and patient is asked to contract the quadriceps. The contraction of quadriceps causes movement of the patella on the trochlear grove against the resistance applied

by the therapist. If the movement of patella produces pain, it is considered as positive for patellofemoral joint osteoarthrosis.

Radiographic Evaluation of Patellar Instability

An axial image, typically a merchant (knee flexed 45 degrees and X-ray beam angled 30 degrees to axis of the femur) or skyline view may be the most significant.

Sulcus Angle: A sulcus angle less than 150 degrees is considered normal. Patients who have sulcus angle more than 150 degrees complain patellar instability. To measure the sulcus angle a line is drawn along the medial and lateral wall of the trochlea. The angle formed between them is termed as sulcus angle (Fig. 24.21).

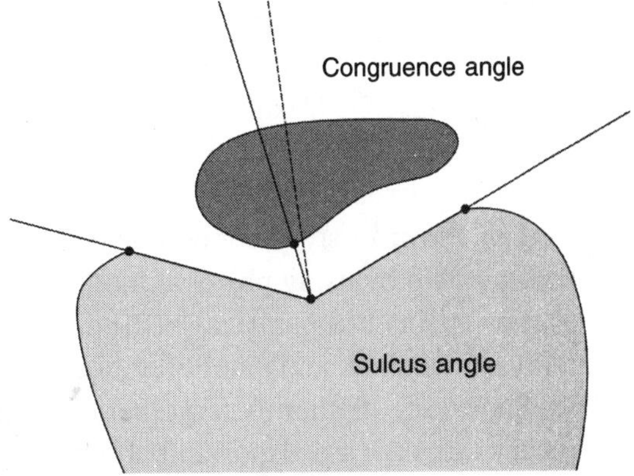

Fig. 24.21: Congruence angle and sulcus angle

Congruence Angle: One line is drawn from the apex of the trochlear groove bisecting the sulcus and second *line is drawn from the apex of the groove, the apex of the patella.* The angle formed between these two lines is the congruence angle which is described as – 6 degrees ± 6 degrees normal.

Patellofemoral Angle: The angle is formed by the two lines. One line is drawn along the lateral wall of the trochlear groove and the second *line is drawn along the articular surface of* *the lateral patella facet.* The lines should roughly be parallel. Divergence of the lines is measured as a positive angle and is considered normal, whereas convergence of the lines is measured as negative and indicates the presence of abnormal patellar tilt (Fig. 24.22).

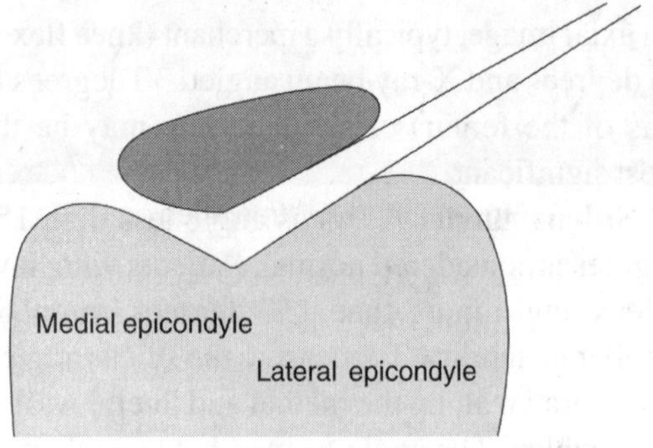

Fig. 24.22: Patellofemoral angle

Treatment

The aims of treatment are of many folds:

1. Approximately, 70% patients with patello-femoral osteoarthrosis improve with conservative treatments.

2. **Relief of Pain:** Firstly treatment is directed to relieve pain by using physical modalities. To relieve pain ultrasound can be used on the lateral retinaculam, and patellofemoral joint line. Shortwave diathermy, cryotherapy and paraffin wax bath are also found effective in patellofermoral dysfunctions.

3. **Stretching Exercises:** The second part of treatment is to improve the patellar tracking which involves stretching of the short muscles. The second part of the treatment is sometimes overlooked but is extremely helpful and important in patients with flexibility deficit. Iliotibial band, quadriceps and hamstrings flexibility deficit are common in these patients, especially in patients with chronic patellofemoral osteoarthrosis. Static structures such as lateral retinaculam and patellar ligaments are also become tight. Restoration

of flexibility can play important role in patients with patellofemoral osteoarthrosis (Figs. 24.23 and 24.24).

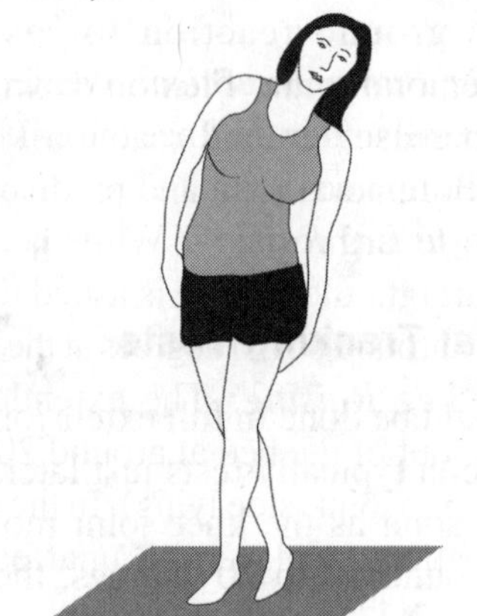

Fig. 24.23: Iliotibial band stretching

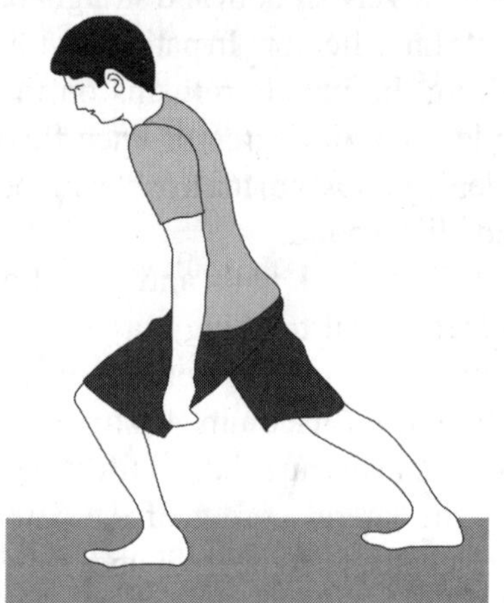

Fig. 24.24: Gastrosoleus stretching

4. **Strengthening Exercises**
   a. **Quadriceps Sets:** In sitting with the knee straight a towel roll is placed under the knee joint. While pressing the towel down the knee is extended fully. The position is held for at least 6 seconds. After 6 seconds of contraction muscles is relaxed. Several repetitions of 15-20 may be performed thrice daily.
   b. **Gluteus Maximus Set:** In sitting with the knee straight a towel roll is placed under the knee joint. The patient is instructed to

press the towel down and hold it for at least 6 seconds. Several repetitions of 15-20 may be performed thrice or twice daily.

c. **Ankle Pump Exercise:** While keeping towel roll under the knee the ankle joint is moved up and down.

d. **Straight Leg Raising:** While keeping the leg straight the patient is asked to raise it above around 60-70 degrees at the hip joint.

e. **Side Leg Raising:** The extended leg is taken out of the bed at around 20 degrees of the hip joint (side lying). In the next step the patient is placed on unaffected side lying and the affected leg is raised upto 70 degrees. Several repetitions are performed.

f. **Vastus Medialis Obliques (VMO):** Vastus medialis obliques inserts on the medial aspect of the patella at 55 degree angles. This muscle is the medial dynamic stabilizer of the patella. Weakness of the vastus medialis may allow lateral stabilizers to pull the patella laterally. This is one of the cause of the lateral maltracking of the patella. In high sitting position a towel roll is placed between the thighs. Patient is asked to press the towel between the thighs (hip adduction) and then extend the knee joint upto the full range. Some studies show that if dorsiflexion is added to the extension more VMO muscle fibers can be recruited. The hip joint is adducted during the extension as the VMO muscle fibers are the extension of the adductor muscle. Adduction of hip joint can strengthen the adductors and helps in improving the strength of the VMO (Fig. 24.25).

g. **Gluteus Maximus Strengthening:** Patient lies prone with both the knees extended. While maintaining the knee extension, hip joint is extended upto full range. The extension is maintained at end

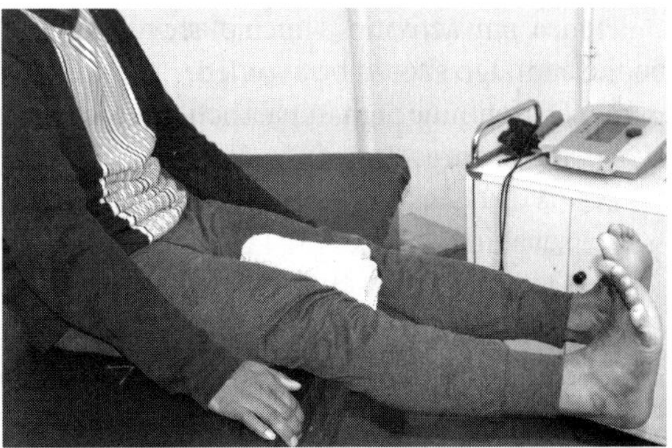

Fig. 24.25: VMO strengthening

range for at least six seconds. 15-20 repetition, twice daily can be performed.

h. **Hip Lateral Rotators Strengthening:** Patient lies prone with knee flexion to 90 degree. Therapist stands at the side, holds the leg at the ankle joint and resists, external rotation of the hip joint.

i. **Mini Squatting:** This is the close kinetic chain exercise which helps in improving the stimulation of the proprioceptors. Therapist must emphasise on the mini squat only upto 15-20 degrees as it does not increase the ground reaction forces significantly. Increase in the angle of knee joint beyond 20 degrees can produce excessive load on the patellofemoral joint underlying surfaces.

5. **General Conditioning and Cross Training:**

   i. Hydrotherapy, aqua exercises, swimming and deep pool running.

   ii. **Cycling:** Initially without resistance or as per tolerance of the patient.

6. **Activity Modification:** The ground reaction forces on the patellofemoral increase during the knee flexion.

   i. **Level Walking:** Negligible body weight.

   ii. **Stair Climbing:** 4 times of body weight.

   iii. **Squatting:** 7-8 times of body weight.

   iv. **Mini Squatting:** 2-3 times of body weight.

Hence, any activities which place more stress on the cartilage should be avoided.

   a. Discontinue high impact activities, change to low impact.
   b. Avoid stair climbing, kneeling, and squatting.
   c. Do not use low chair.
   d. Use western toilets.

HIP JOINT OSTEOARTHRITIS

78% patients show bilateral evidence of the disease. There is non-uniform loss of joint space which is radiographically identified as supralateral migration of the femoral head within the acetabulum. Early osteoarthritic changes affect the superior compartment of the femoral acetabulum. If vacuum phenomenon is produced within the joint, loss of cartilage is seen on the supralateral space of the joint, with maintenance of normal cartilage axially and medially. As the disease progresses (in advanced stage) there may be extensive, non-uniform loss of joint space. Occasionally large subchondral cysts may also be observed which is originated in the acetabulum and they are frequently referred as Egger's cyst. As the result of cartilage loss and migration of the head within the acetabulum the head becomes incongruous with the acetabulum. Osteophytes develop medially on the femoral head to fill the incongruity. A ghost line of the original femoral head is often identified. The weight bearing axis is shifted from its normal position to the medial neck of femur and new bone is added along the medial cortex. The osteoarthritis begin in the roof of the acceptable rather than in the femoral head itself because cysts only appear after denudation of the overlying articular cartilage.

Radiographical Grades of Hip Osteoarthrosis

0 – Normal.

1 – Possible narrowing of joint space medially and possible osteophytes around the femoral head.

2 – Definite narrowing of joint space inferiorly, definite osteophytes and slight sclerosis.

3 – Marked narrowing of joint space, osteophytes, some sclerosis and cyst formation, and deformity of femoral head and acetabulum.

4 – Gross loss of joint space with sclerosis and cysts, marked deformity of femoral head and acetabulum and large osteophytes.

(Adopted from the Council for International Organization of Medical Sciences, 1963)

Cyst formation which may be intrusion or contusion type or both. The intrusion cyst is seen immediately subchorally and may have a wide, narrow or radiographically absent communication with the joint space. The contusion cyst is totally enclosed within the bone and may be farther from the joint space unlike intrusion cyst. A cyst may also be present before there is actual cartilage loss. A cyst may collapse, producing a bizarre configuration of the femoral head.

Secondary Osteoarthritis

The persons with congenital or developmental abnormalities are more prone to the secondary osteoarthritis and the presentation of secondary osteoarthritis is usually 10 years earlier than the usual presentation of the primary osteoarthritis.

Common Conditions are: Hip dysphasias, slipped capital femoral epiphysis, Legg-Calve-Perthes disease, femoral neck abnormalities and primary protrusion acetabulii.

Clinical Features

Patient complaints pain during the activities and stiffness after activities or prolonged rest, which may last for 30 minutes. As the disease progresses the joint range of motion is decreased and there is feeling of instability of the joint. Crepitus and

Overuse Syndromes of the Knee (OSKs): These involve the extensor mechanism and are grouped together under the term Jumpers Knee. Patellar tendinitis is the most common among these patients, typically presenting with pain near the insertion of the tendon at the pole of the patella (Fig. 24.26).

Iliotibial Band Friction Syndrome: The iliotibial band inserts at the Gerdy tubercle on the anterolateral aspect of the proximal tibia. It has small attachments to the lateral patellar retinaculam and to the biceps femoris. During full extension to flexion, the iliotibial band shifts from a position anterior to the lateral femoral condyle to a position posterior to the epicondyle. The transition occurs at about 30 degrees of the knee flexion. In running, the repetitive flexion and extension causes iliotibial band to pass back and forth over the lateral femoral epicondyle. This may cause irritation in the band at the insertion and develop bursitis. The patients with iliotibial band friction syndrome typically presents with pain on anterior to the lateral femoral epicondyle associated with running and jogging (Fig. 24.27).

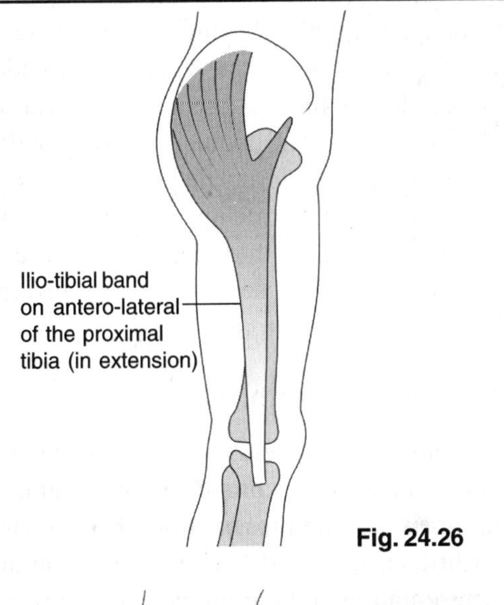

Fig. 24.26

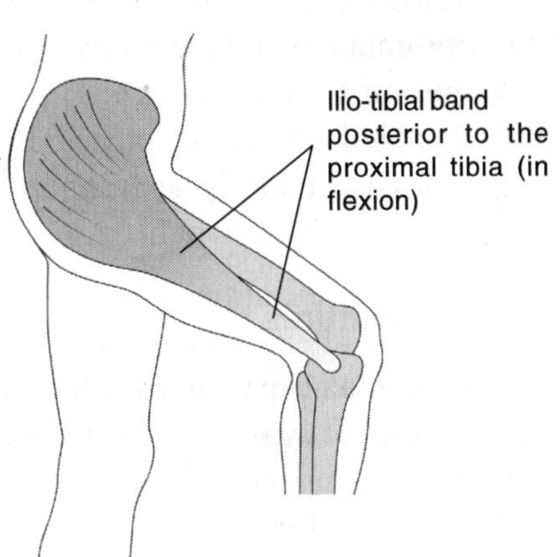

Fig. 24.27

trendelenburg sign, firm swelling and tender points around the joint margin may be present.

Diagnosis

The classical clinical test for hip joint osteoarthritis is internal rotation of the hip joint with flexion which may be limited and painful.

Patrick Test: Also known as figure four test is performed in supine lying. Ankle joint of the leg which is being tested is placed on the thigh of the contralateral leg, the knee joint of the tested side is pushed gently downward. This maneuver may place large stress on the hip joint and patient may experience pain. Test should be avoided on patients with severe osteoporotic changes (elderly).

Management

Reduction of body weight. Obese patients should be advised to reduce the weight so that load on the cartilage can be relieved.

Use of Cane: Cane in the opposite hand can significantly reduce the weight on the hip joint. In normal walk without the cane, the ground reaction forces (resultant force) across the hip joint is three times of the body weight because the force of the hip abductors acts on the greater trochanter to offset body weight and levels the pelvis in single stance.

Use of Supplements: Glucosamine and chondrotin sulphate (cartigen, free flex fort) may be advised, however their efficacy is not proved scientifically.

Modalities: Moist heat therapy, interferential therapy by using the analgesic effect (80 – 100 Hz) and short wave diathermy.

Exercises: Stretching: Abductors and capsule (IR and ER). Strengthening: Gluteus maximus, mediums. Quadriceps and abdominals: Straight leg raising, side leg raising, prone leg raising, knee to chest active, mini squat (30 degrees knee flexion).

Walking: Walking is the safe exercise which strengthens all the muscles of the extremity and also helps in reducing the body weight. One hour walk five times a week is advisable.

Exercises in Water: Exercises in water are beneficial for the patient those have severe symptoms or become non-ambulatory. Initially exercises are started for a short period of time. Non-ambulatory patients are instructed to stand up for a period which is comfortable for them, then rest is given. The ambulation period is increased gradually as per tolerance of the patient. Once the patient gains confidence and feels less pain then partial weight bearing started outside of the pool.

Bicycle Ergo Meter: Initially it should be without resistance for 15 minutes three to four times a week. The resistance is increased as per tolerance of the patient. It helps in improving strength of the lower extremity muscles and cardiovascular stamina.

I.P. JOINTS OSTEOARTHRITIS

Osteoarthritis affects primarily distal and proximal interphalangeal joints with relatively sparing of the metacarpophalangeal joints. There is non-uniform loss of joint space and formation of osteophytes. Osteophytes produces stretching on the periarticular structures. The soft tissue swelling associated with osteophytes in the PIP joints and DIP joint is known as Bouchard node and Heberden's node respectively. Osteophytes project laterally or medially and proximally towards the body and cyst formation is rare.

Management: Patients with PIP and DIP joint osteoarthrosis are managed with superficial heating modalities such as PWB and contrast bath. To restore the strength and ROM, PNF techniques such as hold relax, contract relax and stretching exercises are recommended.

Baker's Cyst

Baker's cyst or popliteal cyst is an accumulation of the fluid in the gastrocnemius and semi-membranosus bursa, was described first, in 1877, by Baker. He noted communication of the cyst with the joint synovium with fluid that leaks into the bursa but cannot return back to the joint. Sometimes the cyst ruptures and releases the fluid into the semi-membranosus and gastrocnemius tendons which produces immense pain in the posteromedial aspect (medial gastrocnemius and semimembranosus tendons). It is, therefore, sometimes confused with the thrombophlebitis.

The popliteal (Backer) cysts are frequently associated with intra-articular pathology or injury such as meniscal tears, rheumatoid arthritis, osteoarthrosis, conditions causing synovitis, Charcot's joints and tuberculosis.

Management

After establishing the cause of the popliteal cyst the treatment should be directed to the cause as well as to the prevention of rupture of the cyst. Patients with rheumatoid arthritis should be advised not to put the weight on the leg. Cryotherapy and interferential therapy may help in relieving pain, swelling and symptoms. Strengthening exercises such as quadriceps sets, gluteus maximus sets, hamstrings and ankle pumps are advised to avoid disuse atrophy of the muscles. Injection of steroids into the cyst may also be recommended.

Patients with meniscal tears who do not respond to the conservative treatment, are advised for arthroscopic intervention or open excision. The recurrence rate of open popliteal cyst excision varies widely, with studies reporting frequent recurrences.

RHEUMATOID ARTHRITIS

Rheumatoid arthritis is a chronic inflammatory disease of the synovium which is characterized by exacerbation and remission. It is a systemic disease which involves heart, lungs, blood vessels and eyes.

Etiology

The cause of rheumatoid arthritis remains unknown but it is believed that an immunological response takes place in the synovial tissues. An unknown, presumably exogenous, antigen enters (encounters) into the defender cell. The lymphocyte, which is transformed into a large plasma cell, secretes (manufactures) antibodies. These antibodies, antigen and complement combine to form a complex, which is also known as immune complex. Scavenger phagocytic cells, contain small enzyme-producing sacs (lysosomes) that destroy the immune complex, however some of the lysosomes escape from phagocytic cells and their proteases attack the cartilage and synovium. The immune complex is responsible for the inflammation in the synovium. The destruction of the tissues (synovium and cartilage) produces some debris which invites further phagocytic activities to remove the debris. Hence, more phagocytic activities leave more enzymes which produce more destruction and further, inflammation, and the arthritic process becomes self-perpetuating.

Pathogenesis and Pathology

Under the examination of electronic microscope of the synovium, the lining of synovium consists of three types of synovial cells, e.g., type A, type B and type C. Type A cells mainly the phagocytic cells are engaged in destroying of complex, in the synovial fluid. Type B, which resembles fibroblast and are believed to synthesize protein and hyaluronic acid. Type C, are also known as undifferentiated cells, have the properties of both A and B.

The early stage of inflammation causes dilatation of the venules and capillaries. The leucocytes pass into the tissue spaces and then into the synovial fluid. This consequence leads to inflammation in the synovium (synovitis). Early hyperemia, cdcma, and swelling occur in the synovium and lining cells proliferate until they are three or more layers (multiply) thick. The underlying tissue is infiltrated with lymphocytes and plasma cells. All these lead to a thickened synovial membrane.

The inflamed synovium forms a pannus a granulomatous mass, that grows over and destroys cartilage, tendon and ligaments. The pannus is formed at the peripheral part of synovium. The pannus of granulation grows progressively and extends over the cartilage surface. In the process of inflammation the cartilage is absorbed (by the pannus) and replaced with the fibrous connective tissue. Vascular granulations are also formed in the marrow which extends into the articular cartilage surface. There is destruction of the cartilage and it becomes thin and deficient. The articular part is mainly covered with the fibrous pannus. The granulation tissue also extend toward the opposite articular cartilage surface bridging the joint with other granulation tissue resulting a fibrous ankylosis (Figs. 24.28 to 24.30).

The synovium also extend into the peripheral part of the joint, putting pressure on the capsule, ligaments and tendons. The ligaments and tendons

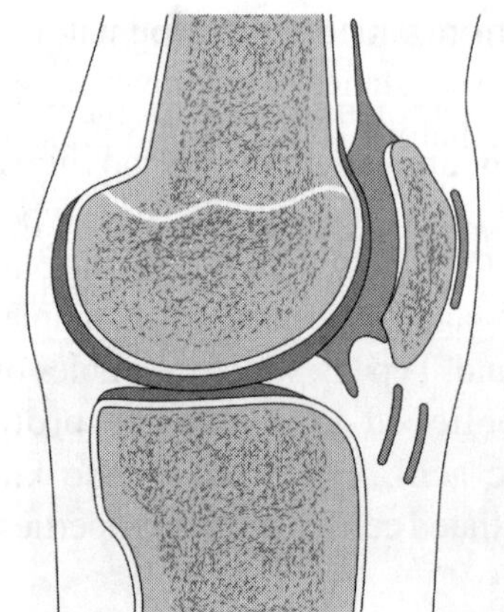

Fig. 24.28: Synovium, cartilage normal

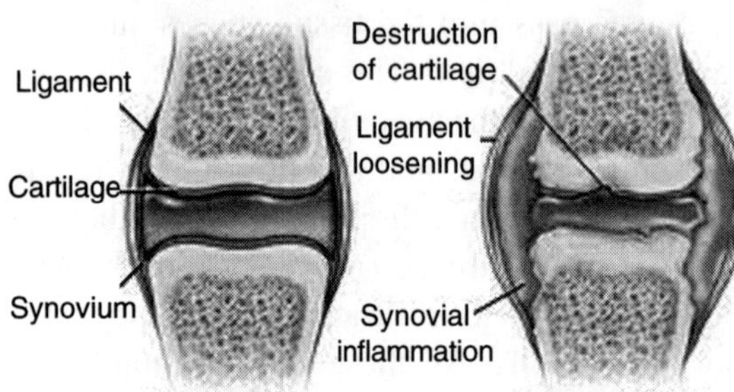

Fig. 24.29: Damaged synovium and cartilage

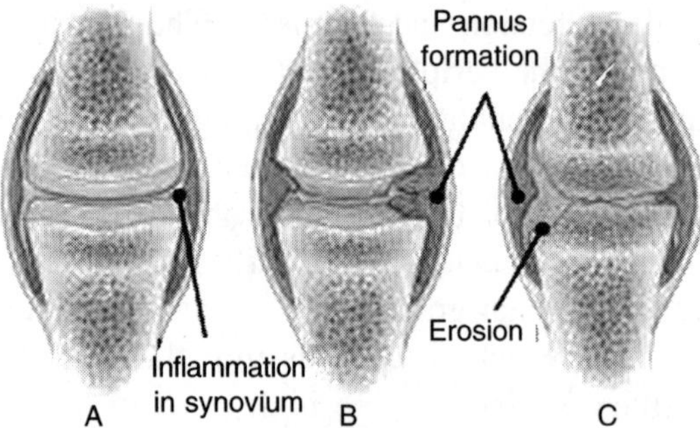

Fig. 24.30: Pannus

may sublux or rupture/tear causing muscular imbalance and joint deformity.

Subcutaneous Nodules: Subcutaneous nodules are composed of a typical basic rheumatoid unit consisting of a central necrotic zone, a surrounding layer of large mononuclear cell radially arranged (pallisade formation), and an outer zone of dense connective tissue with marked round-cell infiltration. Subcutaneous nodules are formed over the extensor surface such as forearm and tibia. They may be present in 20% of patients. Vasculitis is commonly found in rheumatoid arthritis and it is responsible for various skin lesions and may be a feature of early rheumatoid nodule formation (Fig. 24.31).

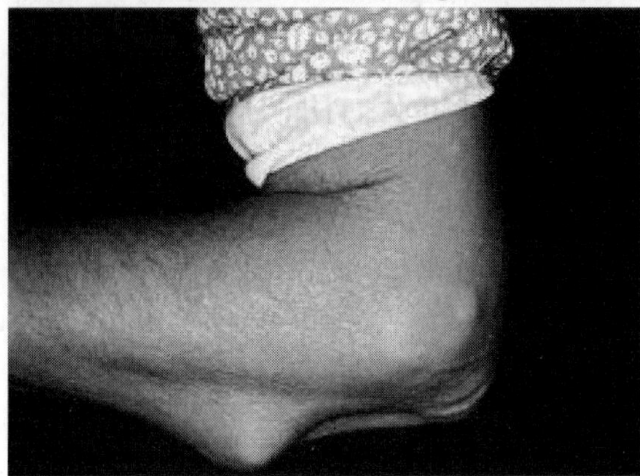

Fig. 24.31: Subcutaneous nodules

Clinical Features

1. Morning stiffness.
2. Pain on movements.
3. Symmetrical joint swelling.
4. Subcutaneous nodules.
5. Increased E.S.R.
6. Positive R.A. factor.
7. Muscle tightness and contracture.
8. Joint deformities.
9. Osteoporosis.

Diagnostic Criteria for Rheumatoid Arthritis

These are given by American Rheumatoid Association.

The diagnostic criteria are mentioned as under:

1. Morning stiffness.
2. Pain on movement or tenderness in atleast one joint.
3. Swelling: It may either be soft tissue thickening or synovial fluid in atleast one joint.

4. Swelling in atleast one other joint.
5. Symmetrical joint swelling with simultaneous involvement of both the sides of the joint. For an example if there is swelling in the left wrist joint the patient should also have swelling in the right wrist joint.
6. Subcutaneous nodules over bony prominences (on the extensor surfaces).
7. X-ray typical of rheumatoid arthritis.
8. Positive RA factor or latex fixation test.
9. Poor mucin clot.
10. Characteristic histologic changes in synovial membrane.
11. Characteristic histologic changes in nodule.

Based on the aforesaid eleven criteria the diagnosis may be classified as classical, definite, probable and possible.

Classical RA: The classical diagnosis cannot be made in the early stages as it requires aforementioned any seven criteria present for six weeks.

Definite: This needs five diagnostic criteria for atleast six weeks.

Probable: This needs three criteria out of eleven and these must be present for four weeks.

Possible RA: This diagnosis needs two of the following criteria which must be present at least for three weeks.
1. Morning stiffness.
2. Tenderness or pain on motion with history of recurrence persistence for three weeks.
3. History of swelling of joint.
4. Subcutaneous nodules.
5. Elevated erythrocyte sedimentation rate.

Laboratory Findings

An ESR is elevated particularly during an active period of inflammation, the rate continue to rise but to a lesser degree.

- Hypochromatic normocytic anemia is frequently associated. The white cell count remains normal.

- Serum from patients with rheumatoid arthritis contain a substance of unknown composition, the rheumatoid factor, in the presence of y globulin, is capable of agglutinating certain strains of streptococci, sensitized sheep cells and latex particles (Figs. 24.32 and 24.33).

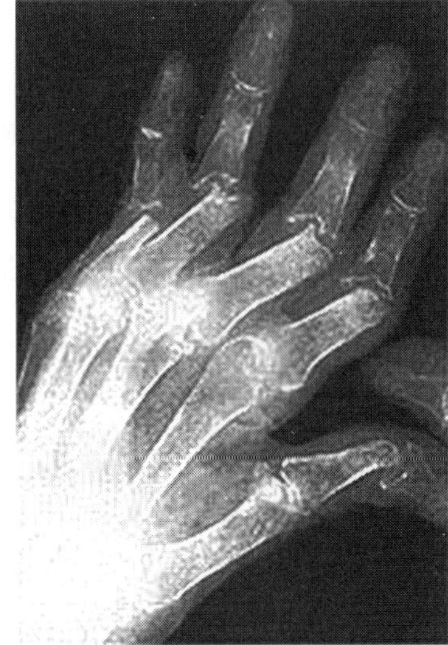

Fig. 24.32: X-ray–Rheumatoid arthritis with destruction of bones

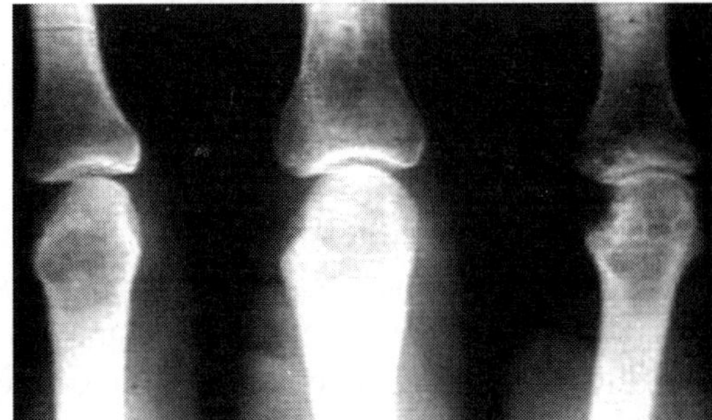

Fig. 24.33: X-rays–RA with destruction of peripheral cartilage and bone

Extra-Articular Manifestations: Apart from intra-articular structures, rheumatic arthritis also involves the other structure, known as extra-articular manifestations. These are not seen in the early stages of disease but as the disease progresses it may cause manifestations in the heart, lungs, blood vessels, eyes, nerves and muscles. These manifestations are as following:

1. **Pulmonary:** Nodules, pleural effusion, bronchitis.
2. **Vascular:** Digital arthritis, ulcer, visceral arthritis.
3. **Systemic:** Fever, weight loss, fatigue, susceptibility to infection.
4. **Musculoskeletal:** Muscle wasting, bursitis, tenosynovitis, osteoporosis, synovitis.
5. **Hematological:** Anaemia, thrombocytosis, eosinophilia.
6. **Cardiac:** Pericarditis, myocarditis, endocarditis.
7. **Nodular:** Sinuses, scleritis.
8. **Neurological:** Cervical cord compression, compression neuropathies, mononeuritis-multiplex.
9. **Ocular:** Episcleritis, sclerotic.
10. **Lymphatic:** Lymphadenopathy, splenomegaly, fatty's syndrome, amyloidosis.

Deformities in Rheumatoid Arthritis

The inflammatory process involves the synovium that becomes edematous and thickened. The synovium forms the pannus which extends over the cartilage and absorbs and replaces it with fibrous connective tissues.

The edematous and thickened synovium extends to peripheral structures such as capsule, ligaments, fibrous sheath and tendons. This process damages and weakens the capsule and supporting structures. There is migration of the fat, pad, capsule and tendons. The joint becomes unstable and predisposes to deformities. The inflammatory process also cause rupture or tear of the tendon which leads to muscular imbalance and deformities. Weakening and lengthening of the static structures (ligaments and joint capsule) and rupture of the muscles in the inflammatory process, produces deformities.

Deformities of Hand and Fingers

The rheumatoid arthritis involves the proximal interphalangeal, distal interphalangeal and metacarpophalangeal joints.

Ulnar Drift: It is the ulnar deviation of the metacarpophalangeal joints. The main cause of ulnar drift is sinovitis. The flexor tendons enter fibrous sheath at angle, exerting ulnar and palmer pull that is resisted in the normal hand. Weakened and elongated joint capsule and ligaments loose the restraining power against the ulnar and palmer pull. Joint capsule and ligaments resistance to displacing force is lost. Extensor tendons are displaced in an ulnar and palmer directions, resulting base of proximal phalanx moves into ulnar and palmer direction (Figs. 24.34 to 24.36).

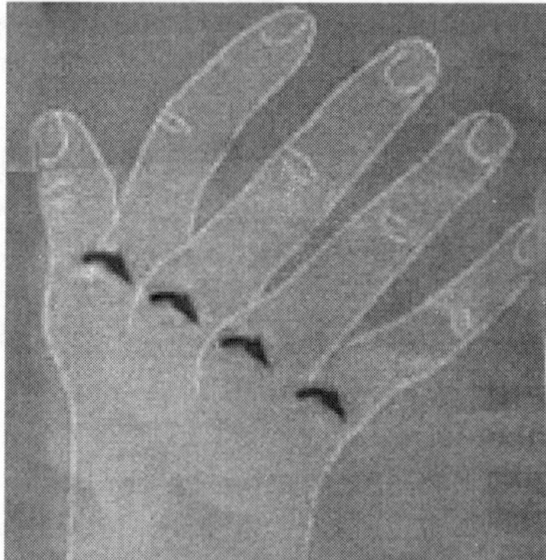

Fig. 24.34: Ulnar drift deformity

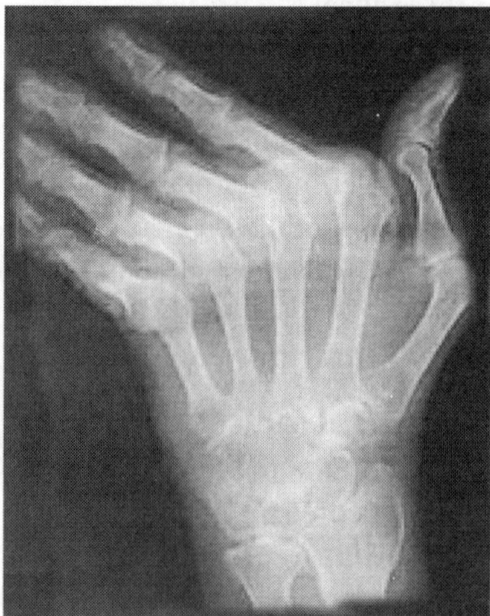

Fig. 24.35: X-ray ulnar drift

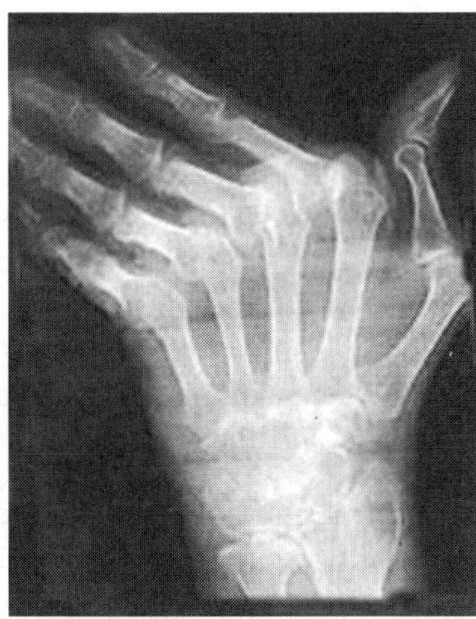

Fig. 24.36: X-ray ulnar drift

The disease affects the joint in two ways:

1. The inflammatory process (inflammatory infiltration) weakens and damages the capsule and supporting structures.
2. Edematous and thickened synovium extends into the extra articular structures and puts excessive load on them. The extensor tendon hoods are loosely fixed and vulnerable to disruption. The ligaments and capsule looses their restraining power against the ulnar forces–allowing tendons to pull across the joint in a way that enhances ulnar deviation and volar subluxation. As resistance to displacing force is lost extensor tendons are displaced into ulnar and palmer directions.

Swan-Neck Deformity (SND)

An SND is a deformity in which the PIP joint goes into hyperextension and DIP joint into flexion. The severity of deformity depends upon the loss of PIP flexion and DIP range of motion. Though SND is very common in rheumatoid arthritis, it may also occur following injury and trauma. The inflammatory process affects the joint in two ways:

i. Synovitis of the PIP may lead to rupture of the flexor digitorum superficial tendon which

allows PIP joint into hyperextension because of muscular imbalance. The hyperextension causes tension in the flexor digitorum profundus which pulls the DIP joint into flexion and predisposes the joint into SND.

ii. The inflammatory process involves the proximal interphalangeal (PIP) joints. Chronic intra-articular swelling due to synovial hypertrophy and fluid places an excessive pressure on the volar and dorsal capsule. There is dorsal migration of the volar band, which produces hyperexten-sion at the PIP joint. Hyperextension at PIP joint causes tension in the profundus tendon that pulls the distal interphalangeal joint into flexion (Fig. 24.37).

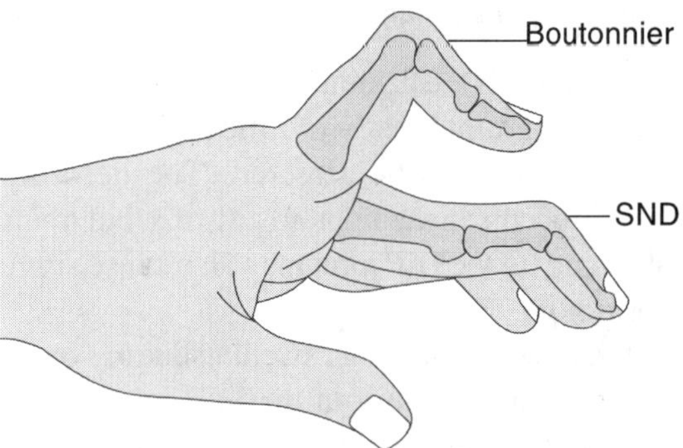

Fig. 24.37: Swan-neck deformity (SND)

Boutonniere or Button-Hole Deformity

Boutonniere deformity is very common after SND in rheumatoid arthritis, may also occur following injury and trauma. The PIP joint goes into flexion and DIP joint into hyperextension.

The main cause of the Boutonniere deformity is the synovitis which usually affects the PIP joint. The inflammatory process damages and weakness the capsule and supporting structures. The edematous (hypertrophied) synovium distends to the dorsal capsule and also displaces the *anterior surface*. There is rupture of the central slip of the extensor digitorum communis that limits the effectiveness of it as an extensor of middle finger. The PIP joint goes into flexion which in turn *increase tension* distal extensor slip, which pulls DIP into hyperextension (Fig. 24.38).

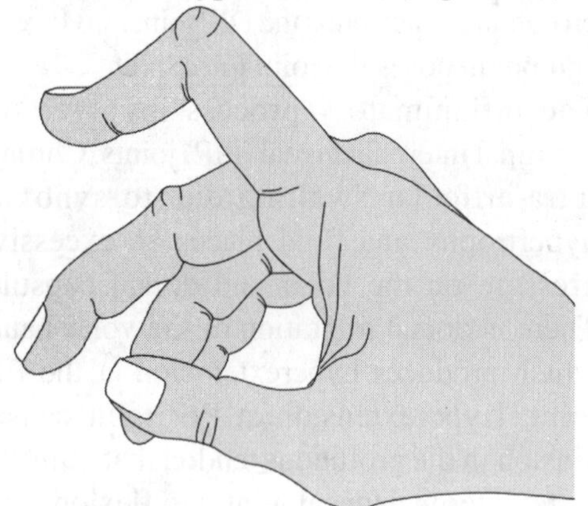

Fig. 24.38: Boutonniere or button-hole deformity

Mallet Finger

Mallet finger is the flexion deformity of distal interphalangeal joint mostly of little finger but other fingers may also be affected. The deformity usually occurs in rheumatoid arthritis, but trauma and injury to the DIP joint may also cause similar deformity.

Chronic intra-articular swelling due to synovial hypertrophy and fluid in the DIP joint extends into the dorsum of the little finger which damages and weaken the capsule and supporting structures. There is pressure on the distal attachment of the extensor tendon, which may lengthen or rupture the extensor tendon and removes the extension force. Due to loss of extension force the flexor digitorum profundus pulls the DIP into flexion (Fig. 24.39). The deformity is graded as mild, moderate and severe which depends on the active loss of flexion range.

Mild: Partial active extension of DIP (Partial rupture of extensor tendon).

Moderate: No active extension of DIP, passive extension possible (Complete rupture of tendon).

Severe: No active and passive extension, fixed DIP flexion (Contractor of profundus).

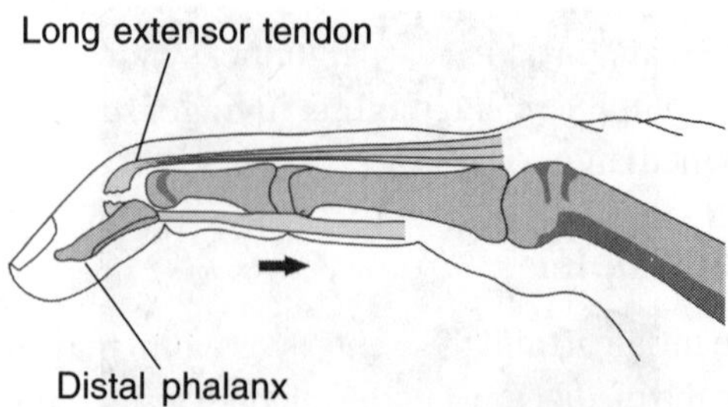

Fig. 24.39: Mallet finger

Wrist

The wrist joint is also involved frequently in rheumatoid arthritis. Initially swelling in the wrist joint is due to synovitis (synovial fluid) but as the disease progresses periarticular synovial thickening swelling may also be seen. Erosions may develop in all the carpal bones.

In the inflammatory process the synovium becomes edematous and thickened and forms the pannus which absorbs and replaces the bones with the fibrous connective tissues. Eventually there is destruction or collapse of the carpal bones at the radial side which will produce radial deviation of the metacarpals. The carpal bones may sublux towards the volar surface, and step like deformity will appear at the wrist joint (Fig. 24.40).

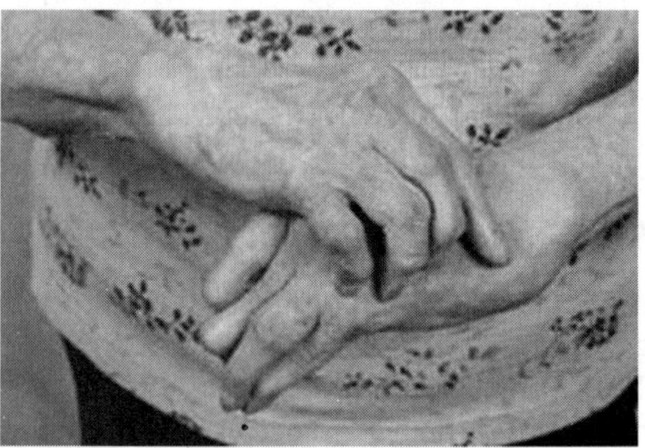

Fig. 24.40: Step deformity

The inflammatory changes also involve the synovium of the flexor tendons which enter into the carpal tunnel with the median nerve. The ischemia and swelling in the synovium of the tendons will increase the pressure within the tunnel and produce carpal tunnel syndrome with pain, numbness and tingling in finger supplied by the median nerve.

Elbow Joint

The inflamed and thickened synovium may bulge into the medial and lateral epicondyles of humerus and olecranon fossa. The olecranon fossa becomes obliterated and limits the extension of the elbow joint. The inflammatory process will destroy the anterior margin of the articular surface of the proximal ulna, allowing the olecranon to migrate in a cephaled direction.

Deformities of Lower Extremity Joint

Fore-Foot-Hallux Valgus, Hammer and Claw Toes: Chronic intra-articular swelling due to synovium hypertrophy and fluid causes broadening of the fore foot and separation of the toes, with capsular and ligamentous laxity. The weight bearing on the inflamed joint can cause dislocation of the metatarsophalangeal joints. The flexor tendons migrate and becomes functional extensors. Proximal phalanges and plantar fat pad are drawn laterally. This progressive muscular imbalance leads to hammer and claw toe deformities of the four lesser toes (Figs. 24.41 and 24.42). The lateral stability of the great toe is decreased. The great toe migrates laterally and develops hallux valgus deformity.

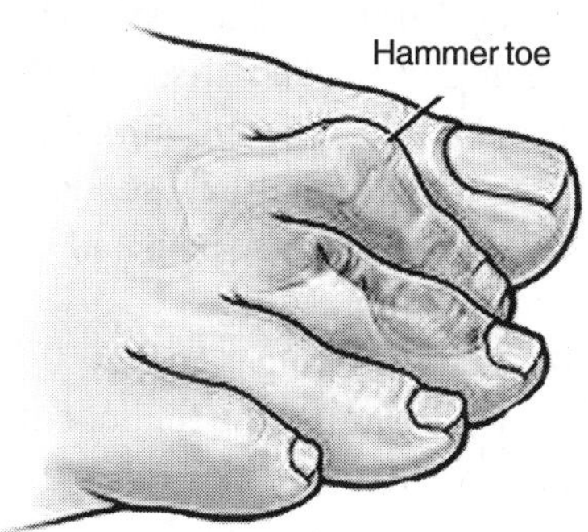

Fig. 24.41: Hammer toes

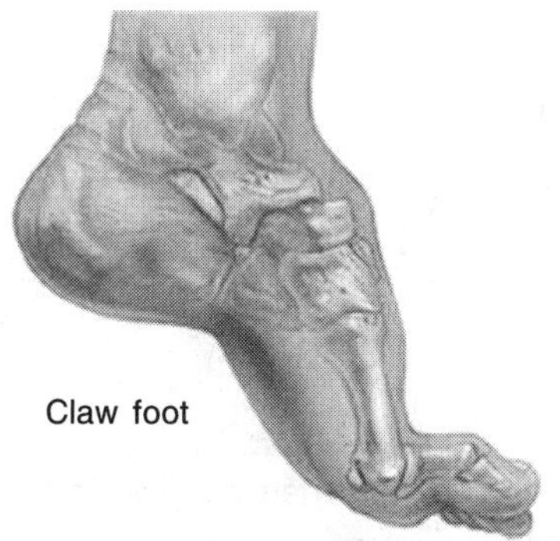

Fig. 24.42: Claw toes

Hind Foot: The hind foot does not develop marked deformities, but the inflammatory process may cause plantar fasciitis, bursitis and spur. The weight bearing on the inflamed and swollen joint may aggravate the symptoms, and may cause excessive pronation.

Ankle: In the early stage of the disease synovitis of the tibialis anterior, peroneii and tibialis posterior are common, however, no clinical evidence is seen but surgical is there. A sausage shaped swelling is seen along the length of the tendon. As the disease progresses it may destruct the cartilage and replace with fibrous connective tissues. The ligamentous laxity produces joint instability. Erosion of the ligamentous insertion can also be seen between tibia and fibula and the talus.

Knee Joint Deformities: The knee joint is frequently involved in rheumatoid arthritis which produces combination of deformities. Potter's knee describes the typical rheumatoid arthritis knee that includes flexion contracture, popliteal cysts, posterior subluxation and dislocation of tibia, valgus and external rotation of the tibia (Figs. 24.43 and 24.44).

- In the early stage of rheumatoid arthritis synovitis alters the centre of motion of the tibiofemoral joint. Intra-articular swelling due to synovitis increases in volume. The weight bearing on the swollen and inflamed knee joint can allow the synovial fluid to pass into popliteal

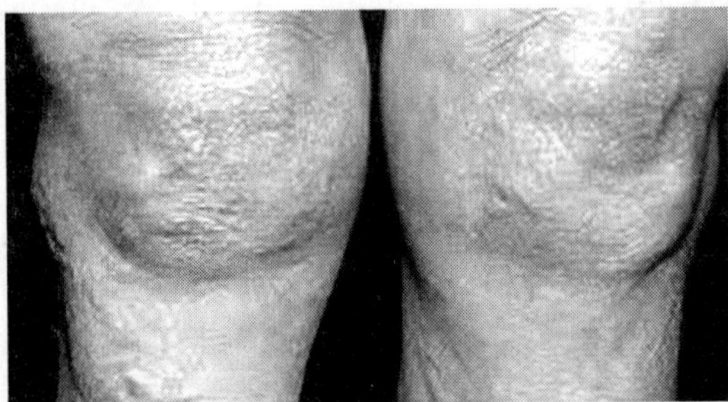

Fig. 24.43: Knee joint swelling

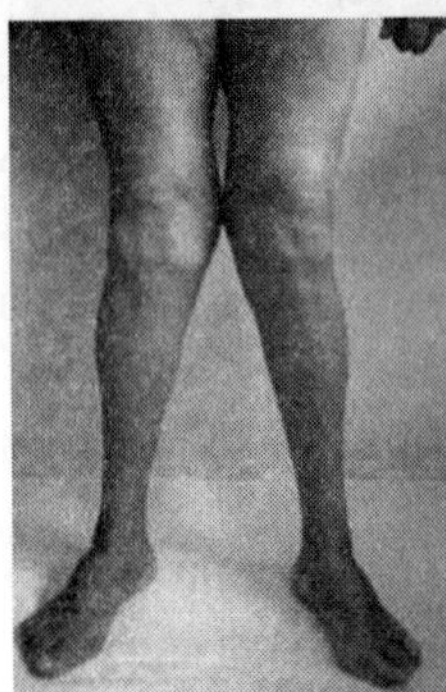

Fig. 24.44: Potter knee deformity

fossa, where it forms a popliteal cyst. Sometimes the popliteal cyst which contains synovial fluid may burst and passes the fluid into the semi-membranosus and semi-tendinosus bursa. This produces intense pain in the posterior knee joint which sometime *mistaken with thrombophlebitis.*

- As the disease progresses the synovium becomes thickened and edematous, and forms pannus that extends into the cartilage (peripheral part) and covers the peripheral part. The pannus absorbs and replaces the cartilage with fibrous connective tissue. The destruction of the cartilage can cause collapse of femoral or tibial condyles. As the cartilage wears crepetus is the evident throughout the movement.
- All components of the knee complex are involved such medial, lateral and patello-femoral joint. Pain and spasm in the hamstrings limit the terminal extension resultant knee joint is maintained slightly in flexion. In non ambulatory patients hamstrings develop contracture which pull the tibia posterior on the femur; this produces subluxation or dislocation of the tibia. Quadriceps becomes weak due to prolong elongation.

- The destruction of the cartilage produces mediolateral instability and knee valgus. The spasm in tensor fascia lata (TFL) pulls the tibia towards lateral rotation and produces tibial external rotation in 50% cases. This causes a shortening of the lateral structure and permanent elongation of medial structures. Therefore, the rheumatoid arthritis affects the knee joint markedly and develops flexion contracture, posterior subluxation and dislocation, valgus and external rotation of the tibia.

Hip Joint: Initially joint destructions are not seen but patients may have complain of pain, stiffness, and limitation in the range of abduction and rotations. Tenderness can be palpated on the posterior and superior aspect of the joint due to trochantric and gluteus maximus bursitis. As the disease progresses patients may develop antaligic gait and Trendelenburg's sign. Swelling may be visible in the groin and femoral triangle.

In advanced cases osteoporosis occurs and the femoral head pieces the acetabulum. Avascular necrosis of the femoral head can cause collapse of the area. Eventually a true leg length discrepancy will occur.

Shoulder Joint: Initially synovial effusion may be seen due to synovitis, which may limit shoulder abduction. The inflammatory changes involve the subacromial and subdeltoid bursa, which will further produce pain and limitation in the range of motion.

The destructive changes and swelling also put an excessive pressure on the rotator cuff muscles. The rupture of the rotator cuff muscles will allow the head of humerus to migrate superiorly to the acromian arch. The suprahumeral space will decrease, supraspinatus and sub-acromial bursa will be impinged (impingement syndrome) between the head of humerus and acromian arch. The range of motion will be limited in all three planes.

Spine: The lumbar and thoracic spine does not involve significantly in rheumatoid arthritis. The most of destructive changes take place at the atlantoaxial joint. The inflammatory changes rupture the transverse ligament which holds the odontoid to the atlas. This will produce vertical subluxation or upward translation of the dens. The subluxation of C_1 and C_2 is a dangerous complication and may lead to compression on spinal cord, the patient may experience numbness and tingling in the arms and legs. The therapist should not advice mechanical traction to the rheumatoid arthritic patients, if X-ray shows subluxation between atlas and axis, patient could be given soft collar or hard collar and be referred to the orthopaedician for surgical intervention such as fusion of C_1 and C_2.

MANAGEMENT OF RHEUMATOID ARTHRITIS

Physical Therapy Assessment

Cardiopulmonary Assessment: Rheumatoid arthritis is a systemic disease which involves not only joints but also other organs such as heart, lungs, blood vessels and eyes, therefore, therapist should assess the functions of vital organs before administering treatment.

Musculoskeletal Assessment: Each joint is to be examined for erythema, warmth, pain, tenderness, temperature, swelling, range of motion, crepetus, contracture, tightness and deformities.

Gait and Posture Assessment: The involvement of hip, knee and ankle joint lead to tightness, contracture and deformities in the lower extremities. In turn, there is reduced range of motion, reduced velocity and increased energy expenditure. The muscles are required to work more for acceleration of swing phase to bring the leg forward. The cadence drops to 72.5 steps per minute or more. The stride length is also reduced. Due to pain patient walks with the stiff knee (antalgic gait) and bending to the same side (Trendelenburg sign).

The Therapist Should Focus on the Following Goals

1. **Education:** The therapist should tell the patient that this is a progressive disease which cannot be cured but it can be prevented to the further progression by taking some measures. Energy conservation principles, work simplification techniques, exercise programs, and joint protection techniques should be taught to the patients. They must learn these management techniques and then continue to practice them through out their life.

   Fatigue is one of the features of rheumatoid arthritis. In order to avoid fatigue patient should be encouraged to organize time, task and rest periods. The position such as sitting which saves upto 25% energy should be preferred over standing. The patient should use large joint and body weight to achieve tasks. Long handled equipments increase the range of hand function and decrease the amount of bending and energy required. Electronic light weight equipments also decrease the amount of time and energy required.

2. **Relief in Pain and Spasm:** The pain and stiffness is mainly of protective in nature. There is overuse (sustained contraction) of the muscles to prevent movement at the joint. The therapist should focus on reduction of muscle guarding by using the cryotherapy and superficial heating modalities such as infra red rays, moist hot packs and paraffin wax bath.

PNF techniques of slow reversal, reciprocal inhibition, hold relax and contract relax may be found of valve in reduction pain and spasm. Exercises in water not only help in relief of pain but also play important role in improvement of range of motion and muscle strength. In patients with acute pain where ESR is extremely high and patients find difficultly in doing hold relax and contract relax they may be taught reciprocal inhibition; as it consists isometric contraction of antagonistic muscles that is useful in relaxing the agonists group of muscles. The electrotherapy modalities such as short wave diathermy should not be advised as it may increase inflammation especially during the excrebatory phase. Instead of SWD, pulsed diathermy or curapulse is advised. Interferential therapy of analgesic mode 80-100 Hz helps in relieving pain and muscle spasm.

The physiotherapeutic management in relief of pain should be considered as temporary but it is the crucial step that helps in preventing tightness; contracture and deformities. Patients should learn and receive the treatment such as cold pack, hot pack, PWB and muscle relaxation exercises at home in order to prevent muscles guarding, tightness and contractures.

3. **Protection of Joints:** Activities of daily living may put excessive pressure on the painful and swollen joints. These joints become more vulnerable to damage and instability. Hence, activity that produces pain lasting more than 1-2 hours indicates joints are being overstressed and needed to be protected. To provide the dynamic stability to the inflamed joints, these joints should be supported well with work splint particularly when muscle strength is inadequate. For activities of daily living the patient should be advised to use the body weight and large joints to push the large objects instead of hands. Patient should also be advised to maximize the effect of gravity (e.g., use a laundry chute to eliminate carrying and stairs) for daily activities and office work. The following points should be taught to the patient to protect the joint:

a. Respect the pain: Pain occurs during an activity is an important indication of joint protection.

b. Maintain adequate muscle strength and range of motion.

c. Avoid holding one position for any undue length of time.

d. Use correct patterns of movements.

e. Avoid the position in which deformity occurs.

4. **Prevention of Deformities:** Development of deformities in patients with rheumatoid arthritis is very common, as pain, swelling and muscle spasm encourage the patient to adopt the posture which relieves symptoms. Later there will be change in the length of muscle fibers, periarticular structures and decrease strength of muscle. The muscle strength is essential to support damaged joint. Pain, however, should not be ignored as doing so can lead to further damage and discomfort. Rheumatoid arthritis affects interphalangeal joints of hands, wrist and foot swelling in 90 percent of patients. Deformities are mainly caused by swelling and proliferation of the synovium into the particular structures. This, in turn, causes destruction of cartilage, erosion of bones, ligamentous laxity and rupture or tear of the muscle tendons. This lead to muscular imbalance and deformity. To prevent muscular imbalance and deformities the joint should be held in such a position that not only reduces load on the muscle tendon but also helps in relieving pain and symptoms; especially during an acute phase. The splints, proper positioning, and passive stretching, play

crucial role in preventing deformities and relieving in pain and symptoms.

Splints

These are very useful in acutely inflammable joints. Improved biomechanical designs and the introduction of light weight, strong, low temperature material that are resistant to wear have provided the client with a wide array of splints. There are two types of splints–resting and dynamic.

Resting Splints: These are very effective in reducing the protective muscle guarding that is responsible for deformity. The resting splints should be worn at night and predetermined periods during the day. Splint use should continue full time for duration of flare and removed at least once a day for skin hygiene and gentle active movements. The splint should be well fitted, padded over the bony prominences to avoid pressure. These are usually made of plaster of Paris which are easy to apply. The therapist should explain the application procedure to the patients and in case of redness, pressure sores they should use soft materials between the splint and treatment part. The weight of splint also puts an additional stress on the extremity and may cause pain and fatigue, hence, the splint should be as light weight as possible.

Generally, for the upper extremity, splint is applied in 10-30° wrist extension, slight lunar deviation, interphalangeal joint in 5° flexion, meta-carpophalangeal joint should be just off full flexion. Thumb should be abducted and opposed. However the position of hand and wrist may vary somewhat by practitioners (Fig. 24.45).

Wrist splint–Neutral or slight extension, Unlar deviation–5°, Ulnar drift–Should be corrected, Meta carpophalangeal joints–Should be just off full flexion, Thumb–Abducted and opposed.

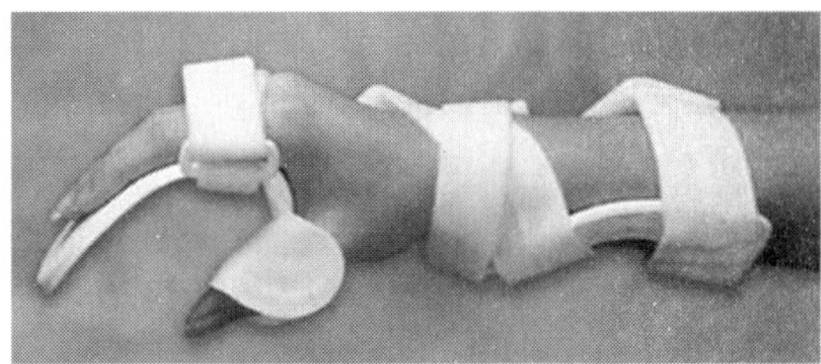

Fig. 24.45: Wrist (resting) splint

Swan Neck Splint: To restrict unwanted PIP hyperextension and to prevent swan neck deformity a proximal interphalangeal hyper-extension block splint is used. The patients with swan neck deformity usually finds difficulty in performing activities with the hand. The swan neck splint not only blocks the PIP joint in slight flexion but also allows patient to flex the PIP joint more efficiently which helps in performing activities with the hand. For short term or trial purposes a custom fabricated thermoplastic material can be used but for long term use an adjacent finger, commercial products made from metal or polypropylene are often recommended as they are more durable, less bulky, more easily cleaned, and more cosmetically appealing (Figs. 24.46 a-b).

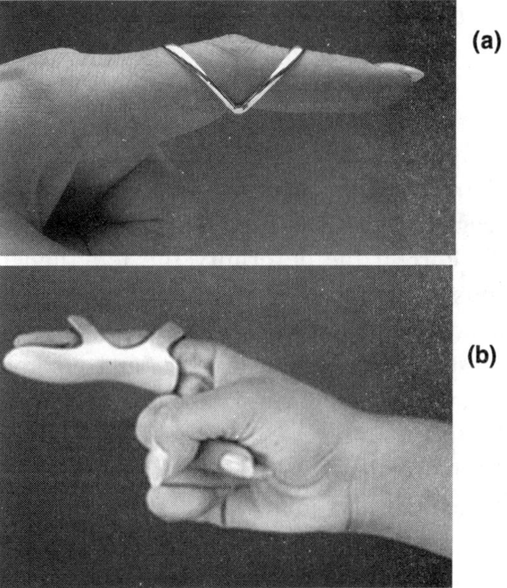

(a)

(b)

Figs. 24.46a-b: Splints for swan neck deformity

Boutonniere Splint: To prevent the boutonniere deformity the proximal interphalangeal joint is blocked in the extension and distal interphalangeal joint is left free to flex. The splint is very useful in prevention of deformity if the deformity is flexible (Fig. 24.47).

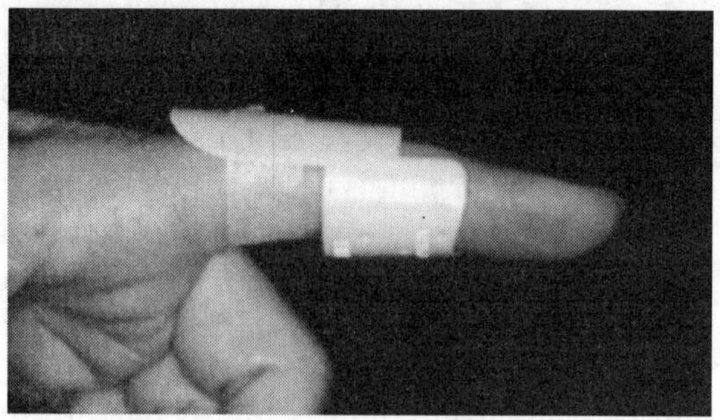

Fig. 24.47: Boutonniere splint

Knees: The knee is kept straight in 5° of flexion and then a back slab is applied from distal ischial tuberosity to the proximal heal.

Ankle and Foot: To prevent the deformities at ankle joint, a back slab is applied which extends from the neck of fibula to the tip of toe. The ankle joint should be at neutral with no valgus or varus.

5. **Correction of Deformities:** Rheumatoid arthritis is a progressive disease which develops deformities in the later stages; however, efforts are made in prevention of deformities. Once the deformity is established there is shortening (concave side) and lengthening (convex aspect) of the soft tissues. To correct the deformity the lengthened muscles are required strengthening and shortened muscles require stretching. Serial plaster, serial splinting, orthoses and dynamic splints are used to correct the deformities.

Serial Plaster: To correct the flexion contracture of the knee joint, a POP cast is applied over the deformed joint. The cast is split after 2-3 days on the concave (popliteal) side and separated as far as possible using the uncut POP on the convex side as a hinge. After cutting on the concave side the knee joint is extended as much as possible (as per tolerance of the patient) and wedges are inserted on the split POP to maintain the achieved position. The whole part is secured by a POP bandage. It is repeated once before the entire plaster has to be replaced.

Orthosis: Swelling due to synovitis and synovium hypertrophy places stretch on the periarticular structures such as ligaments, tendons and capsule that may rupture or lengthen. This whole phenomenon produces ligamentous laxity and joint instability. The orthosis provides not only passive stability to the joint but also holds the joint in functional position (Fig. 24.48).

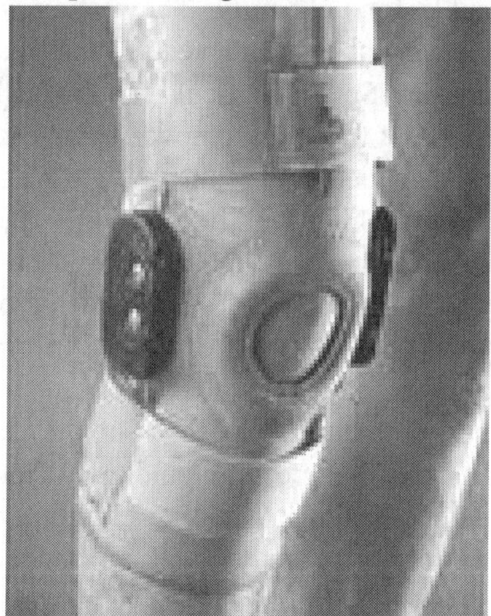

Fig. 24.48: Knee orthosis

6. **Maintenance and Restoration of Joint Range of Motion:** During exacerbatory period active assisted, hold relax, and contract relax exercises are advised to maintain the range of motion. Passive movements may increase the pain and symptoms therefore these should be avoided. Hold relax, contract relax and slow reversal exercises are found effective in increasing range of motion of the joint. For an example to improve the flexion contracture, the therapist extends the knee joint as much as possible and holds it firmly. The

patient is asked to contract the hamstrings against the resistance of at least six seconds, followed by rest of same period. This exercise helps in lengthening of the hamstrings and increasing in extension of the knee joint. Several repetitions of hold relax or contract relax may be performed until a significant improvement in the range is achieved. The exercise in water (hydrotherapy) also helps in improving range of motion.

7. **Maintenance and Improvement of Posture:** Core strengthening, upper back extensors and peripheral muscle strengthening, should be taught to the patient to improve posture. Exercises in water also help in improving posture.

Surgical Management

If pain and symptoms are not relieved with a fair trial of conservative treatment including drugs then patient may be elected for surgical intervention. Relief in incapacitating pain, restoration of joint stability and improvement in activities of daily living are the main objectives of the surgery. The progression of the stages of the rheumatoid arthritis decides the choice of surgery. Synovectomy, arthroplasty and arthrodesis are the common surgical procedures recommended to the patients with rheumatoid arthritis.

Synovectomy: The removal of the synovium relieves pain in almost all rheumatoid joints and at least temporarily halts progression of the local disease. The procedure is usually recommended in early stages of the disease where other structures of the joint remain intact except of synovium. In synovectomy the site of immuno-globulin synthesis is removed to prevent the formation of immune complexes that cause tissue destruction by activating lysosomal hydrolases. This will also decrease in the synovial rheumatoid factor, IgG/Igm ($7^s/19^s$ complex). The removed synovium usually regenerates completely within 60 days. The regenerated synovium once again capable of secreting synovial fluid, but the synovial function is considerably reduced. The regenerated synovium is again susceptible to inflammation (synovitis).

Post Operative Synovectomy: Breathing exercises, intensive coughing, hold relax, general strengthening exercises are initiated to improve posture and gait. The synovectomy is usually recommended to the knee, MCP wrist and elbow joint. To achieve the range of motion, an ice towel can be placed on the spasmodic muscles, and contract relax exercises are performed. For an example, to improve flexion of knee joint an ice pack is placed along the length of quadriceps and knee is flexed as much as possible. The therapist holds the leg firmly and asks the patient to extend the leg. The contraction is held at least for six seconds followed by relaxation. After relaxation new flexion range is achieved and same procedure is repeated. Several repetitions are performed to improve the range of motion. In case of severe muscle spasm reciprocal inhibition helps in improving flexion range of knee joint. As the spasm decreases in severity contract relax exercises may also be performed. Passive movements often increases protective muscle spasm, therefore, should be avoided.

Arthroplasty

It is the removal of one or both of the articular surfaces with or without a foreign implant. There are four types of arthroplasty:
- Excision arthroplasty.
- Interposition arthroplasty.
- Partial joint replacement (arthroplasty).
- Total joint replacement (arthroplasty).

Excision Arthroplasty: The aim of excision arthroplasty is to reduce pain in the joint. The surgery is rarely done at the hip and knee joint except salvaging procedure. If the procedure is advised for knee joint, it is usually associated with arthrodesis.

The excision arthroplasty involves the rejection of periarticular bone and the space thus formed becomes (created by surgical procedure) filled with scar tissues during the healing process. The procedure creates unstable joint due to reduction intention of the ligaments and joint capsule.

The excision arthroplasty has a great benefit in the rheumatoid foot as it completely relieves persisting pain, disability, metatarsalgia and subluxation of the metatarsophalangeal joint. For excision of the metatarsal head and proximal part of proximal phalanx a fowler's compression excision arthroplasty is performed. For hallux valgus keller's excision arthroplasty is the choice of surgical procedure.

Post Operative Excision Arthroplasty: The emphasis is given on the footwear. The therapist should assess the foot accurately and review footwear. The weight bearing should be as per tolerance and as advised by the surgeon. Strengthening exercise of intrinsic muscles may be initialled after first week of operation. The faradic foot bath should be started after one month of the surgery. It helps in strengthening of the intrinsic muscles as well as in reducing the swelling of the foot. In cases of swelling in the ankle and foot faradism under pressure may also be used.

Interposition Arthroplasty: Interposition arthroplasty involves debridement of joint. In this procedure the space created with debridement is filled with fat pad, fascia or foreign material, which cover only one joint surface. The procedure is usually done at shoulder joint as replacement of shoulder is unlike hip and knee joints. Pendular exercises are initiated in the first week of the surgery upto 3 weeks. After three weeks isometric exercises may be initiated if advised by the concerned surgeon.

TOTAL HIP REPLACEMENT

It is the replacement of both the articular surfaces of the joint with the foreign implants. The pain is eliminated completely by replacing both the articulating surfaces. The restoration of hip motion improves gait and reduces stress on the back and knee joint (Fig. 24.49).

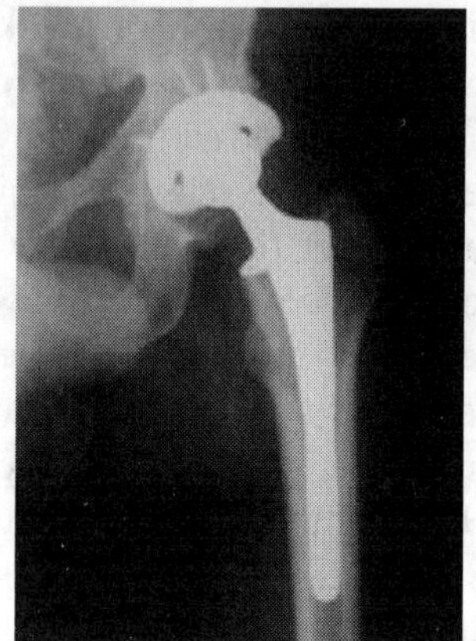

Fig. 24.49: Total hip replacement

Indications of THR

1. Persistent and debilitating pain with destruction of joint surfaces and with gross deterioration in activities of daily living and a fair trial of conservative treatment fails to improve the symptoms.
2. Failure of prior surgery.
3. Avascular necrosis.
4. Neck of femur fracture.
5. Hip arthrodesis in a poor functional position associated with increase in back or knee pain.
6. Osteoarthrosis-grade-4.

Contraindications of THR

1. Acute infection in the joint.
2. Systemic infection.
3. Malignant tumors that do not allow adequate fixation of the components.
4. In adequate bone mass.

Relative Contraindications of THR: Absent or relative insufficiency of the abductor mechanism, and progressive neurologic deficit.

Approaches: The hip joint can be approached from anterior, lateral and posterior view. All three approaches have advantages and disadvantages; but lateral approach is preferred over other.

> **Osteotomy:** The patients who have leg length discrepancy may require osteotomy of the femur. It may be done for alignment correction, either angular or rotational shortening, such as a calcar episiotomy or sub-trochanteric shortening; or *exposure, such as trochanteric osteotomy or slide.* These patients should not be allowed to do SLR and side SLR unless and until the concerned surgeon advises.

Who Can Be Elected for THR? The implant used in the surgery has a projected life span of less than 20 years, hence the patients of more than 60 years are usually elected for the THR. Younger patients may also be elected for the THR if their functional status is severely compromised and persistent pain becomes intolerable. As the young patients demand more physical activities, therefore the life span of the implant is reduced further (less than 20 years). These patients require a revision surgery later in their life (after 20 years of THR).

Types of Implants

There are three types of prosthesis–Cemented, non-cemented and hybrid.

Cemented: Cement is placed between the bone and the prosthesis, therefore, stability is provided by the cement. The cemented prosthesis is as strong as it will ever be 15 minutes after insertion. The cemented components can support weight immediately after surgery. The implant achieves an adequate stability to allow an immediate full weight bearing with a cane or walker. However, some surgeons believe that weight bearing restriction should be there at least upto 6 weeks, as the bone is damaged by mechanical and thermal trauma during the surgery.

Non-Cemented Prosthesis: The implant tends to be more expansive and technically demanding to implant; however, they are easier to revise when they fail. The implant is inserted into the bone by press fit method. The stability is usually achieved by tissue on growth or in growth into the implant. The maximum stability is achieved in the 6 months of the surgery.

Weight Bearing Restrictions: The patients with non-cemented are allowed to toe touch weight bearing with the walker for at least 6 weeks. The walker is removed after 6 weeks and stick is advised further unless and until patient archieves good hip abductor mechanism and also confidence. It usually takes 4-6 weeks. These patients may do stairs by the end of 3 months, however, stair climbing may be allowed before 3 months, if the concerned surgeon permits.

The patients with cemented implant may be allowed full weight bearing with the walker as soon as they come out of the operation theater. The walker may be removed after 4-6 weeks and a stick is given. Patients can do the stairs after 6 weeks of the surgery, however, it should be advised by the concerned surgeon.

Precautions

- No cross leg sitting.
- No internal rotation.
- No hip adduction.
- No hip flexion beyond $100°$.
- No low chair (>22 inches) (Figs. 24.50a-g).

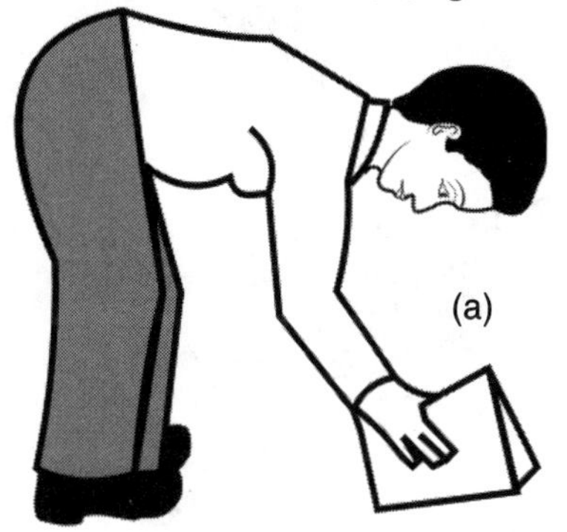

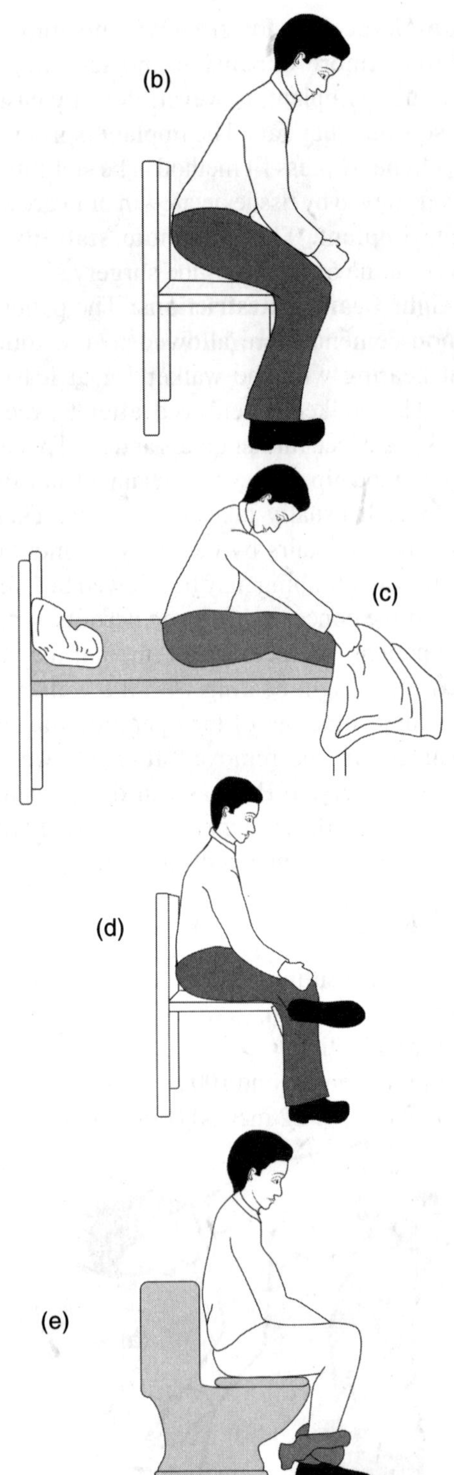

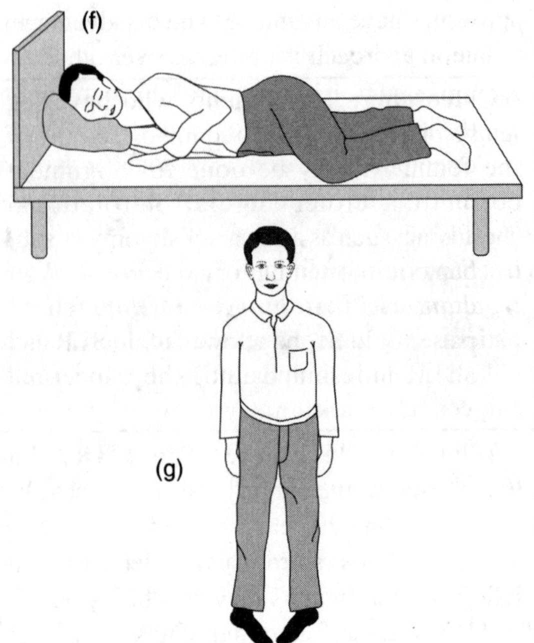

Figs. 24.50a-g: Prevention following THR

Post Operative Total Hip Replacement Management

Brace: The hip joint is guarded in the orthosis or wedge to prevent adduction of the hip as the joint is more vulnerable to dislocation in adduction. The brace may be removed during the exercise; however, it should be worn at night and predetermined period of day.

Exercises: The following exercises are initiated from day one:

i. *Quadriceps Sets:* For 6 weeks.

ii. *Gluteus Maximus Sets:* For 6 weeks.

iii. *Ankle Pump Exercises:* For 6 weeks.

iv. *Straight Leg Raising:* This exercise can produce very large *out-of-plane* loads on the hip, hence, it should be avoided, however, if it is advised, it should be performed with assistance in the first four weeks.

v. *Side SLR:* The exercise has an important role in improving abductor mechanism; initially it should be done in the supine position by bringing the leg out of the edge of the couch with assistance by the therapist. As the strength improves therapist may resist the movement. Exercise may be progressed to the side lying. In case of trochanteric osteotomies, the exercises should be avoided unless and until the concerned surgeon advises.

vi. ***Stairs:*** Stair climbing and descending also depends upon the type of implant. The patients with cemented implant may be allowed to climb the stairs after 6-8 weeks. Whereas patients with non-cemented implant should do stairs after 3 months only.

vii. ***Sitting on Chair:*** Both cemented and non-cemented patients are advised to use a chair of at least 22 inches height (for an average height person). Low chairs allow the hip to flex beyond 100 degrees, that may cause dislocation of the joint.

viii. ***Weight Bearing:*** Full weight bearing with the walker is allowed to the patients with cemented implant, whereas patients with cement less implant are advised to touch weight bearing with the walker for at least 6 weeks. Weight bearing on the operated side may also be limited if the greater trochanter is removed. The walker is removed and stick is advised till the patient gains confidence and abductor mechanism. It is usually given after 4-6 weeks (four weeks for the cemented and six to eight weeks for the cementless patients).

ix. ***Stretching:*** The hip flexors are of tonic muscles, and have tendency of getting shortened. *Thomas Stretch:* To stretch the iliopsoas muscles, the patient is placed in supine position and the unaffected leg is flexed at hip and knee joint as fully as possible. This will stretch the opposite iliopsoas muscles (extended leg). To stretch the iliopsoas muscles, the therapist should not extend the operated hip joint as it may cause implant to dislocate.

x. ***Exercises to Improve Hip and Knee Flexion:*** After hip joint arthroplasty there is severe reflexive spasm in the quadriceps muscles which limit the hip and knee flexion. In supine ICE towel or ICE pack is placed along the length of the quadriceps muscles and reciprocal inhibition is started. The technique is very much effective particularly in severe muscle spasm conditions where contract relax or hold relax are not possible. In this technique, to break the spasm in the quadriceps, the knee and hip is flexed as much as possible. The position is held and simultaneous strong isometric contraction of hip extensor and hamstrings are also performed. These isometric contractions will help in relieving quadriceps and iliopsoas muscle spasm, which improves hip and knee flexion. After 3-5 days of significant improvement in quadriceps muscle spasm, the reciprocal inhibition is progressed to hold relax and contract relax exercises. Passive stretching sometimes increases the muscle spasm hence, should be administered with caution.

CHAPTER-25

Shoulder Injuries

STABILITY OF THE SHOULDER

Shoulder is a complex of 20 muscles, 3 bony articulations, 3 soft tissue moving surfaces (functional joints) that permit the greatest mobility of any joint area found in the body. The large humeral head articulates with the glenoid fossa. The support and stabilization of the shoulder joint primarily depends upon the static and dynamic stabilizers. The static stabilizers are the non-contractile structures such as—coracohumeral ligament, glenohumeral ligament, joint capsule and labrum itself. The dynamic stabilizers are the contractile structures basically rotator cuff muscles. These stabilizers (static and dynamic) keep the head of humerus in the glenoid fossa and prevent the excessive translation to the anterior, posterior and superior directions. The mobility is however at the expense of structural stability (Figs. 25.1a-c).

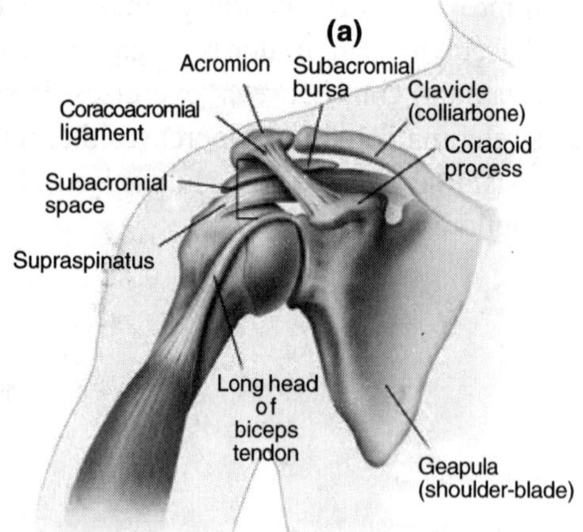

Fig. 25.1a: Static stabilizers of shoulder

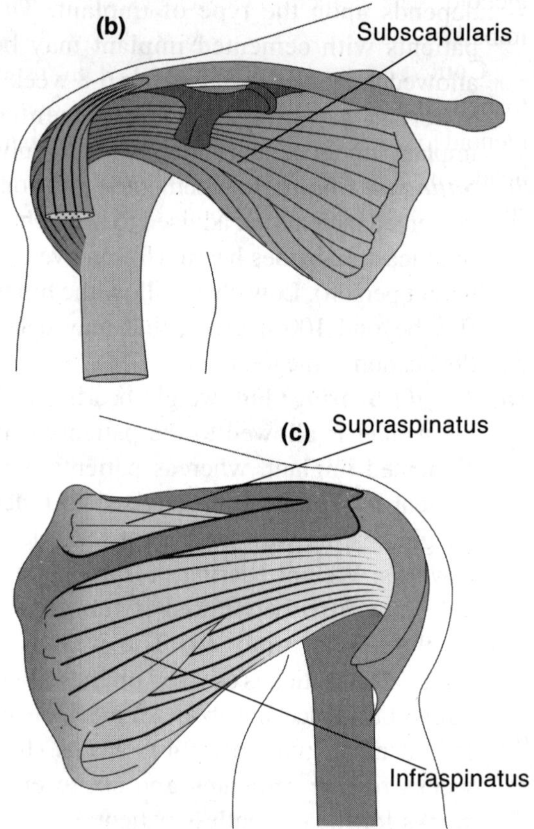

Fig. 25.1b-c: Dynamic stabilizers

Masten *et al*. describe following concepts of the stability of the shoulder: balance, concavity and compression, superior stability, adhesion-cohesion, glenohumeral suction cup, limited joint volume and capsuloligamentous constraints.

Balance: Balance refers to the passage of the net joint-reaction forces on the humeral head through the center of the glenoid fossa. The key components of balance include alignment of the humerus with the glenoid center line, facilitated by the surface arcs and areas of the glenoid and humeral head and by the muscles that position the glenoid and humerus relative to each other—namely, the rotator cuff and scapular stabilizers. The balance can be affected by the area of the glenoid, malalignment of the scapula and muscular imbalance.

Concavity and Compression: This refers to the stabilizing effect of the depth of the concave glenoid fossa on translation of the convex humeral head. The concavity and compression concept is strengthened by the three factors:

a. Increased thickness of the glenoid articular surface at the periphery of the glenoid relative to its center.

b. Glenoid labrum; and

c. Compressive forces produced by the rotator cuff muscles on the joint.

Superior Stability: It refers to the superior stability of the glenoid cavity, that plays major role in resisting proximal migration of the humeral head. During elevation of the arm the deltoid pulls the head of humerus up and superiorly which is resisted by the rotator cuff muscles and the superior stability of the shoulder. Therefore, even with a torn rotator cuff muscles (supraspinatus) this component can resist the upward migration of the head of the humerus. The superior stability of the shoulder can be affected by the deficient superior glenoid and the biceps labral anchorage.

Adhesion-Cohesion: Adhesion-cohesion is a mechanism by which fluid on coated articular surfaces provides an intrinsic adherence between the articular surfaces. The adhesion-coherent mechanism may be affected by changes in the fluid chemistry due to inflammatory disease, loss of thickness of the articular surfaces due to degenerative disease, and alterations in the contact areas.

Glenohumeral Suction Cup: The glenohumeral suction cup effect depends upon the tendency for matched concave and convex surfaces with a flexible periphery to center and stabilize after expressing any intervening air and fluid, thereby forming a seal. Deficiencies of the glenoid labrum or of the margin of the glenoid can adversely affect this stabilizing mechanism.

Limited Joint Volume: The normal glenohumeral joint is a potential space which has minimal synovial fluid and has an inherent negative pressure. A sealed joint ensures an increase in this negative pressure with attempted distraction, thus increasing the joint reactive force independent of other muscular forces. The stability of the shoulder is decreased if the synovial fluid is increased due to trauma, inflammation, and laxity of the capsule.

Capsuloligamentous Restraints: The joint capsule and ligaments surrounding of it provides static stability not only during the elevation but also during the rest when the arm is at side. The other concepts of Masten and *et al.* (balance, concavity and compression, superior stability, adhesion-cohesion, glenohumeral suction cup, and limited joint volume) contribute to the stability particularly during the midrange but the capsuloligamentous restraints contribute to the stability throughout the range of motion. The glenohumeral ligaments are ideally positioned thickenings within the capsule that serve to check large forces encountered within the capsule during specific arm positions and activities. The laxity of the capsuloligamentous restraints produces instability.

Movements

The shoulder permits greatest mobility in almost all directions. The mobility is, however, at the expense of structural stability. The following important movements take place in the shoulder during overhead activities mentioned in Table 25.1.

Table 25.1

Movement	Plane	ROM	Muscles
Flexion	Sagittal	0°-180°	Prime movers - Deltoid (anterior) secondary movers-Biceps brachii, Pectrolis major
Extension	Sagittal	0°-45°	Prime movers - Deltoid (posterior) Secondary movers - Latissimus dorsi
Abduction	Frontal	0°-180°	Prime movers - Deltoid middle secondary movers - Supraspinatus
Adduction	Frontal	180°-0°	Prime movers - Latissimus dorsi secondary movers
External rotation	Transverse	0°-90°	Prime movers - Supraspinatus, infraspinatus
Internal rotation	Transverse	0°-80°	Prime movers - Subscapularis
Horizontal adduction		90°-45°	Prime movers - Pectoralis major

Rarely does a single muscle act in isolation at the shoulder complex. Muscles work in "Teams" to produce a highly coordinated action that is expressed over multiple joints. Because of the nature of the functional relationship among muscles, paralysis or weakness of any muscle often disrupts the natural kinematics sequencing of the shoulder.

Scapulohumeral Rhythm

In 1934, the term scapulohumeral rhythm was introduced by Codman to describe the smooth, integrated movement of the humerus, scapula and clavicle.

During elevation of the arm smooth coordinated 120 degrees movement occurs at the humerus and 60 degrees at the scapula to the total movement of 180 degrees of elevation of the arm (Fig. 25.2).

Scapulohumeral rhythm is divided into three phase as initial phase (0 and 60 degrees), middle phase or critical phase (60 to 140 degrees) and final phase (140 to 180 degrees).

Initial Phase of Elevation: The initial phase of elevation is referred as setting phase of the elevation. The instantaneous centre of rotation (ICR) is located near the root of the scapula. The relative contribution from scapula rotation during this phase is considerably less than from glenohumeral (3.29:1). The pull of deltoid produces an upward shear force on the humeral head, which is counteracted by the transverse

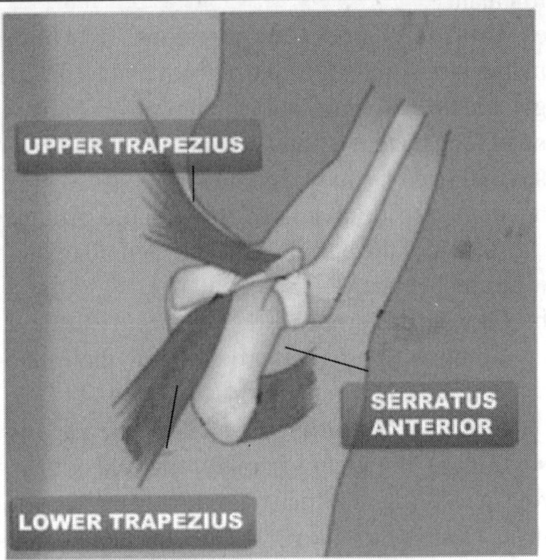

Fig. 25.2: Scapulohumeral rhythm

compressive forces of the rotator cuff muscles (primarily by the subscapularis). The sternoclavicular joint permits movement at the scapula by rotating 4 degrees for each of 10 degree rotation of the shoulder abduction. Movement in the acromioclavicular joint occurs in the thirty degrees of the initial phase, thereafter; it ceases and reoccurs at 135 degree of elevation.

Middle Phase of Elevation: This phase is also known as critical phase as shear and transverse forces are generated at the peak level in this phase. The deltoid continues to produce upward shear and noted maximum at 110 degrees. Supraspinatus activity peaks at 100 degrees of elevation and rapidly diminishes thereafter whereas subscapularis activity decreases substantilly after 130 degrees. In addition to that the movement at the scapula takes place more than the humeral rotation.

The resultant acting force at 90 degrees of elevation with shear and compressive forces equal. The greatest relative motion at scapula occurs between 80 and 140 degrees of arm abduction and the rotation of glenohumeral to scapulohumeral has been calculated to be 71 to 1 in the critical phase of elevation. This important external rotation of the scapula during critical phase is mainly provided by the force couple generated by trapezius upper fibers and levator scapulae (upper portion) and serratus anterior and lower fibres of trapezius (lower portion). During the middle phase of elevation and ICR of scapula begins to migrates towards the acromioclavicular joint. Movement in the acromioclavicular joint reoccurs after 135 degrees.

Final Phase (140-180 degrees): The movement at the scapula decreases considerably during this phase and mostly movement occur at the glenohumeral joint at the ratio of 1:3.49. the ratator force arm of the upper trapezius muscles are just supportive at this stage, however lower trapezius muscles and serratus anterior continues to increasease in activity during the final phase of elevation acting as upward rotator and opposing the force of the upper and middle trapezius.

ANTERIOR INSTABILITY

The term "shoulder instability" constitutes a spectrum of disorders that includes dislocation, subluxation and laxity. Anterior instability is the most common form of glenohumeral instability and may be associated with nerve injury. The shoulder may dislocate anteriorly, posteriorly or inferiorly. Multidirectional instability is the combination of two or more than one instability.

Laxity: Laxity is defined as an unwanted translation of the head of humerus with symptoms. However, laxity may be considered as a normal translation of the head of humerus in the glenoid fossa if it is asymptomatic.

Subluxation: Subluxation is a partial loss of the articulation to the degree that symptoms are produced. It is caused by repetitive trauma, or direct blow to the shoulder.

Dislocation: Dislocation is defined as complete loss of the humeral articulation with the glenoid fossa as a result of acute trauma or seizures. The shoulder may dislocate anteriorly, posteriorly or inferiorly.

Anterior Laxity or Instability in Overhead Athletes

During elevation of the arm the head of humerus is maintained in the glenoid fossa by the static and dynamic stabilizers. The shoulder sacrifices stability for the mobility and, as a result is the most common unstable joint, with over 90% instability occurring to anteriorly. Anterior instability is an unwanted translation of the head of the humerus anteriorly with respect to the glenoid fossa.

Over 90% instability of shoulder occur anteriorly, usually with the arm in abduction and external rotation. This position (abduction and external rotation) represents the "weakest position" of the glenohumeral biomechanically and is the "classic position" for anterior instability.

Overhead athletic activities require repetitive motions with the arm in at least 90° of flexion or abduction with an external rotation of the shoulder.

The throwing motion and its related biomechanics is divided into its six stages— windup, early cocking, late cocking, acceleration, deceleration and follow through. In late cocking when the body rapidly moves forward, the dominant shoulder achieves maximal abduction and external rotation. Significant torque and forces are placed on the anterior stabilizers of the shoulder. At the extreme elevation (flexion/

abduction) with external rotation head of humerus pushes anterior stabilizers (anterior joint capsule, anterior glenohumeral and coracohumeral ligaments). Prolonged repetitive stresses on the anterior stabilizers can cause hyperlaxity of the capsule and glenohumeral ligament (anterior stabilizers) and eventually there is an excessive anterior translation of the head of humerus. The posterior capsule becomes tight which limits the internal rotation (Fig. 25.3).

Due to anterior instability the rotator cuff muscles develop secondary inflammatory response (rotator cuff tendinitis). Rotator cuff tendinitis produces pain in the shoulder. The stabilizing ability of the rotator cuff muscles decreases. At the end, the shoulder joint looses its static and dynamic stability; there is excessive translation of the head of humerus, further contributing to the instability.

Clinical Features

Athletes usually complain pain in the anterior aspect of the shoulder joint. In the late cocking phase they experience apprehension and sometimes hold the shoulder with the non-dominant hand in the adduction position. Pain may radiate down the lateral arm. The internal rotation is decreased due to posterior joint capsule tightness. In neglected cases the range of motion may decrease in all three planes.

SHOULDER COMPLEX ASSESSMENT

Observation of the Shoulder Girdle: The shoulder girdle is observed from anterior, posterior and lateral views.

Anterior View: The shoulder girdle is viewed from anterior for:

(i) Swelling, subluxation and dislocation of glenohumeral, sternoclavicular, and acromio-clavicular joints; and

(ii) Wasting of pectoralis major, deltoid and biceps brachii.

Lateral View: The examiner should observe excessive protraction of the scapula and sulcus sign. A depression between humeral head and acromian arch indicates inferior subluxation of the head of humerous. The position of the head on the cervical spine is also viewed from lateral view.

Posterior View: The shoulder girdle is viewed from back for:

(i) Scapulothoracic joint: The medial border of the scapula extends from spinous process of second thoracic vertebra to spinous process of seventh vertebra. The inferior angle and medial border of the scapulae should be equidistance from the spine. The scapula rests on the thoracic wall. Weakness of serratus anterior allows medial border of scapula to move away from the thoracic wall which is known as winging of the scapula. Sometimes the parascapular muscles are not developed

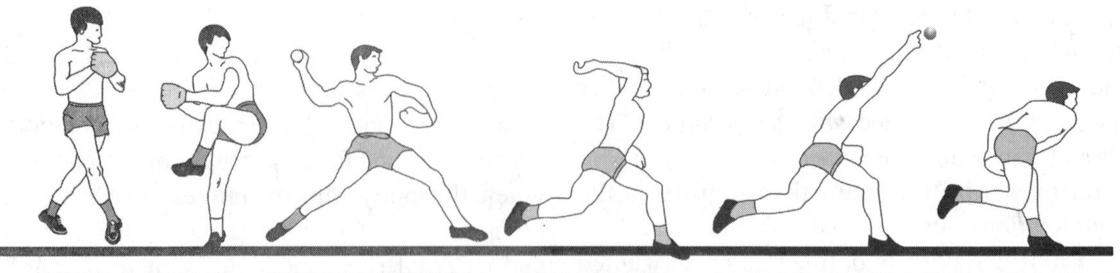

Fig. 25.3: Throwing phases

fully or they are replaced by fibrous band; allows scapula to displace superiorly (high), the condition is termed as Sprengel's scapula (high) or descended scapula. Usually affected scapula is smaller and medially rotated than normal.

(ii) Wasting or weakness of scapular muscles supraspinatus, infra spinatus and parascapular muscles serratus anterior muscle, rhomboid, trapezius middle and lower fibres is also viewed from posterior view.

Observation of Active Movements: Active range of motion of the glenohumeral and scapulothoracic joints should be observed carefully.

Glenohumeral: It is the most mobile joint of the body. Movements occur in all the three planes:

Resisted Isometric Movements: To reproduce the symptoms, the muscles are contracted isometrically against the resistance. Isometric movements elicit pain if there is tendinitis or impingement.

Passive Movements: Passive movements are performed to reproduce the symptoms if active movements fails to do so. The passive movements are performed to examine the end feel, muscle tightness and contracture. The movements are performed in relaxed position with proper stabilization of the scapula as lot of trick movements are possible in the shoulder joint.

Palpation: The glenohumeral, sterno-clavicular and acromioclavicular joints are examined for tenderness. Therapist can use thumb or pisiform aspect of the wrist to apply pressure on the joint, if patient complains pain the site is suspected for possible area of pain and symptoms.

Test for Anterior Instability: Stability of the shoulder is provided by static and dynamic stabilizers. Static stabilizers are the non-contractile structures such as coracohumeral ligament, glenohumeral ligament, acromioclavicular ligament, joint capsule and labrum itself. The dynamic stabilizers are basically rotator cuff muscles such as supraspinatus, infraspinatus, teres minor and subscapularis. Weakness or laxity of these stabilizers may cause shoulder instability and may produce symptoms such as pain, anxiety and apprehension. The following maneuvers are performed to test the stability of the shoulder:

- **Apprehension Test (Crank Test):** This test is performed to evaluate the anterior stability of the shoulder. Test may be performed in supine, standing or sitting position but supine lying is preferred over standing and sitting as patient feels more comfortable and relaxed (Fig. 25.4).

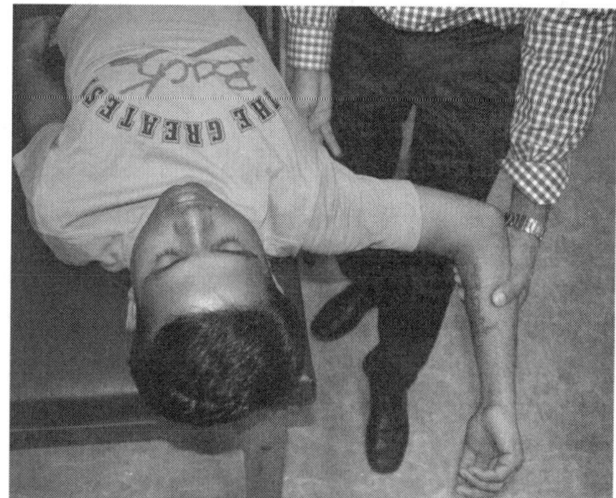

Fig. 25.4: Anterior apprehension test (crank test for anterior instability of the shoulder joint)

Position of Patient: Supine, shoulder at the edge of table.

Position of Examiner: Stands at the side of the shoulder which is being examined. The examiner holds the elbow of the patient at 90° of flexion and abducts the shoulder to 90° with slight horizontal abduction.

Procedure: While maintaining the above position the examiner brings the shoulder into external rotation, and further, abduction and horizontal abduction is added. This position simulates the most common position of sublaxation or dislocation in the patient with symptomatic anterior instability. In case of anterior instability the patient reacts by expressing concern or anxiety or apprehension, and sometimes, prevents the external rotation with other hand. This test produces pain in patients with subtle cases of anterior instability, but it does not produce true anxiety or apprehension. Pain is a suggestive but not diagnostic of anterior instability. For diagnosis of anterior instability patient must complain apprehension; therefore the test has modified into relocation and release test.

- **Relocation Test:** It is the extension of the anterior apprehension test. To perform this test the examiner places the shoulder joint in the apprehension position (abduction, horizontal abduction and external rotation). Until the patient feels apprehension or pain. While maintaining this position the examiner places the free hand on the anterior aspect of the shoulder joint and then the head of humerus is pushed posteriorly into the glenoid fossa. This relocates the head of humerus from subluxed position to glenoid fossa. If patient reports reduction or resolution in apprehension, then it confirms the anterior instability. After pushing the head of humerus into the glenoid fossa the apprehension disappears and now the shoulder can be abducted externally rotated and extended further (Fig. 25.5).

  Release Test: It is the sequence of the relocation test. When the posterior directed force is released gradually the symptoms of apprehension returns which further confirms the anterior instability of the shoulder joint (Fig. 25.6).

- **Anterior Drawer Test: Position of Patient:** Sitting with the arm hanging loosely.

  Position of Examiner: Standing at the side of shoulder joint. To test the right shoulder joint the examiner stabilizes the scapula with left hand and holds the head of humerus with right hand. While maintaining the position the

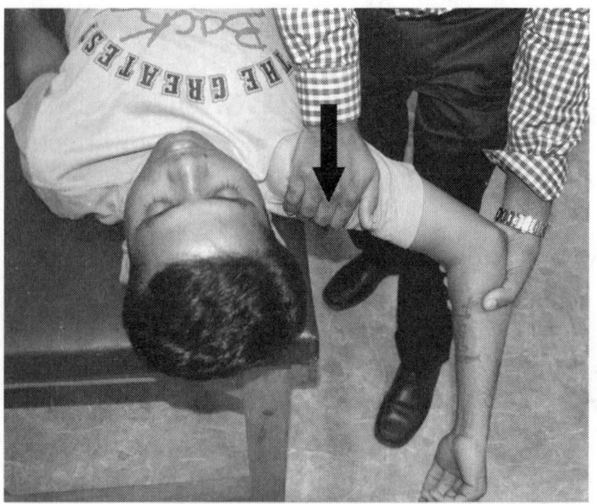

Fig. 25.5: Relocation test

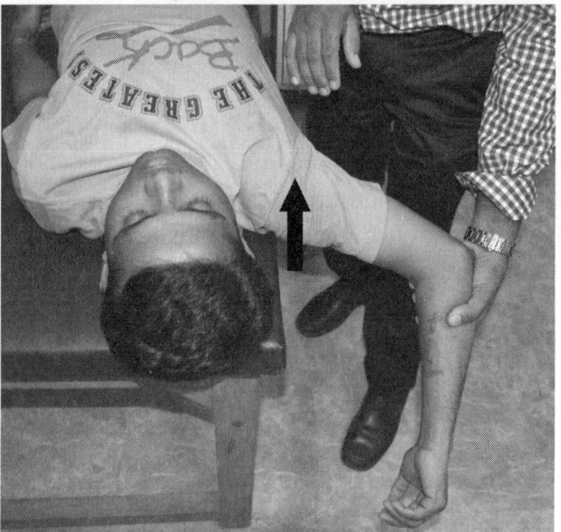

Fig. 25.6: Release test

head of humerus is pushed anteriorly. In normal subject the head of humerus may be translated anteriorly upto 25% of the width of the glenoid. If the head of humerus can be translated more than 25% of the width of the glenoid then test is considered positive for anterior instability. Patient may complain apprehension. To test the posterior instability a posterior directed force is applied to translate the head of humerus posteriorly. In normal subjects the head of humerus can be translated posteriorly upto 50% of the width of the scapula. In case of more than 50% translation of the width of the glenoid a posterior instability may be considered (Fig. 25.7).

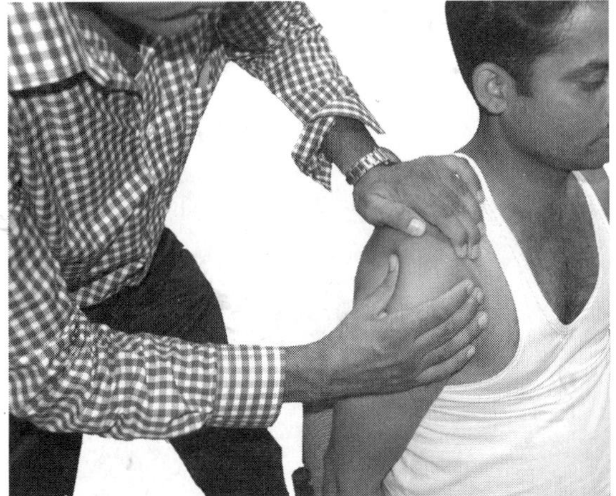

Fig. 25.7: Anterior drawer test

- **Load and Shift Test:** This test is similar to the anterior drawer test but it is performed in supine position with slight abduction range. **Position of Patient:** Supine, shoulder is slightly out of the plinth with slight abduction and extension. **Position of Therapist:** Standing at the side which is being examined, facing the shoulder joint (anteriorly). To examine the patient's right shoulder, the examiner stabilizes the scapula (glenoid) with the left hand, and grasps the head of humerus with right hand (Figs. 25.8a-b).

Procedure: While maintaining above position (slight abduction and extension) an anterior directed force is applied with the right hand to translate anteriorly. The amount of translation is assessed as in the anterior drawer test. The position of shoulder may be changed until the position of greatest laxity is found. For posterior instability the head of humerus is pushed posteriorly and an amount of translation is assessed as in the posterior drawer test. The test may be performed in various position until the position of greatest laxity is found.

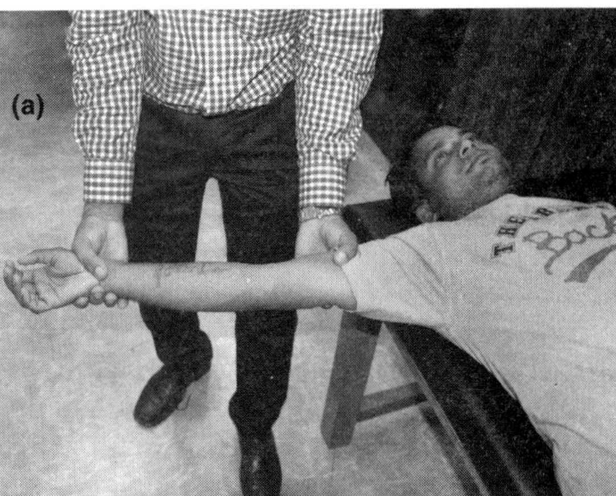

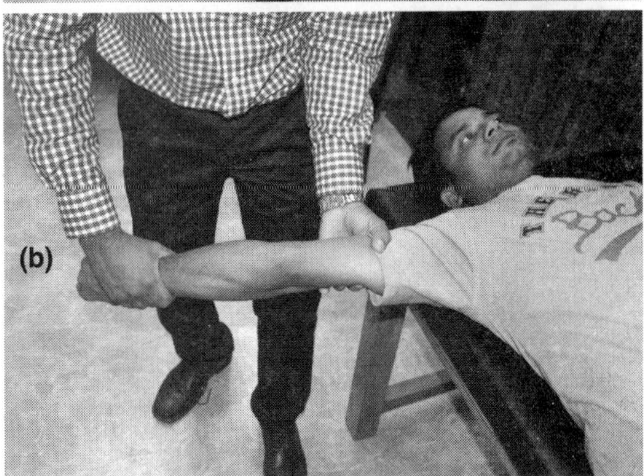

Figs. 25.8a-b: Load and shift test

Management

The goals of the therapist are of restoring shoulder stability (static and dynamic), and reducing pain, apprehension and improving strength of rotator cuff and parascapular muscles.

Immobilization: The patients with anterior instability rarely require shoulder immobilization. It may be advised if the patients complaint pain and apprehension in the painful arc with rotator cuff tendinopathy. The shoulder is immobilized in the sling just to avoid the overhead activities. However, passive range of motion may be performed throughout the range of motions.

Precaution: The athlete must take precautions to avoid stress on the anterior stabilizers of the shoulder such as anterior joint capsule, anterior glenohumeral ligament and coracohumeral ligament. Patient must avoid extreme ranges of elevation with external rotation until shoulder achieves pain free stability. Shoulder hyperextension is contraindicated as it stretches the anterior stabilizers.

Relief of Pain: To decrease pain, cold packs or hot packs can be used for 15-20 minutes per treatment session, thrice or twice daily. Interferential therapy with the frequency of 80-100 Hz over the shoulder may be beneficial in relieving pain and symptoms.

Strengthening Exercises

Sub maximal isometric exercises of biceps, deltoid, rotator cuff muscles, and parascapular muscles are started in pain free range. These muscles may also be strengthened with the surge faradic currents.

Rotator Cuff Strengthening: Rotator cuff strengthening should be started in the pain free range of motion. Isometric exercises in arm adducted position should be preferred over the overhead. For external rotators patient stands close to the wall with elbow flexion to 90 degrees. The dorsal aspect of the hand and forearm rests on the wall. While maintaining the position in the shoulder adduction patient rotates the shoulder externally against the wall for six seconds. Several repetitions of isometric contraction may be performed to strengthen the supraspinatus and infraspinatus muscles. To strengthen the subscapularis muscle (internal rotator) the patient places the palmer aspect of hand and forearm on the wall. While maintaining the shoulder in adduction, the patient rotates the shoulder internally against wall. Several repetitions of isometric contractions may be performed (Figs. 25.9a-h).

With the improvement in the sign and symptoms the exercise is progressed to the open kinetic chain exercise with the tubing, dumbbells or theraband. In standing position the therapist

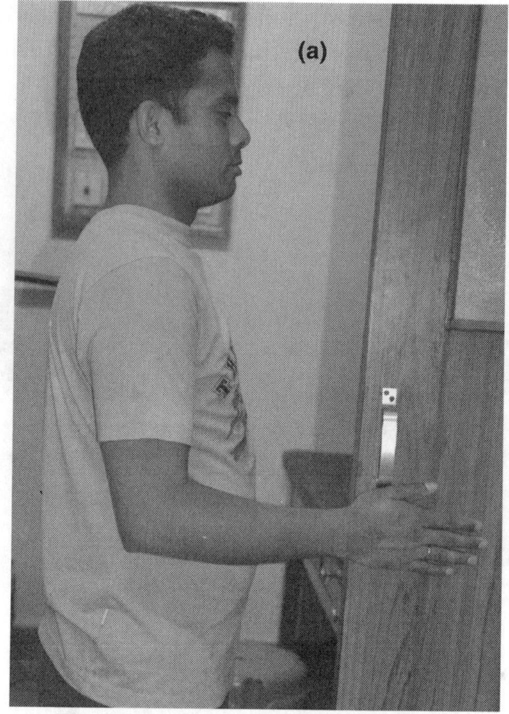

Fig. 25.9a: External rotators isometric strengthening against the wall in standing

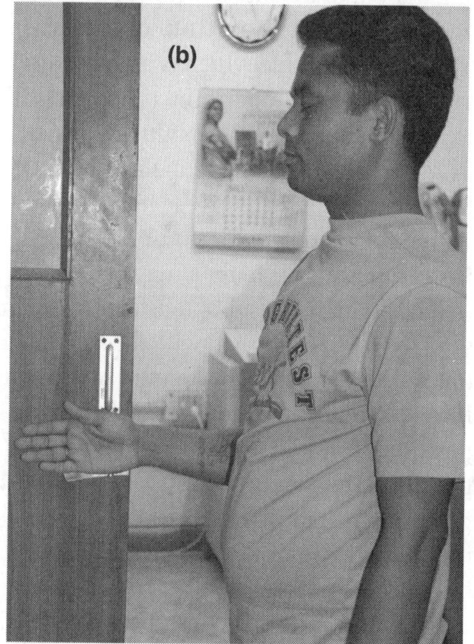

Fig. 25.9b: Internal rotators isometric strengthening against the wall in standing

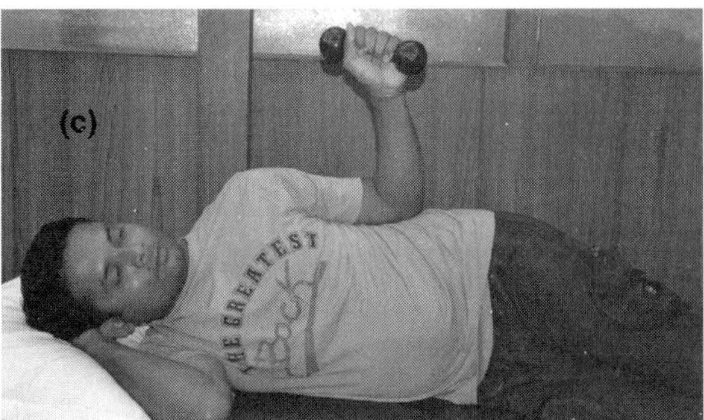

Fig. 25.9c: External rotators strengthening in side lying with dumbbell

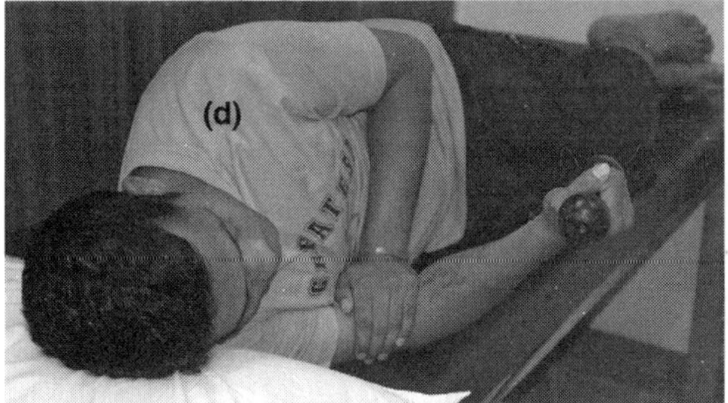

Fig. 25.9d: Internal rotators isometric strengthening in side lying

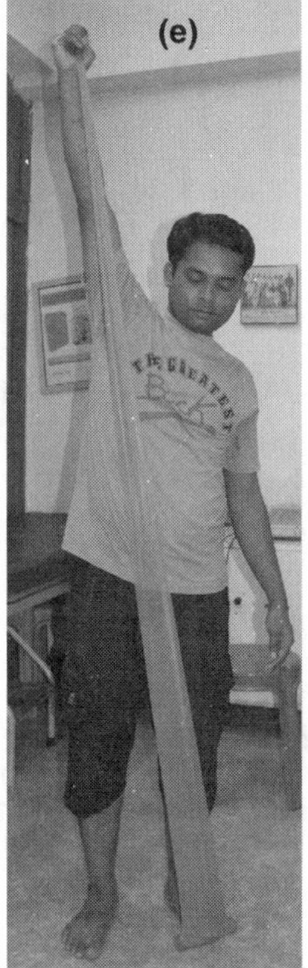

Fig. 25.9e: Di flexion pattern with theraband

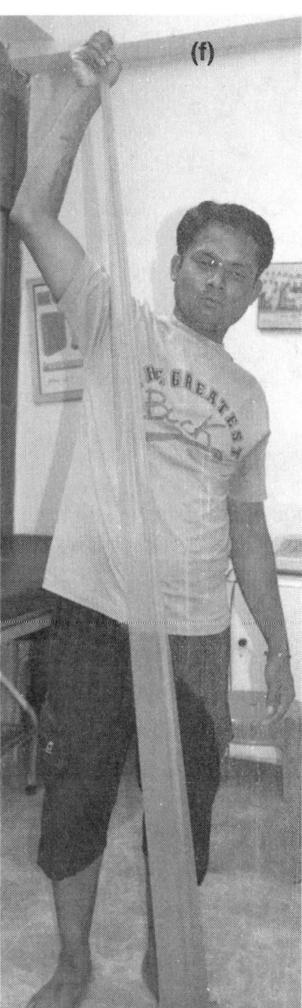

Fig. 25.9f: Diextension pattern with theraband

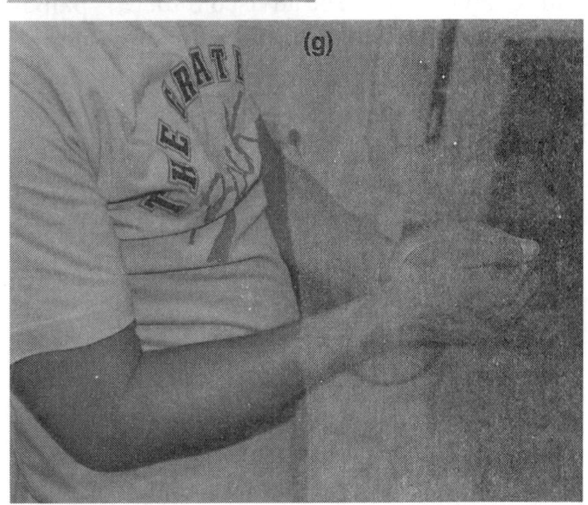

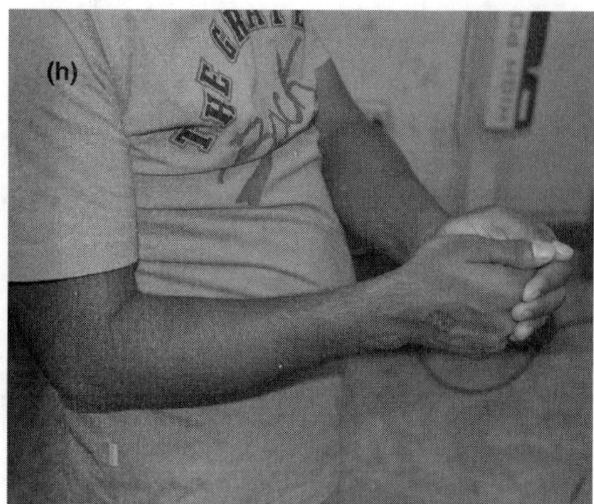

Fig. 25.9g-h: Self strengthening with resistance in sitting with elbow flexion. Other hand grasps the distal forearm

places one end of the theraband under the opposite foot and holds the other end of the theraband. While maintaining the position the shoulder is flexed, abducted and rotated externally in the diagonal 2 pattern. Several repetitions may be performed.

Scapula Stabilizers Strengthening: To strengthen the levator scapulae, trapezius and rhomboids the patient lies in a sitting position with both the arms at the side of body. Patient holds the elbows with the hands. While maintaining the position the patient retracts both the shoulders. This exercise should be advised if there is pain in the overhead activities. As the symptoms improve the exercise is progressed to the prone lying. Patient lies prone with the shoulder out of the edge of the plinth and arm hanging downward. While maintaining the position patient elevates the arm in sagittal plane upto full range. The end range is held for at least six seconds followed by relaxation. In the next step the exercise is performed in the scaption plane, and then in the horizontal. Several repetitions are performed until the muscles go in a fatigue state. Exercises of both the scapula stabilizers may be performed in the same position with little modification. In prone

position the head is taken out of the plinth. While maintaining the position of the head in line with the spine, both the shoulders are elevated in the scaption plane. With improvement of the strength the exercise may be performed with the light dumbbell (Figs. 25.10a-g).

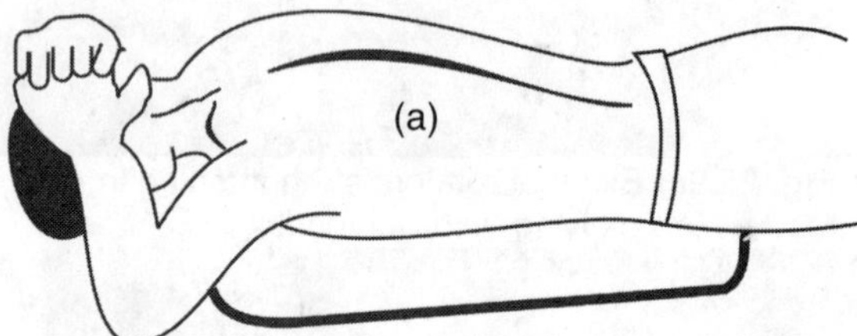

Fig. 25.10a: Trapezius and rhomboids strengthening, a-prone, head slightly out of the couch and hands on the occiput. Patient raises the elbows above the shoulder level and holds for the count of six. Thirty repetitions with brief rests between each ten repetitions. This exercise helps in strengthening of the rhomboid and middle trapezius

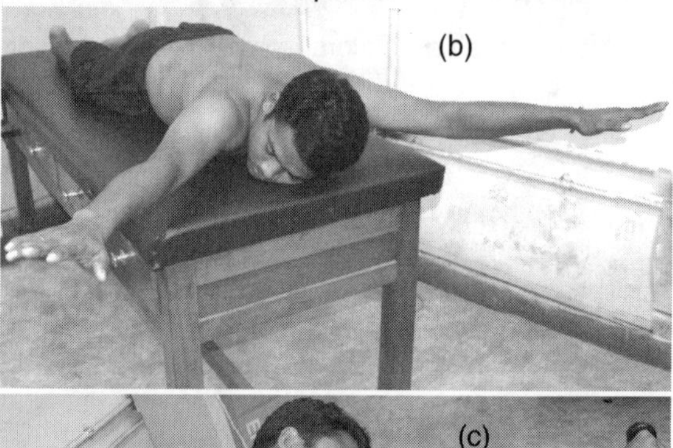

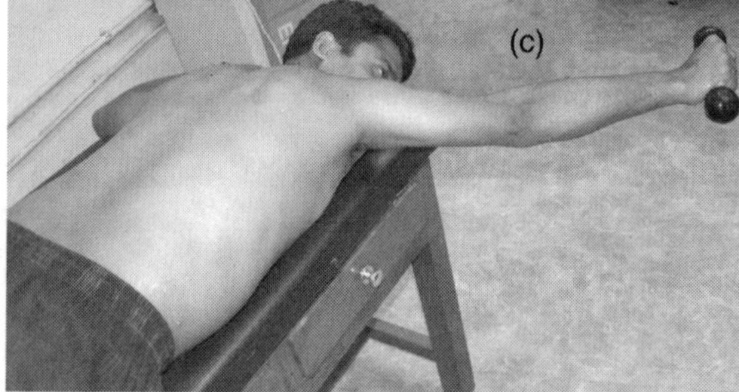

Fig. 25.10b-c: Prone, head is slightly out of the edge of the couch, shoulders are raised in a scaption plane with elbow extension. With the improvement over the time in the strength of the muscles the patient can lift the shoulders in scaption plane with the dumbbell. Thirty repetitions with brief rests between each ten repetitions

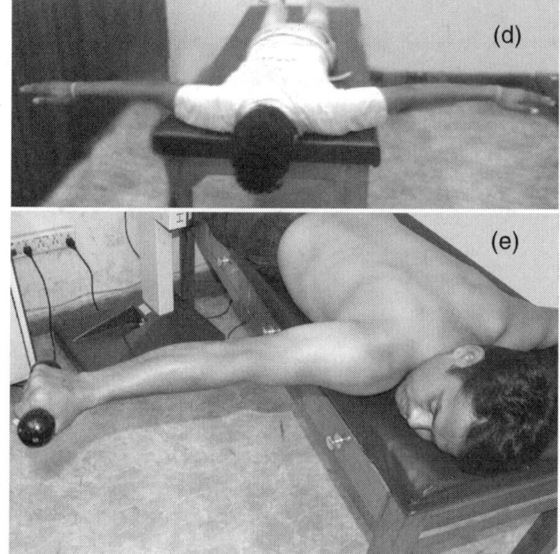

Fig. 25.10d-e: Prone, head is slightly out of the edge of the couch. Shoulders are raised horizontally to the level of shoulder blades. Thirty repetitions with brief rests between each ten repetitions. This exercise helps in strengthening of the middle trapezius. With the improvement over the time in the strength of the muscle the exercise can be done with the dumbbells

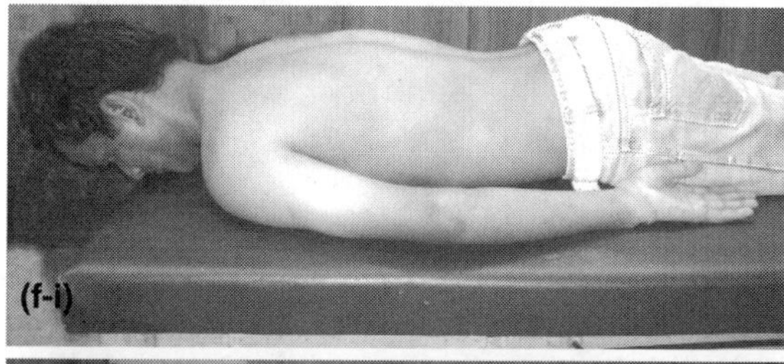

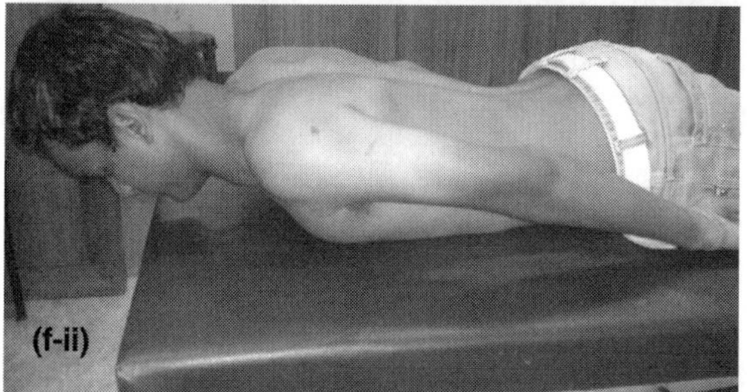

Fig. 25.10f(i-ii): Prone with both the hands at the side of the body. Patient retracts the shoulders as much as possible without changing the position of the hands. With the improvements in the strength, the therapist can apply resistance against the retraction. Thirty repetitions with brief rests between each ten repetitions

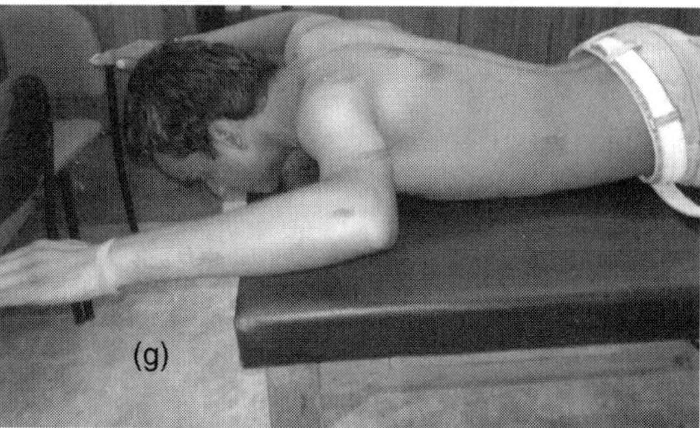

Fig. 25.10g: Prone with head slightly out of the edge of the couch. Elbows flexed to 90 degrees. Patient raises the shoulder horizontally above the shoulder blade level

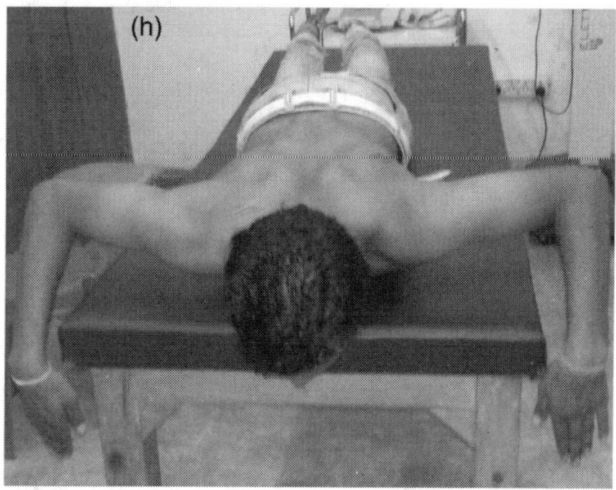

Fig. 25.10h: Rowing, rhomboid strengthening

Strengthening of the serratus anterior muscle is one of the major goals of the rehabilitation as its function is not only the stabilizing scapula on the thoracic wall but also plays important role in external rotation of the scapula. To strengthen the serratus anterior muscle the exercise should progress from minimal load. The patient lies in a quadruped with the hips and shoulders directly on the knees and hands respectively. Then the patient lifts the opposite hand off the plinth bringing to the level of the shoulder. The supported shoulder should not alter any position. While maintaining the quadruped position patient moves hips and shoulders forward on the knees and hands and then the opposite hand is lifted off the ground upto the level of the shoulder. In further progression patient is positioned in a quadruped position and hips are brought to the neutral by bending the knees while the shoulders remain on the hands. In the last step of exercise the patient assumes the quadruped position and then brings the hips and knees to the neutral position, now patient stationed on the hands and toes. The chest is brought to the floor by bending the elbows. Several repetitions are performed till the muscles fatigue (Figs. 25.11a-i).

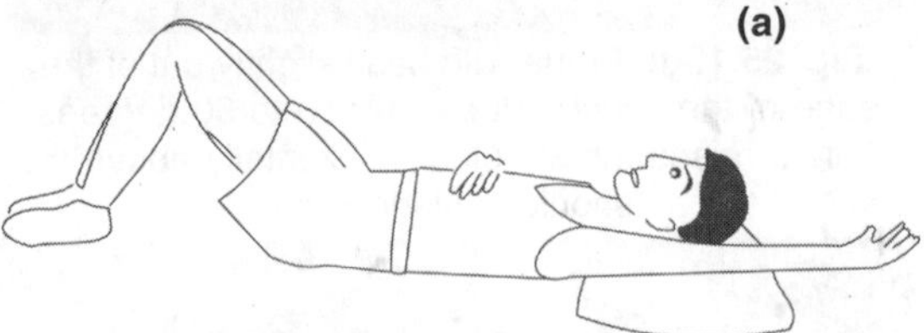

Fig. 25.11a: Serratus anterior strengthening, a-supine with knees flexion. Patient flexes and extends the shoulders alternately throughout the range of motion in a controlled manner

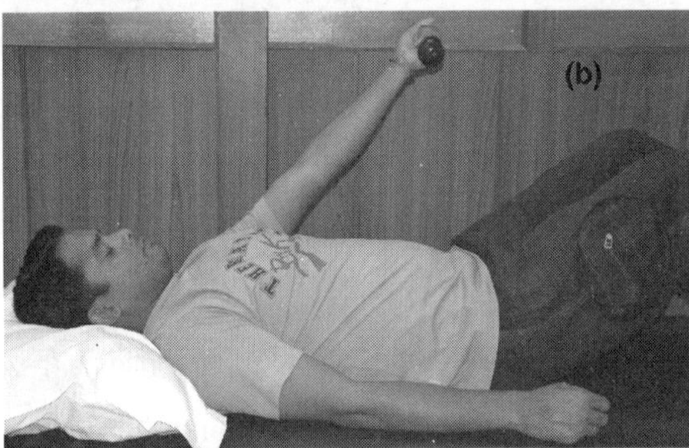

Fig. 25.11b: Supine with knees flexion. Patient flexes and extends the shoulder joint throughout the range of in a controlled manner with the dumbbell

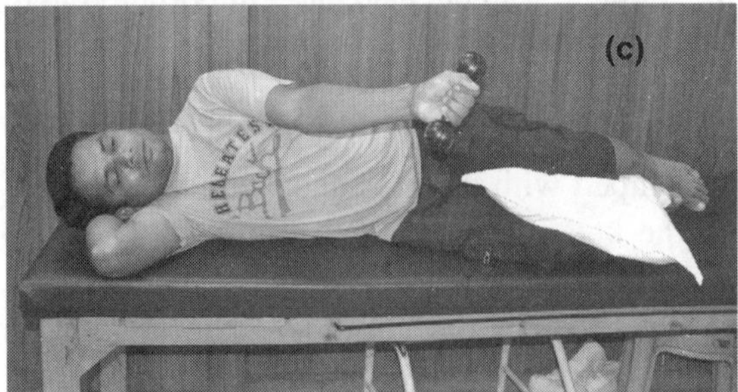

Fig. 25.11c: Side lying with pillows under the uppermost leg flexed. Patient flexes and extends the shoulder joint throughout the range of in a controlled manner in a scaption plane

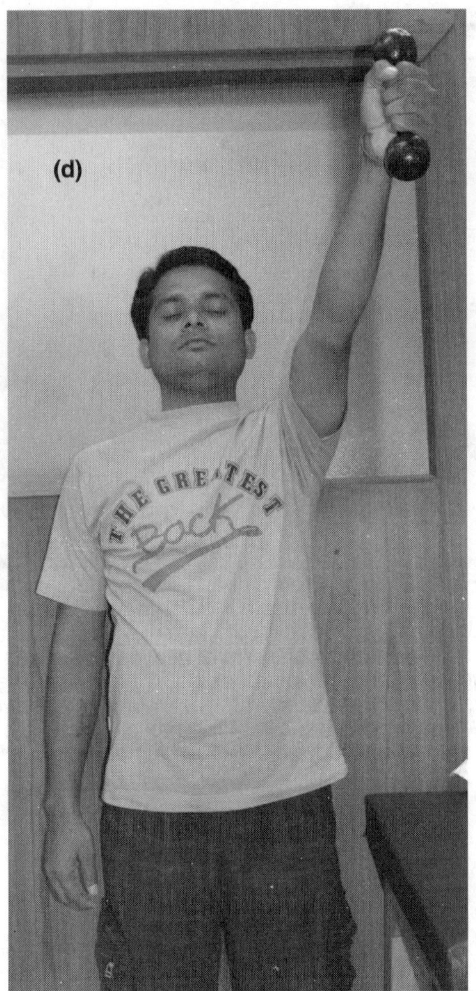

Fig. 25.11d: Sitting or standing with back supported on the wall. Patient flexes and extends the shoulder joint throughout the range of in a controlled manner with the dumbbell

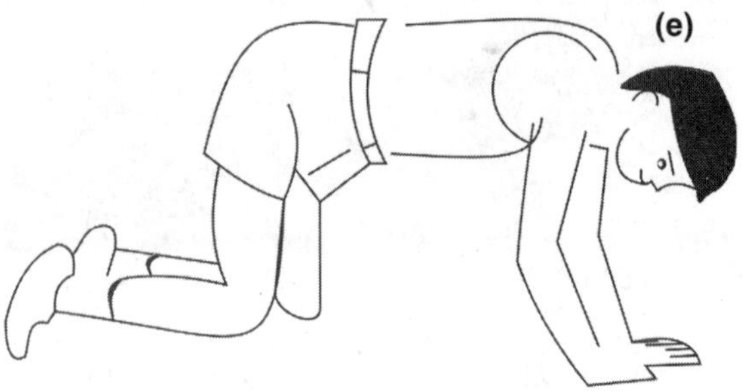

Fig. 25.11e: Quadruped position with hips directly over knees and shoulders directly over the hands

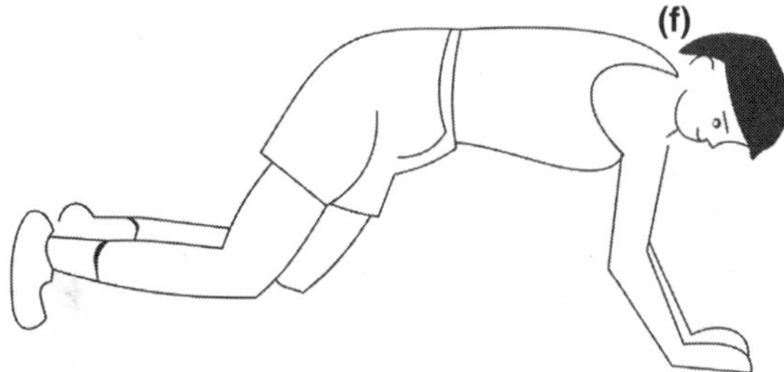

Fig. 25.11f: Quadruped position with hips slightly in front of the knees and shoulders directly over the hands

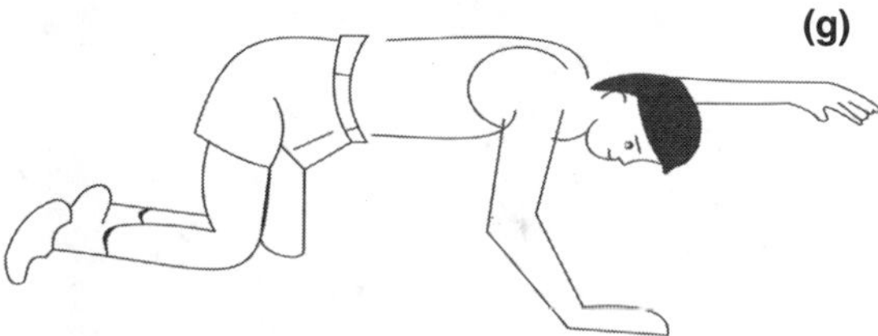

Fig. 25.11g: Quadruped position with hips slightly in front of the knees and shoulders directly over the hands and patient raises the arms alternately to the level of the shoulder

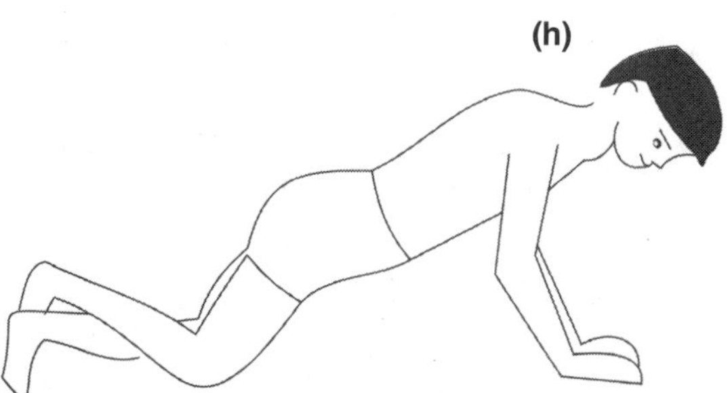

Fig. 25.11h: The weight of the body remains on the knees and hands

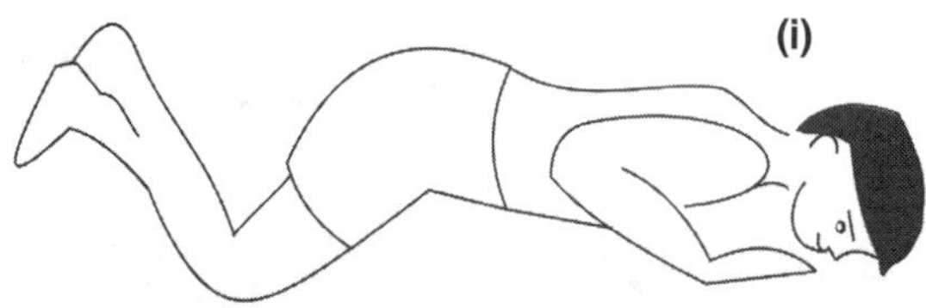

Fig. 25.11i: Push ups, while maintaining the position of the spine and hips at neutral, the patient slowly lowers the body towards the floor by flexing the elbow joints

Deltoid Strengthening: In standing position the patient abducts the shoulder with or without the dumbbell (Figs. 25.12a-e).

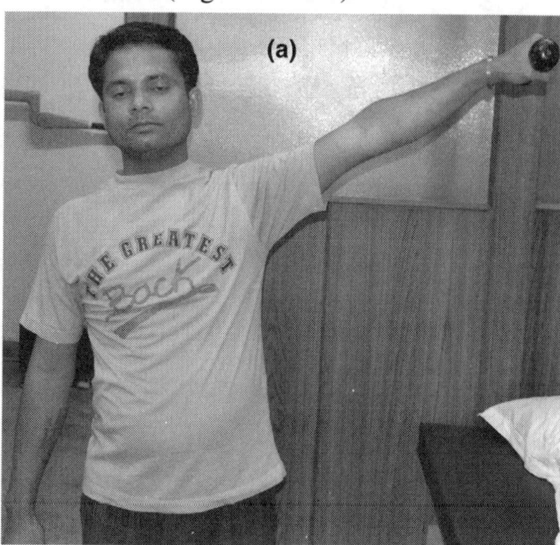

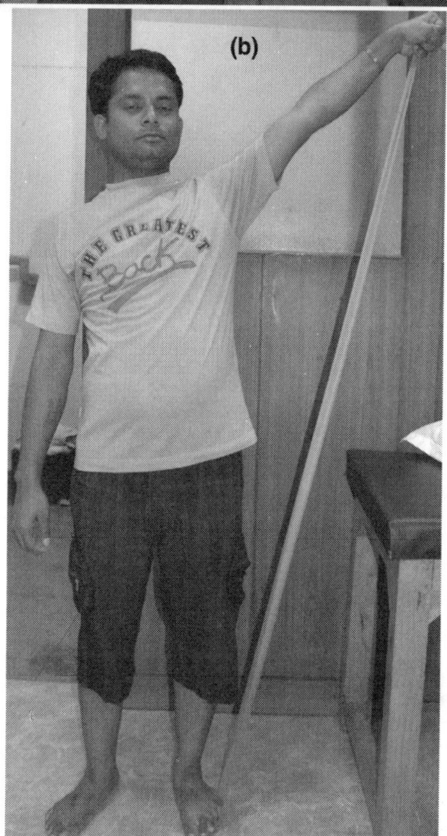

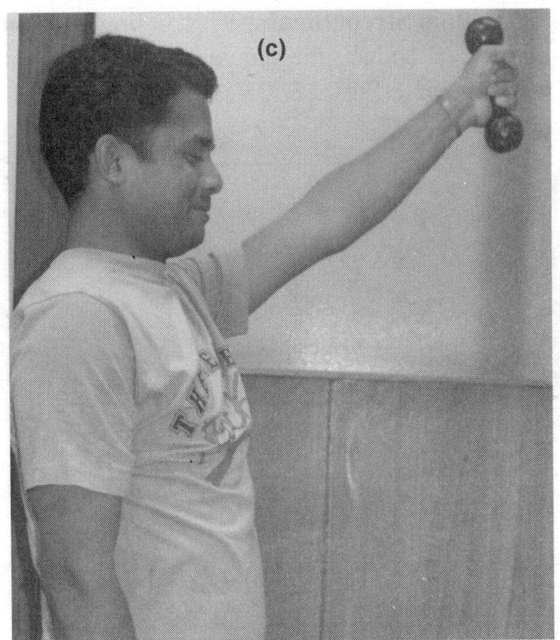

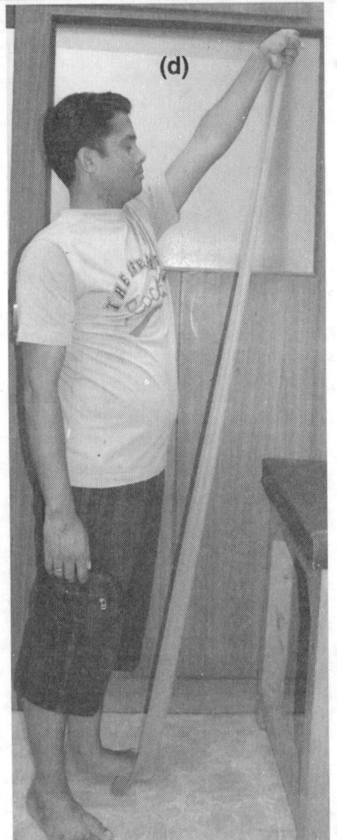

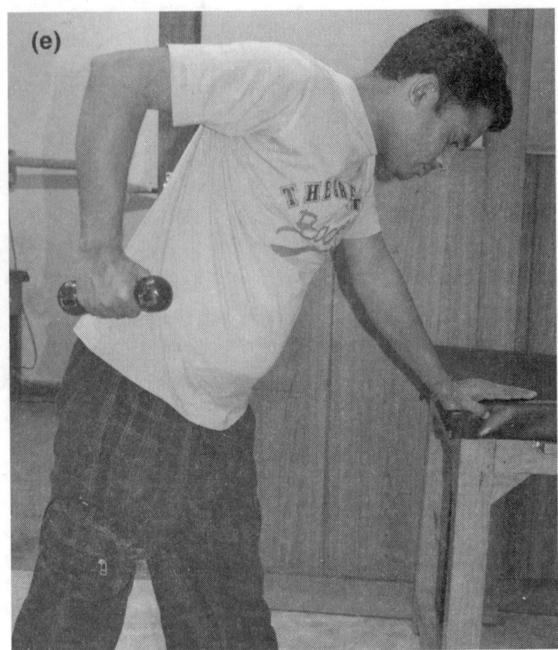

Figs. 25.12(a-e): Deltoid strengthening

Biceps Strengthening: In standing or sitting position with the arm adducted the elbow joint is flexed with the appropriate weight of dumbbell (Figs. 25.13a-b).

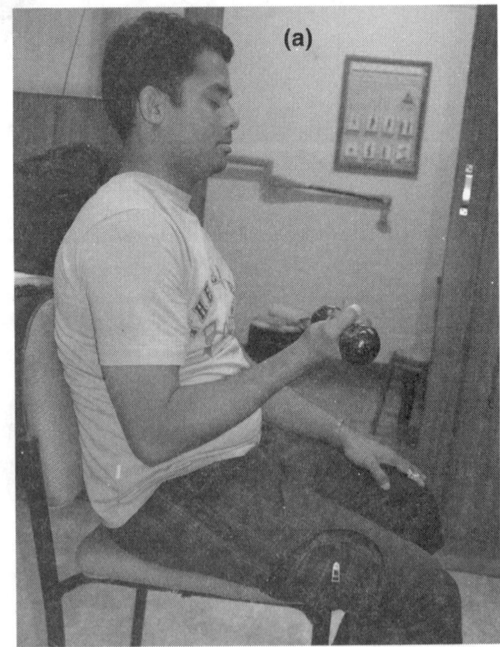

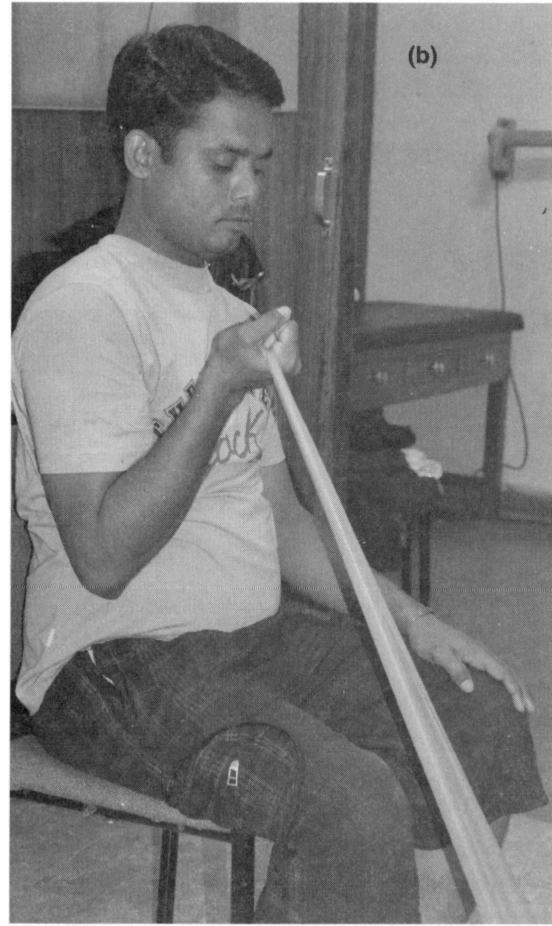

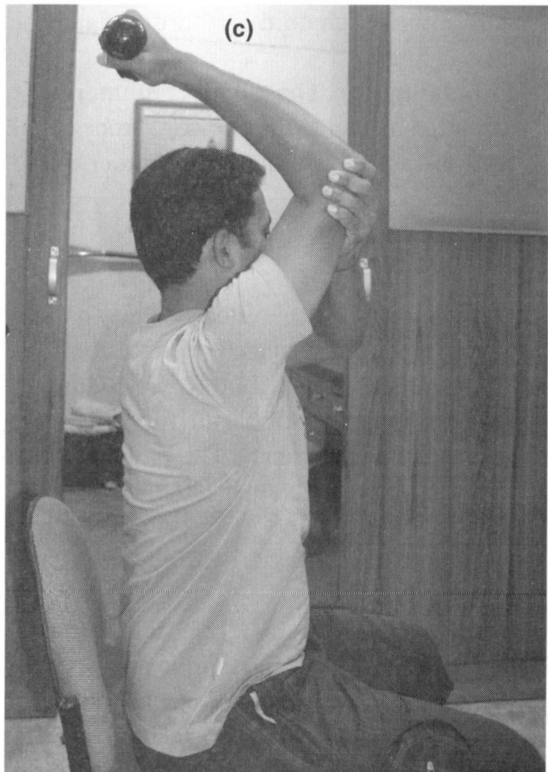

Figs. 25.13(a-b): Biceps strengthening

Triceps Strengthening: In standing or sitting position with shoulder full flexion the elbow joint is extended and flexed with the appropriate weight of dumbbell (Figs. 25.13c-d).

ANTERIOR DISLOCATION OF SHOULDER

Anterior dislocation of the shoulder is complete loss of articulation between the head of humerus and glenoid fossa. The head of humerus is displaced anteriorly as the anterior stabilizers of glenohumeral joint disrupts. Anterior dislocation is of three types as described below:

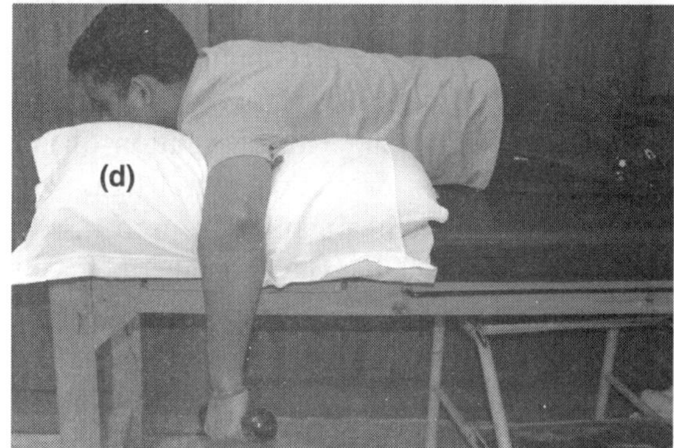

Figs. 25.13(c-d): Triceps strengthening

a. **Sub-Coracoid:** It is the most common type of anterior dislocation in which humeral head is displaced anteriorly with respect to the glenoid, and inferior to coracoid process.

b. **Subglenoid:** The head of humerus is displaced anteriorly below the glenoid fossa. These types of dislocations are associated with either a glenoid fracture or anterior glenoid rim.

c. **Subclavicular:** The head of humerus is displaced medial to the coracoid process and rests just inferior to the lower border of the clavicle.

Pathophysiology

The patients with shoulder dislocation may present with many findings, such as Bankart lesion, Hill Sachs lesion, anterior glenoid rim damage, capsular redundancy, subscapularis deficiency, and glenoid fossa deficiency. These findings can occur alone or in combination with other lesions. Sometimes few patients may present with a history of anterior dislocation with absence of any pathological findings.

a. **Bankart Lesion:** In 1923, Bankart had described the "essential lesion" in patients with post traumatic anterior glenohumeral instability as the "detachment of the capsule from the fibrocartilaginous glenoid ligament". Avulsion of the anteroinferior glenoid labrum at its attachment to inferior glenohumeral ligament (IGHL) causes an obligatory concomitant capsular disruption, with elongation of an IGHL. The inferior glenohumeral ligament heals in redundant position in upto thirty percent patients; but no healing takes place in the disrupted avulsed anteroinferior glenoid labrum, which is the primary cause of recurrent dislocation of the shoulder. However, no single lesion is responsible for the recurrent dislocations of the traumatized shoulders. Baker *et al.* advised a system of classification for the Perthes-Bankart lesion as follows:

- Type I-Pure capsular lesion.
- Type II-Partial labral detachment.
- Type III-Complete detachment of the inferior glenohumeral labral complex.

b. **Hill Sachs Lesion:** This type of lesion occurs upto 40% in patients with anterior dislocation

and upto 80% of recurrent anterior dislocations. The indentation fracture of the posterolateral humeral head occurs during this type of anterior dislocation of the shoulder. The head of humerus impacts against relatively hard anterior glenoid. Sometimes this lesion is confused with the normal bare area of the posteroinferior aspect of humeral head (Fig. 25.14).

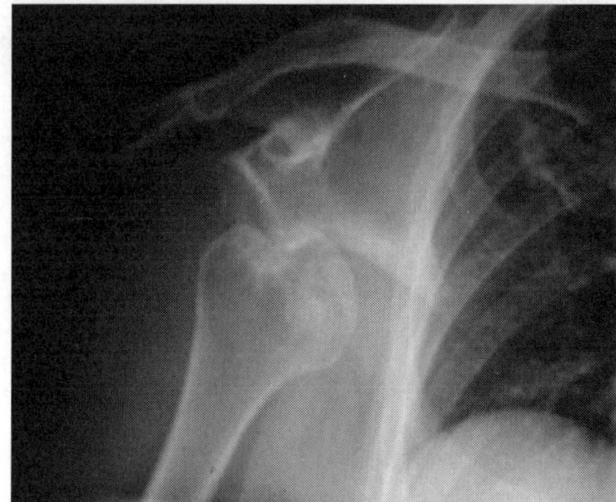

Fig. 25.14: Hill Sachs lesion

Epidemiology

First time shoulder dislocation can occur at any age although they tend to occur most frequently in the second and sixth decades. However, an average age of initial shoulder dislocation is in early thirties. Twenty-five percent patients with shoulder dislocation present with the family history of the similar problem (Fig. 25.15).

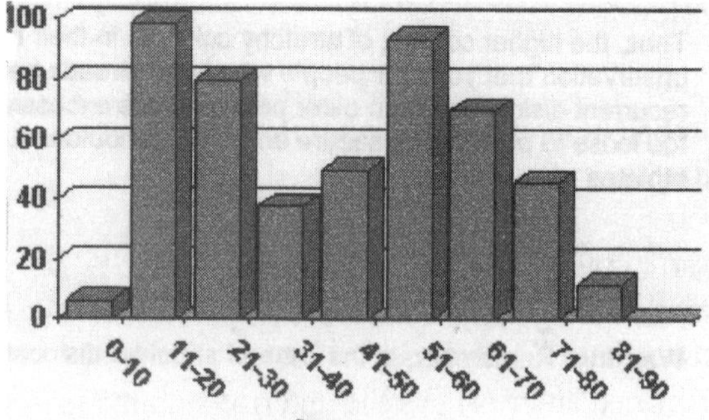

Fig. 25.15: Rate of shoulder dislocation according to the age

Mechanism

The shoulder joint may dislocate when a strong force such as a traumatic injury puts an excessive load on the labrum, capsule and ligaments. Ninety-five percent shoulder dislocations are resulted from a sudden wrenching movement during sport, by falling on to an outstretched arm, and from motor vehicle accidents. An individual falls on an outstretched hand, forcing the arm into abduction and external rotation, levering the humeral head out of the glenoid fossa. This is the most vulnerable position of the shoulder for dislocation.

Clinical Features

Patient usually complaints apprehension or instability and often feel that he or she is at the risk of shoulder dislocation. They learn the positions that reproduce and ease the symptoms and tend to lean towards the affected side. The arm is held in the adduction and internal rotation positions by the contralateral extremity.

Patient experiences pain in the anterior aspect of the shoulder joint. It aggravates in abduction with external rotation and slight extension. These positions put excessive load on the joint capsule and ligament (IGHL). In long standing cases weakness and atrophy of the scapular and para-scalar muscles with loss of motion in all three planes may also be seen.

Physical Examination

The shoulder joint is examined for pain, swelling, erythema, temperature, crepitus and range of motion. To test the anterior instability, anterior apprehension (crank test), relocation release, and anterior drawer tests should be performed as these tests are having good sensitivity. The cross chest adduction test is also helpful in diagnosing anterior dislocation. In patients with anterior shoulder dislocation cross chest adduction will be limited and painful.

Imaging Studies

X-rays are taken in three views such as true AP view also known as Grashey view, scapula view and axillary view to confirm the anterior dislocation. Internal and external rotation views may also be taken as these provide oblique visualization of the shoulder joint, with the humeral head overlapping the glenoid rim. Stryker-Notch view is taken to confirm the Hill Sachs lesions. It is obtained with the patient supine. This view provides good details of the posterolateral margin of the humeral head. MRI is the choice of the imaging modality for soft tissue injury. It has 91% sensitive in detecting capsule-labral injury in the early post-dislocation phase (Fig. 25.16).

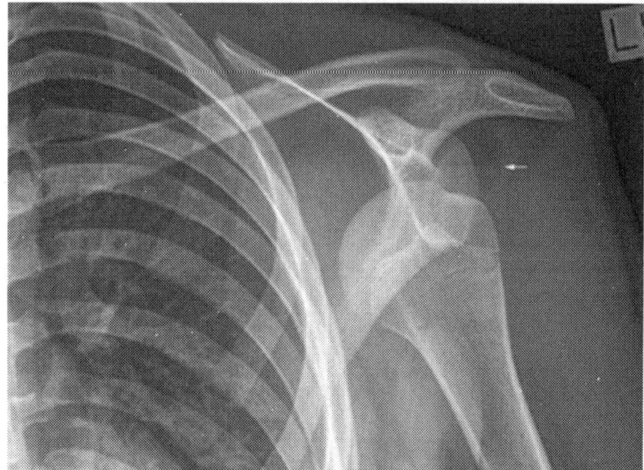

Fig. 25.16: X-ray anterior shoulder dislocation

Management

1. **Shoulder Reduction:** The dislocated shoulder is reduced as soon as possible. There are several techniques of reducing the shoulder. Early treatment of the shoulder dislocation should be directed to eliminate the static structure stretch, compression on the nerves, and muscle spasm. Some patient's shoulder reduced without the medication while others require muscle relaxants or anaesthesia. Many techniques have described by the physicians since hippocrates to reduce the shoulder dislocation few techniques are described as under:

a. *Hippocrates Technique*: Hippocrates described the technique where physician placed his foot on the chest wall and used it as a counter traction. The arm is rotated internally and externally to disengage the head of the humerus.

b. *Stimson's Technique*: The patient is positioned prone with the dislocated arm hanging freely out of the edge of the table. Approximately 5-6 pound weight is tied on the wrist. The shoulder is reduced after 15-20 minutes.

c. *Milch's Technique*: The patient is positioned on the back. The dislocated arm is flexed and externally rotated. The therapist places his thumb on the head of humerus and gently pushes the head of humerus into the glenoid fossa (Fig. 25.17).

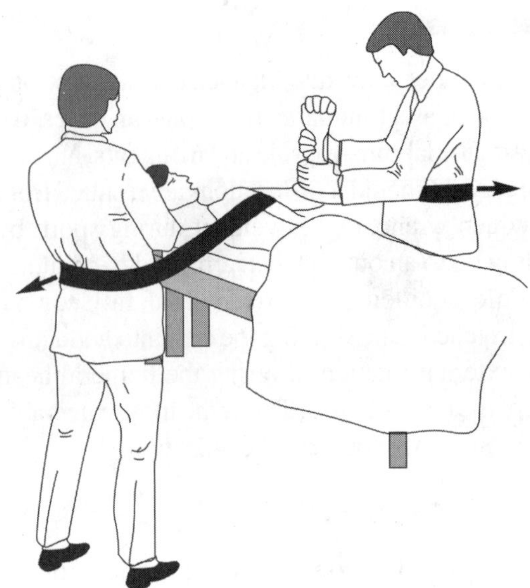

Fig. 25.18: Matsen's preferred method

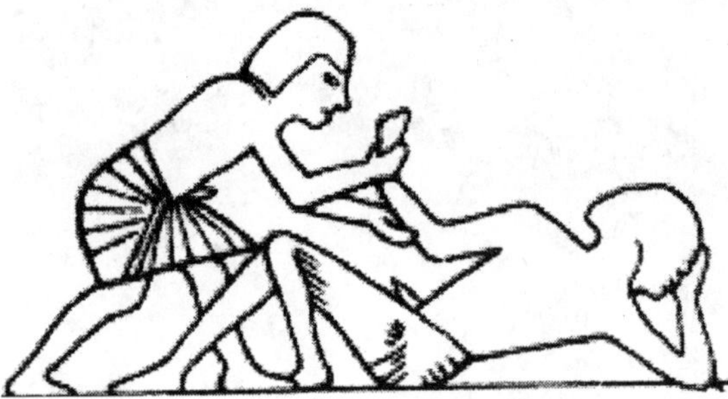

Fig. 25.17: Milch's technique of shoulder reduction

d. *Matsen's Preferred Method*: The patient lies on the back. An assistant stands at the normal shoulder. A belt is wrapped around the chest of the patient and waist of the assistant. The practitioner stands at the dislocated shoulder near the waist of the patient. The practitioner holds the patient's elbow with flexion at 90°. A second belt is wrapped around the practitioner's waist and looped over the patient's forearm. While maintaining the position the practitioner leans backward against the belt. A steady traction along the axis of the forearm usually causes shoulder reduction (Fig. 25.18).

2. **Immobilization:** After reduction, the shoulder is immobilized in a sling, which may be removed during the exercises. The immobilization depends upon the age of the patient (Fig. 25.19).

i.   Below 20 years : Shoulder is immobilized for 3-4 weeks.

ii. Between 20 and : Shoulder is immobilized 30 years for 2-3 weeks.

iii. Between 30 and : Shoulder is immobilized 40 years for 10 days to 2 weeks.

iv. Above 40 years : Shoulder is immobilized for 3-5 days.

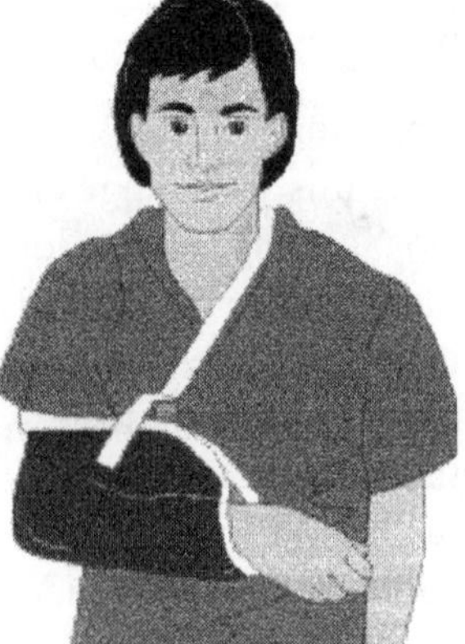

Fig. 25.19: Shoulder immobilization in sling

Recurrent Dislocations

One of the complications of primary dislocation is recurrence dislocations of the shoulder. Row found significantly higher recurrence rate in young patients. The recurrence rate of shoulder dislocation is decreased as the age is increased.

i. Those younger than 10 years had a recurrence rate of 100%.

ii. The recurrence rate is decreased to 94% in patients aged between 10 and 20 years.

iii. Between 20 and 30, the recurrence rate is found 79%; and

iv. Between 30 and 40, the recurrence rate is found 50%.

Some authors found that the recurrence rate is higher in athletes than the non-athletes. Most of the studies found that the recurrence rate of shoulder dislocation is higher in younger patients than the older patients. This is because of the arrangements of the collagen fibers and change in collagen that occurs as people grow older. In newborn, type III collagen is produced and the fibers formed from this type of collagen are supple and elastic. As the age progresses the collagen producing cells make less type III collage fibers and convert to synthesizing another form of collagen type I fibers. The type I collagen fibers contain sulfur groups that have a high tendency to cross link and form bridges between the collagen filaments, causing the fibers they comprise to be relatively tough and non-elastic. This changing ratio of collagen type I and III throughout the body is so reliable that the chronological age of an individual can be determined by analyzing the collagen type III content of a skin sample (Fig. 25.20).

3. **Exercises:** The exercises are divided into four phases:

   i. *Phase I: 01 week to 03 weeks*: This phase is crucial for maintaining the strength and range of motion in pain free range. Hold

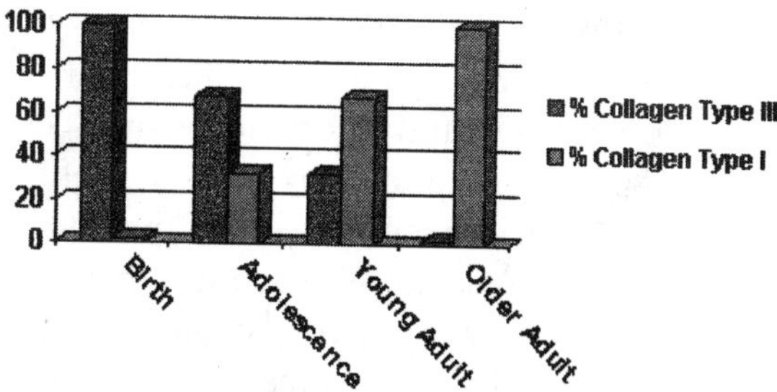

Fig. 25.20: Distribution of collagen fibers I and type II according to the age

relax or isometric exercise of deltoid muscles, rotator cuff muscles, and para-scapular muscles (scapular stabilizers) such as serratus anterior, rhomboids, and trapezius muscles are initiated. Elevation with external rotation and hyperextension must be avoided as these movements place greater stress on the anterior stabilizers of the shoulder.

ii. *Phase II: 3 weeks to 4 weeks*: The exercises may be progressed to the contract relax or isotonic and closed kinetic chain exercise of the deltoid, rotator cuff muscles and scapular stabilizers.

iii. *Phase III: 4 weeks to 8 weeks*: The closed kinetic chin exercises are progressed to the open kinetic chain exercises and light isotonic dumbbell exercises of the deltoid, rotator cuff muscles and scapular stabilizers.

iv. *Phase IV: 8 weeks to 12 weeks:* The aim of physiotherapist here is to improve the strength, power, endurance, range of motion and proprioceptive neuromuscular control of the shoulder and shoulder girdle musculature. The open kinetic and isotonic dumbbell exercises remain same as phase III. Upper body ergometer, proprioceptive training of the joints and proprioceptive neuromuscular facilitation patterns are initiated to achieve the aims.

v. *Phase V*: The aim of the treatment at this phase is to prepare for gradual return to functional and sport activities. The therapist explains exercises such as plyometric exercises to the patient to perform at home. When patient returns to the sport or office he should take brief period of rest during the sport activities. The maximum improvement is expected by 6 weeks.

4. **Operative Options:** The patients who experiences three or more episodes of recurrence of the shoulder dislocation after primary dislocation are the right candidates for the surgical intervention. A relative indication for the surgical intervention is young population; especially professional athlete who is participating sports activities actively. The early surgical intervention will reduce the risks of the recurrent instability and allow the athletes to return to sport at the earliest. There are several surgical interventions for the anterior dislocation of the shoulder. The traditional open Bankart repair is the standard of core of open stabilizing procedure with a recurrence rate of less than 5%. The recurrence rate of arthroscopic stabilization is highly variable from 0 to 45%. Few operative options are mentioned as under:

a. *Bristow Procedure*: A small fragment of the coracoid process is removed and is attached with the anterior scapular neck. Active and passive range of motion may be initiated after 4 days of the procedure.

b. *Putti Platt Procedure*: The procedure basically tightens the anterior capsule and subscapularis muscle with subsequent loss of the external rotation. It has been described as a "vest over pants" fashion along with a "double-breasted" technique. The lateral part of the subscapularis muscle is cut vertically and removed from its insertion part. The remaining medial stump of the subscapularis is attached to the lesser tuberosity of the humerus with thick absorbable mattresses sutures across the stumps so that they overlap on tightening the medial stump lying over the lateral one. The arm is immobilized in full internal rotation for three weeks. Full external rotation is never regained. In 1976, Morrey and Janes reported an 11% recurrence of dislocation following surgical repair. A 10-year follow-up was completed by Salomonsson *et al.* and identified that of the thirty patients who returned the questionnaire, 15 had had an episode of instability defined either as a redislocation or a subluxation. The studies have reported that Putti Platt procedure alters the forces on the glenohumeral joint. This increases the load on the posterior aspect of the joint with potential to create an abnormal posteroinferior humeral head subluxation. This also contributes to the secondary osteoarthritis of the glenohumeral joint.

c. *Eden-Hybinede Procedure*: This procedure is similar to Bristow. About 2 cm × 3 cm bone graft is removed from the coracoids process and attached to the anterior surface of the scapula. The arm is immobilized in the adduction and internal rotation. No external rotation for at least 3 weeks is allowed.

d. *Bankart Arthroscopic Procedure*: The torn edges of the labrum are removed to reveal fresh labrum. A small hole is drilled into the bone to receive the anchor. The anchor is pushed into the drilled hole. Four sutures are attached to the anchor which is used to reattach the labrum to the glenoid. A guide wire is passed under the labrum. A suture and guide wire is retrieved through the cannula to be knotted together. The suture is then safely pulled under the labrum by the guide wire. The sutures are knotted to close the Bankart lesion and the ends of the suture are then cut. The procedure is repeated until the labrum is completely reattached to the glenoid. In the due course of time the sutures are dissolved and the static stability of the shoulder is restored by the Bankart arthroscopic procedure.

Post Operative Management After Anterior Stabilization Procedure

Phase-1 : 0-4 Weeks

a. *Sling*: Shoulder is immobilized in a sling, in adduction and internal rotation, especially at night. Sling can be removed for exercises.

b. *Range of Motion*: Flexion is increased gradually and achieved upto 140 at the end of 4th week. No external rotation and active internal rotation.

c. *Control of Pain*: To control pain ice pack can be used around the shoulder for 20 minutes per session.

d. *Strengthening*: Grip strengthening, external rotator cuff strengthening (within the prescribed range of motion), no internal rotators strengthening.

Phase-2 : 5-8 Weeks

Criteria to Progress to Phase 2: Patient should have minimal pain and discomfort with the exercises. No sensation or finding of instability.

a. Shoulder sling is discontinued.

b. Ice packs to control pain and symptoms.

c. Patient can progress to forward flexion upto 160, external rotation 50 and abduction 70.

d. Rotator cuff and scapular stabilizer strengthening. Exercises are progressed to the open kinetic chain exercises with theraband. No internal rotator strengthening.

Phase-3 : 8-12 Weeks

Criteria for Progression: The patient should have minimal pain and discomfort with exercises. Significant improvement in the strength of the rotator cuff and scapular stabilizers.

a. Pain is relieved by ice packs.

b. *Range of Motion*: At this phase patient achieves full active and passive range of motion equal to the contralateral shoulder. Capsular stretching may be beneficial in case if range of motion is not regained.

c. *Strengthening*: Similar to the phase II rotator and scapular stabilizers. Upper body ergometer for upper extremity endurance and PNF patterns for proprioceptive training may be added. Plyometric exercises with the ball to improve the functional activities are beneficial in this stage.

- **Maximum improvement after anterior stabilization is expected by 12 months but patients can return to sports by 6 months.**

POSTERIOR DISLOCATION OF THE SHOULDER

Posterior instability may be described as a symptomatic excessive posteriorlly and laterally translation of the head humerus with respect to the glenoid fossa. On the axial X-ray the head of humerus is displaced toward the acromian or away from the ribs. The posterior instability may be ranged from abnormal translation to the subluxation and dislocation. The posterior instability is far less common than the anterior instability becouse of significant stability from muscular and static stabilization (glenoid fossa).

Posterior instability can either be a traumatic or atraumatic. Traumatic instability typically follows a distinct history of true dislocation, or subluxation, sustained during a significant injury. Traumatic posterior instability (posterior dislocation) of the shoulder is very rare, it typically stems from episodes of generalized muscle contraction, such as seizure or severe electric shock. Following posterior dislocation there is strong sustained contraction of the adductors and internal rotators, which keep the shoulder at lateral chest wall with internal rotation. Patients with a traumatic posterior instability donot reveal any history of traumatic injury but these patients fall into younger age side and associated with sports activities such as throwing, tennis, bowling in cricket, rugby and swimming. These activities place significant stress on the static stabilizer that eventully cause laxity of the joint capsule, ligaments and labrum. Subsequent posterior instability produces pain in the shoulder that limits range of motion and diseases strength of the rotator cuff muscles. The weakness of the rotator and parascapular muscles contributes further to the posterior instability of the shoulder.

Clinical Features: The posterior dislocation patient usually presents with shoulder adduction and internal rotation along with prominence of the humeral head on the posterior shoulder. Athletes with posterior instability complaint pain in the posterior aspect with exercising posterior translation of the head of humerus with respect to the glenoid and jerk. Sometimes posterior instability may be confused with subacromial bussities as pain occurs in the flexion with internal rotation.

Evaluation: The traumatic posterior dislocation is less commoner than the anterior dislocation, however, episodes of seizure, electric shock and strong contraction of the muscles especially adductors, and internal rotators can cause posterior dislocation of the shoulder. Standard shoulder radiographs do not demonstrate posterior displacement of the humeral head. Therefore, this diagnosis is missed acutely about 50 percent of the time. The loss of external rotation is the main clinical feature of the

dislocation. The athlete involved in repeated overhead sports activities may complaint weakness of the posterior rotator cuff muscles which is in turn causes posterior instability. Offensive linemen are particularly vulnerable to this injury because of the forward-flexed and internally rotated shoulder position needed for blocking (Figs. 25.21a-b).

(a)

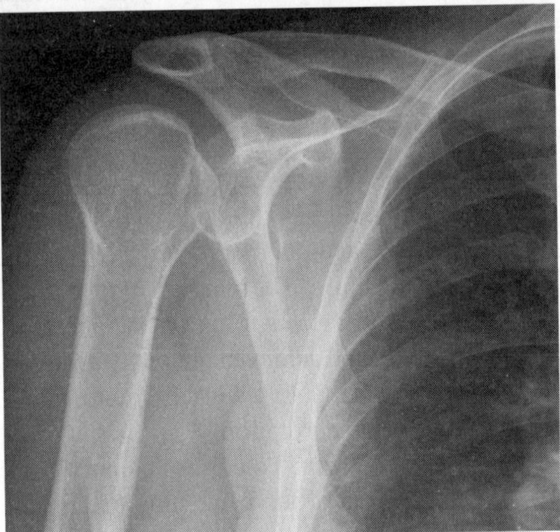

(b)

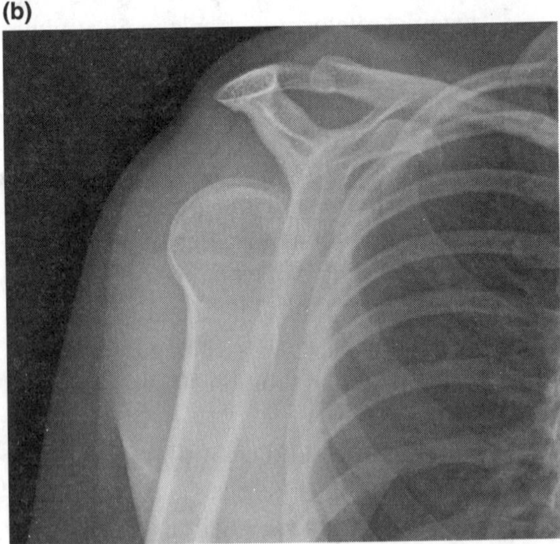

Figs. 25.21a-b: X-ray posterior disloc00ation of the shoulder

Tests for Posterior Instability

There are two provocative tests to reproduce the symptoms of the patient if posterior instability is present.

Jerk Test: Position of Patient: Sitting with shoulder and elbow flexion to 90°, and full medial rotation.

Position of Examiner: Standing, facing the patients shoulder (anterior aspect). The examiner holds elbow with one hand and places other hand on the same side of scapula of the patient. A posterior directed force is applied through the elbow, and then the arm is moved horizontally across the body. If therapist feels sudden jerk, then the test is considered positive for posterior instability. A second jerk is felt as soon as the arm returns to the starting position (Fig. 25.22).

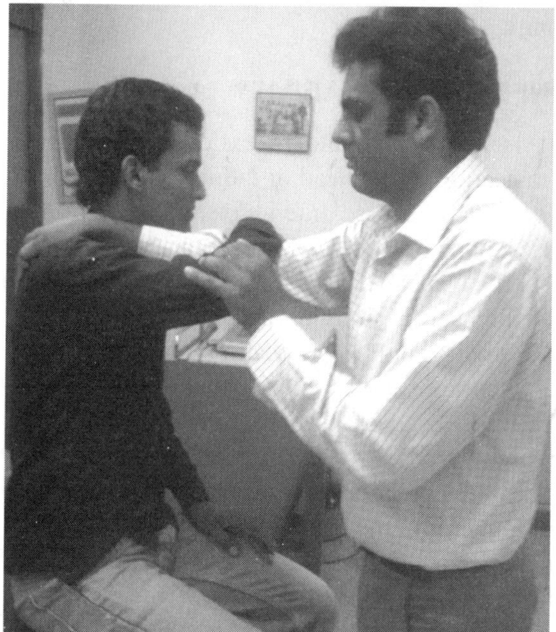

Fig. 25.22

Circumduction Test: Position of Patient: Standing.

Position of Examiner: Stands behind the patient, places one hand on the top of the shoulder and grasps the arm of the patient with other hand.

The examiner initiates circumduction by bringing the patient's shoulder into extension and slightly abducted position. The examiner brings the patient's arm on the top and then the front of the patient into flexion and adduction position. This is the position of risk for posterior dislocation and in patient's with posterior instability the head of humerus is subluxed posteriorly or produces the symptoms of pain and apprehension (Fig. 25.23)

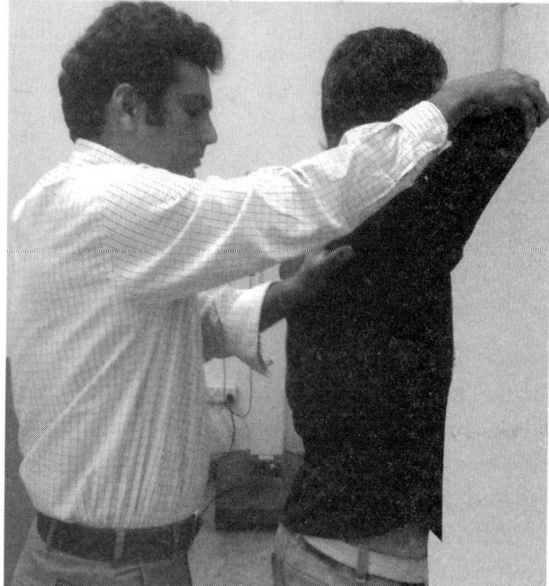

Fig. 25.23: Circumduction test for posterior dislocation of the shoulder

Posterior Apprehension Test: The test is similar to the jerk test. The patient lies supine and shoulder and elbow is flexed to 90°. The examiner holds the elbow joint with one hand and stabilizes the scapula with other hand. While maintaining the above position a posterior directed force is applied through the elbow. The patients with posterior instability complaints pain or apprehension in the posterior directed force (Fig. 25.24).

Management

Reduction: In sitting positions, the hand is placed on the lumbar spine with elbow flexion. Therapist

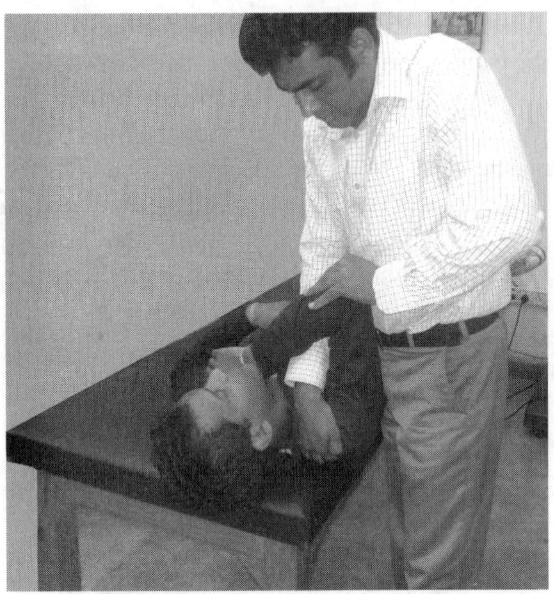

Fig. 25.24: Posterior apprehension test for posterior dislocation of the shoulder

places one hand on the posterior aspect of the head of humerus and other hand grasps the flexed elbow joint. While maintaining the position of elbow, an anterior directed force is applied on the humeral head to bring it to the glenoid fossa.

After reduction the shoulder is immobilized in a sling or brace in an externally rotated position. Internal rotation and horizontal cross chest adduction places stress on the posterior joint capsule, therefore, these should be avoided. Pendulum exercises should be initiated in a painfree range of motion. Submaximal isometric of deltoid (anterior, middle and posterior) external and internal rotators in the adductition are beneficial in improving the strength.

- With significant improvement in the range of motion and pain, the submaximal isometric exercises should be replaced with isotonic with therabands and tubing. Rowing in prone and wall press in standing help in strengthening parascapular muscles.
- As soon as patient gains full painfree range of motion in all three planes the aforesaid

exercises are added with plyometric training and D2 flexion and extension patterns.

The athletes with posterior instability due to repeated trauma to the posterior capsule demanded by the sports activities usually respond to the conservative treatment. These patients rarely require sling, but elevation with internal rotation, cross chest adduetion and extreme extension should be avoided to accelerate the posterior capsule healing. The exercises for athletes with posterior instability are mainly of strengthening of deltoid, rotator cuff muscle, parascapular (serratus anterior, rhomboids, trapezius (all fibers), which are explained as of above for poserior dislocation.

Failure to respond to the conservatve treatment, may require, surgical intervention; capsular suture plication, and posterior capsule shift.

INFERIOR INSTABILITY

It is the symptomatic excessive, inferior translation of the head of humerus with respect to the glenoid fossa. Inferior instability can either be subluxations or dislocation of the shoulder. Inferior humeral dislocation also known as luxatio, is extrensely uncommon, accounting for less than 1% of all shoulder dislocations. Forceful hyper abduction of the shoulder causes impingement between head of humerus and acromian and places extreme stress on the inferior joint capsule. The inferior joint capsule disrupts and allows head of humerus to dislocate inferiorly. The shoulder may also dislocate posteriorlly if there is an axial force on the abducted shoulder.

The patients with inferior shoulder dislocation presents with severe pain and pain is aggravated in movements. The affected arm "locked" in varying degrees of abduction. Classically the shoulder is hyperabducted with the elbow flexion and resting on top of or behind the head. The head of humerus can be palpated over the lateral chest wall. Standard closed reduction is not done as it may cause humeral shaft or neck fracture and injury to the vessels. Surgical open reduction is the choice of reduction of inferior shoulder dislocation.

Complications

1. 50-60% patients will have brachial injury.
2. Axillary artery injury, thrombosis.
3. Rotator cuff tears.
4. Glenohumeral and inferior capsule disruption.
5. Fracture of humeral shaft or head.

Test for Inferior Laxity or Instability:
Position of Patient: Sitting with the arm hanging loosely.

Position of Examiner: Stands or sits behind the patient, places one hand on the superior aspect of the shoulder. The other hand groups the distal arm of the patient.

Procedure: The examiner pulls the patients arm downwards. In normal subjects when the arm is distracted downward no sulcus or gap is formed between the acromian arch and head of humerus. The presence of sulcus indicates inferior laxity or instability (Fig. 25.25).

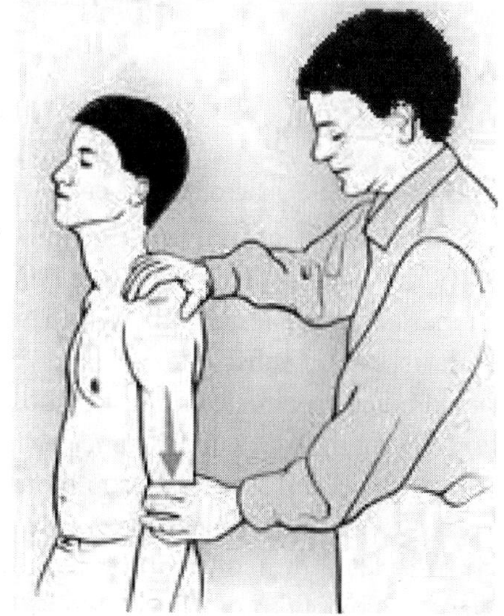

Fig. 25.25: Sulcus sign for inferior instability

MULTIDIRECTIONAL INSTABILITY

It is the symptomatic instability in more than one directions: anterior, posterior and inferior. However, there may be a predominance of one direction, typically anteroinferior or postero-inferior. Patients with generalized laxity of the ligaments associated with weakness of the rotator cuff usually demonstrate multidirectional instability.

Patients with multidirectional instability complaints pain, weakness and instability in overhead activities. These patients often report history of laxity in other joints demonstrated by frequent ankle sprain or recurrent patellar dislocation. Labral grind, SLAP (superior labrum from anterior to posterior), and anterior apprehension tests are helpful in diagnosing the multidirectional instability.

Management

Conservative: The conservative treatment is focused on the strengthening of the rotator and scapular stabilizers.

Surgical Intervention: The surgical intervention is considered if an extensive trial of exercises for at least 6 months fails to relieve the sign and symptoms. The patients with multidirectional instability are recommended for open inferior capsular shift.

Open Inferior Capsular Shift: The purpose of this approach is to balance tension on all sides of the glenohumeral joint and surgically reduce capsular volume. The procedure is effective particularly in patients with multidirectional instability as it reduces the laxity of the capsule in all the directions. The capsule is reflected from the subscapularis in a medial to lateral direction. It is then incised from the glenoid margin forming a T shaped incision. The inferior capsule leaf is shifted to the superiorly and superior capsule is shifted to inferiorly and attached to the respective margins by various types of the fixation devices.

Post Operative Open Inferior Capsular Shift

Phase-I : 0-6 Weeks

a. *Immobilization*: The shoulder is immobilised in a sling or gunsling orthosis during day and night for 6 weeks.

b. *Relief of Pain*: To control pain and symptoms ice packs can be used for 20 minutes per session.

c. *Range of Motion*: No active and passive range of motion is permitted throughout the Phase I. Active and passive range of motion of other joints such as elbow and hand is initiated.

d. *Strengthening*: The isometric exercises in sling of rotator cuff and scapular stabilizers may be initiated in a closed kinetic chain positions.

Phase-II : Weeks 07-12

a. *Range of Motion*: Patient achieves upto 140 degree flexion, 40 degree external rotation and 70 degree abduction.

b. *Strengthening*: Rotator cuff, scapular stabilizers and deltoid strengthening are progressed to the open kinetic chain with the theraband or tubing.

Phase-III : 3-6 Months

a. *Range of Motion*: Patient achieves full range of motion. Glides to stretch the capsule may be initiated with precaution if range is limited.

b. *Strengthening*: Upper body ergometer for upper extremity endurance and PNF patterns for proprioceptive training may be added. Plyometric exercises with the ball to improve the functional activities are beneficial in this stage.

IMPINGEMENT SYNDROME

The term shoulder impingement syndrome (SIS) was introduced by Neer in 1972, which described as "impingement of long head of biceps and supraspinatus tendon" between the head of humerus and acromial arch.

Subacromial Space: Subacromial space or suprahumeral space is formed between the superior surface of the humeral head and inferior arch of the acromian process. The tendons of supraspinatus and long head of biceps and subacromial bursae lie in the subacromial space. In healthy shoulders the normal subacromial space is considered as 10 mm. A distance (between head of humerus and acromian arch, subacromial space) of less than 6 mm is considered pathologic for impingement (Fig. 25.26).

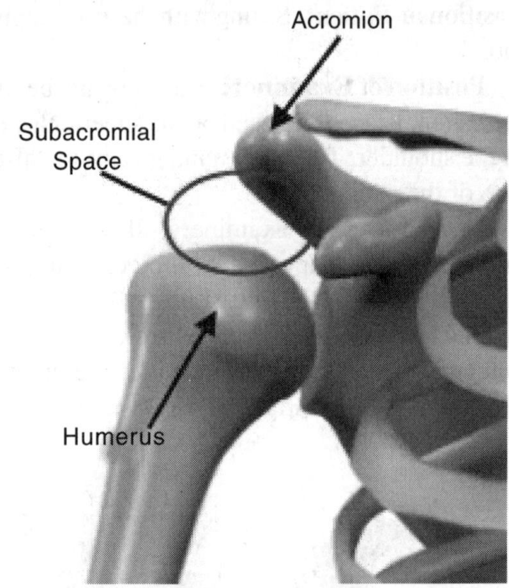

Fig. 25.26: Subacromial space

Coracohumeral Compartment: This space is identified by Patte. This is the space between greater tuberosity and lesser tubercle in which subscapularis bursa, subscapularis tendon and subcoracoid bursa are situated. In resting position with arm rotating medially, the distance between tip of the coracoid and the most prominent part of the lesser tubercle has been measured to be approximately 8.7 mm in healthy shoulders. Decreased in coracohumeral space to 6.8 mm is considered to be potential for the coracohumeral impingement, the space may be decreased due to trauma or fracture of the tip of the coracoid process.

Mechanism

In overhead activities the rotator cuff muscles spin, rotate, and depress the head of humerus, thus maintaining the suprahumeral space. Overuse of these muscles in overhead activities may cause weakness. The weak rotator cuff muscles fail to spin, rotate, and depress the head of humerus adequately. Therefore, the head of humerus migrates superiorly to the acromion arch, decreasing the subacromial space and causing compression of the soft tissues such as: tendon of supraspinatus and long head of biceps and subacromial bursa between superior surface of the humeral head and inferior arch of the acromion process.

The parascapular muscles protract and rotate the scapula during overhead activities which provides room for the rotating humerus, thus maintaining the subacromial space. The excessive use of the shoulder girdle muscles may cause weakness of the parascapular muscles, resulting in inadequate external rotation of the scapula. Therefore, during overhead activities there is elevation of the arm but no external rotation of the scapula which leads to decrease in subacromial space. Eventually compression of the soft tissues such as: tendon of supraspinatus and long head of biceps and subacromial bursa between superior surface of the humeral head and inferior arch of the acromion process.

Factors Contribute to the Impingement

Several factors can contribute equally to the impingement, which are divided into extrinsic and intrinsic:

A. Extrinsic: These factors affect the suprahumeral space from outside. The extrinsic factors may include anteroinferior one third of the acromion, muscular imbalance, postural changes and precipitating factors including training errors and occupational or environmental hazards.

i. *Acromion Anomaly*: The anteroinferior one third of the acromion is thought to be the causative factor in mechanical wear of the rotator cuff through a process called impingement. Neer believed that the tendon of supraspinatus and long head of biceps are repeatedly compressed when the arm is elevated in the forward flexion (functional arc of elevation of the arm). There are three types of acromian, namely flat, curved and hooked. Neer has found no impingement with the flat acromian; most of impingement patients (70%) were present with hooked acromian.

ii. *Muscle Imbalance*: The movements of the scapula and humerus in elevation are primarily controlled by the scapular and parascapular muscles. There are two force couples formed in the upper corset to control the movements are termed as scapula force couple and glenohumeral force couple. ***Force couple:*** A force couple is defined as two forces of equal magnitude but in opposite direction that produces rotation on a body. ***Scapula force couple:*** The scapula force couple is formed by the two portions of parascapular muscles. The upper portion is formed by the upper fibers of the trapezius, and the levator scapulae. The lower portion of the scapula force couple is formed by the lower fibers of the trapezius and lower fibers of the serratus anterior. Simultaneous contraction of these two groups of muscles produces a smooth rhythmic motion to rotate and protect the scapula along the posterior thorax during elevation of the arm. This external rotation of the scapula provides not only a room for the rotating humerus but also a stable base of support for the rotating humerus to allow the humeral head to maintain its normal pathway or rotation along the glenoid. Weakness of these parascapular muscles may lead to inadequate elevation of the scapula (external rotation of the scapula) which in turn does not provide room for the rotating humerus. The greater tuberosity will stuck to the acromion and the suprahumeral space is compromised which in turn compresses the tendons of supraspinatus and long head of biceps (Figs. 25.27a-b). *Glenohumeral force couple:* The glenohumeral force couple is formed by the scapular muscles. One portion of the force couple is formed by the lateral fibers of the deltoid and other portion is formed by the rotator cuff muscles. Simultaneous contraction of these two groups of muscles causes elevation of the humerus with an intact suprahumeral space. The result is that the rotator cuff muscles in effect "steer" the head of humerus along the glenoid during the elevation of the arm. The force generated by the middle fibers of the deltoid pulls the head of humerus upward which in turn is resisted by the strong contraction of the rotator cuff muscles thereby the suprahumeral space is maintained throughout the range of motion. Weakness of the rotator cuff muscles fails to counteract the force of the middle fibers of the deltoid, therefore, the center of rotation of the humeral head migrates 6 mm or greater to the superior direction. The suprahumeral space is compromised and the tendons of supraspinatus and long head of biceps and subacromial bursa are impinged (Fig. 25.28).

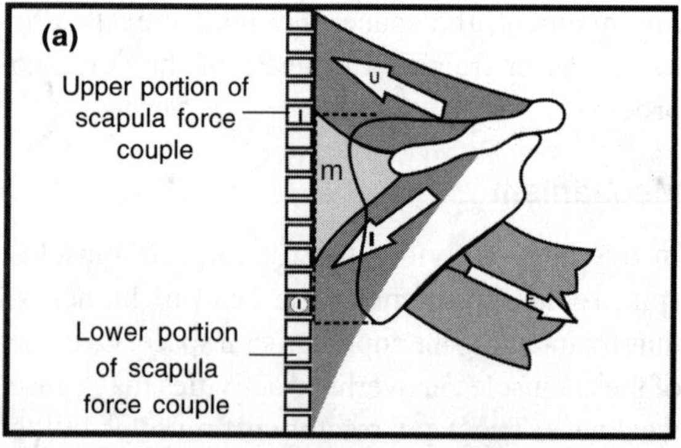

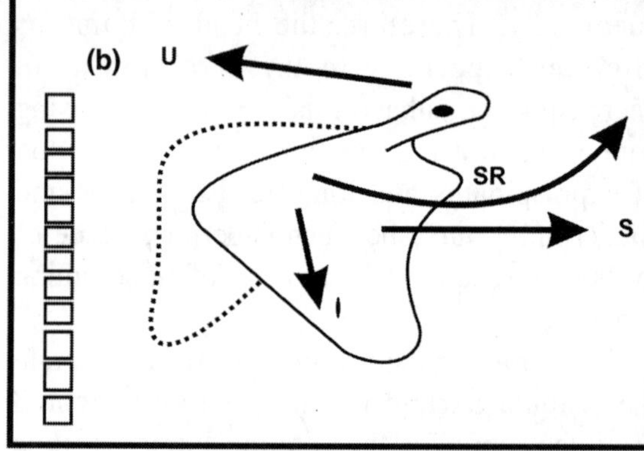

Fig. 25.27a-b: a-Scapula force couple muscles, b-Scapula external rotation following contraction of the scapula muscles

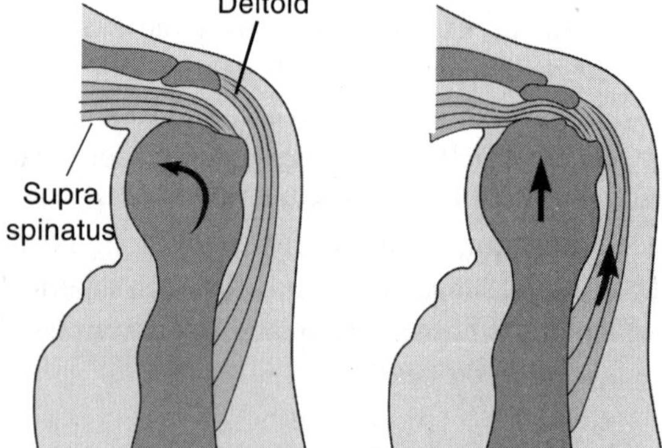

Fig. 25.28: Glenohumeral force couple muscles

iii. Postural Changes: The postural changes seen in the upper corset can adversely affect the force couple mechanism about the shoulder with potential patho-mechanical changes. The common postural changes associated with shoulder are protracted and rounded shoulders with internal rotation and forward head posture typically seen in upper crossed syndrome.

iv. Precipitating Factors: The individuals involved in overhead activities such as baseball pitching, painting, cricket bowling, and tennis (overhead shots) are in the risk of the impingement syndrome. These activities may weaken the rotator cuff muscles as of overuse and thereby the rotator cuff muscles fail to depress the head of humerus downward during the elevation.

B. Intrinsic Factors: These are the changes which take place within the joint and contribute to the reduction of the joint space. Glenohumeral joint is a synovial joint which is involved in the degenerative process. There is loss of the thickness of the articular surfaces, in turn osteophytes are formed. The subacromial bursa and tendons get impinged as the subacromial space is compromised by the formation of the osteophytes. Degenerative changes in the acromioclavicular joint cause osteophyte formation, which may project to the glenohumeral joint and reduce subacromial space. Furthermore, the vascularity of the rotator cuff muscles may also contribute to the impingement. Approximately 1 centimeter medially to the insertion of the supraspinatus tendon is believed to be relatively avascular. Codman has referred this as a *"critical zone"*. The studies have suggested that the most of degenerative changes of the supraspinatus tendon take place in this zone and this is intensified by aging.

Types of SIS

Primary Impingement Syndrome: This type of impingement is common in older than 40 years and less commonly found in the athlete population. These patients complain pain in the shoulder and arm particularly in the anterior aspect of the shoulder and lateral aspect of the arm with inability to sleep on the affected side. As the condition progresses they also complain pain and weakness in the overhead activities. The common causes include:

a. Degenerative changes (osteophyte formation) in the glenohumeral and acromioclavicular joints (Fig. 25.29).

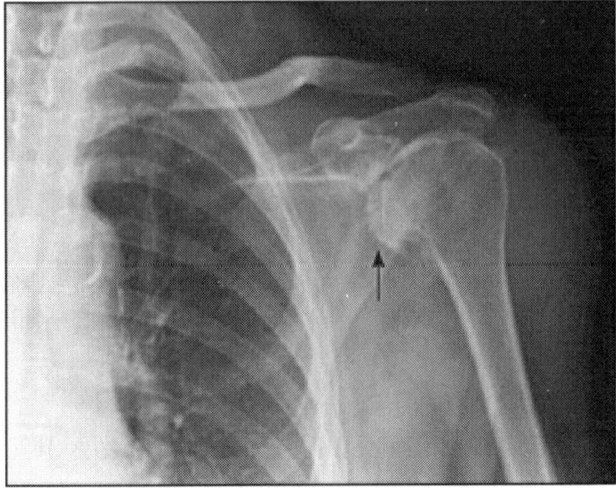

Fig. 25.29: Degenerative changes (osteophyte formation)

b. Congenital hooked acromian process (Fig. 25.30).
c. Congenital prominent tuberosity.
d. Rotator cuff tendon thickening from calcific deposit or after trauma/surgery.

Secondary Impingement Syndrome: This type of SIS is more usual in younger population between 20 and 40 years. These patients are involved in the overhead sports activities such as cricket bowling, baseball, swimming, volleyball and tennis. The symptoms remain same as primary SIS but weakness of the shoulder girdle muscles is most dominant. Patient's experience a feeling of the arm going dead. The common causes include: weakness of the rotator cuff muscles and scapular stabilizer. These muscles provide dynamic stability to the glenohumeral and scapulothoracic joint.

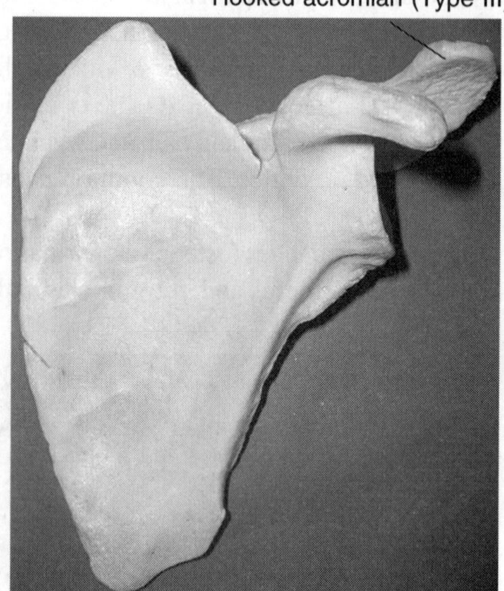

Fig. 25.30: Congenital hooked acromian process

Progressive Stages of SIS

Stage-I: Edema and Inflammation

Typical Age:
- Younger than 25 years but may occur at any age.

Physical Signs:
- Tenderness over the greater tuberosity and along the anterior-ridge/acromion.
- Painful arc of abduction between 60° and 120°.
- Positive impingement sign.
- Decrease ROM with significant subacromial inflammation.

Stage-II: Fibrosis and Tendinitis

Typical Age:
- Between 25 and 40 years.

Physical Signs:
- Crepitus of soft tissues.
- Catching sensation with the lowering of the arm at approximately 100°.
- Limitation of active and passive range of motion.
- Inability to participate in overhead activities.

- Symptoms of Stage I.

Clinical Course: Not reversible by modification of activity.

Stage-III: Bone Spurs and Tendon Ruptures

Typical Age:
- Greater than 40 years.

Physical Sign:
- Atrophy and weakness of shoulder girdle muscles.
- Limitation of active range of motion is more pronounced.
- Significant restriction in use of affected upper extremity.
- Biceps tendon involvement.
- AC joint tenderness.

Clinical Course: Not reversible.

Internal Impingement: Internal impingement is the compression of the rotator cuff tendons between postero-superior edge of the glenoid labrum and head of humerus. It occurs in younger athletes who participate in overhead sports such as swimming, baseball, or tennis. The late cocking phase abduction, external rotation and extension places large loads and casuses microtrauma to the posterior capsule of the shoulder joint. The posterior capsule becomes scarred, tight, and painful and causes the humeral head to migrate superiorly in a higher position than usual in the cocking phase of throwing or when abducted and rotated. This unwanted superior transalation of the head of humerus cause impingement of rotator cuff muscle between the head of humerus and posterior glenoid. In the later stages of the condition the posterior capsule become tight which reduces the internal rotation of the shoulder, causing stiffness, pain and increasing the risk of developing injuries to the under surface of the rotator cuff or superior shoulder labrum (SLAP lesions) by a "peel back" mechanism. Athletes with internal impingement are considered at risk to develop a superior labrum from anterior to posterior (SLAP) lesion.

Clinical Features: The diagnosis of internal impingement is based on the subjective assessment including careful observation of the shoulder and history, and objective assessment. **Posterior Shoulder Pain:** Chronic-diffuse posterior shoulder girdle pain is the chief complaint in the throwing athletes with internal impingement, but the pain may also be localized to the joint line. The patient may describe the onset of posterior shoulder pain, particularly during the late cocking phase of throwing. **Decrease in Throwing Velocity**: A progressive decrease in throwing velocity or loss of control and performance in the overhead athlete. **"Dead Arm"**: Some signs of the pathologic process include a so-called "dead arm", the feeling of shoulder and arm weakness after throwing, and a subjective sense of slipping of the shoulder. **Muscular Asymmetry**: Overhead athletes and throwers in particular often have muscular asymmetry between the dominant and the non-dominant shoulder. **Muscular/ Neuromuscular Imbalance**: A common finding is muscle imbalances in the shoulder complex as well as improper neuromuscular control of the scapula. **Increased Laxity**: A patient with isolated internal impingement may have an increase in global laxity or an increase in anterior laxity alone of the dominant shoulder. **Anterior Instability**: Patients may have instability symptoms, such as apprehension or the sensation of subluxation with the arm in a position of abduction and external rotation.

Test for Impingement Syndrome

- **Impingement Sign:** The examiner flexes the shoulder passively, at the end of flexion range, if patient complaints pain, the possible cause of pain is considered as impingement.

  In the next step of test leidocaine is injected to subacromial space and then the passive shoulder flexion is performed. If pain is relieved by injecting leidocaine, the test is considered positive.

- **Impingement Test:** The examiner flexes the shoulder passively upto the full range of motion. If patient complaints pain at the end range of motion the test is considered positive for impingement syndrome (Fig. 25.31).

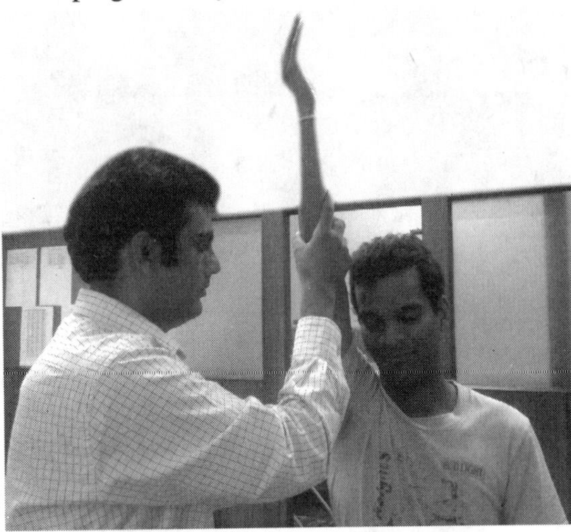

Fig. 25.31: Neer impingement test

- **Modified Impingement Test:** Neer has modified its previous test and added the internal rotation to the flexion. The internal rotation brings the head of humerus under the acromion arch. If the internal rotation provokes the symptoms, the test is considered positive for impingement syndrome (Fig. 25.32).

- **Howkins Kennedy:** In sitting or standing position to patient is asked to flex the elbow and shoulder to 90°. Examiner stands at the side which is being examined, stabilizes the shoulder with one hand and holds the flexed arm at the elbow joint. The shoulder is rotated medially. Reproduction of pain and symptoms indicates impingement syndrome. The medial rotation brings the greater tuberosity under the acromion arch and reproduces symptoms in case of inflamed bursa or tendon. This test has a good sensitivity; hence, it is preferred over impingement test (Figs. 25.33a-b).

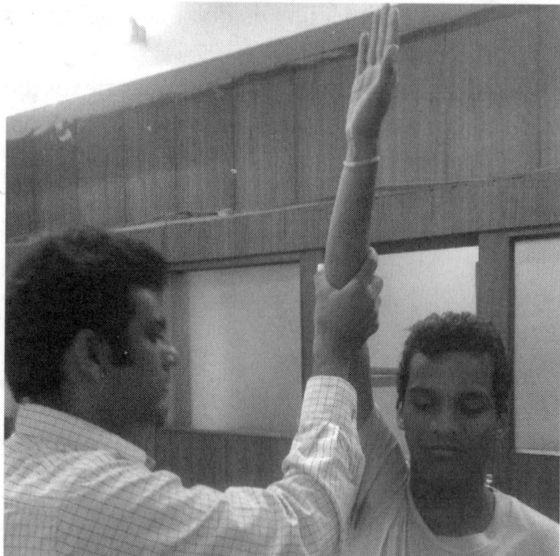

Fig. 25.32: Modified impingement test

(a)

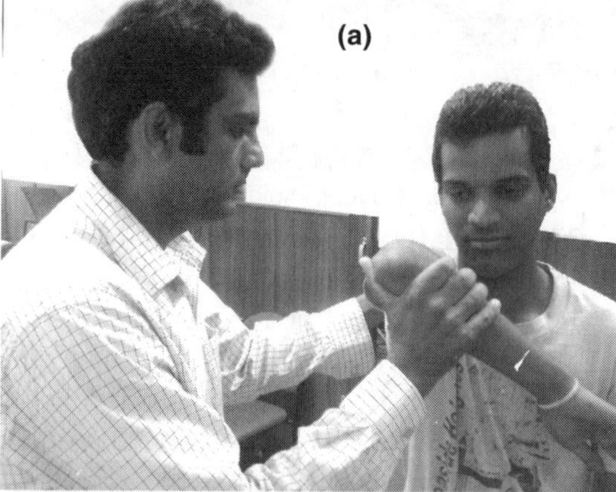

(b)

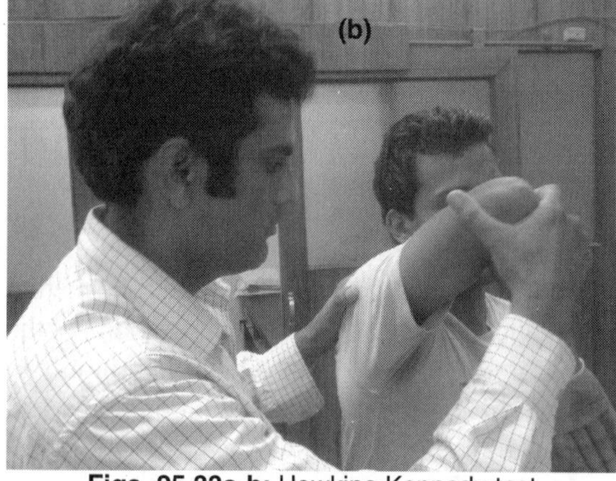

Figs. 25.33a-b: Howkins Kennedy test

- **Drop Arm Test:** In standing the patient's arm is abducted passively to 180° by the therapist, then patient is asked to lower the arm passively in a controlled manner. After 100° patient can not control the arm and drops it suddenly. This indicates supraspinatus tendinitis. Sometimes patient tries to hold the arm with other hand to control it.
- **Empty Cane:** The patient stands comfortably with both the shoulders elevated to 90° in scaption plane (between flexion and abduction) and full internal rotation (thumb pointing downwards). The therapist stands in front of the patient and holds both the hands of the patient. The patient is asked to elevate the shoulder in the scaption plane against the resistance applied by the therapist. The test is positive if the maneuver aggravates pain in the shoulder (Fig. 25.34).

Fig. 25.34: Empty cane test

Management

Conservative Non-operative: The conservative management for both primary and secondary impingement syndromes are same. The aim of treatment is to relieve pain, improve range of motion, improve posture, correct the abnormal kinematics and strengthen the shoulder girdle muscles.

Immobilization: Usually not required.

Precautions: Loss of dynamic stability of the shoulder allows head of humerus to migrate superiorly to the acromian process that impinges the soft tissues between the head of humerus and acromian arch. Hence, overhead activities may require absolute restriction, however, to maintain the range of motion passive exercises are performed throughout the range.

Relief of Pain: To relieve pain, patients can use hot water bag or cold pack for at least 15 minutes twice daily for 2-3 weeks or till the symptoms improve. Hot pack can be followed by cold pack (10 min. each).

Shoulder Girdle Conditioning Program: Prolong pain in the shoulder may cause disuse atrophy of the shoulder girdle muscles. The muscles unable to produce adequate force to perform movements of the body. The functional performance such as activities of daily living, instrumental activities of daily living, recreation, leisure activities, and sport are compromised grossly. The conditioning program of all the major group of muscles helps in improving in the strength of the shoulder girdle muscles.

Strengthening Exercises: Pain and stiffness decrease the contraction of the muscles which in turn can reduce the strength of the muscles. Initially strengthening (sub maximal isometric) exercises are started in pain free range of motion. The closed kinetic exercises are preferred over the open kinetic chain exercises. As the patient reports improvement in the sign and symptoms the open kinetic chain exercises can be started but these should be with the minimal resistance in pain free range. The progressive resistive exercises are started with the dumbbells (10 repetitions X 03 sets daily for 5 days a week). The resistance is increased every week, till the muscles gain good strength or equal to contralateral extremity. The shoulder girdle muscles such as rotator cuff, serratus anterior, rhomboids, trapezius all fibers and levator scapulae are required to be strengthen.

Following strengthening regime can be used:

1. Diagonal pattern (D2) Flexion and Extension.
2. Dumbbell exercises for deltoid and supraspinatus. The initial abduction is provided by the supraspinatus upto 30°. Abduction beyond 30° is provided by the deltoid middle fibers. All fibers of deltoid may be strengthen with the dumbbell.
3. Prone shoulder abduction for rhomboids diagonal pattern (D2) flexion.
4. Prone shoulder extension for latissimus dorsi.
5. Internal and external rotation at 90° abduction.
6. Biceps strengthening with dumbbell.
7. Dumbbell exercises for triceps and wrist extensors.
8. Serratus anterior strengthening.
9. Press ups.
10. Rowing.

Stretching Exercises

Pain in the shoulder joint limits the range of motion. The joint capsule, ligaments and muscles become tight. With the time the range of motion will be limited in all three planes. Patients find difficulties in combing, fastening bras and reaching overhead activities. To improve range of motion the therapist should work on flexibility of the joint capsule, ligaments and muscles. These structures are required to stretch either by the patients themselves or by the therapist. Following self-stretching exercises may be performed.

Mobilization

To place significant force on the capsule, ligaments and muscles the joint is mobilized with the glides.

Internal Rotation: Internal rotation is commonly decreased in patients with impingement and anterior instability as posterior capsule becomes tight. To improve right side internal rotation the patient lies supine position with the shoulder abduction and elbow flexion to 90°. The therapist stands at the side of the patient. Superior aspect of the shoulder rests on the therapist thigh. Therapist holds the elbow with the right hand and places his left hand on the anterior aspect of the shoulder. The shoulder is abducted to 90° and rotated internally as much as possible with the elbow flexion to 90°. At the range where further movement is not possible because of pain, and tightness of the posterior capsule it is maintained at this position. While maintaining the position the therapist glides the head of humerus posteriorly with the left hand. Several glides are performed to place significant stretch on the posterior capsule (Figs. 25.35a-b).

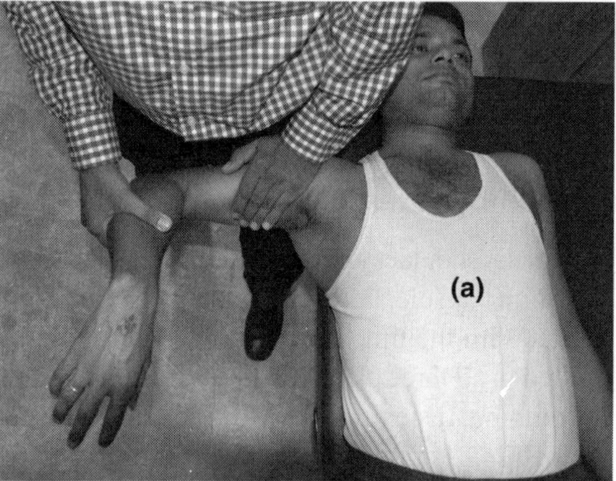

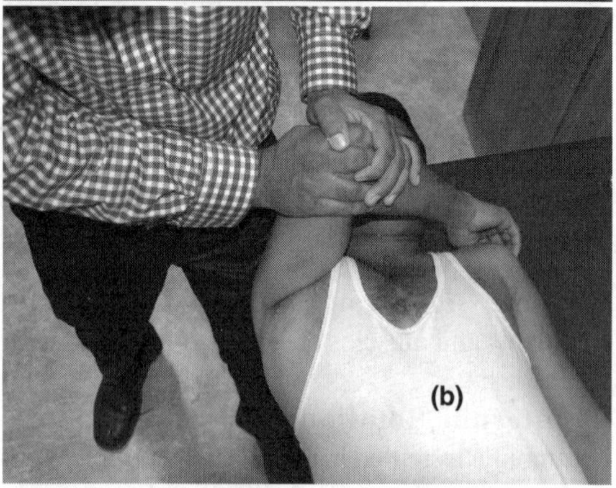

Figs. 25.35a-b: Posterior capsule stretching to improve internal rotation of the shoulder

External Rotation: External rotation is not affected severely in patients with impingement syndrome, but in Stage III it is also limited. To improve external rotation the patient lies supine position with the shoulder out of the edge of the couch. The therapist stands at the side of the patient. For right shoulder the therapist stands at the right side and places right hand on the anterior and posterior aspect of the shoulder. Patient's elbow is held with the left hand. The shoulder is abducted to 90°. While maintaining the position the shoulder is rotated externally as much as possible and at the point where limitation starts the head of humerus glided anteriorly. The shoulder should be stabilized with the right hand to prevent protraction. Practically anterior glide is not effective hence, it is rarely applied (Fig. 25.36).

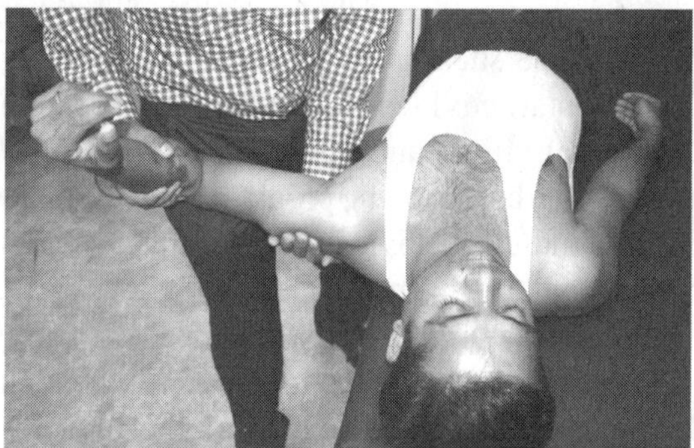

Fig. 25.36: Posterior and inferior capsule stretching to improve external rotation of the shoulder

Abduction: To improve abduction range the patient lies supine. For right side abduction the therapist stands at the right side and places left hand on the top of the shoulder. The left hand grasps the arm firmly. The shoulder of the patient rests on the thigh of the therapist. The shoulder is abducted as much as possible and then the head of humerus is glided inferiorly. Several repetitions are performed to place significant stretch on the inferior capsule.

Flexion: The patient lies in a supine with the shoulder out of the edge. Therapist stands at the side of the patient. Shoulder is flexed with the one hand as much as possible. The other hand glides the capsule anteriorly and inferiorly (Fig. 25.37).

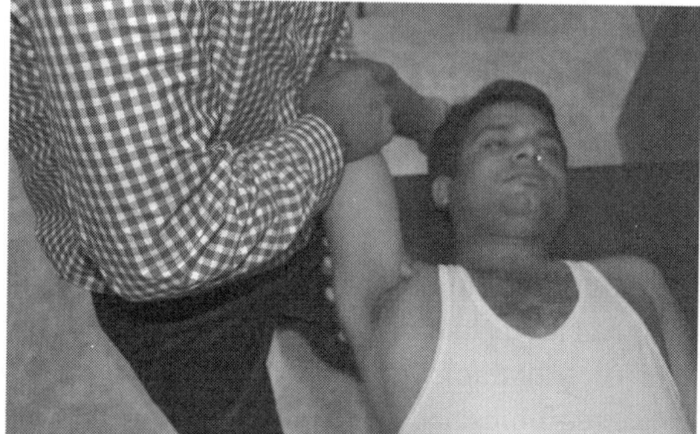

Fig. 25.37: Inferior capsule stretching to improve abduction of the shoulder

Surgical Intervention

Patients with impingement syndrome usually respond to the conservative treatment. Surgical intervention is required if a fair trial of conservative treatment at least for one year fails to improve the symptoms. Main aim of the surgery is to increase the subacromial space. Surgical procedure involves removal of the subacromial spurs and anterolateral acromion.

ROTATOR CUFF INJURIES

The rotator cuff muscles are a group of muscles which includes supraspinatus, infraspainatus, subscapularis and teres minor. This group of muscles help in depressing, rotating and gliding the head of humerus in the glenoid fossa during elevation of the arm. The tendons of these muscles are situated in the subacromial space between head of humerus and inferior surface of the acromian arch. The tendons injured due to decrease in the subacromial space, weakness of the parascapular muscles, overuse of the scapular and parascapular muscle and in the process of degeneration. Rotator cuff injuries are mainly tendinopathies and tear that can either be partial or full thickness. A rotator cuff injury can include any type of irritation or damage to the rotator cuff muscles or tendons.

Rotator Cuff Tears: A rotator cuff tear may be of one or more of the tendons of the four rotator cuff muscles. The tendon of the rotator cuff muscles are commonly torn and of the four the supraspinatus most frequently affected as it passess between the acromian arch and head of humerus. Supraspinatus and infrasponatus tendons fuse 1.5cm proximal to their insertion. Tears in supraspinatus is more commoner and they are more frequently found near to the tendons bony insertion. As the tear in the supraspinatus increase in size it involves the infraspinatus tendon also due to their common insertion. Tear usually occurs at its insertion at the greater tuberosity. Many patients with rotator cuff tear remain asymptomatic. The frequency of rotator cuff tear is increased with age. There is a progressive mechanical failure of the trendon to meet the physical demands placed upon it (Figs. 25.38a-b).

The rotator cuff tears are may be partial or full thickness. Partial tears are often appears as fraying of an intact tendon. Full thickness tears are "through-and-through". These tears can either be pin point, or large button hole with involvement of majority of tendons, where the tendons still remains substatially attached to the humeral head and thus maintain functions. If full thickness tears detach from the humeral head it may cause loss of motion and function of the shoulder.

Mechanism: The tear of rotator cuff tendons may either be acute or chronic. Acute tears occur as a result of sudden, high stress motion or impact, such as a fall on the outstretched arm, or a heavy lift with a jerky motion. Chronic tears are mainly as the result of wear that occurs gradually over time as a natural part of degenetration. Initially dominant shoulders show partial tears without the symotoms but as the age progresses the non dominant shoulders may also involve in the process

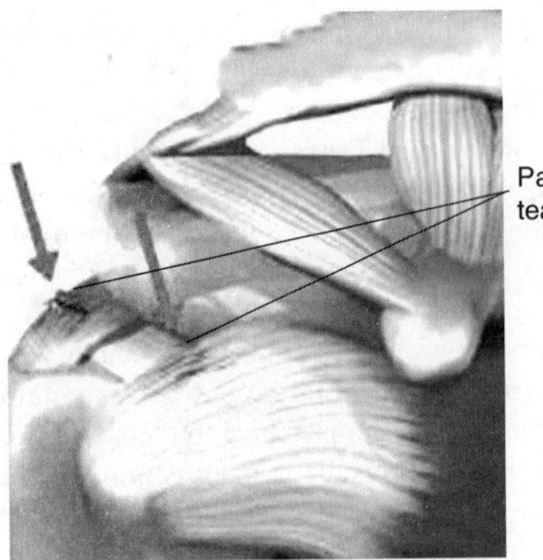

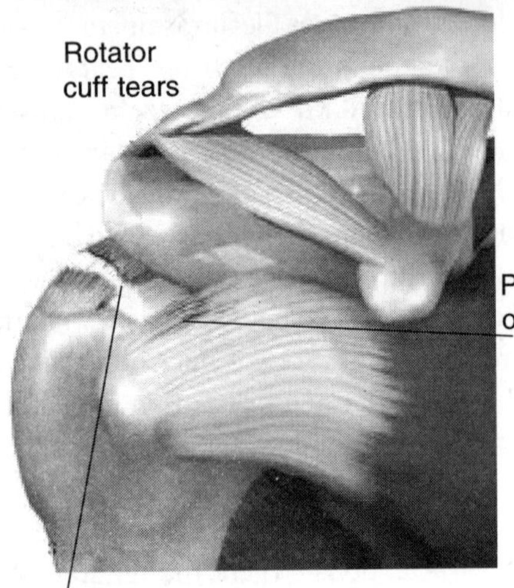

Figs. 25.38a-b

of degeneration and show tears which increase in size over the time. Number of factors contribute to the rotor cuff tear but degenerative changes and gradual repeatititve micro trauma or stresses are the most common causes of the tear. Overhead activities such as throwing, rowing, weight lifting painting etc produces microtrauma to the joint capsule, and subacromial bursa which predisposes rotator cuff muscles to the degenerative changes and tear. The tear may progress to the full thickness over the time.

The second major cause of the rotator cuff tendon tear is impaired blood supply to the tendon of the rotator cuff especially supraspinatus tendon. In old age the blood supply to the rotatoe cuff tendons considerably decreases which impaires the natural ability of repairing of the tendons especially in the individual involved in the overhead activities. Eventually this leads to microtear or partial tear of the supraspinatus tendon.

The third cause of the tear is the impingement of the tendons that may cause micro tear, partial tear or full thickness tear. The tendon of the rotator cuff muscles especially supraspinatus may get iminged between the head of humerus and the acromian arch. The nature of mechanical activities such as bowling in cricket, swimming, tennis, baseball, and throwing are the most common activities contribute to the impingement. Rotator cuff tears following secondary impangement usually begins in the fourth decade of the life. This cause of tear is considered as an extrinsic factor whereas other factors such as degeneration, impaire blood supply are considered as intrinsic factors.

Pathophysiology: The pathogenesis of rotator cuff tear is multifactorial and likely results from a combination of intrinsic, extrinsic and enviromental factors. The small tears of the rotator cuff show features consistent with an attempt to heal such as increase fibroblast cellularity, blood vessel prolifiration and the presence of a significant inflammatory component. However these features of attempting healing (reparative and inflammatory changes) diminishes as the size of tear and amount of tendon degeneration increases over time. As the degenerative changes progress the tendons show thinning of the collagen fibers, a loss of collagen structure, myxoid degeneration chondroid metaplasia, and fatty infiltration. Marked edema and degeneration was seen in large and massive tears, wich more often showed chondroid metaplasia and amyloid deposition. Tissue from large and massive tears is of such a degenerative nature that it may be a significant cause of re-rutpture after surgical repair and could make healing improbable in this group.

The normal supraspinatus tendon has the proteoglycans or glycosaminoglycans of tendon fibrocartilage which suggests that it has capacity of adaptation to mechanical force (tension, compression, and shear), act on the rotator cuff tendons in the shoulder. This functional adaptation may have an important consequences for the structural strength of the supraspinatus tendon and to influence the ability of the tendon to repair after injury. Unfortunately in old age it has been noticed that there is decreased in concentration of glycosaminoglycans, chondroitin sulphate and dermatan.

As the tear increases in size, the total colagen contents decrease, while there is a significant increase in the proportion of type II and type III collagen relative to type I collagen. This changes in collagen composition continues with a transformation of matrix from large organized fibrils to smaller disorganized fibrils with decreasing mechanical and physical properties of the collagen fibers. Eventully disintegration begins in the collagen fibers and proteoglycans and they fail to resist the repititive microtrauma.

Clinical Features: The patients with acute rotator cuff tears usually reveal the history of mechanism of injury. Pain in the shoulder with or without radiation to the lateral arm. difficulty in lifting arm above the shoulder level, and weakness of scapular and parascapular muscles are the common features of rotator cuff tear. External rotation with resistance increases pain and symptoms. Passive movements may be full and pain free but in long standing cases these would be limited in all three planes with disuse atrophy of the shoulder girdle muscles.

Patients with chronic rotator cuff tear often present with gradual onset of pain in the shoulder with difficulty in moving the arm above the shoulder level. Passive motion is full intially in three planes but it may be associated with subacromial crepitus. Patient finds difficulty in lowering the arm actively from over head position. Weakness of scapular and parascapular muscle with atrophy in the supraspinatus and infraspinatus fossa may also be seen. Patients complaint of pain in the empty can test. Howkins Kennedy and Neer impingement may also be beneficial to perform as these tests detect the impingement syndrome with or without tear of the rotator cuff.

Ultrasonography (US) has been shown to be an effective imaging modality in the evaluation of both rotator cuff and non-rotator cuff disorders, usually serving in a complementary role to magnetic resonance imaging of the shoulder. US technique for shoulder examination depends on patient positioning, scanning protocol for every tendon and anatomic part, and dynamic imaging. The primary US signs for rotator cuff supraspinatus tendon tears are tendon non visualization for complete tears, focal tendon defect for full-thickness tears, a hypoechoic defect of the articular side of the tendon for an articular-side partial-thickness tear, and flattening of the bursal surface of the tendon for a bursal side partial-thickness tear. Secondary US signs such as cortical irrregularity of the greater tuberosity and joint and subacromial-subbeltoid bursal fluid are helpful when correlated with the primary signs. Tendon degeneration, tendinosis, and intrasubstance tears are demonstrated as internal heterogeneity.

An MRI examination of the shoulder may help to demonstrate a rotator cuff tear, its size and degree of retraction.

Plane radiographs may show degenerative changes in the articular cartilage, calcification of the tendon and collapse of the bone associated with rotator cuff tear.

Management: Conservative: The patients with chronic rotator cuff tear follow a fair trial of conservative treatment for at least six months. These patients do not require surgical repair until and unless there is a acute tear of a chronic injury.

1. **Precautions:** Following precautions should be taken to avoid excessive stress on the rotator cuff muscles.
   i. No exercises in scapular (empty can) plane.
   ii. No overhead elevation with internal rotation.
   iii. No hyperextension.
2. **Immobilization:** The chronic rotator cuff tears patients do not require sling or braces to immobilize the shoulder however, this may be advised for comfort for short period.
3. **Control of pain:** To relieve pain moist heat therapy and cryotherapy may be used alternately.
4. **Restoration of range:**
   i. Codman pendulum exercises
   ii. Passive internal and external rotation in the arm adducted position
   iii. Passive elevation with external rotation
   iv. Capsular stretching
5. **Restoration os strength:**
   i. Sub-maximal isometric strengthening of rotator cuff muscles in arm adducted position to avoid strain in the tendons.
   ii. Rowing in prone for retractors.
   iii. Wall press for serratus anterior
   iv. Sub maximal Isometric contraction of the deltoid muscles

These exercise are progressed to the isotonic with tubing/theraband, open kinetic chain and functional exercises such as plyometric after four weeks.

a. Light weight (isotonic) dumbbell exercises of deltoid in pain free range
b. PNF Di flexion and extension pattern in pain free range.
c. Plyometric exercises
d. Exercises in quadruped position with alternate body forward and backward on the hands and knees.
e. Scapula stabilizers strengthening in quadruped position with raising of hands to the shoulder level alternately
f. Scapula stabilizers strengthening in quadruped position with raising of hands and legs to the shoulder and hip level respectively.

Surgical Management: There are three surgical approaches commonly recommended for rotator cuff tear-arthroscopic, mini open, and open surgical repair. Patients with small tear or partial tears can be treated very well with the arthroscopic approach while large or massive tears require open surgical repair. Now a days arthroscopic approach is being used for repair of even the large tears and for mobilizing many of the retracted tears. The procedure is painless and allows patients to recover with a short period. The following patients may be elected:

i. The patients with chronic (partial or full thickness) tear, who do not respond to the fair trial of conservative treatment and
ii. Acute tear patients below age of sixty years.

The rotator cuff tears following impingement and bone spur require subacromial decompression with repair. Subacromial decompression consist removal of anterolateral (hooked) acromian. This will reduce the compression on rotator cuff tendons and promote healing and recovery; but physically subacromial decompression does not repair the rotator cuff tear, therefore, arthroscopic subacromial decompression is recently combined with mini open repair of the rotator cuff tears.

A complete full thickness tear involves tissue sutures. An anchor is placed in the bone at the insertion of the tendon and torn tendon is re-sutured to the anchor. In case of chondroid metaplasic and amyloid deposition, mesh (collagen, artelon or degradate material) may be used to reinforce the repair. The mini open technique is preferred over open surgical approach as it requires tear through a deltoid splitting approach, which causes minimal injury to the deltoid muscles and produce better results. The open surgical repair procedure requires detachment of a portion of the deltoid.

Post Arthroscopic and Mini open Repair Management: The rehabilitation of rotator cuff tears repair consist immobilization, relief in pain, restoration of range of motion, restoration of strength and functional strengthening.

Phase I 0 to three weeks

i. **Immobilization:** Sling is recommended to immobilise the shoulder during the day for one week and at night at least for 6 weeks. The sling is removed for the exercises.

ii. **Mobilization:** Pendulum exercises started within 48 hours of the operation in the pain free range of motion. Passive internal and external rotation in painfree range with the arm adducted and elbow flexed to 90 degrees.

iii. **Restoration of strength:** Sub maximal isometric contraction in pain free range of deltoid (anterior, posterior and lateral), rotator cuff muscles and parascapular muscles.

Phase II Four weeks to six weeks

i. Sling continue at night

ii. Progress isometric exercises with theraband or tubing or dumbbell as per weight tolerance within the pain free range of motion.

iii. Rowing in prone for retractor muscles strengthening

iv. Wall press for serratus anterior strengthening

Phase III Seven weeks to three months (early intermediate phse)

i. Continue strengthening exercises of rotator cuff with tubing, rowing in prone for retractors with dumbbells and wall press.

ii. Anterior, posterior and inferior glides to stretch the capsule and increase range of motion.

iii. Progress to light functional activities.

Phase IV Three months to six months (Advanced strengthening)

i. Functional activities

ii. Plyometric exercises

iii. Swimming

iv. Return to play with warm up and conditioning exercises.

Prognosis: Rotator cuff tears is the degenerative process which affects people often in the fifth decade of life. Many studies have shown the people with rotator cuff tear remain asymptomatic, however, micro tears are progressed to the partial and large rotator cuff tears over the time, and 20% patients of whose tears enlarges remain asymptomatic and 80% patients eventually develop symptoms gradually. The high rate of tear prevalence in asymptomatic individuals suggests that rotator cuff tears could be considered a "normal process of degeneration" rather than of an apparant pathological process.

ADHESIVE CAPSULITIS

Adhesive capsulitis is a condition of glenohumeral joint in which the non-contractile structure joint capsule becomes inflamed and tight. In 1946, Naviaser had surgically explored 10 cases of stiff shoulders, and found absence of glenohumeral synovial fluid and redundant axillary fold of the capsule, as well as thickened and contracted joint capsule which had become adherent to the humeral head, thus he used the term adhesive capsulitis. On microscopic examination he found reparative inflammatory changes in the capsule.

Etiology: The etiology of adhesive capsulitis or frozen shoulder remains unknown, however, evaluation of anatomic, histologic, and surgical specimens from patients with idiopathic frozen shoulders demonstrate that the disease often involves inflammation in the glenohumeral joint capsule. Although, most of authors describe that limitation in the range of motion of glenohumeral joint in chronic phase is not due to capsular adhesions. Instead, pathologic data confirm an active process of hyperplastic fibroplasia and excessive secretion of type III collagen fibers, that cause tightness in the coracohumeral ligament, soft tissues in the rotator interval, the subscapularis muscle, and the subacromial bursae.

The contractures in patients with frozen shoulder are identical to those seen in a Dupuytren contracture of the hand. These contractures have a classical feature of progressive loss of range of motion of the joint. Despite these histopathologic similarities, the favourable and regressive outcome of adhesive capsulitis differ from the unfavourable and progressive outcome of Dupuytren disease. The studies have also found presence of autonomic sympathetic dysfunction in the upper extremities in patients with isolated idiopathic frozen shoulder. The studies have found similar histologic findings in joints affected by complex regional pain syndrome and frozen shoulder. Both the conditions have similar risk factors such as trauma, diabetes, thyroid disease and dyslipidemia.

Epidemiology: The prevalence of adhesive capsulitis in the general population is reported to be 2%, however, the unselected individuals with diabetes may have prevalence rate of upto 11%. The most significant association with insulin dependent diabetic patient is the risk of developing of adhesive capsulitis in their life is approximately 40%. The disease may affect bilateral shoulders in as many as 16% of patients. Both the shoulders may be affected, either simultaneously or sequentially. The contralateral shoulder is usually affected within 5 years of disease.

Adhesive capsulitis is also associated with medical conditions such as, hyperthyroidism, ischemic heart disease, inflammatory arthritis and cervical spondylosis.

Adhesive capsulitis affects females more than males with the female to male ratio of about 1.4:1. The females are affected somewhat earlier than the males; with the mean age of onset are 52 years for females and 55 years for males. There is no racial variation seen in the patients with adhesive capsulitis.

Clinical Features: Stiffness and pain with progressive loss of both active and passive movements are the dominant features of adhesive capsulitis. Initially patients with adhesive capsulitis complaint pain at night with sleep disturbance but in the advance phase pain decreases in intensity and also patients feel less discomfort in sleeping, however active and passive range of motions are decreased in all three planes. The loss of range of motion occurs in a typical capsular pattern-external roation, abduction and flexion and internal rotation. Reverse scapulohumeral rhythm is the classical feature of the adhesive capsulitis in late phases. Pain may radiate down the lateral aspect of arm. The symptoms of adhesive capsulitis usually progress gradually over a number of months or years. The symptoms may also vary greatly from person to person. Adhesive capsulitis is classically characterized by three phases which can sometimes be difficult to distinguish.

Freezing Phase: Patients typically experience stiffness and dull ache, deep situated pain that may increase to a sharper with certain movements or activities. The pain is usually more severe at rest and at night and often aggravates when the patients turn side on the affected shoulder. This keeps the patient awaken for hours. To relieve pain, patient uses hot water bag. The range of motion is not limited in this phase. This phase lasts upto 2-9 months.

Frozen Phase (3-18 months): This phase is also known as progressive stiffness phase in which range of motion decreases gradually over the time. Progressive limitation in range of motion occurs in a capsular pattern, such as external rotation, abduction, flexion and internal rotation. The intensity of pain is decreased gradually but pain at night remains a common complaint especially when the patient turns on the affected side. The intensity of referred pain from shoulder to lateral arm also decreases. The activities of daily living are grossly compromised, patient finds difficulty in combing hair, reaching into the back pocket, washing the opposite shoulder, taking off the inner wears and fastening the bra.

Thawing Phase: It is the last stage of adhesive capsulitis characterized by minimum pain, gross limitation in range of motion and slow recovery in range. Patients may demonstrate reverse scapulohumeral rhythm.

Differential Diagnosis: It is not easy to differentiate the adhesive capsulitis from other conditions as pain stiffness, and loss of range of motion are present in all the shoulder conditions. However, based on some clinical and radiological findings adhesive capsulitis can be differentiated from other shoulder conditions. Rest pain, night pain, sleep disturbance with loss of external rotation are the distinguished features of adhesive capsulitis, moreover, all the resisted movements of shoulder remain pain free.

Impingement Syndrome: External rotation is not limited in the initial phase. End range flexion with internal rotation elicits pain. Painful arc, empty cane and Hawkins Kennedy tests are positive in patients with impingement syndrome. These tests are negative in adhesive capsulitis.

Rotator Cuff Tendinitis: Resisted movements are painful. Painful arc syndrome will also be positive. Patients complaint pain in the mid range. The passive flexion may be full and pain free.

Anterior Instability: Patient feels instability rather than pain. Pain is present in the posterior deltoid because of overuse and eccentric contraction to prevent anterior translation of the head of humerus. There is no limitation in external rotation, instead of that internal rotation is decreased as posterior capsule becomes tight.

Therapist asks the chief complaint to the patient and establishes a pleasant relationship so that he or she can take history. Therapist asks questions related to the complaint, which helps in making a provisional diagnosis.

Special Test: These tests are performed on the patient to put the load on the structure so that the injured structure can reproduce the symptoms.

i. **Biceps Tendinitis Evaluation: Yargason Test:** It is performed to test the bicipital tendinitis. Patient sits comfortably on stool with the elbow flexion to 90° and forearm fully pronated. The therapist holds the hand and elbow and simultaneously resists the forearm supination and elbow flexion. If the maneuver reproduces pain in the shoulder joint, it suggest bicipital tendinitis (Fig. 25.39).

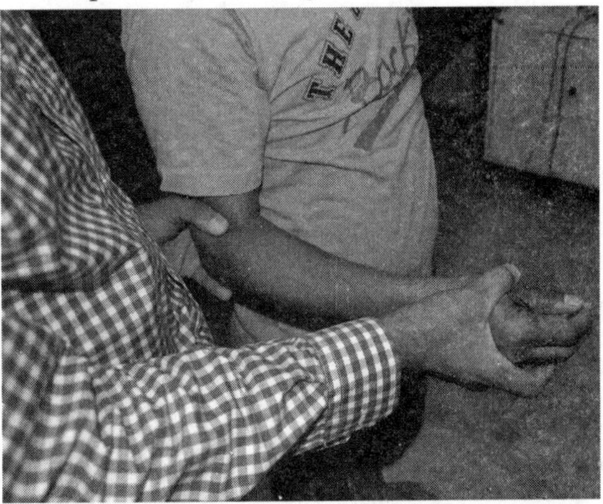

Fig. 25.39: Yargason test for bicipital tendinitis

ii. **Speed Test:** The patient stands comfortably with both the shoulders flexed to 90° in scaption plane and forearm fully supinated. Therapist holds both the hands and resists the shoulder elevation with forearm supination (Fig. 25.40).

iii. **Biceps Load Test for SLAP:** The patient lies supine with the shoulder abduction to 90°. The examiner stands at the side of the shoulder which is being examined; and grasps the arm at the elbow and hand. The shoulder is rotated externally till the patient feels apprehension. When the patient becomes

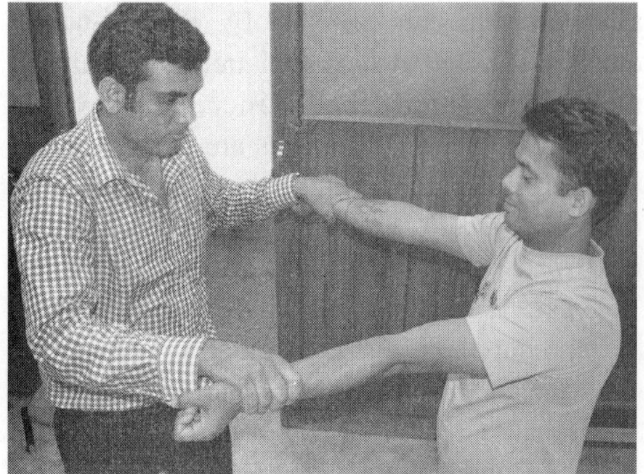

Fig. 25.40: Speed test for bicipital tendinitis

apprehension during external rotation, the examiner stops the external rotation, and asks the patient to flex the elbow against the resistance. If apprehension is exchanged and becomes more painful, the test is considered positive for SLAP lesion (Figs. 25.41a-b).

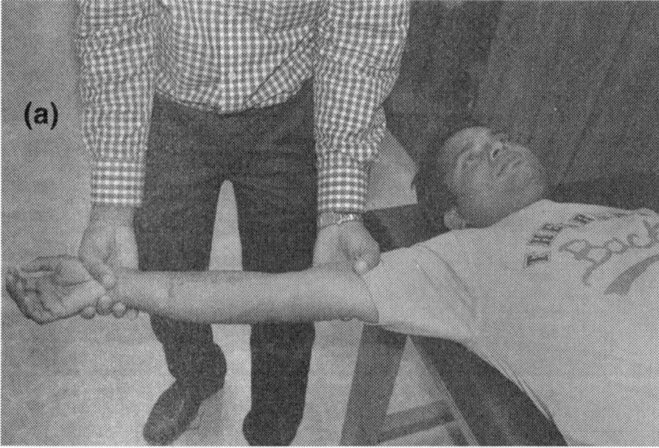

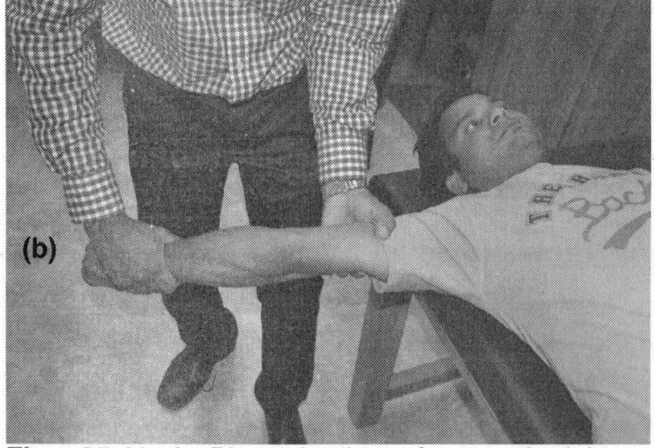

Figs. 25.41a-b: Biceps load test for superior labrum from anterior to posterior

iv. **Painful Arc Syndrome:** In an active flexion and extension, patient feels pain between 120 and 100 degrees. This particular arc is painful because in this range load on the shoulder during active flexion and extension increases. The test is considered positive for impingement syndrome (Fig. 25.42).

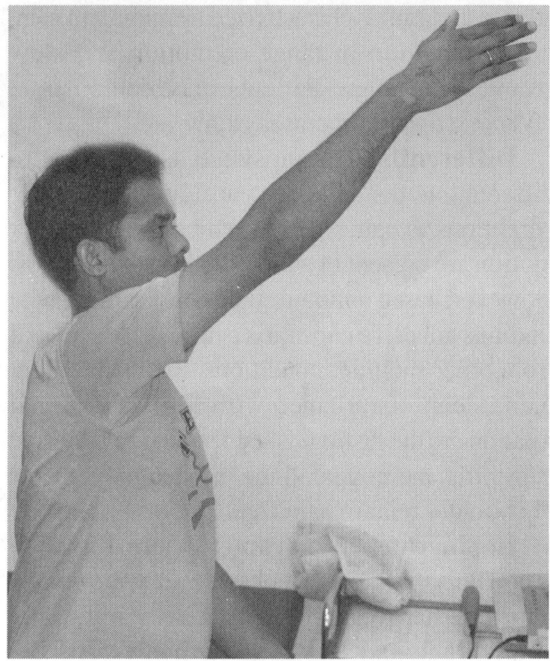

Fig. 25.42: Painful Arc syndrome

v. **Apley's Scratch Test:** The test is performed to assess the shoulder external and internal rotations. The patient stands comfortably, places one hand on the opposite shoulder and tries to touch the superior aspect of the opposite scapula. In the next step the hand is placed on the back and slides up to touch the inferior angle of the scapula. If patient can reach to the scapula the external and internal rotations are considered normal (Figs. 25.43a-b).

vi. **Test for Infraspinatus and Teres Minor Tendinitis:** Patient stands comfortably. Position of patient remains same as Emply cane test with the arm at the side (adducted)

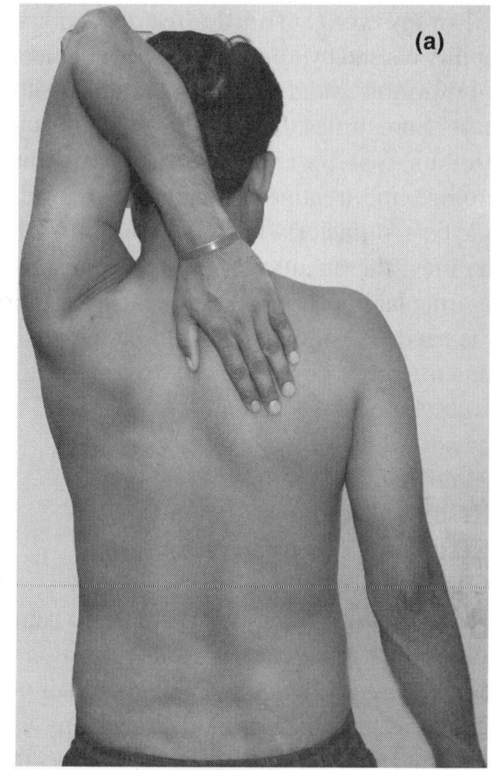

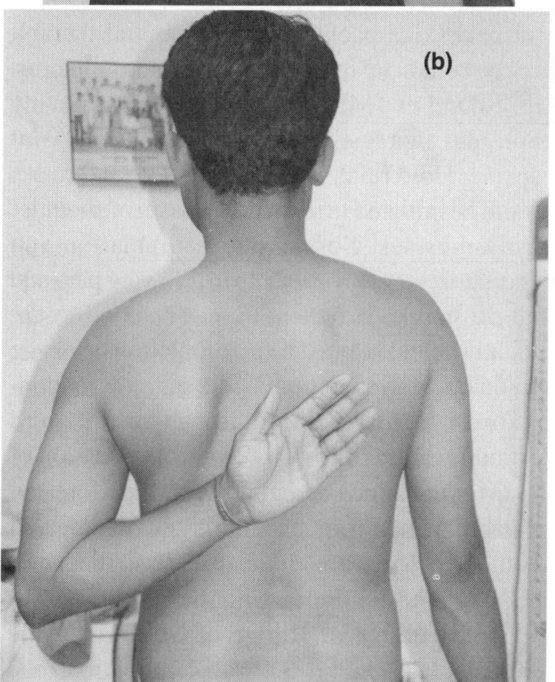

Figs. 25.43a-b: Apley's scratch test

and elbow flexion to 90°. Examiner stands at the side and resists the external rotation of the shoulder. If the patient complaints pain against the resistance of external rotation of the shoulder, it indicates tendinitis of infraspinatus or teres minor (Fig. 25.44).

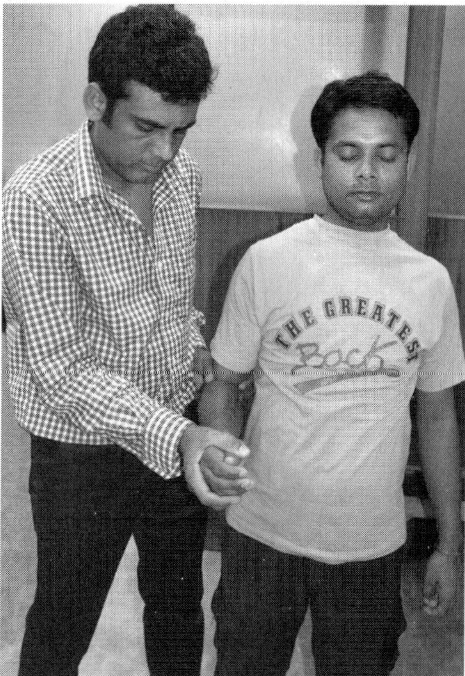

Fig. 25.44: Infraspinatus and teres minor tendinitis test

vii. **Test for Subscapularis Tendinitis (Lift Off Test):** Patient sits comfortably on the stool with the hand (dorsum aspect) on the lower back region (lumbar spine). Patient is asked to lift the hand off the back. Inability to lift the hand off the back suggests injury to the subscapularis muscles. The test cannot be performed on the patients who have limitation in the internal rotation. For these patients modified lift off test is performed. In this version patients places the hand (palmer aspect) on the abdomen and rotates internally against the resistance. If patient complaints pain, it suggest subscapularis tendinitis (Figs. 25.45a-b).

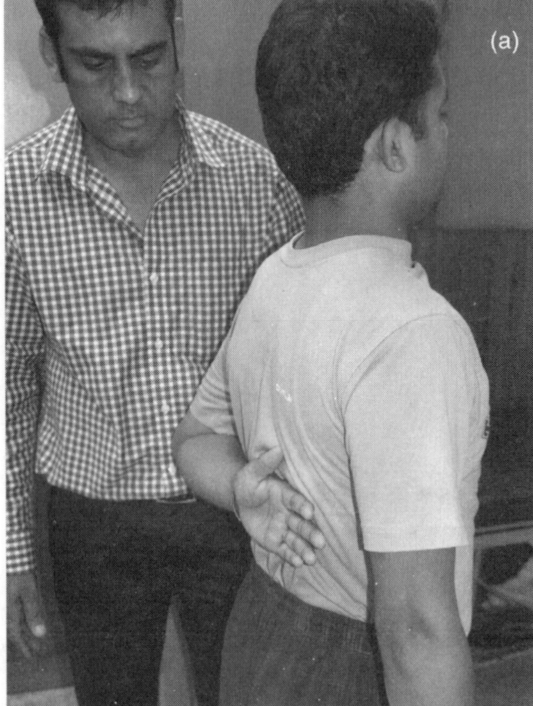

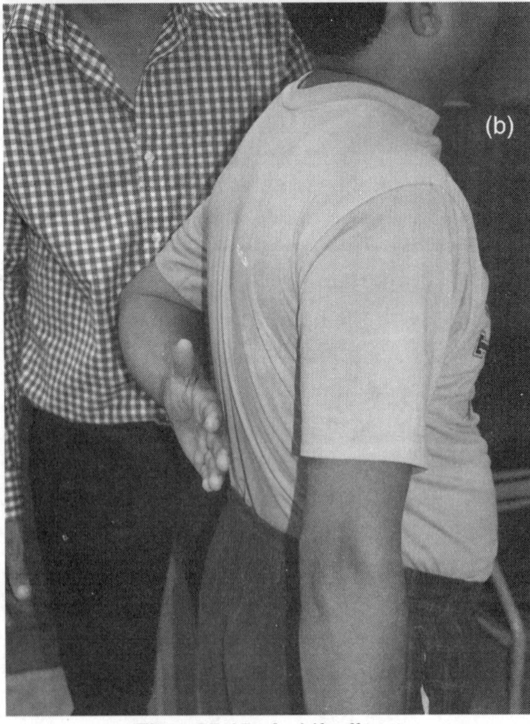

Figs. 25.45a-b: Lift off test

Management: The degree of pain and disability caused by idiopathic frozen shoulder is highly variable and depends on the stages of the disease. Sometimes the physical modalities and exercises fail to improve the symptoms. Therefore, the treatment to adhesive capsulitis should be multifactorial. It should consist physical modalities, therapeutic exercises, medications, intra-articular injections and surgical intervention if it is needed. Following should be the goal of treatment:

1. Relief of pain.
2. Maintenance of range of motion.
3. Maintenance of muscle strength.
4. Restoration of range of motion.
5. Restoration of muscle strength.
6. Correction of posture.

Relief of Pain: Adhesive capsulitis is a painful condition that often causes great frustration for both patients and clinicians. Pain progresses over time, hence, the physical modalities being used for relieving pain may not be effective at one time. Hot packs, ice packs and interferential therapy may be beneficial in relieving pain and symptoms. Ultrasound of 1MHz may also help in relieving pain, and increasing extensibility of the joint capsule. Hold relax and contract relax exercises should be initiated to reduce the spasm of shoulder girdle muscles. Soft tissue manipulation and pendulum exercises also help in relieving pain and muscle spasm. If patient do not respond to the modalities and soft tissue manipulation he or she should be referred to orthopedic surgeon for non-steroidal anti-inflammatory drugs and corticosteroids. Unfortunately the progression of the disease cannot be halted with the aforesaid treatments, therefore, patient should be educated about the progression of the disease so that he or she should be continued with the treatment.

Maintenance of Range of Motion: In the freezing phase pain is the main complaint of the patient. The limitation in the range of motion is not the usual feature of freezing phase. But because of pain, patient starts avoiding end range movements, that can limit the range of motion of joint in the frozen phase. Hold relax, contract relax and passive range of motion, gentle glides and pendular exercises should be started to maintain the range of motion. Exercises to maintain the range of motion should be continued unless and until there is significant improvement in pain and sumptoms.

Maintenance of Muscle Strength: Isometric exercises of rotator cuff muscles and scapular stabilizers are initiated to maintain the strength of muscles.

Restoration of Range of Motion: Range of motion is limited because of tightness of the muscles, ligaments and joint capsule. To improve range of motion muscle relaxation technique and glides are administered to increase the flexibility of muscles, ligaments and joint capsule.

PNF Techniques: Hold Relax and Contract Relax: These techniques are beneficial in relaxing the muscles. To improve the external rotation, patient is placed in a comfortable position, and shoulder is rotated externally as much as possible. With an appropriate stabilization the internal rotators (subscapularis muscle) are allowed contract isotonically (contract relax) against the resistance. Several repetitions of contract relax are performed to improve external rotation.

To improve flexion, patient lies in a comfortable position, and shoulder is flexed as much as possible. With an appropriate stabilization, the extensors are contracted against the resistance (contract relax). Several repetitions of contract relax are performed to improve flexion range.

To improve abduction, the patient lies in a comfortable position and shoulder is abducted as much as possible. With an appropriate stabilization the shoulder is adducted isotonically against the resistance (contract relax). Several repetitions are performed to improve abduction range.

To improve internal rotation, the patient lies in a comfortable position, and shoulder is rotated internally as much as possible. With an appropriate stabilization the shoulder is rotated externally against the resistance. Several repetitions of contract relax may be performed to improve internal rotation.

The muscle relaxation techniques are followed by muscle stretching and capsule glides to achieve maximum results.

Hold relax and reciprocal inhibition techniques may also be performed to relax the muscles in case of severe muscle spasm.

Mobilization

The patients with adhesive capsulitis usually present with capsular pattern. Initially the anterior capsule adheres to the humerus followed by inferior and posterior. To improve range of motion, the capsule must be stretched. To stretch the capsule the joint is distracted and glided with significant force.

Capsule Stretching: The loss of range of motion in patients with adhesive capsulitis is mainly due to tightness in the capsule. Initially anterior joint capsule becomes tight which limits the external rotation of the shoulder but as the disease progresses inferior and posterior part of capsule also becomes tight. The joint capsule can be stretched with the glides after placing the joint in an extreme limitation range.

CHAPTER-26

Cervical Spine

CONCISE ANATOMY

The cervical spine is comprised seven vertebrae. C_1 vertebra also known as atlas does not have body and spinous process and it serves as a ring or washer that the skull rests upon and articulates in a pivot joint with the dens or odontoid process of C_2. The atlas is composed of two arches anterior (thick) and posterior arch (thin), and two prominent lateral masses. Each lateral mass has a superior and inferior articular facet joint. Superior articular facets are kidney shaped, concave, and face upward and inward, these articulate with the occipital condyles. The inferior lateral articular facet joints are relatively flat face downward and inward and articulate with the superior facets of the axis. According to Steele's rule of thirds, at the level of the atlas, the odontoid process, the subarachnoid space, and spinal cord each occupy one third of the area of the spinal canal.

C_2 vertebra also known as axis has a large body which contains the odontoid process (dens). The odontoid process to the atlas is held in place by the transverse ligament. The apical, alar, and transverse ligaments, by allowing spinal column rotation, provide further stabilization and prevent posterior displacement of the dens in relation to the atlas. Fifty percent rotation (45 degrees) of the cervical spine occurs at the atlano-axial joint.

Stability

The static stability of the upper cervical spine is mainly provided by the external and internal ligaments. The external ligaments consist of the

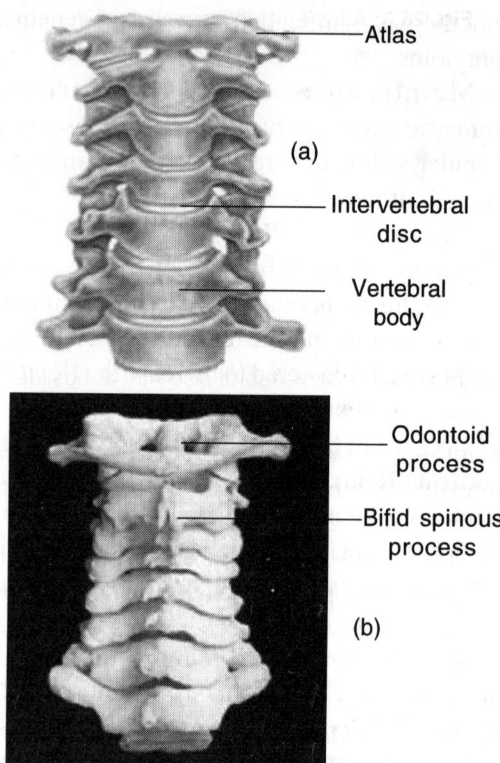

Figs. 26.1a-b: Cervical spine: a. Anterior view b. Posterior view

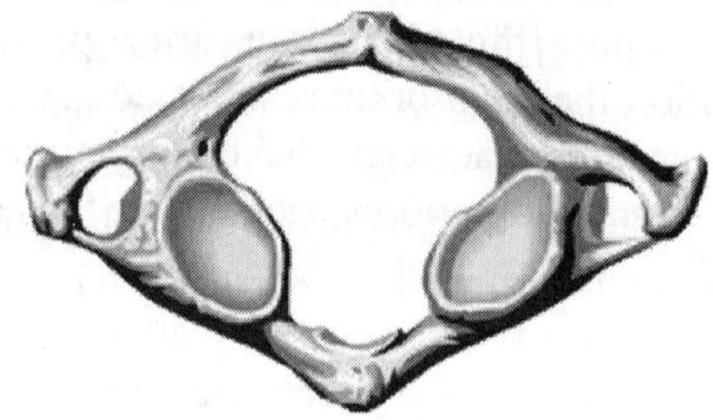

Fig. 26.2: Atlas

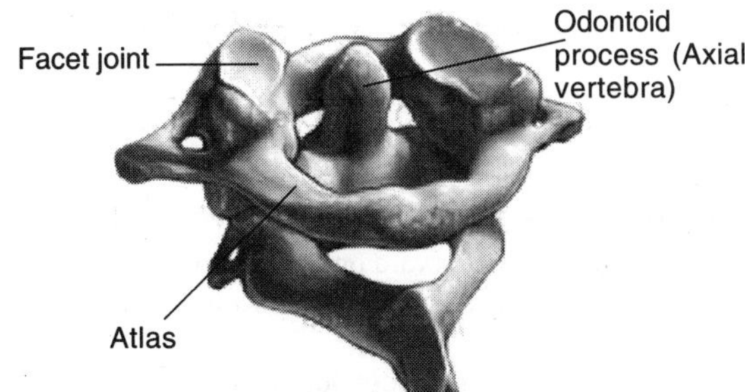

Fig. 26.3: Atlas articulation with axial vertebra superior view

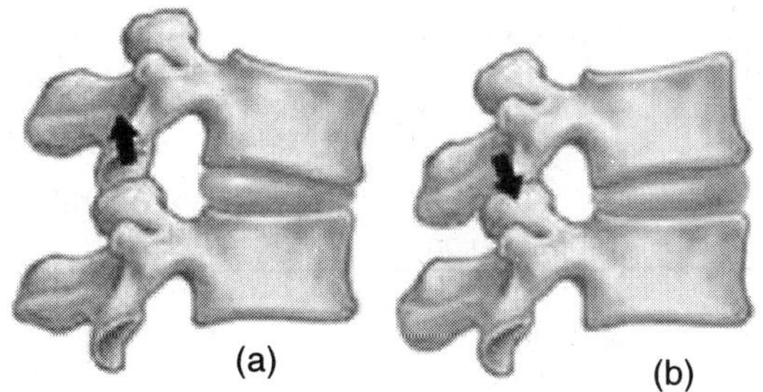

Fig. 26.4: Intervertebral disc with a. upslide, b. down slide of the facet joints

atlanto-occipital, anterior atlanto-occipital, and anterior longitudinal ligaments. The internal ligaments have 5 components:

i. The transverse ligament holds the odontoid process in place against the posterior atlas, and prevents anterior subluxation of C_1 on C_2.

ii. The accessory ligaments arise posterior to and in conjunction with the transverse ligament and insert into the lateral aspect of the atlanto-axial joint; the apical ligament lies anterior to the lip of the foramen magnum and inserts into the apex of the odontoid process.

iii. The paired alar ligaments secure the apex of the odontoid to the anterior foramen magnum.

iv. The tectorial membrane is a continuation of the posterior longitudinal ligament to the anterior margin of the foramen magnum.

v. The 3 cm × 5 mm accessory atlantoaxial ligament not only connects the atlas to the axis but also continues cephalad to the

occipital bone; functionally, it becomes maximally taut with 5-8° of head rotation, lax with cervical extension, and maximally taut with 5-10° of cervical flexion.

The lower cervical spine is made up of five vertebrae from C_2 to C_7. Each vertebra from C_2 to C_7 has a body which is concave on its superior surface and convex on its inferior surface. The spinous processes of C_3 to C_6 are usually of bifid, whereas the spinous process of C_7 is nonbifid and somewhat bulbous at its end.

Facet Joints

The facet joints in the lower cervical spine are most noticeable near the pedicles. These are diarthrodial synovial joints with fibrous capsules surrounded by a capsule of connective tissue and produces synovial fluid to nourish and lubricate the articular cartilage. The C_0-C_1 and C_1-C_2 joints are innervated by anterior rami of the first and second cervical spinal nerves, whereas, C_2-C_3 facet joint is innervated by two branches of the posterior ramus of the third cervical spinal nerve. Each C_3-C_4 to C_7-T_1 is innervated by the medial branches above and below.

Movements: Movement in the cervical spine occurs in all three planes as flexion, extension and rotation, these are mentioned in the Tables 26.1 to 26.4.

PROLAPSED INTERVERTEBRAL DISC

Intervertebral Disc

The intervertebral disc is the largest avascular structure in the body which is situated between two vertebral bodies. It is composed of annulus fibrosus (AF), and a nuclease pulposus (NP). It is reinforced peripherally by an end plate. As it is the largest avascular structure in the body its nutrition depends on diffusion. It receives its blood

**Table 26.1: Movements of the facet joints
of cervical spine**

Movement	Plane of movement
Flexion	The upper facet slides up and forward on the lower facet
Extension	The upper facet slides down and back on the lower facet
Side flexion	The upper facet slides down and back on the same side and up and forward on the opposite side
Rotation	The upper facet slides down and posterior on the same side and up and anterior on the opposite side

Table 26.2: Approximate range of motion of cervical spine (Craniocervical region)

Joints	Flexion	Extension	Axial rotation	Side flexion
Atlanto-occipital	5	10	Negligible	5
Atlanto-axial	5	10	40-45	Negligible
Intracervical region (C_2-C_7)	35	70	45	35
Total range of motion at craniocervical region	45	90	90	40

Table 26.3: Muscles of the craniovertebral region

Muscles	Action(s)
Rectus capitis posterior minor	Atlanto-occipital extension
Rectus capitis posterior major	Craniovertebral complex extension
Superior oblique	C_0-C_1 ipsilateral side flexion and extension
Inferior oblique	C_1-C_2 ipsilateral rotation
Rectus capitis lateralis	C_0-C_1 joint ipsilateral side flexion
Rectus capitis anterior	C_0-C_1 joint flexion

Table 26.4: Muscles and their action/movements of lower cervical

Muscles	Action (s)/ Movement (s)
Longus coli	Flexion, ipsilateral rotation, ipsilateral side flexion
Longus capitis	Flexion, ipsilateral rotation
Scalenes anterior	Flexion, contralateral rotation, ipsilateral side flexion
Scalene medius	Ipsilateral side flexion, contralateral rotation
Scalene posterior	Ipsilateral side flexion, contralateral rotation
Sternocleidomastoid	Flexion, contralateral rotation, ipsilateral side flexion and extension
Trapezius upper fibers	Ipsilateral side flexion, contralateral rotation and extension
Levator scapula	Ipsilateral side flexion and ipsilateral rotation
Splenius, capitis and cervicis	Extension, ipsilateral rotation and ipsilateral side flexion
Spinalis, capitis and cervicis (inconsistent—blends with semispinalis)	Extension
Semispinalis, capitis and cervicis	Contralateral rotation and extension
Longissimus, capitis and cervicis	Extension, Ipsilateral rotation and ipsilateral side flexion
Iliocostalis cervicis	Extension and ipsilateral side flexion
Interspinalis	Extension
Multifidus	Extension, contralateral rotation
Rotators	Extension and ipsilateral rotation
Intertransversarii	Contralateral rotation

supply from the two closest vessel sources, which are those beneath the vertebral end plate and those at the periphery of the annulus fibrosus. Certain movements possible those in and out of the flexion, may facilitate nutrition of the disc (one of the benefit of exercise may be to facilitate the nutrition of the intervertebral disc). The intervertebral disc has a blood supply upto 8 years, thereafter, they are dependent for their own diffusion of tissue fluids. As the intervertebral disc is an avascular and its nutrition depends upon the diffusion and movements its healing transpires, but complete healing takes months to years (Fig. 26.5).

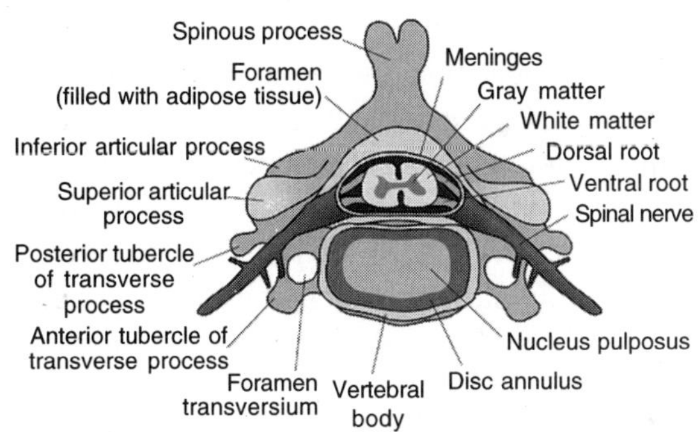

Fig. 26.5: Normal disc image

Pathomechanics

Disc herniation is the protrusion of the nucleus pulposus of the disc through the annulus fibrosus. The nucleus pulposus is a non compressible gelatinous material of the disc which absorbs and transfers the weight to the adjacent vertebra. As the load of the body comes on the nucleus pulposus it may protrude anteriorly, posteriorly, or laterally but fortunately it is prevented by the annulus fibrosus. The annulus fibrosus is strengthened and reinforced by the end plate. Therefore, in spite of protrusion to the anteriorly or posterolaterally that the nucleus pulposus transfers the weight to the adjacent vertebra. Unfortunately, forward bending of the cervical spine places excessive load on the

posterior annulus fibrosus and on the end plate. If the movement is combined with jerk, twist or injury it may rupture the annulus fibrosus and end plate and the nucleus pulposus may protrude through the ruptured annulus fibrosus to the posterolaterally, where it can put significant pressure on the nerve roots.

Disc herniation in the cervical spine occurs most commonly at the C_5-C_6 and C_6-C_7 vertebral levels, and radicular symptoms are experienced in the course of C_6 and C_7 nerve roots. There are two mechanisms which may cause disc herniation. First, the disc herniation may result from general wear and tear, such as when performing jobs that require constant sitting or involves forward bending movements. Such types of activities elongate and weaken the annular fibrous and end plate, which may in turn later stages allow the nucleus pulposus to herniate through the annulus fibrosus. This is a slow process of the disc herniation. The second mechanism, involves the jerk or sudden injury to the disc which causes nucleus pulposus herniation through the annulus fibrosus posterolaterally that may put pressure on the nerve roots to produce radicular symptoms. Since there is not a lot discs material (size of the disc) between the vertebral bodies in the cervical spine, the discs are not usually very large. The size of the vertebral foramen from where the nerve roots pass are also not that great, which means that even a small cervical disc herniation may impinge the nerve and cause significant radicular symptoms (Fig. 26.6).

Clinical Features

A cervical herniated disc may produce pain either in the cervical region or in the arm or both that depends upon the severity of the disc herniation and pressure on the nerve roots. In case of

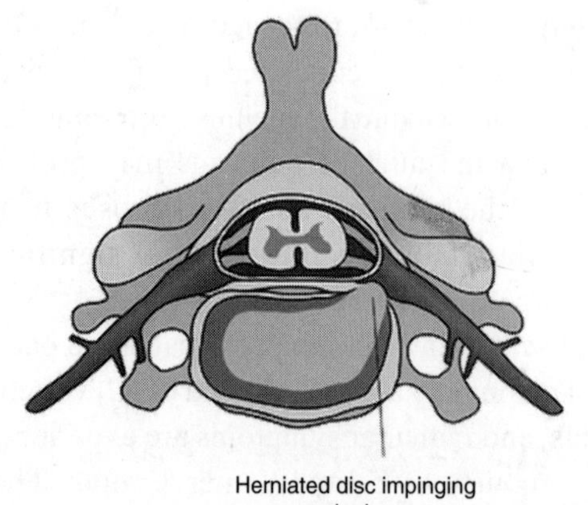

Herniated disc impinging
on spinal nerve

Fig. 26.6: Intervertebral disc herniation causing nerve compression

posterolateral herniation with significant nerve root compression the area of symptoms will be as below:

1. **C_4-C_5 Intervertebral Segment:** Pain and weakness will be in the course of the C_5 nerve root (deltoid region) it usually does not cause numbness and tingling sensation.

2. **C_5-C_6 Intervertebral Segment:** It is one of the most common sites, involves C_6 nerve root. Pain numbness, tingling sensation may be experienced in the course of the C_6, i.e, thumb of the hand. Adequate pressure on the C_6 nerve root can cause weakness in the biceps and wrist extensor muscles. The biceps jerk may diminish.

3. **C_6-C_7 Intervertebral Segment:** Pain, numbness and tingling sensation is experienced in the course of the C_7 nerve root, i.e., posterior aspect of the arm and middle finger. It may cause significant weakness in the triceps and finger extensors. This is also one of the most common levels for a disc herniation. Triceps jerk may diminish.

4. **C_7-C_8 Intervertebral Segment:** This may produce weakness in the finger flexors and numbness and tingling sensation in the forearm (ulnar side) to the little finger of the hand.

Assessment

Symptoms: Patients experience more pain and symptoms in the arm and shoulder. To avoid pain and stretching in the nerve the patient keeps the shoulder elevated, which further contributes to the spasm in the upper fibers of trapezius muscle of the same side. Diffused type of tenderness may be present on the neck. The patient bends the cervical spine to the opposite side to avoid pressure on the nerve roots which in turn produces cervical scoliosis or list. In patients with acute radiculopathy the symptoms such as pain, parasthesia, numbness and tingling sensation are the common symptoms. Weakness and loss of jerks may also be present in long standing cases. Patients report that their symptoms decrease when they place their hand on the top of the head, as this position decrease the tension in the nerve roots. The symptoms are aggravated by the neck movements particularly by flexion which opens the posterior intervertebral space that allows disc to protrude posteriorly. Sneezing and coughing also aggravate the symptoms.

Observation: The chin should be in line with the sternum (manubrium), the ears should be in line with the shoulders and the forehead vertical in the cervical spine. Deviation such as side flexion and rotation due to torticolis or muscle spasm should carefully be observed from anterior view. Other postural deviations such as Klippel Feil syndrome (fusion of the some cervical vertebra usually C_3-C_5), forward head posture (poking chin), torticolis should also be observed. *Shoulder Elevation:* Usually the dominant shoulder will slightly be lower than the non-dominant side, spasm or injury can cause elevation of the shoulder to provide protection and relief in the symptoms. *Shoulder Protraction:* Shoulders may be protracted due to weakness of the depressors and retractors (rhomboids). *Scapula Winging:* The medial border of the scapula may also be raised on thoracic wall due to weakness of the serratus anterior. ***Rounded Shoulders:*** The rounded shoulders may be associated with forward head posture. It is common in long standing and chronic cases. ***Muscle Wasting:*** Muscle wasting usually does not seen but in long standing cases it may be observed on the scapular, para-scapular and muscles supplied by the corresponding nerve root. The motion may be limited and painful in all three planes in later stages. ***List:*** It is the most common feature of the prolapsed intervertebral disc which can be observed in acute and chronic cases. The patient bends the neck to the opposite side to relieve the pressure on the nerve roots. In long standing cases the muscles of the concave side becomes tight and produces scoliosis in the cervical spine (Figs. 26.7a-e).

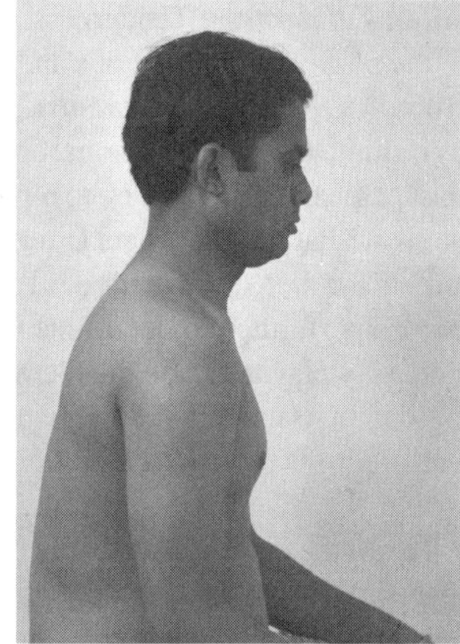

Fig. 26.7c: Lateral view

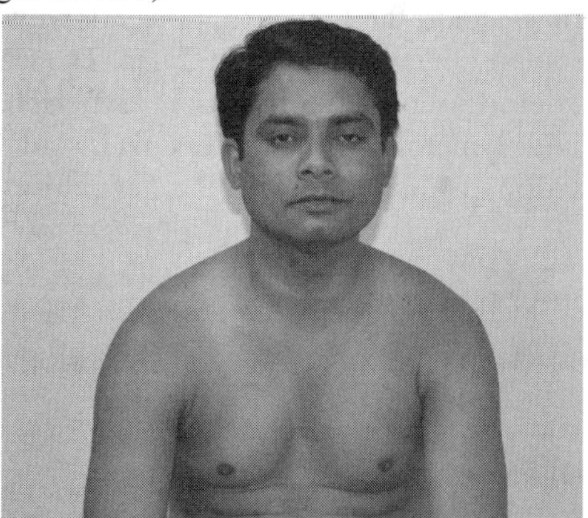

Fig. 26.7a: Anterior view

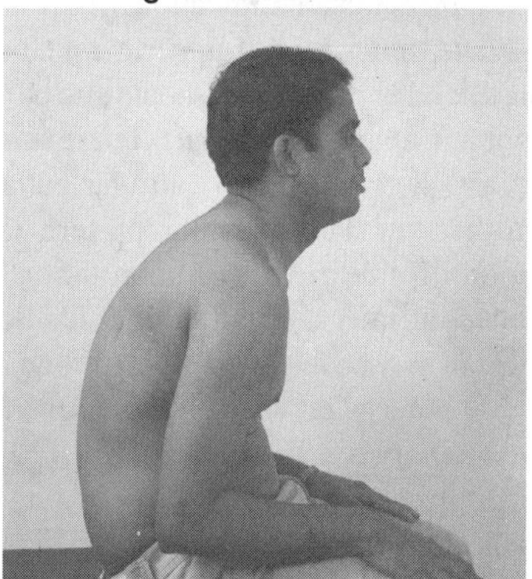

Fig. 26.7d: Forward head posture

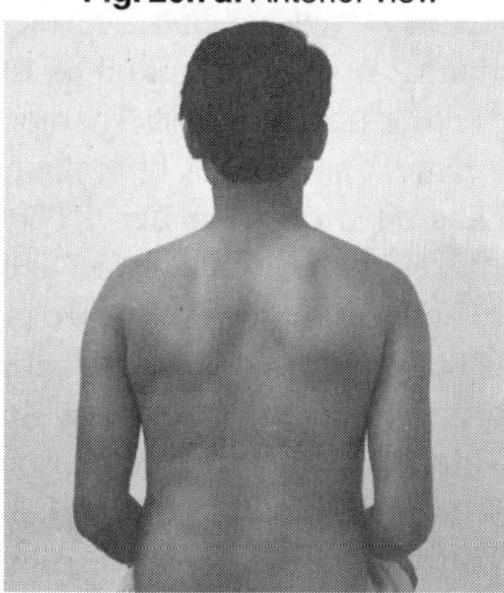

Fig. 26.7b: Posterior view

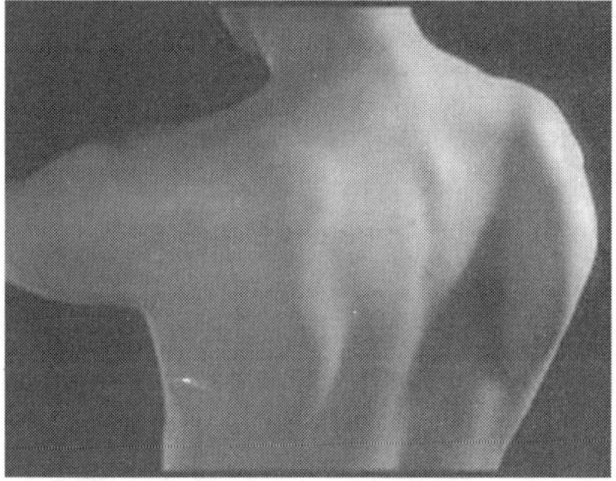

Fig. 2.3e: Winging of the scapula

Palpation: *Tenderness:* Tenderness may be present on the para-vertebral regions and on the spinous processes. *Passive Movements:* Passive ranges may be limited with the abnormal end feels. The therapist palpates each structure to reproduce the symptoms so that the site where from pain is originated may be determined. Passive movements are performed to determine the end feel. Patients may play tricks on the therapist by performing compensatory movements at other joints, therefore, to determine the motion at the cervical spine the distal segments should be stabilized. To test the flexion at the cervical spine the examiner should first flex the upper cervical spine and then (while maintaining it), the lower cervical spine is flexed. Limitation in the range of motion determines loss of upper cervical spine flexion. The other movements should also be tested passively. *Capsular Pattern:* The examiner should also note whether a capsular pattern is present or not. The capsular pattern is the limitation of side flexion with rotation. The movements at each segment during side flexion and rotation may be felt by palpating the adjacent transverse process on each side. *Identification of the Transverse Process of the C_1:* The examiner places the thumb and index finger on each side of the mastoid process and then moves the finger and thumb inferiorly and anteriorly until a hard bump is palpated on each side (usually below the ear lobe and just behind the jaw) (Fig. 26.8). *Identification of the C_7 Vertebra:* The spinous process of the C_7 vertebra is very prominent and it can easily be identified by placing the thumb on the spinous process.

If the passive movements with over pressure fail to reproduce the symptoms, the examiner may with great care, progress to the combination of movements.

Special Tests: Special tests are performed to reproduce the symptoms.

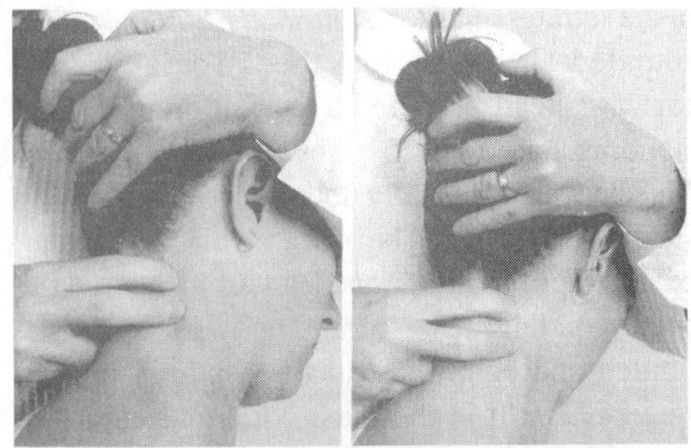

Fig. 26.8: Identification of the transverse process of the C

Foraminal Compression and Distraction: Patient sits on the stool with both arms hanging at the side of the body. Therapist stands behind the patient and places both the hands on the top of the head of the patient. While maintaining the neck in neutral position the therapist applies downward pressure through the body to the head. The test is considered as positive if patient experiences radicular symptoms with the pressure. It suggests radiculopathy due to soft disc herniation or degenerative changes putting pressure on the nerve roots. If symptoms such as pain aggravates in the cervical spine without radiation it may be due to arthritic changes without radiculopathy (Figs. 26.9 and 26.10).

Spurling Test

Also known as quadrant test is very useful in reproducing the symptoms in the cervical spine. Patient remains in sitting position as foraminal distraction and compression test. Therapist stands behind the patient and places both the hands on the top of the head of the patient. The head is extended, flexed to the affected side, and rotated (same side) and a downward pressure is applied through the body and arms. The test is considered positive if it reproduces radicular symptoms to the same side. This suggests radiculopathy due to soft disc herniation or degenerative changes causing compression on the nerve roots. If the test aggravates pain on the same side of the side

Table 26.5: Approximate range of motion of cervical spine (craniocervical region) (Fig. 2.3)

Joints	Flexion	Extension	Axial rotation	Side flexion
Atlanto-occipital	5	10	Negligible	5
Atlanto-axial	5	10	40-45	Negligible
Intracervical region (C_2-C_7)	35	70	45	35
Total range of motion at craniocervical region	45	90	90	40

flexion and rotation without radicular symtoms, it suggests changes in the facet joints and outer part of the disc to the same side (Figs. 26.11a-c).

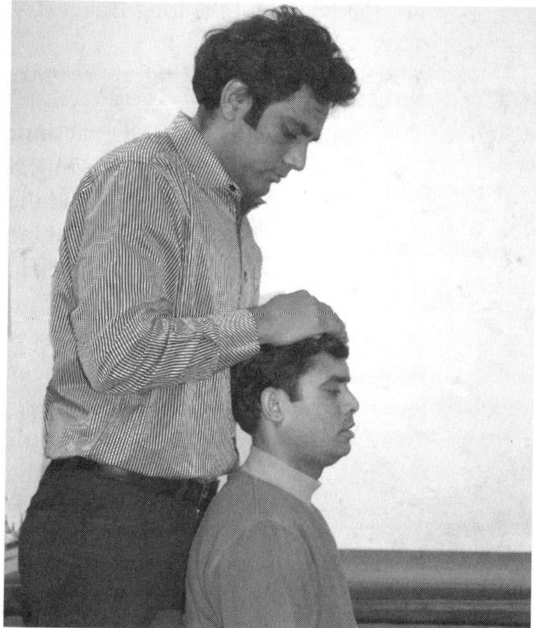

Fig. 26.9: Foraminal compression test

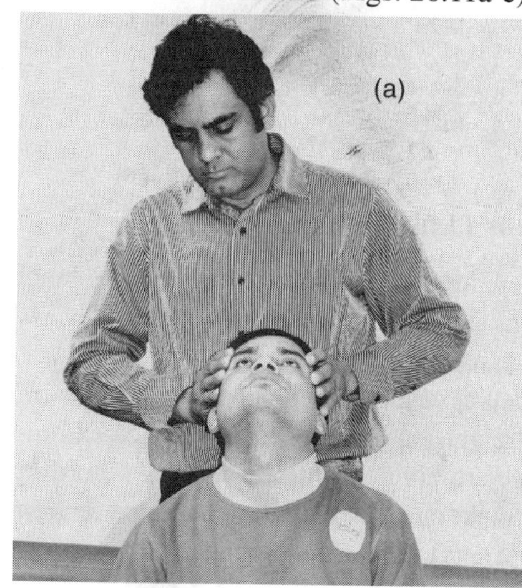

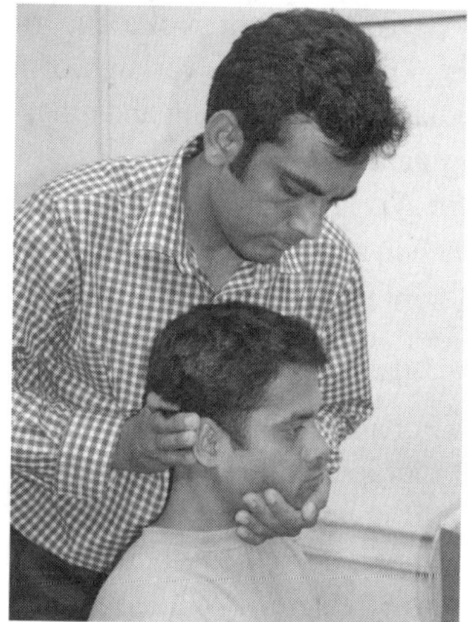

Fig. 26.10: Foraminal distraction test

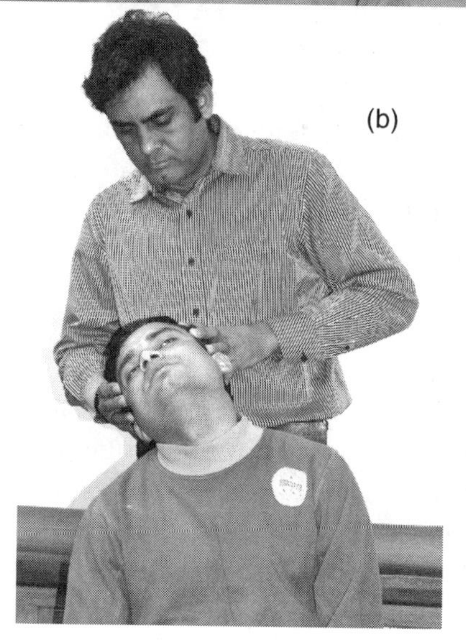

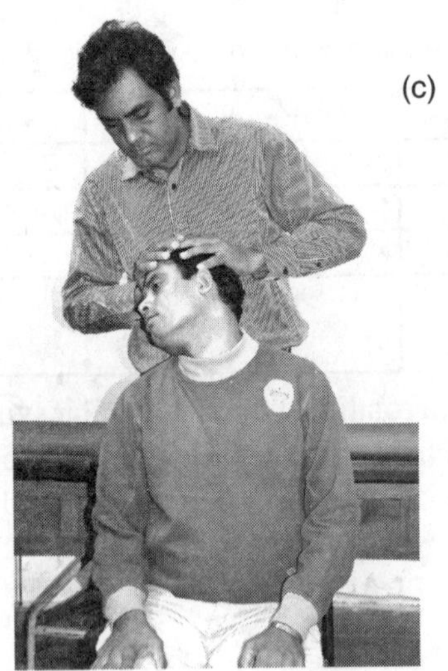

Figs. 26.11a-c: Spurling test

Upper Limb Tension Tests

Upper limb tension tests are known as brachial plexus tension tests were first described by Elvey. The tests were designed to put the pressure on the neural structure of the upper extremity similar to straight leg raising test for lower extremity. These are divided into three tests according to the course and distribution of the upper extremity spinal nerves (brachial plexus).

Upper Limb Tension Test$_1$: This test is also known as median nerve dominant test. It is designed to test the median nerve roots of C_5, C_6 and C_7. Patient is positioned in a supine lying and therapist stands at the side of the patient which is being tested. For an example, to test the right side, the therapist holds the right hand of the patient with his right hand and grasps elbow joint with the left hand. Therapist depresses the shoulder with the thigh. The shoulder is brought into the 110 degree abduction. While maintaining the shoulder depression with the right hand, the fingers, wrist and elbow are extended, followed by supination of the forearm. The neck is bent first to the affected side and then to the opposite side. The test is considered positive if the neck

bending toward the affected side relieves the symptoms, and neck flexion to the opposite side aggravates the symptoms.

The true radicular involvement would radiate the symptoms to the lateral arm deltoid and mid arm (C_5), down the dorsal radial aspect of the forearm to involve the index finger and the thumb (C_6), and centrally down the forearm to involve the dorsum of the hand and the long finger (C_7) (Fig. 26.12).

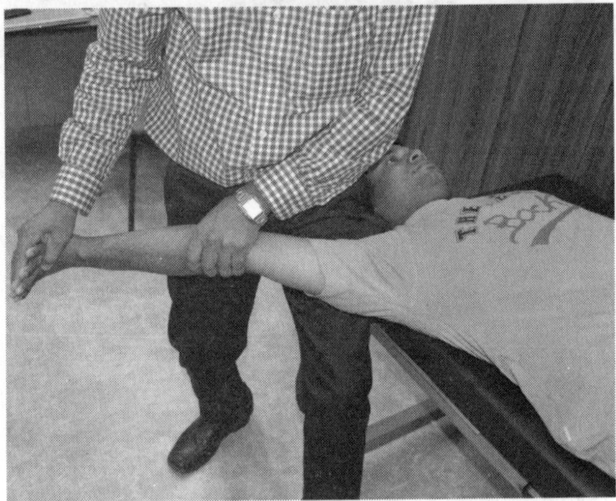

Fig. 26.12: Upper limb tension test$_1$, median nerve dominant

Upper Limb Tension Test$_2$: This test is designed to place significant tension on the nerve roots of C_6 or C_7 to provoke the radicular symptoms. There are two variants of this test, one is median nerve dominant and other is radial nerve dominant.

Median Nerve Dominant Test: The patient is positioned in supine with the scapula out of the edge of the table. The therapist stands close to the shoulder joint which is being tested. The shoulder is depressed with the help of the thigh inferiorly. For an example, to test the right median nerve the therapist holds the arm of the patient with the left hand and the hand with the right hand. The joint is depressed, abducted and rotated externally to 90 degrees. While maintaining the above position the therapist extends the wrist joint.

The test is considered positive if the maneuver produces radicular symptoms to the course of C_6 and C_7 nerve roots (Fig. 26.13).

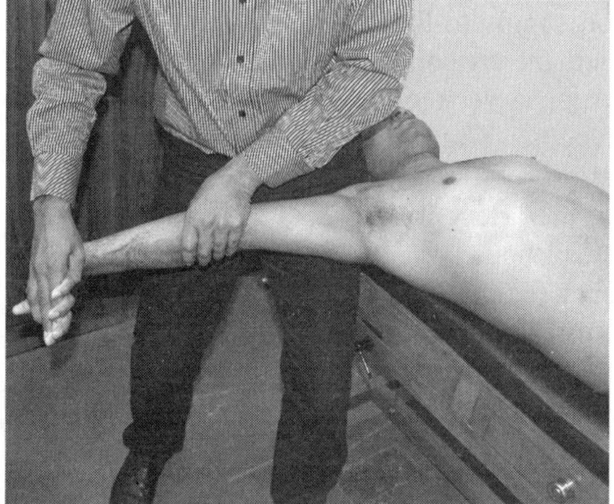

Fig. 26.13: Upper limb tension test$_2$, medial nerve dominant

Radial Nerve Root Dominant Test: The position of patient, therapist and arm remains same as median nerve dominant test. Shoulder is abducted to 10-20 degrees and rotated medially instead of externally as was in median nerve dominant test with wrist flexion. The test is considered positive if the radicular symptoms are produced particularly to the radial nerve distribution (Fig. 26.14).

Upper Limb Tension Test $_3$: The upper limb tension test 3 is designed to place the tension on the nerve roots of the ulnar nerve C_8 and T_1. It is also known as ulnar nerve dominant test. The patient is positioned in supine and therapist stands at the side of the patient, facing the shoulder. To test the right ulnar nerve the therapist stands toward the same side and places right hand on the top of the patient's shoulder and grasped the left hand of the patient with his or her left hand. The patient's flexed elbow rests on the anterior thigh of the therapist. While maintaining the shoulder depression and elbow flexion the therapist abducts the shoulder joint upto 90 degree with external rotation. At the last an extension of the wrist is added to the above maneuver to place significant tension on the ulnar nerve. The test is considered positive if the radiating symptoms aggravate down the arm past the elbow to the ring and little finger (C_8) or into the axilla (T_1) (Fig. 26.15).

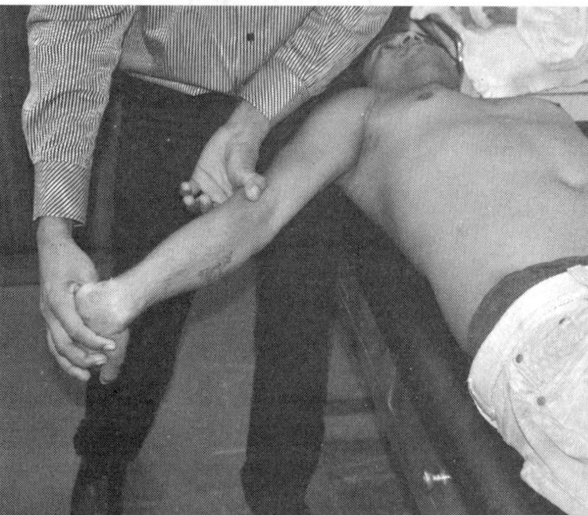

Fig. 26.14: Upper limb tension test$_2$, radial nerve dominant

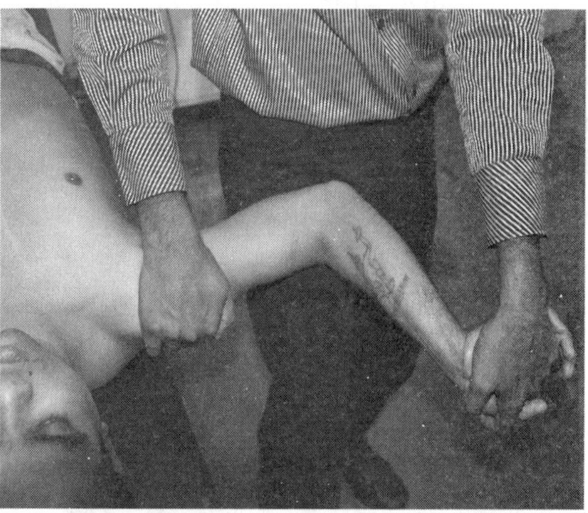

Fig. 26.15: Upper limb tension test$_3$, ulnar nerve dominant

---

Box 2.1 : Vertebro Basillary Insufficiency

Disc and facet joint degenerative changes may project the osteophytes laterally and posterolaterally or anteriorly, which can compress and distort the vertebral artery. Compression on one side vertebral artery rarely produces the symptoms because blood supply to the brain is compensated by the other vertebral artery. Osteophytes which project to both the vertebral arteries and caused significant compression and distortion can produce symptoms such as vertigo or giddiness dysarthria, visual symptoms (diplopia) and ataxia with episodes of syncope. The symptoms are aggravated by the neck movements particularly by extension with rotation.

Due to its close proximity to cervical vertebra, the artery is at risk of kinking with neck motions, especially in the presence of degenerative changes.

Course: The vertebral artery enters at the C_6 vertebral foraman and runs through it to C_2.

Examination: Patients present with the symptoms of vascular such as drop-attack, diplopia, dizziness etc. Headache is not the dominant feature, however, pain may be felt in the cervical spine due to degenerative changes. The movements of the cervical spine will aggravate an VBI symptoms.

Test: The test must be performed prior to any manipulative technique specially if there are the symptoms of VBI. The patient is placed in supine position with the head off of the edge of the couch. Therapist stands at the top of the head of the patient and places both hands on either side of the patient's head. The head is rotated to the right side followed by side flexion and extension. The patient is instructed to keep the eyes open and hold the position for atleast 10-15 seconds. During this period the therapist may busy the patient in simple conversation rather than asking the symptoms of the VBI. In case of positive VBI, patients will complain dilatation of pupil, nystagmus, distress, dizziness, slurred speech, visual disturbances or any other untoward occurrence.

Note:
- Test must be performed with cautious, sometimes it may be fatal and can cause death by blocking/kinking the artery.
- Positive VBI is the absolute contraindication of any kind of joint manipulation, such as thrust at the end etc.
- Therapist may administer aspirin or raise the legs in case of positive test to avoid unwanted danger.

Muscle Strength Testing/Myotomes (Figs. 26.16a-i)

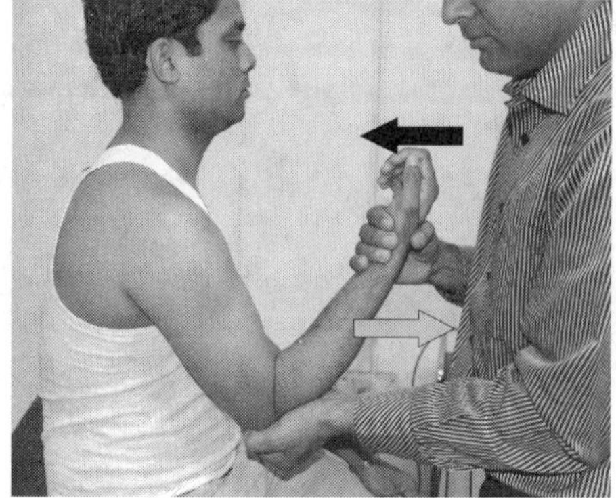

Fig. 26.16a: Biceps

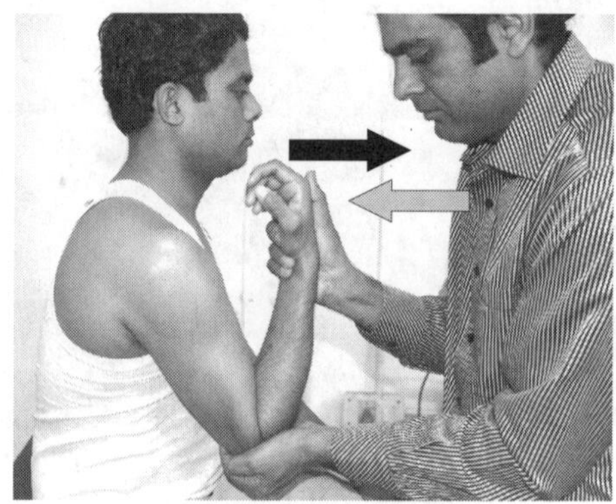

Fig. 26.16b: Triceps

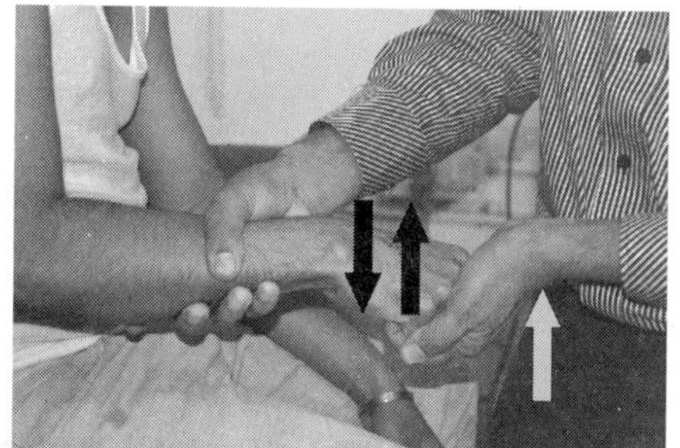

Fig. 26.16c: Wrist flexors

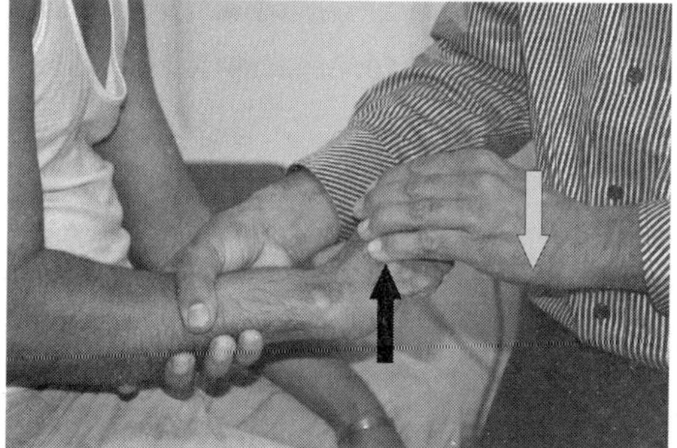

Fig. 26.16d: Wrist extensors

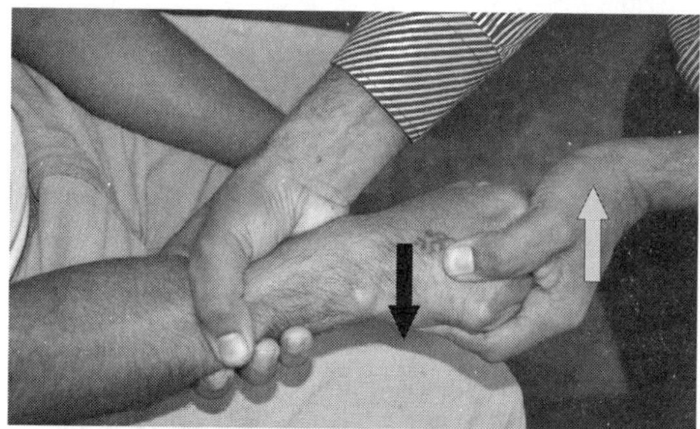

Fig. 26.16e: Wrist ulnar deviators

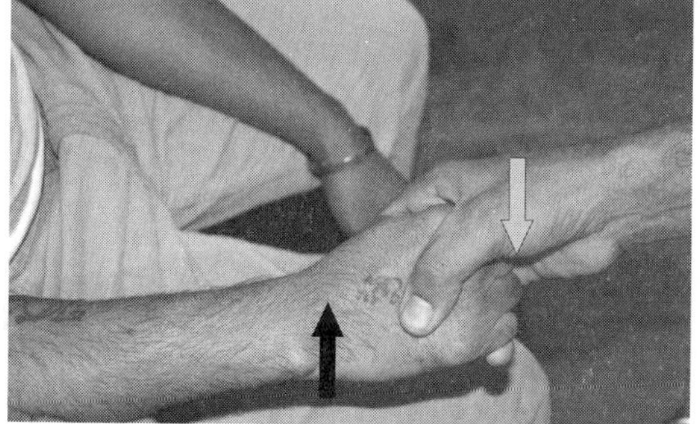

Fig. 26.16f: Wrist radial deviators

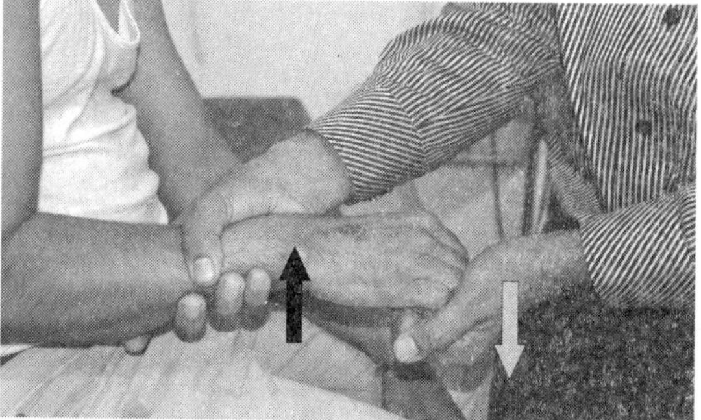

Fig. 26.16g: Finger flexors

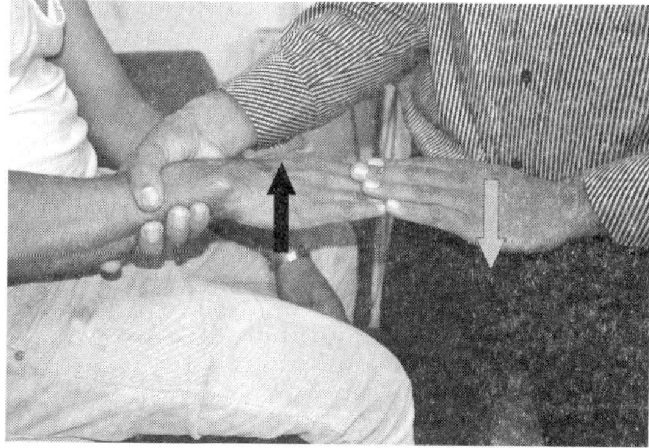

Fig. 26.16h: Finger extensors

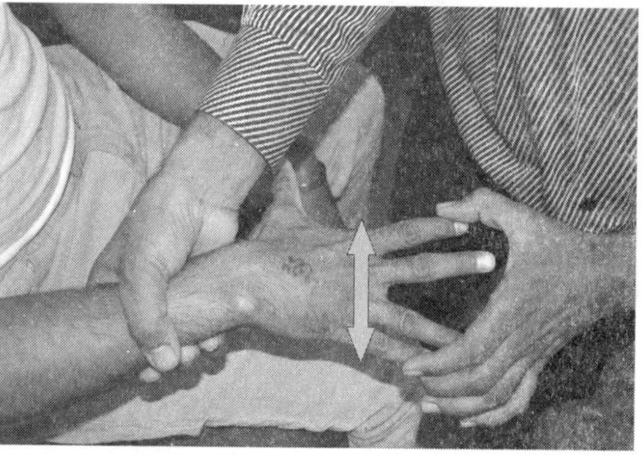

Fig. 26.16i: Finger abductors

Deep Tendon Reflexes: Biceps, triceps or supinator jerk may be diminished or lost (Figs. 26.17 to 26.19).

Dermatomes: Sensation may be decreased or lost of a particular dermatome in longstanding cases (Fig. 26.20).

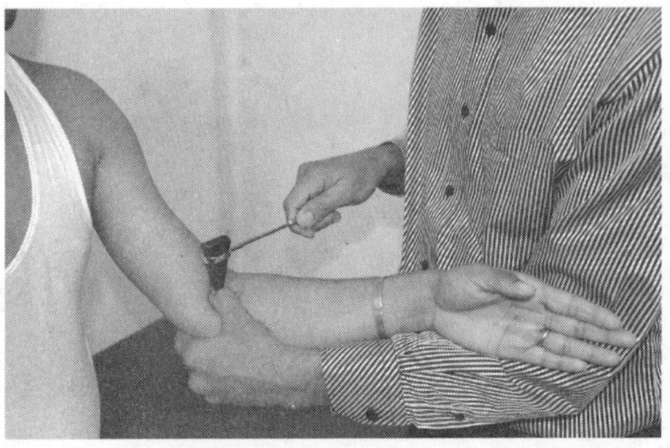

Fig. 26.17: Biceps jerk

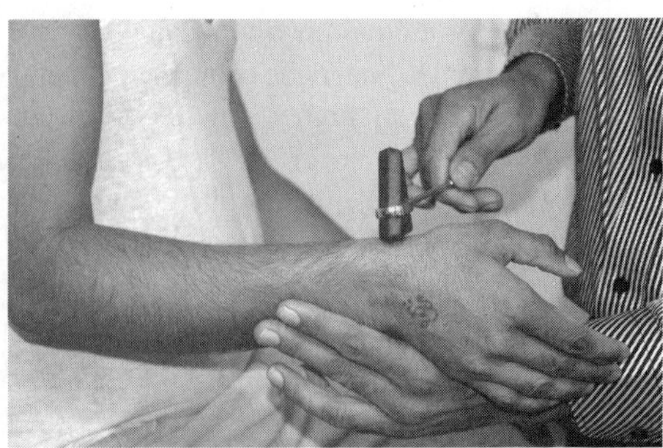

Fig. 26.19: Supinator jerk

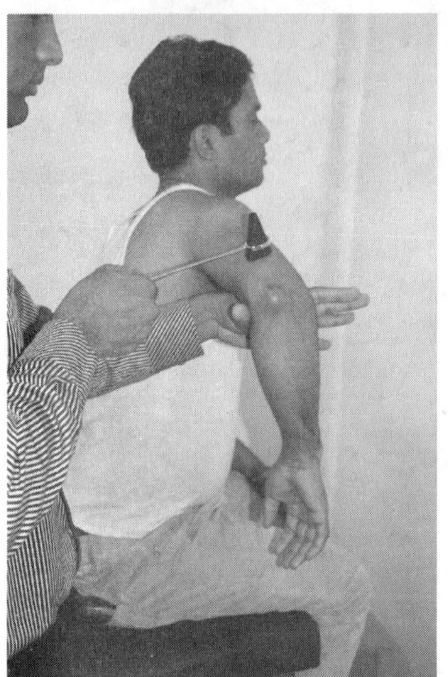

Fig. 26.18: Triceps jerk

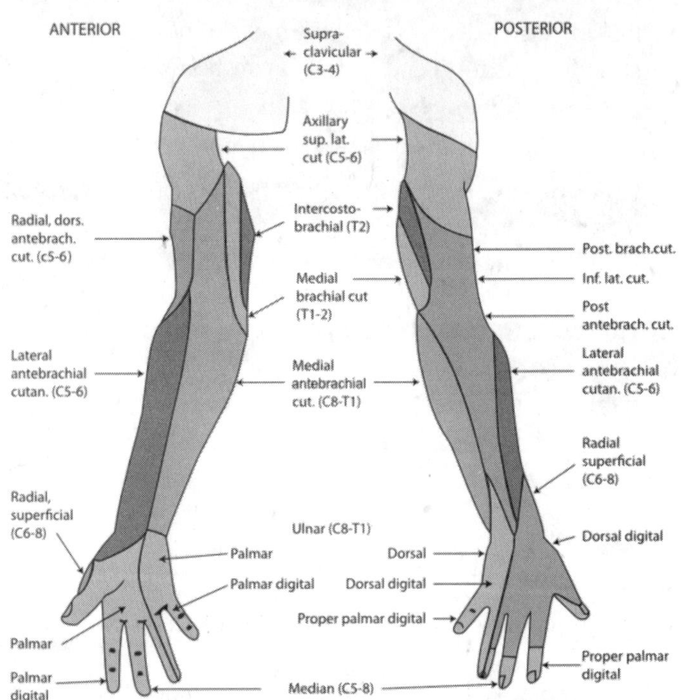

Fig. 26.20: Dermatomes upper extremity

Management

1. **Spontaneous Resorption of Sequestrated Intervertebral Disc:** Acute radiculopathy improves rapidly with conservative treatment. This is because the soft disc herniation, with time and treatment can shrink (resorption) and disappear. Orief T, Orz Y, Almusrea KA conducted the study on radicular pain due to sequestrated disc herniation of cervical and lumbar disc. The patients were managed conservatively. All patients recovered from their radicular pain within three to four weeks and it was correlated with resorption of their sequestrated intervertebral disc herniation as documented in their follow up magnetic resonance imaging (MRI) at 4-6 months. They found that sequestered disc herniation has

potential for regression which can clearly be demonstrated by magnetic resonance imaging because of having higher water content, and therefore, may regress through both dehydration and inflammation-mediated resorption. They suggested conservative treatment in the initial course of the sequestrated of disc herniation for at least two months before recommending the surgical intervention unless severe neurological deterioration take place.

2. **Control of Pain and Spasm:** Moist heat therapy which helps in relieving muscle spasm should be recommended and it can be used by the patient twice or thrice daily for atleast 15-20 minutes per session at workstation or house. Transcutenous Electrical Nerve Stimulation (TENS) (pocket type) which stimulates A large diameter and blocks the A delta fibers at gelatinous is also beneficial. However it is less recommended now-a-days.

3. **Immobilization of Cervical Spine:** The patients with acute radiculopathy are advised cervical collar (soft or hard). The cervical collar which distracts the intervertebral joints helps in reducing the intradiscal pressure and protrusion of the nucleus pulposus on the nerve roots. In case of moderate disc prolapse soft collar is advised to prevent the movements at the cervical spine, thus preventing the intervertebral disc to further prolapse. But in case of severe disc prolapse and involvement of more than one segment (constant symptoms not relieved by placing the hand on the head or by other measures), hard collar is advised which provides immobilization and keeps the cervical spine in distracted position thus helps in reducing the pressure on the nerve roots and shrinking of the protruded disc (Figs. 26.21 and 26.22). The use of cervical collar for prolong period of time can

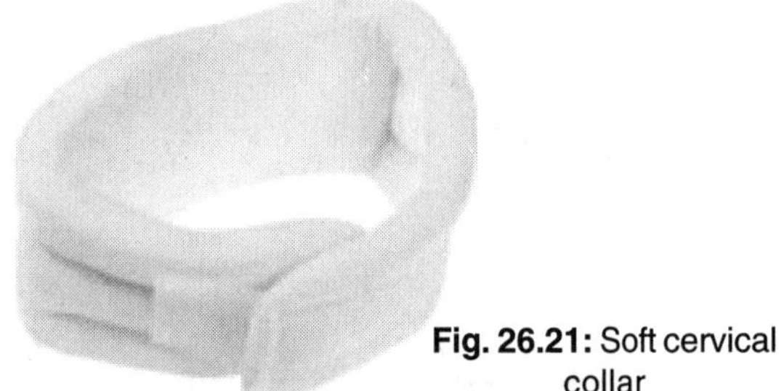

Fig. 26.21: Soft cervical collar

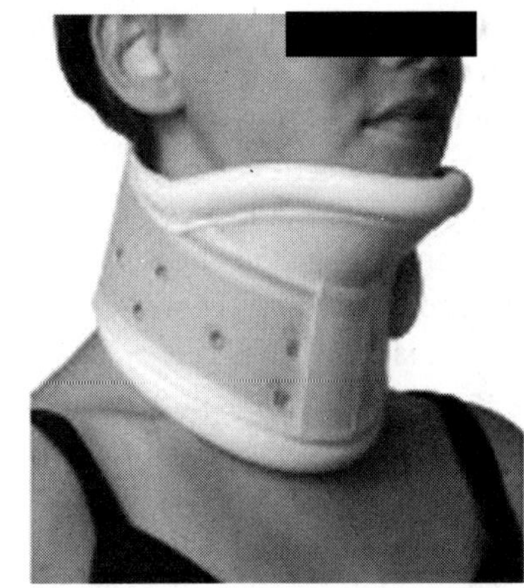

Fig. 26.22: Hard cervical collar

cause adverse effects such as disuse atrophy of the muscles hence, it should be advised only for short period of time.

4. **Stress Reduction:** Emotional and physical stresses can increase tension in the neck muscles and interfere with or delay the recovery process. Patient should be advised to eliminate stress as much as possible by placing the non-urgent jobs on hold, obtaining counseling for major life stresses and seeking support from family, friends and health providers.

5. **Cervical Pillow:** In case of straightening of the cervical spine due to spasm, an H-shaped pillow is placed under the nip of the neck to maintain the cervical lordosis. The patients with forward head posture require a small towel roll under the head instead of neck. (Figs. 26.23a-b).

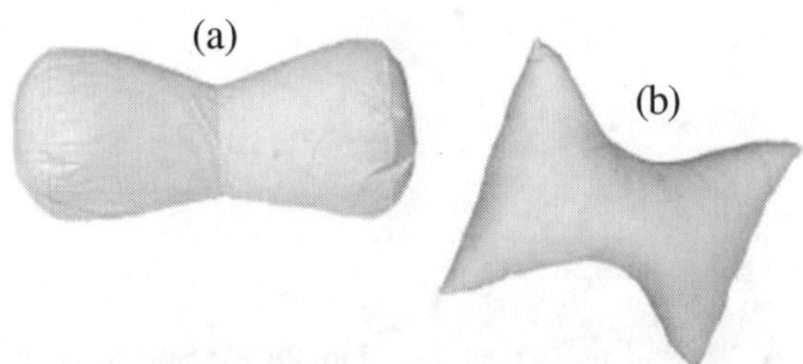

Figs. 26.23a-b: Cervical pillows

6. Activity Limitation and Posture Modification:

a. Avoid sitting posture in the same position for prolonged period of time.

b. Maintain good posture by holding head up and keeping shoulders back.

c. Use the chair arm rests to keep the shoulder slightly shrugged.

d. Sleep with neck in a neutral position.

e. Place small pillow under the nape of the neck to maintain the cervical lordotic curve.

f. Place enough pillows to keep the neck straight in line with body (side lying).

7. Traction:
It is one of the most important treatments for an acute radiculopathy. Traction is the most effective means to stretch the supporting ligaments of the neck. Distraction of the intervertebral joint by the mechanical device helps in relieving the symptoms. It should be recommended in the flexed position approximately 15-20°, as flexion will open the intervertebral foramen that will allow disc to shrink back to its normal position. Some patients find difficulty in attending the clinics therefore; they may be advised cervical traction at home. They can purchase a cervical traction kit available in the market. The kit is placed on the wall and patient should use it in slightly neck flexed position. Intermittent traction may help in reducing circulatory congestion and relieve pressure on the dura, blood vessels and nerve roots in the intervertebral foramen. Removing pressure on the blood vessels will improve the blood circulation, remove noxious chemical irritants and decrease pain and other symptoms (Figs. 26.24a-b).

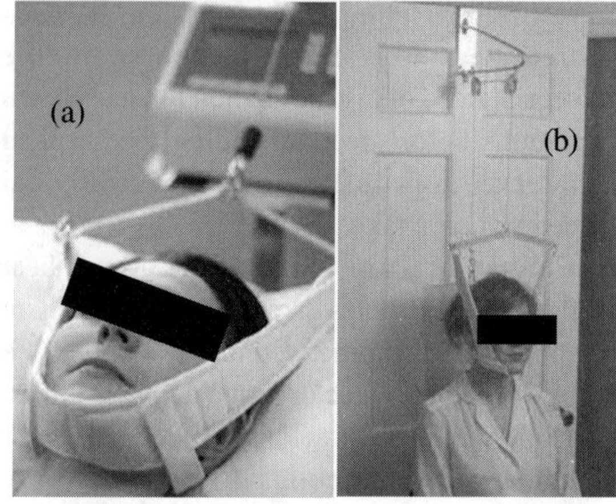

Figs. 26.24a-b: Traction (a) lying (b) sitting

8. Exercises:
Exercises should begin as the acute pain starts subsiding. The collar is removed and exercise which relieves the symptoms should be repeated several times. The therapist must note that any movement particularly flexion which aggravates the symptoms must be avoided. Repeating exercises in pain free range helps in centralizing the symptoms. Patients with severe degree of disc prolapsed will also have malalignment of the facet joints. These patients will improve with the conservative treatment but pain will persist at the end ranges of motion especially in flexion and side flexion. Sustained natural apophyseal glides may help in improving the pain and range of motion but it should be advised at the stage where radicular symptoms subside.

a. ***Strengthening:*** The weak muscles such as deep neck flexors, rhomboids, serratus anterior and trapezius middle and lower fibers are strengthened (Figs. 26.25 and 26.28).

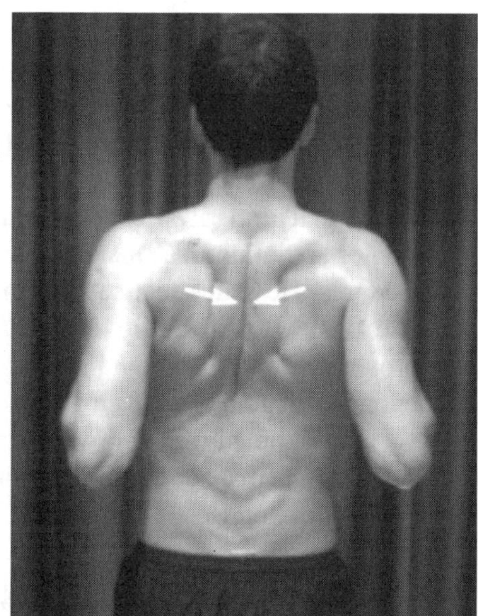

Fig. 26.25: Rhomboids and trapezius middle in standing

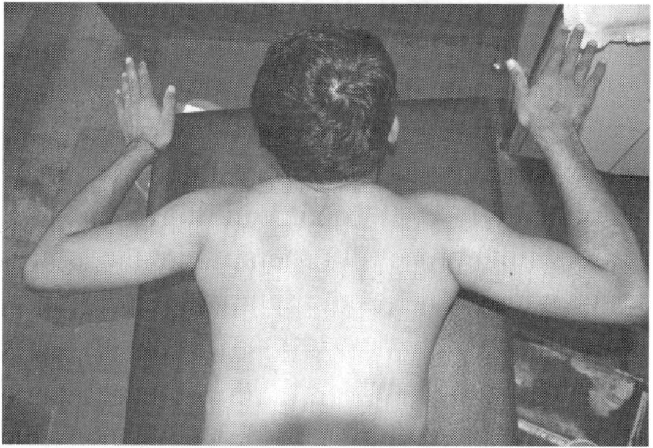

Fig. 26.26: Rhomboid in prone

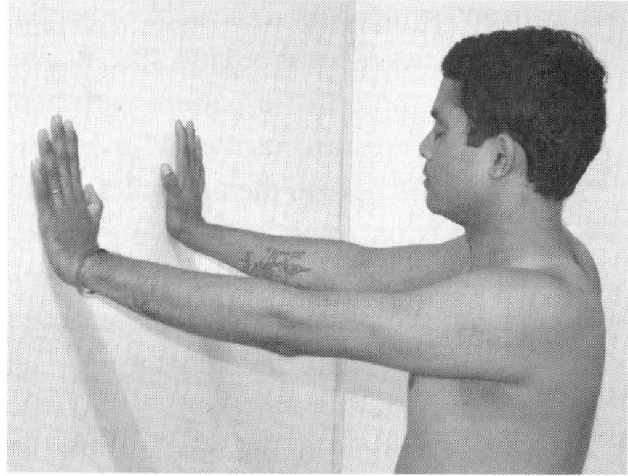

Fig. 26.27: Serratus anterior

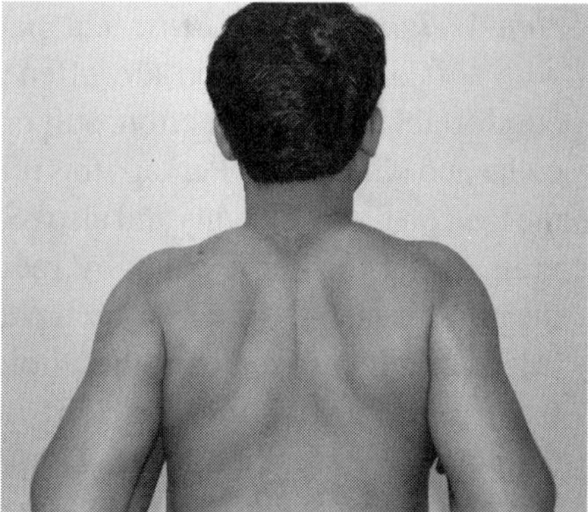

Fig. 26.28: Trapezius middle in sitting

b. ***Stretching:*** The tight muscles such as levator scapulae, trapezius upper fibers, erector spinae, and pectoralis major should be stretched to improve the flexibility (Figs. 26.29 and 26.30).

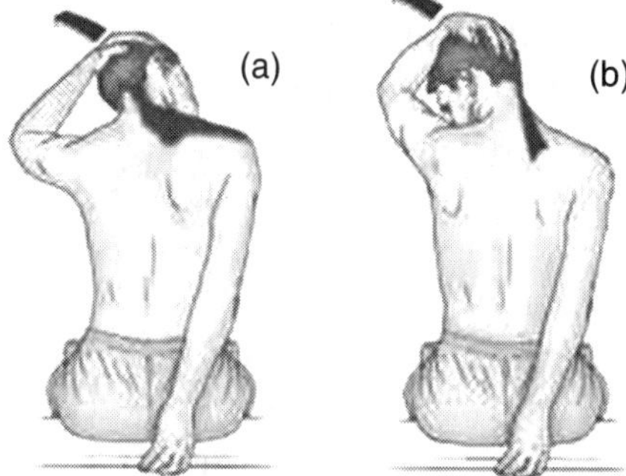

Figs. 26.29: Stretching a. Levator scapulae b. Trapezius upper

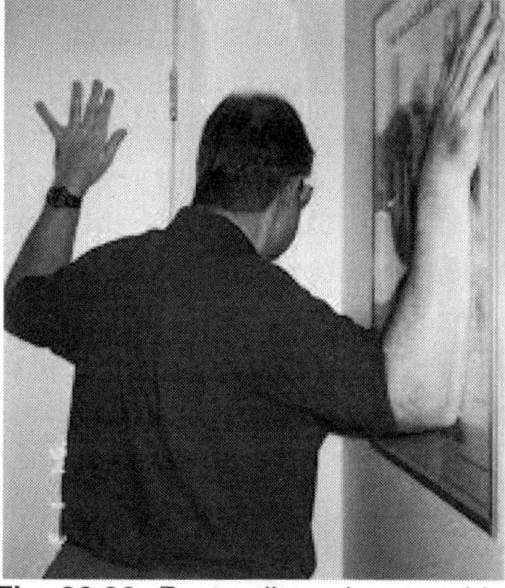

Fig. 26.30: Pectoralis major stretching

c. ***Non-Weight Bearing Bias:*** The patients with soft disc herniation are often more comfortable with the traction, soft or hard collar and lying down. Perhaps this relieves the load on the facet joints and also reduces pressure on the nerve roots by reducing the intradiscal pressure. For such patients traction and rest may be the choice of treatment until the patient feels comfortable in weight bearing. The patient is progressed to weight bearing as healing improves and he or she begins to tolerate weight bearing.

d. ***Adverse Effects of Rest:*** Rest in collar increases intradiscal pressure with the time; the nucleus potentially can absorb more water contents to equalize pressure (imbibition). On the other hand, lying with flexed spine allows the imbibed fluid to accumulate posteriorly in the intervertebral disc where there is greater space. When patient stands, pain and symptoms from a disc protrusion are accentuated, because, accumulated fluid in the disc spaces will increase the intradiscal pressure. Therefore, to avoid exacerbating symptoms absolute rest during acute phase should not be advised. Rest for 1-2 days may be advised, but it should be interrupted with short intervals of exercises.

e. ***Extension Exercise Bias:*** Patients with cervical disc protrusion are often comfortable and may have partial or full relief with extension of the neck. The patients with extension bias often assume a flexed posture with or without neck side flexion. The impairment may be due to a contained intervertebral disc lesion, fluid stasis, injury to the facet joints, or a muscle imbalance from a faulty flexed posture.

f. ***McKenzie:*** New Zealand based physical therapist Robin Anthony McKenzie had developed and launched the concept in 1981 which he called Mechanical Diagnosis and Therapy (MDT). An MDT is a system encompassing evaluation, diagnosis, and treatment for the spine and extremities. It primarily uses self treatment strategies and minimizes manual therapy procedures. He states that self treatment is the best way to achieve a lasting improvement in the sign and symptoms. The long term goal of McKenzie concept is to teach the patients how to treat themselves and manage their own pain for life by using exercises.

In the process of diagnosis he performs repeated movements on the cervical spine or lumbar spine and finds the movement which relieves the symptoms from distal to proximal part of the area. As an example, for soft disc herniation (acute radiculopathy) there are the movements which relieve and aggravate the symptoms. The movements which relieve the symptoms become the diagnostic tool. In the process of therapy the movement which relieves the symptoms from distal to proximal is performed repeatedly, while the movement which aggravates the symptoms is discarded. The goal of the therapy part is to centralize the patient's pain and symptoms in the neck rather than treat pain that is localized in a specific area. As an example, for a patient with acute cervical radiculopathy, whose chief complaint is pain in the arm and forearm, the extension movement of the neck is performed repeatedly to decrease the radicular symptoms from forearm, arm, to the neck rather than directing the treatment to the arm and forearm.

The mechanical diagnosis and therapy concept categorizes the clinical presentations of the patients into subgroups which are not based on anatomy. Based on the categorization the patient is instructed on specific exercises to gradually decrease the pain and symptoms. There are mainly three types of syndromes— Postural, Dysfunction and Derangement Syndrome.

i. **Postural Syndrome:** It is the result of positions or postures those place significant stress on the intervertebral discs, ligaments, capsule and muscles. The pain is localized and not reproduced with the movements, but if the movements at end ranges are maintained for sustained periods of time may reproduce the pain and symptoms. The postural syndrome is very much common in the population whose job requires prolong sitting. Posture is worst while working on the computers, reading and even driving. People who work on computer in slouch posture and read or drive with a forward head posture create enormous stresses on the muscles, ligaments, tendon, discs and facet joints of the cervical spine. 8-10 lbs weight creates no stress on the neck if the head is on the midline of the neck (normally the ears position directly over the tip of the acromion process). If the head moves one inch forward to the midline it can create an extra 10 lbs stress on the neck. Hence, the patients with forward head posture carry an extra weight between 10 lbs and 30 lbs or more. Imagine if you hold the 30 lbs dumbbell at 90 degree shoulder flexion with elbow straight for an hour what it would be with your arms? The forward head posture leads to long term muscle strain, disc herniations and nerve root compression. McKenzie consists a set of exercises for this syndrome which include chin tuck or neck retraction, neck extension and expansion in sitting, and neck extension and expansion in standing.

a. ***Chin Tuck or Neck Retraction:*** This exercise is also known as double chin exercise. The head is drawn backwards without the chin lifting up. The patient keeps the chin tucked in and down and draws it back as far as it can be done comfortably. The position is held for six seconds at the end range. Exercise is repeated ten times. This exercise will align the neck itself with the rest of the spine, and releases the pressure on the muscles, ligaments and discs (Fig. 26.31).

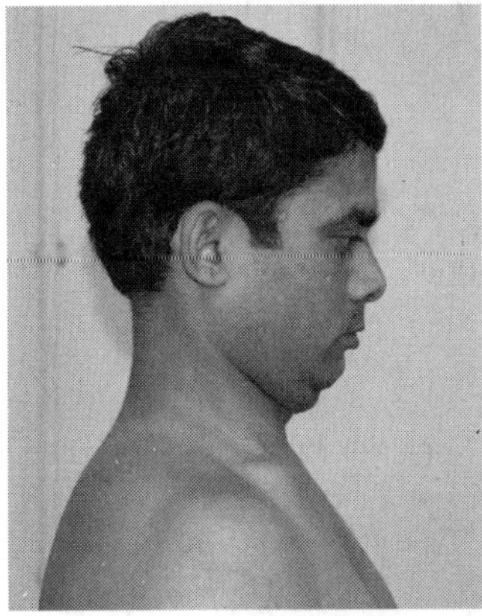

Fig. 26.31: Chin tuck or neck retraction

b. ***Neck Retraction and Expansion in Sitting:*** The exercises not only releases the pressure occurs in slouched posture but also releases the strain on the muscles. This exercise produces the movement at the discs which helps in lubrication of the fluid and nutrition to the discs. The neck retraction and expansion in sitting is the extension of the chin tuck exercise. The patient sits on the stool comfortably and draws the head backwards without lifting the chin up. The chin tucked in position is drawn back as far as it is possible. Patient looks up gradually toward the roof as far as possible. It is essential to keep the chin stays down and in, even during the head tilts. After holding this position for five seconds, the patient relaxes the muscles and brings to the starting position. The exercise can be repeated ten times. In the next step of the exercise as the symptoms improve, the head is turn side to side with the neck retraction and expansion. Ten repetitions can be performed. Patient should be taught to breathe and relax during the exercise (Figs. 26.32 and 26.33).

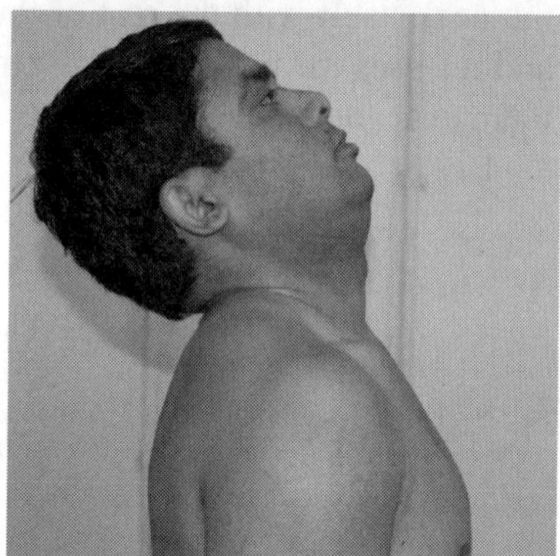

Fig. 26.32: Neck retraction and expansion in sitting up

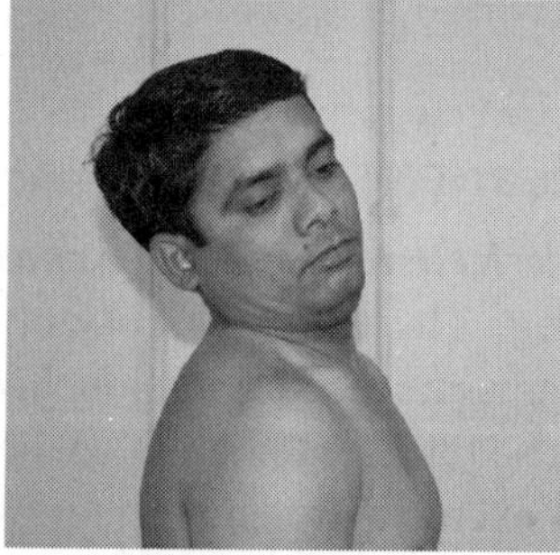

Fig. 26.33: Neck retraction and expansion with side flexion in sitting

c. *Neck Retraction and Expansion in Supine:* This exercise is recommended to the patients who find difficulty in performing the chin tuck exercise in sitting positions. The patient lies supine, head is taken out of the edge of the table. Head is drawn back on the neck as far as possible and the position is held at least for five seconds. It can be repeated ten times 2-3 times daily (Fig. 26.34).

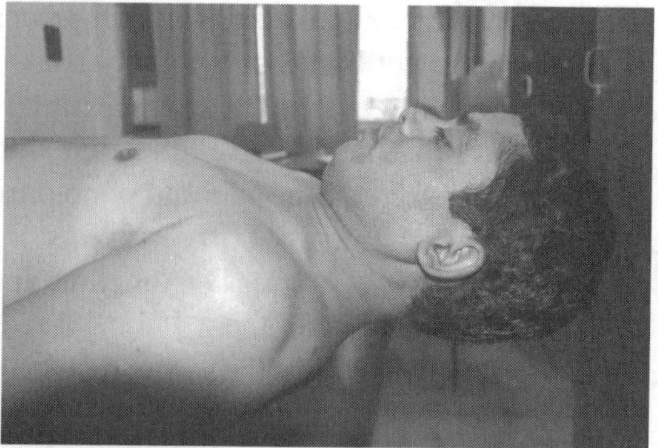

Fig. 26.34: Neck retraction in supine

ii. **Dysfunction Syndrome:** In this syndrome patients present with pain and limitation in the motion at the end ranges. Due to poor posture there is shortening or scarring or adherence of the connective tissues which limit the motion at the end ranges. A dysfunction may be intermittent or chronic, but its hallmark is a consistent movement loss and pain at the end range of motion. The movements hardly produce pain and symptoms in the initial and mid range. Exercises which can stretch the muscles or break the adhesions are usually effective. Treatment is focused on tissue remodeling which require regular exercises. The improvement in the sign and symptoms is slow because the process of tissue remodeling progresses slowly. In addition to the stretching exercises the postural correction exercises are the cornerstone of the dysfunction syndrome.

iii. **Derangement Syndrome:** This category is the most common syndrome that presents clinically. Hallmark of derangement syndrome is its sensitivity to certain movements and its preference for particular movement pattern. When these movements such as flexion and or extension are performed, the symptoms either aggravate or relieve. The derangement syndrome is very common after the prolapsed intervertebral disc. The radicular symptoms which are originated from the neck are experienced in the arm and forearm. It is not uncommon for the patient to experience rapid reduction in the radicular symptoms immediately during the assessment. Treatment for the patients with derangement syndrome, as with the postural and dysfunction syndromes, is directly guided by the patients response to these provocative assessment movements.

iv. **Manual Therapy:** Manual mobilization such as maitland and mulligan can also be started as patient shows improvement in the radiculopathy symptoms. The techniques are explained in cervical spondylosis/disc degeneration.

SPONDYLOSIS (CERVICAL DISC DEGENERATION)

The disc is relatively a non-compressible gel, comprises proteoglycans, collagen fibers and water. The physical ability to absorb the weight of the body depends on its proteoglycan water complex. The disc degeneration is a gradual process which begins usually after fourth decade of the life but in some cases such as traumatic or pathological, it may commence even in fourth decade of the life. The degenerative changes in the disc increases as the life progress, but it is not essential that these changes will produce symptoms. Some people remain asymptomatic throughout their life though degenerative changes can be seen on X-rays. On the other hand people with minimal degenerative changes may have symptoms and seek intervention. This depends upon the adaptability of the body. As the disc degeneration is a slow process, the body adapts the changes hence, no symptoms are produced in the due course of time, but a trauma or injury to the cervical spine can cause stress on the changes and the symptoms are reproduced.

In the process of degeneration the nucleus pulposus looses its water binding capacity and becomes compressible and less able to absorb and transfer the weight or load to the annulus. In turn the annular collagen fibers break down and cease to function as weight absorber, the result

is desiccation of the nucleus with fragmentation and tear or fissuring of the annulus (Figs. 26.35 to 26.37).

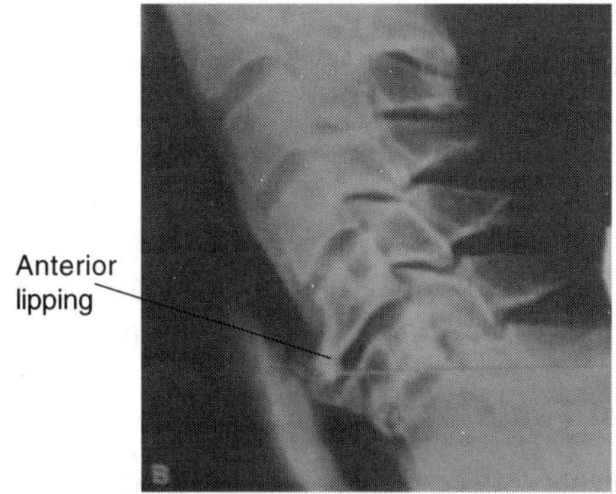

Fig. 26.35: Spondylosis with anterior lipping

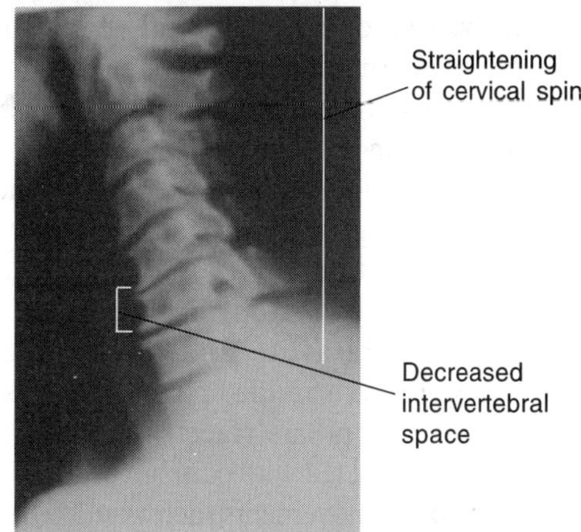

Fig. 26.36: Disc degeneration with reduced intervertebral space between C_5-C_6 and C_6-C_7 and anterior lipping

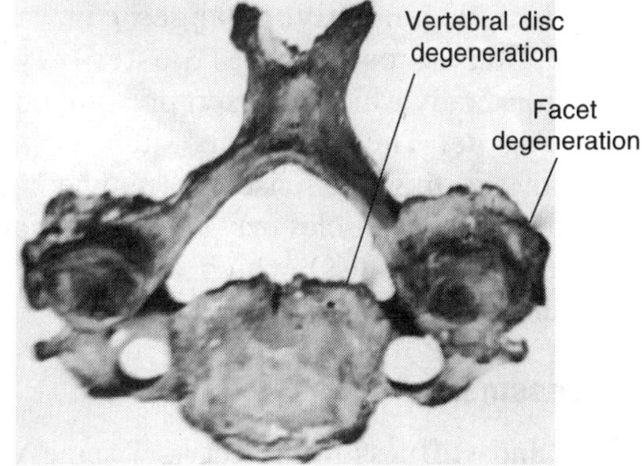

Fig. 26.37: Disc degeneration with facet joint degeneration

Due to fragmentation, desiccation and fissuring, the height of the disc is decreased. The annular fibers bulge may into the nerve roots and cord territory and abnormal movement occurs in the mobile segment due to instability. In an attempt at repair and stabilization, fibrotic changes occur in the nucleus. Stabilizing osteophytes occur at the margin of the disc spaces. In the next process of disc degeneration, the desiccated nuclear material may or may not rupture through a tear in the annulus to cause nerve root or cord pressure.

Clinical Features

The patients with cervical spondylosis experience pain in the cervical spine which may be in the central part or on paravertebral region of the cervical spine. Initially pain is localized but may radiate down the arm or forearm and hand. Activities which hold the neck in extension such as shaving, painting, putting on shoes and shocks, knitting, reading with bifocals or half moon glasses, using telephone or even excitedly watching cricket match on television may precipitate, aggravate and perpetuate the symptoms. These activities put excessive stress on the posterior pillars (facet joints). Initially extension is restricted with pain but as the disease progresses other movements such as sided flexion, rotation and forward flexion will also be painful and restricted. The forward flexion may be limited initially due to spasm in the posterior neck muscles.

Gross degenerative changes can cause projection of osteophytes posteriorly or posterolaterally which can exert pressure on the nerve roots. The symptoms such as pain, parasthesia, tingling sensation, numbers and weakness of the muscles may be felt at the arm, forearm and hand(s) which are termed as radiculopathy (chronic).

Assessment

Pain and stiffness in the cervical spine with restriction of extension and other range of motion

---

Flowchart 2.1: The normal disc

The normal disc is composed of collagen – Proteoglycan complex and fluid which maintain its physical properties such as height, shape and structure

↓

As the age progresses, disc loses its water binding capacity and becomes compressible

↓

The disc loses its physical properties (height, shape and structure), and the intervertebral space is decreased (instability). Load is transferred to the posterior pillars (facet joints). Dysfunction and subluxation of the facet joints, facet joint synovitis/capsulitis occurs

↓

Patients experience localized pain and limitation in the movements. Muscle guarding (muscle spasm) further contribute to the limitation in the range of motion

↓

Formation of osteophytes which may project anteriorly, posteriorly and posterolaterally. The osteophytes project to the nerve roots may cause significant pressure on the neural tissues

↓

Neural tissue compression, numbness, tingling sensation, radicular pain, down the arm. Decrease biceps or triceps jerks(s), decrease muscle power

---

are the common complaints of the patients with cervical disc degeneration or spondylosis. Middle aged group people are generally involved. Disease progresses with gradual onset.

Observation: The chin should be in line with the sternum (manubrium); the ears should be in line with the shoulders and the forehead vertical on the cervical spine. Deviation such as side flexion and rotation due to muscle spasm should carefully be observed from anterior view. Other postural deviations such as Klippel Feil syndrome (fusion of the some cervical vertebra usually C_3-C_5), forward head posture (poking chin), should also be observed.

Usually the dominant side shoulder will slightly be lower than the non-dominant side, spasm or injury can cause elevation of the shoulder to provide protection and relief in the symptoms. The rounded shoulders may be associated with forward head posture. *Muscle Wasting:* Muscle wasting may be seen in long standing cases it may be observed on the scapular and para-scapular region. Shoulders may be drooped and protracted due to weakness of the depressors and retractors (rhomboids), the medial border of the scapula may also be raised on thoracic wall due to weakness of the serratus anterior. Extension is limited initially but other movements may also be limited and painful in all three planes in later stages.

Special Tests

A. Foraminal Compression and Distraction: Patient sits on the stool with both arms hanging at the side of the body. Therapist stands behind the patient and places both the hands on the top of the head of the patient. While maintaining the neck in neutral position the therapist applies downward pressure through the body to the top of the head. If patient experiences radicular symptoms with the pressure it suggests chronic radiculopathy and the test is considered positive. If symptoms such as pain aggravates in the cervical spine without radiation it may be due to osteoarthritic changes in the cervical spine.

B. Spurling Test: Also known as quadrant test is very useful in producing the symptoms in the cervical spine patient. Position of patient remains sitting as foramen compression and distraction test. Therapist stands behind the patient, places both the hands on the top of the head of the patient. The head is extended, bent and rotated to the affected side (same side) and a downward pressure is applied through the body and arms. If it aggravates pain on the same side of the side flexion and rotation, it suggests degenerative changes in the facet joints and outer part of the disc to the same side. If the test reproduces radicular symptoms, it suggests chronic radiculopathy due to degenerative changes causing compression on the nerve roots. The spurling test has good sensitivity to the radiculopathy.

C. Alar-Odontoid Integrity: Patient is positioned in a comfortable sitting with arms hanging freely on the sides. Therapist stands on the same side of alar-odontoid ligament and places the thumb of one hand lateral to the spinous process of C_2 vertebra and other hand on the top of the head. *Procedure:* To test

Table 26.6: Stages of intervertebral disc degeneration

Stages	Nucleus pulposus	Annulus fibrosus	Facet joint	Result
Normal	Proteoglycan/water	Collage fibers structure with high tensile strength	Smooth gliding	Nucleus absorbs forces and transfers to annulus. Smooth pain free movement
Stage I	Loss of water, breakdown of proteoglycans	Fissuring and tearing of fibers	Synovitis, hypomobility	Intermittent axial pain
Stage II	Nuclear protrusion	Fissuring, disc resorption	Capsular laxity and subluxation	Axial and radicular pain
State III	Desiccation and narrowing	Osteophyte formation	Osteophyte formation	Minor axial pain and neurological compromise

the left ligament the therapist bends the patients head to the left side (same side). The side flexion of the head should produce immediate and simultaneous rotation of C_2 to the same side as of side bending, which is palpated as movement of spinous process of C_2 in the direction opposite of the side bending (Fig. 26.38). A test is considered as positive if the motion of C_2 spinous process is absent. It is the indication of rupture or lax of alar ligament or fracture of the odontoid process (Fig. 26.38).

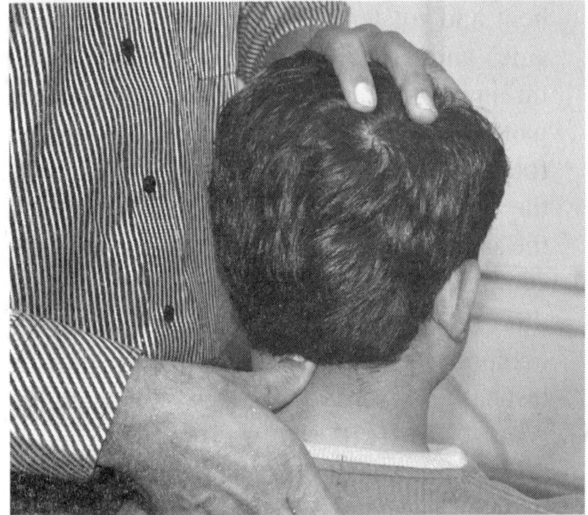

Fig. 26.38: Alar odontoid integrity test

D. Transverse Ligament Test: In case of lax or ruptured transverse ligament, it is recommended to have the patient perform the self test, as it is a very serious condition and can be a fatal. For self testing, patient sits comfortably on the stool with both the hands hanging freely at the sides. Patient is asked to gently nod the head. Therapist looks for any signs or symptoms of cord compression such as nausea, bilateral arm symptoms etc.

E. Sharp Purser Test: The patient sits comfortably, and therapist stands at the side of the patient. Therapist places stabilizing hand on the occiput and forearm around the temporal region. The thumb of the mobilizing hand is placed on the spinous process of axis. *Procedure:* The patient actively performs forward bending to his or her comfort. Therapist applies a posterior to anterior force on the axis. A positive test is the feeling of occiput and atlas sliding back on axis, often with a click sound, indicating reduction of subluxation of occiput and atlas (Fig. 26.39).

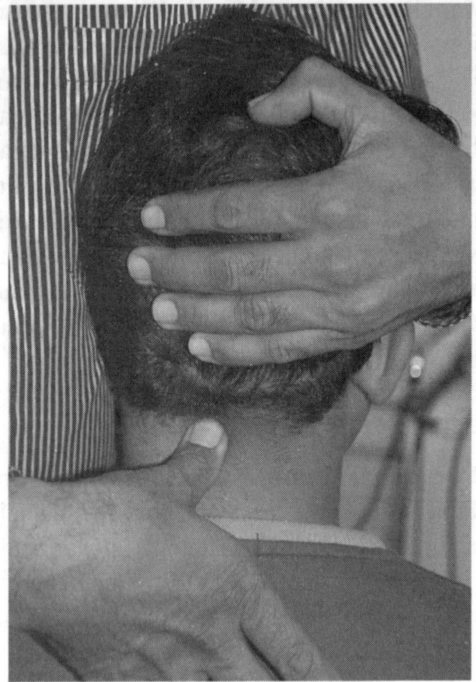

Fig. 26.39: Sharp purser test

Differential Diagnosis

Acute Radiculopathy: Patients with acute radiculopathy (soft disc herniation, a sudden process) experience more symptoms in the arm, forearm and hand, while patients with chronic radiculopathy (degenerated disc herniation, a gradual process of disc degeneration) experience more pain and symptoms in the neck rather than in the arm and forearm. Moreover, acute radiculopathy is commoner in young age group with onset of unilateral symptoms. On the other hand the chronic radiculopathy occurs in the middle aged group of patients.

Thoracic Outlet Syndrome

Introduction: Thoracic outlet syndrome is a compression of the brachial plexus or subclavian artery or subclavian veins in the outlet formed by the scalene muscles on three sides and cervical rib on the fourth side at the upper thorax. The subclavian veins are rarely involved in the syndrome as they pass beneath the thoracic outlet.

Causes: The neurovascular bundle which passes through the thoracic outlet gets compressed if the outlet is narrowed due to spasm in the anterior and middle scalene muscles, or if the shoulder girdle is depressed. The common causes of thoracic outlet syndrome include physical trauma from a car accident, repetitive injuries from a job such as frequent non-ergonomic use of a key board, sports-related activities, anatomical defects such as having an extra rib and pregnancy. The athletes who frequently raise their arms above the head such as swimmers, volleyball players, shuttlecock players, baseball pitchers, and weightlifters may be at the risk of thoracic outlet syndrome.

Types: There are three types of thoracic outlet syndromes classified according to the involvement of the structures. The compression can occur in three anatomical structures (arteries, veins and nerves), can be isolated, or-more commonly-two or three of the structures are compressed to greater or lesser degrees.

a. **Neurogenic Thoracic Outlet Syndrome:** It accounts 95% of all cases of thoracic outlet syndrome. This type of syndrome includes the compression of brachial plexus. The symptoms are of pain, parasthesia, tingling sensation and weakness of the thenar and hypothenar muscles.

b. **Arterial Thoracic Outlet Syndrome:** It is due to compression of the subclavian artery.

c. **Venous Thoracic Outlet Syndrome:** This type of syndrome occurs due to subclavian vein compression.

Sometimes the thoracic outlet syndrome is classified by the name of the structure which produces compression on the neurovascular bundle.

Scalenus Anticus Syndrome: The spasm in the scalene muscles particularly anterior and middle scalene can reduce the outlet and can put significant compression on the brachial plexus or/and on the subclavian artery.

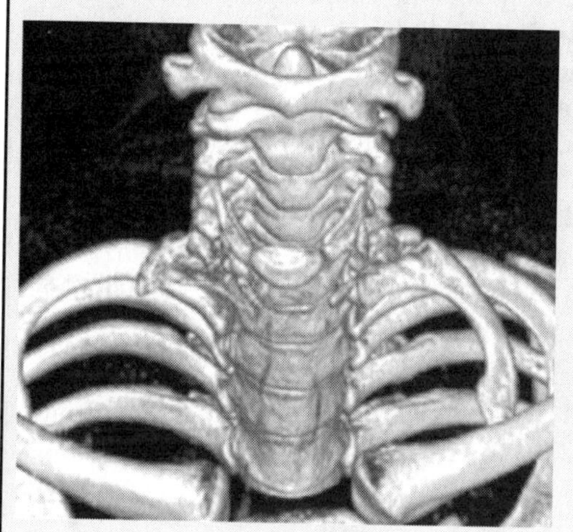

Cervical Rib Syndrome: Some people are born with an extra incomplete and very small cartilaginous rib. It is known as cervical rib because it is originated from the cervical (seventh) vertebra. This rudimentary rib causes fibrous changes around the brachial plexus nerves, inducing compression and causing the symptoms and signs of thoracic outlet syndrome.

Costo-clavicular syndrome: The thoracic outlet is narrowed between the clavicle and the first rib and the symptoms of neurovascular bundle compression are produced.

Symptoms: The symptoms either neurogenic or vascular or both types be present. Thoracic outlet syndrome mainly affects the upper extremity. The

Contd.

Contd.

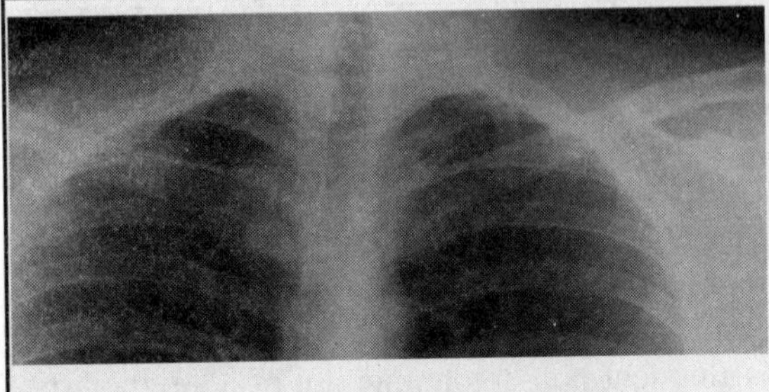

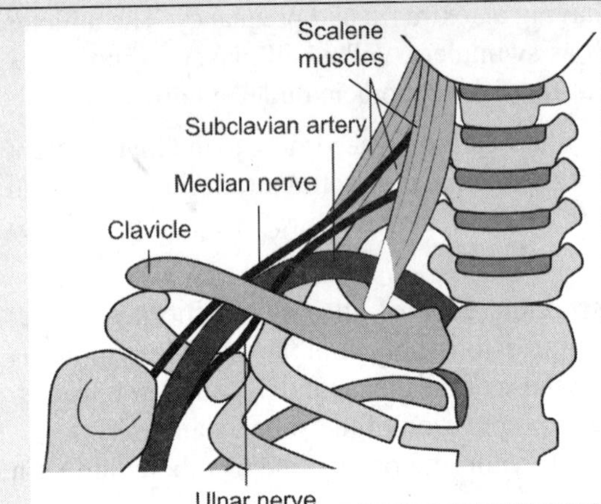

neurogenic symptoms such as pain, parasthesia, numbness are almost always present, and can be sharp, burning, or aching. It can involve only part of the hand (as in the 4th and 5th finger only), all of the hand, or the inner aspect of the forearm and upper arm. Pain can also be felt in the side of the neck, the pectoral area below the clavicle, the axillary area, and the upper back (i.e., the trapezius and rhomboid area). Tenderness on the anterior scalene muscle (pectoral area) may also be present. The vascular symptoms such as discoloration of the hands (one hand colder than the other hand), swelling, and weakness of the hand and arm muscle are commonly present. A painful, swollen and blue arm, particularly when occurring after strenuous physical activity, could be a sign of a venous compression or subclavian vein thrombosis called Paget-Schroetter Syndrome.

Examination: The patients with thoracic outlet syndrome usually complaints pain, weakness, heaviness and swelling in the hand. The symptoms are aggravated after the activities. Patients commonly find difficulty in performing overhead activities. A cervical rib may be seen on the X-rays.

a. **Adson's Test:** The patient sits on the stool with both the hands hanging freely on either side. The neck is rotated and flexed to the opposite side. Therapist stands behind the patient and palpates the radial pulse with one hand. While keeping the pulse palpated the extremity is abducted and extended to the 30 degrees. The patient is instructed to take the deep breath. The test may be considered positive, if the therapist finds diminished or feeble radial pulse.

b. **Roos Test:** In a comfortable sitting position, the patient is asked to abduct the shoulders at 90 degrees with elbows flexion to 90 degrees. Patient is instructed to open and make the fist of both the sides as fast as possible at least for three minutes. The test is considered positive if patient complaints heaviness and finds difficulty in keeping the arms at 90 degrees. The affected arm will drop gradually while the normal side will be maintained. In case, where, both the sides are affected, the patient will start dropping both the arms gradually after one minute.

c. **Doppler Arteriography:** With probes at the fingertips and arms, tests the force and "smoothness" of the arterial flow through the radial arteries, with and without having the patient perform various arm maneuvers (which causes compression of the subclavian artery at the thoracic outlet). The movements can elicit symptoms of pain and numbness and produce graphs with diminished arterial blood flow to the fingertips, providing strong evidence of impingement of the subclavian artery at the thoracic outlet.

Management: The patients with thoracic outlet syndromes are managed with the conservative treatment. This includes mostly exercises but for symptomatic relief in pain and symptoms the heat

Contd.

Contd.

modalities may also be advised. If the patients do not respond to the fair trial of conservative treatment, surgical intervention is the last choice, which may include resection of cervical rib.

Conservative treatment: This includes stretching, strengthening exercises and heat therapy. The muscles which keep the shoulder girdle elevated and retracted such as trapezius (upper, middle and lower) fibers, rhomboids, serratus anterior are need to be strengthened in order to avoid pressure on the neurovascular bundle. The core muscle strengthening also plays important role in the management of thoracic outlet syndrome as it helps in correcting kyphotic anomaly of the upper back. The pectoralis major, scalene (anterior, middle and posterior) and extensors of cervical should be stretched. Continuous mode of ultrasound therapy of 1Mhz over the scalene muscles with the intensity of 1watt per centimeter square may be useful in increasing the extensibility of the scalene muscles. Hot pack may also help in decreasing the muscle spasm.

Neural Tissue Mobilization: The patients with thoracic outlet syndrome often involve compression of a large cluster of nerves, typically resulting in motor and/or sensory impairment throughout the arm, forearm and hand. Neural tissue mobilization given by David Buttler, Australian based physical therapist also known as neural gliding or buttler neural tissue mobilization is considered to be very effective in terms of stretching and mobilizing affected nerve fibers. It is performed in a similar manner of D2 flexion pattern of proprioceptive neuromuscular facilitation (PNF). The patient lies supine with the shoulder out of edge of the couch. The therapist stands at the side and grasps the hand of the patient and elbow joint. The shoulder joint is depressed appropriately and arm is rotated externally with the elbow extension. While maintaining the aforesaid position the therapist abducts and flexes the extremity over the shoulder.

Surgical Management: It may be advised to the thoracic outlet syndrome patients who presents with cervical rib. It involves removal of the cervical rib, scalene muscles and any compressive fibrous tissue which causing pressure on the neurovascular bundles. However, no surgical option should be considered until all non-invasive approaches have been exhausted.

Anzina Pectoralis: Similar symptoms of radiculopathy are produced but patients with anzina pectoralis experience pain on the left anterior chest. The symptoms are relieved by taking isosorbite trinitrate drugs orally.

Thoracic Outlet Syndrome: Patients with thoracic outlet syndrome present with mixed type of symptoms (neurovascular). In addition to neurological symptoms patients also experience heaviness and swelling. These patients present with drooped shoulders and tenderness on the anterior chest (over the anterior scalene muscle) X-ray findings may reveal cervical rib.

Manual Therapy

A. Distraction of Occipito-Atlanto and Atlanto-Axial Joints:

Position of Patient: Sitting on the treatment table. *Position of Therapist:* The therapist stands at the side of the patient opposite to the joint being mobilized. To mobilize the right side facet joint of OA and AA the therapist stands at the left side of the patient and places right hand (stabilizing) on the transverse process of the atlas for OA or articular rim of axis for AA facet joint. The mobilizing hand is around the base of the occipital. The therapist stands with 30-40° knee flexion. *Procedure:* The therapist cradles the head between the mobilizing hand and stabilizing hand on the chest and extends the knees to produce cranial force or distraction of facet joints of OA and AA (Figs. 26.40 and 26.41).

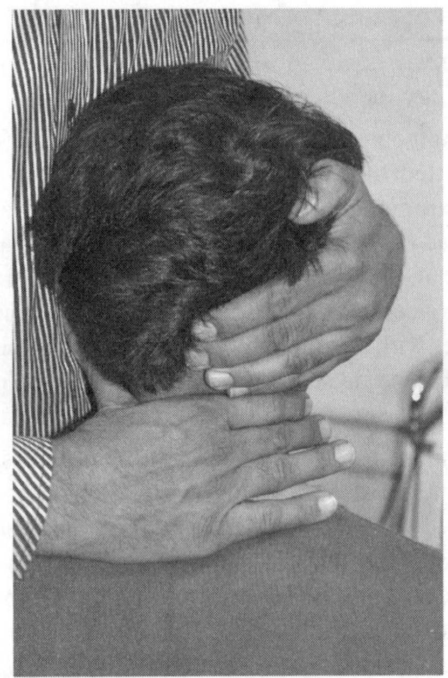

Fig. 26.40: Position of hands

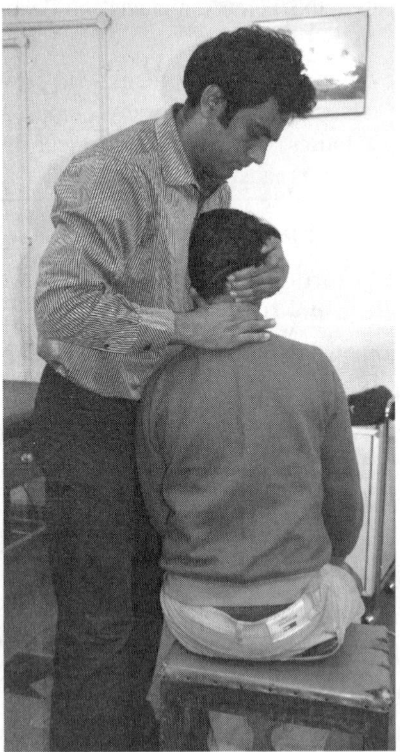

Fig. 26.41: Occipito-atlanto and atlanto axial distraction

B. Mobilization (Maitland): Maitland mobilization is one of the conventional mobilization techniques which is always performed in a relaxed position. *Position of Patient:* Supine, head remains off of the couch, arms at the side of the body. *Position of Therapist:* Therapist stands at the top of the head. Left hand grasps the occiput and right hand holds the chin. The patients head rests on the belly of therapist. A paper or napkin may be placed between the head and belly for cosmetic purposes. Therapist stands with slight knees bent (Figs. 26.42 to 26.46).

a. Distraction: While maintaining the above position the therapist distracts the head with the help of body. End range may be held for at least 6-10 seconds. 10-15 repetitions may be performed (Fig. 26.42).

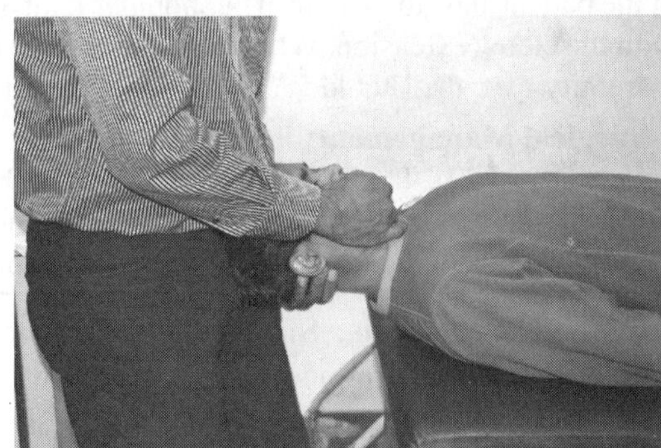

Fig. 26.42: Distraction

b. Side Flexion: While maintaining the traction the head is taken to the left side up to the full range or till the restriction starts and then to the neutral position, the pressure may be released. Then the head is taken to the right side with the traction. The traction is maintained throughout the range of motion till the head comes to the neutral position. When the head is taken to the left and to the right the therapist should have wide stance and should move the body with the head without changing the stance (Fig. 26.43).

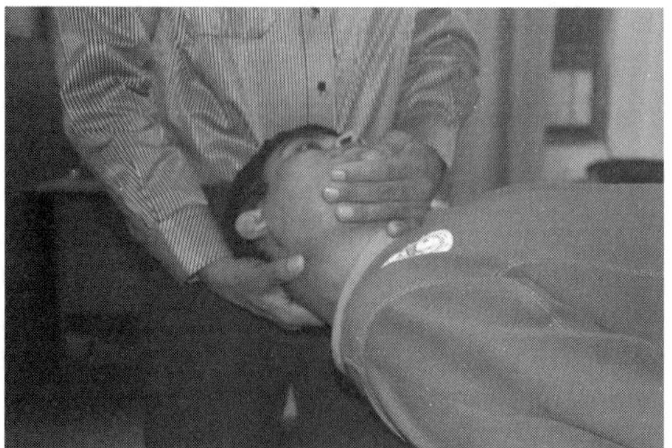

Fig. 26.43: Side flexion

c. ***Rotations:*** While maintaining the traction in the neutral position the head is rotated to the left and then to the neutral and to the right. The traction is maintained throughout the range until the head is brought to the neutral position (Fig. 26.44).

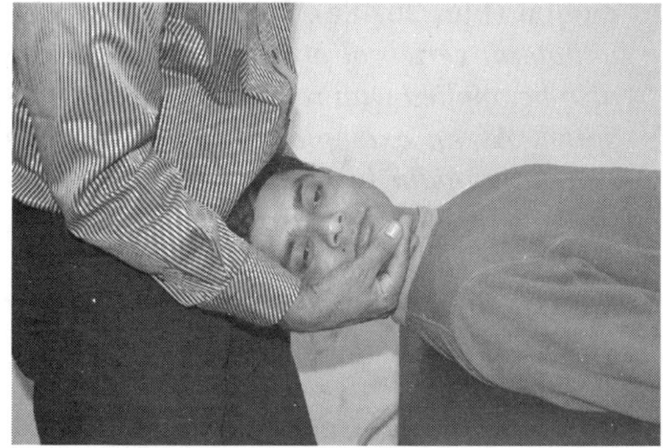

Fig. 26.44: Rotation

d. ***Forward Flexion:*** In neutral position traction is applied with both the hands and the head is taken to the forward flexion in full range of motion. The traction is maintained throughout the range of motion until the head comes to the neutral position (Fig. 26.45).

e. ***Extension:*** While maintaining the traction the head is taken to the extension in the full range of motion or till the restriction starts. The traction is maintained throughout the range of motion (Fig. 26.46).

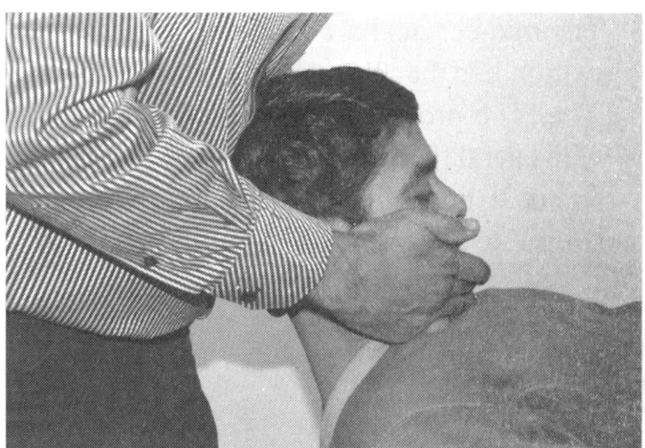

Fig. 26.45: Forward flexion

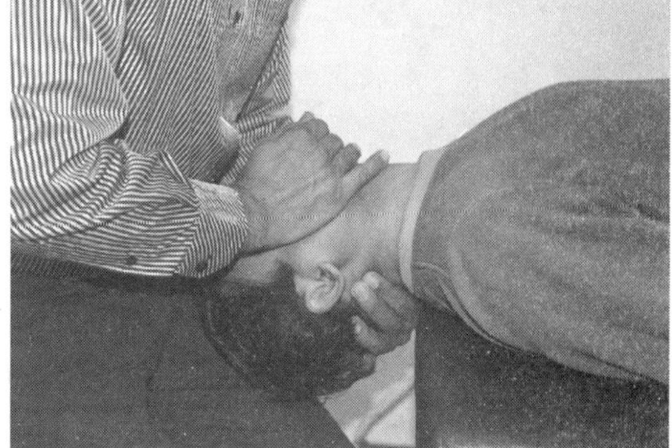

Fig. 26.46: Extension

C. Posterior Anterior Central Vertebral Pressure: To mobilize the vertebral column pressure is applied on the spinous process with the thumbs. *Position of Patient:* Prone, forehead rests on the palm of the hand of the patient. Chin is tucked fully in particularly for C_1, C_2 and C_3 vertebra. *Position of Therapist:* Therapist stands at the head of the patient. Thumbs are held in opposition and back to back (to reinforce). The tip of the thumb pad is placed on the spinous process of the vertebra which is being mobilized. The fingers are placed on either side of the neck. *Procedure:* While maintaining the position of neck and the hands, the therapist applies gentle pressure through the arms and body to the spinous process which will produce oscillatory movements in the mobile vertebral segment.

The mid-cervical area requires less pressure to mobilize than the upper and lower cervical area. The procedure can also be performed with lateral flexion and rotation of the cervical spine. It is termed as combined technique (Figs. 26.47a-c).

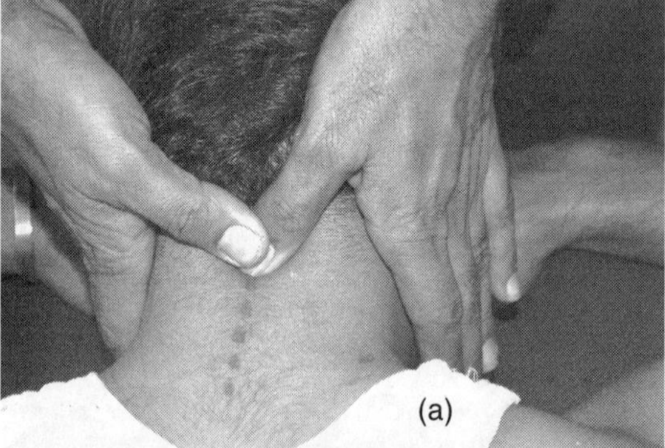

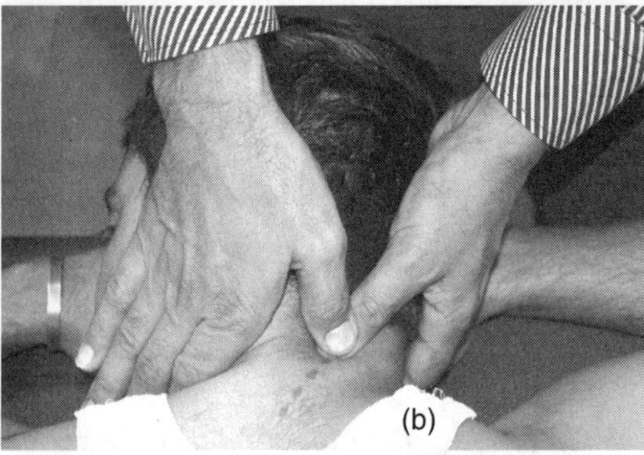

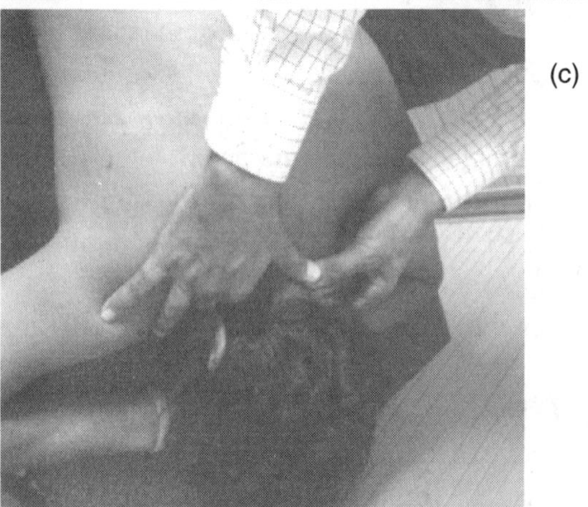

Figs. 26.47a-c: PA central pressure technique, a. in neutral, b. in rotation, c. side in flexion

D. Posteroanterior Unilateral Vertebral Pressure: To mobilize the vertebral column pressure can also be applied on the transverse process with the thumb through the body. *Position of Patient:* Prone, forehead rests on the hands of the patient with chin tucked well in. *Position of Therapist:* The therapist stands at the side of the neck of the patient, places one thumb on the posterior surface of the articular process to be mobilized. The fingers may rest on the neck of the patient. *Method:* While maintaining the above position of the neck and thumb a gentle pressure is applied through the arms and body to the posterior surface of the articular process; which produces oscillatory movement at the mobile vertebral segment. The technique is useful in unilateral pain with limitation in the range of motion (Fig. 26.48a). *The posteroanterior unilateral vertebral pressure technique can also be applied with rotation of the cervical spine. As an example for a patient who complains pain in the cervical spine and the origin of that is from the C_2 and C_3 segment. The patient's neck is turned to the left at 30 degree rotation; therapist places the thumb on the left posterior surface of the articular process of the C_2 vertebra. The pressure is directed through arms and trunk to the articular surface which produces oscillatory movement at the C_2 and C_3 segment. This helps in increasing the range particularly symptoms arising from the $C_2/_3$ mobile segment. It is usually performed on the side of the pain or restriction* (Fig. 26.48b).

E. Transverse Vertebral Pressure: To mobilize the vertebral column; pressure is applied on the lateral aspect of spinous process with the thumb. *Position of Patient:* Prone with forehead rests on the hands of the patient. The chin is tucked in (moderate degree) to reduce the cervical lordosis.

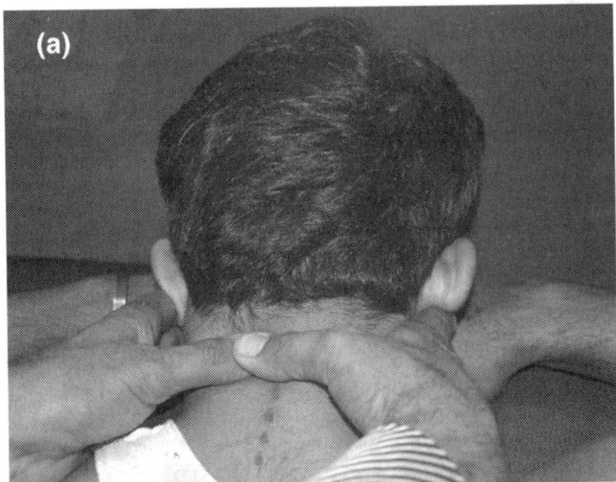

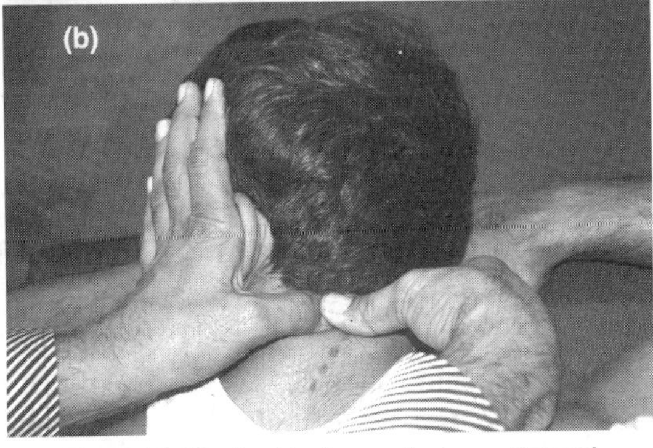

Figs. 26.48a-b: Posteroanterior unilateral vertebral pressure a. in neutral b. in rotation

Position of Therapist: The therapist stands at the side of the patient. The thumb of one hand is placed on the lateral side of the spinous process of the vertebra, while thumb of other hand is placed on the thumb of first hand to reinforce it. The fingers rest on the neck and head. *Procedure:* A gentle pressure is applied through the trunk and arms to the lateral side of the spinous process which produces oscillatory movements at the mobile segment. The technique is useful in unilateral painful conditions particularly originated due to degenerative changes in the vertebral column. The pressure is directed from the non-painful side to the painful side. For an example if patient has pain and symptoms on the right side, then the therapist stand at the left side and place thumb on the left lateral side of the spinous process (Fig. 26.49).

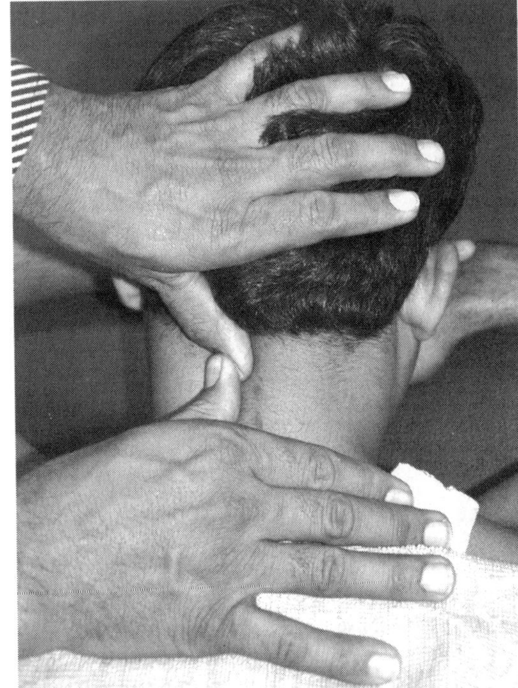

Fig. 26.49: Transverse vertebral pressure—left thumb on left side of spinous pressure

F. Sustained Natural Apophyseal Glides (SNAGs): *Position of Patient:* Sitting on a height adjustable stool. *Position of Therapist:* The therapist stands at the side of the patient. For an example; for a C_2/C_3 vertebral segment; the therapist stands on the right side of the shoulder of the patient. The right index and middle finger is placed on the base of the occiput; the middle phalanx of right little finger is placed over the spinous process of axial vertebra. The thenar eminence of the left hand is placed on the left little finger. *Procedure:* While stabilizing (cradling) the head between the therapist right arm and the chest a gentle pressure through the left hand is applied to the (left little finger) spinous process of the axial vertebra for at least 5-10 seconds. Similar glides of 8-10 repetitions may be performed. The pressure created from left arm and thenar eminence to the little finger thrusts the second vertebra (axial) anteriorly on the first (atlas) and if pressure is sufficient it may also thrust the first vertebra (atlas) forward on the occiput (Fig. 26.50).

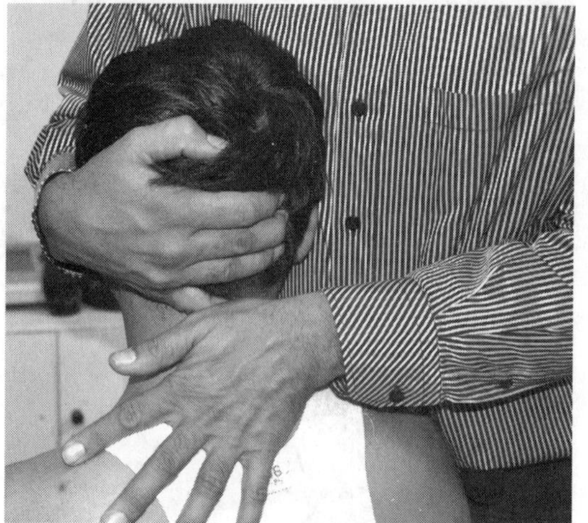

Fig. 26.50: SNAG to improve pain and range of motion at C_1 and C_2 mobile segment

Strengthening Exercises

1. **Deep Neck Flexors (Nodding or Chin Tuck Exercise):** This exercise is the cornerstone for the cervicogenic headache patients with forward head posture. *Position of Patient:* Sitting on a stool. *Position of Therapist:* Therapist sits on the stool and faces the patient. He demonstrates the exercise to the patient. Therapist can place one hand on the chin and other hand on the head to facilitate the movement. *Procedure:* The patient is instructed to tuck the chin in. Some patients find it difficult to perform in the desired direction, therefore, the therapist stabilizes the head with the right hand and pushes the chin back as much as possible with the left hand. The chin tuck exercises produce flexion at the upper cervical spine. At the end range of motion (full flexion) the patient is asked to hold the position for atleast six seconds. Three sets each of ten repetitions may be performed twice or thrice daily till the

hyper extension of the upper cervical spine is corrected. The exercise should be an active in order to strengthen the deep neck flexors (Fig. 26.51).

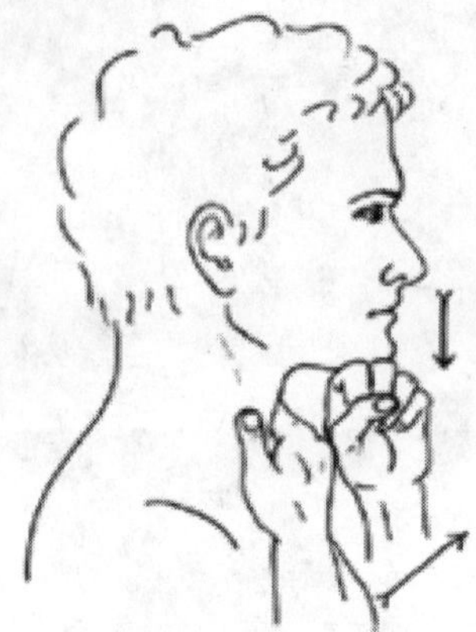

Fig. 26.51: Deep neck flexors exercises

2. **Trapezius (Middle and Lower Fibers) and Rhomboid (Retractors):** These muscles are the stabilizers of the scapula and play important role in keeping the scapula on the thoracic wall. The trapezius muscles (middle and lower) contribute to the force couple during the elevation of the arm. In sitting position with arms at side and hands resting on the thighs, the patient is asked to take the shoulders girdle back as much as possible without changing the position of hands. Therapist may stand behind the patient and place the hands on the patient's shoulder blades (scapula). The patient is asked to take the shoulders back against the resistance applied by the therapist (Fig. 26.52).

3. **Serratus Anterior:** The patient stands against the wall flexes both the shoulders to 90° and places both the hands on the wall. Wall is pushed without changing the position of the hands. This may be repeated several times twice or thrice daily until the scapula is stabilized on the thoracic wall properly. Weakness of serratus anterior muscle can cause winging of the scapula (Fig. 26.53).

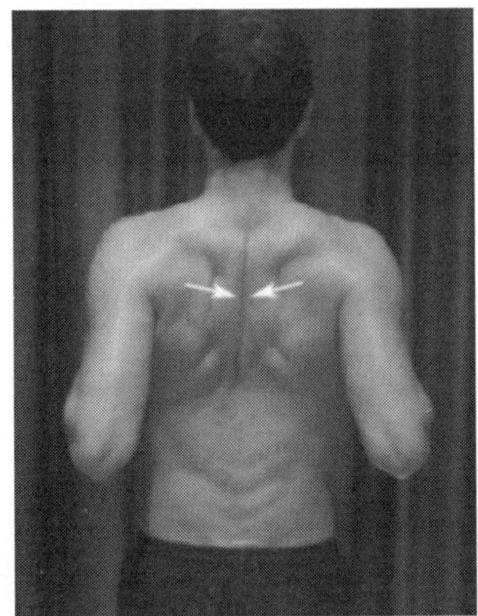

Fig. 26.52: Trapezius and rhomboids strengthening

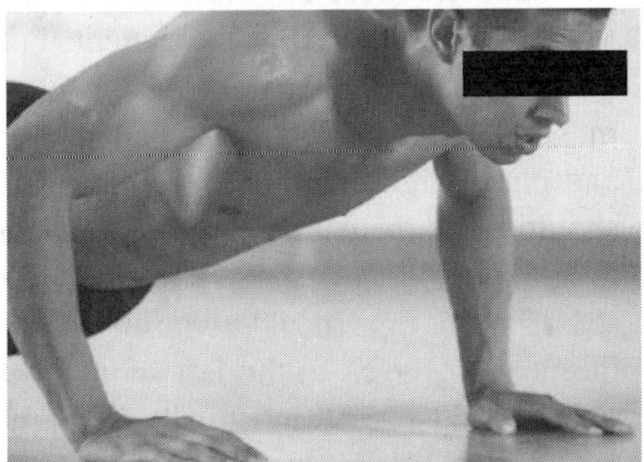

Fig. 26.53: Serratus anterior strengthening

4. **Upper Thoracic Extensors or Erector Spinae Muscles:** The upper thoracic erector spinae muscles are the phasic type of muscles which are having tendency of weakness and lengthening. *Position of Patient:* Prone lying with both hands at the side of the body. Patient is instructed to raise the head and upper thoracic spine and hold at least for six seconds (Fig. 26.54).

5. **Trapezius Upper Fibers:**Trapezius upper fibers are the tonic type of muscle fibers which

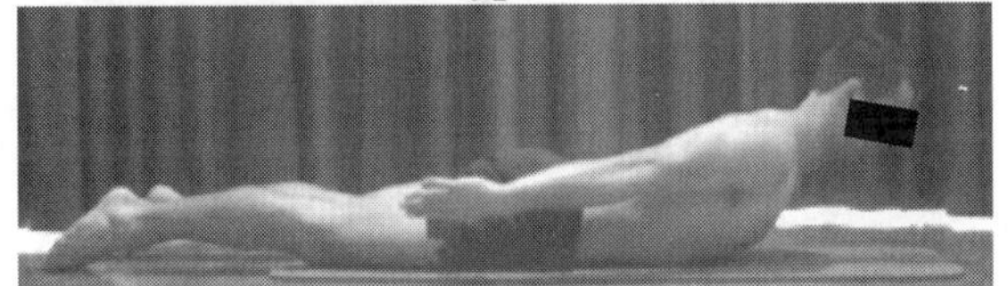

Fig. 26.54: Upper thoracic extensors strengthening

are having tendency of shortening; however, in some postural problems such as drooped or protracted shoulders or rounded shoulders the muscles go in the lengthening position. To correct the posture the trapezius upper fibers are also need to be strengthened. In sitting position patient places both hands on the thigh and elevates the shoulders as much as possible which is held at end range at least for six seconds. Therapist can place both hands on the top of shoulders and can resist the shoulder elevation (Figs. 26.55a-b).

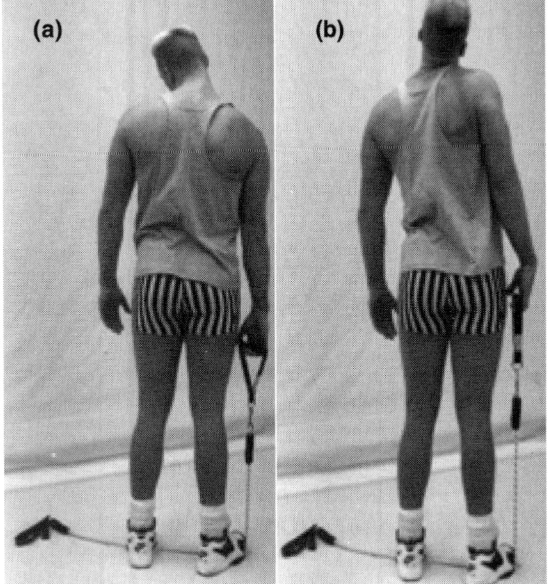

Figs. 26.55a-b: Trapezius upper fibers strengthening

6. **Multifidus, Gluteus Maximus and Transverse Abdominis Strengthening:** See core strengthening program.

Stretching Exercises

1. **Posterior Neck Muscle Stretching:** These are the tonic muscles which become shortened and cause hyperextension at the cervical spine (upper) following degenerative changes and pain. *Position of the Patient:* Supine lying.

Position of Therapist: Stands at the end of the plinth (at head of the patient). The patient's head rests on the therapist thigh. The therapist grasps the occiput with the left hand and the chin with the right hand. Therapist bends the knees slightly to allow the COG to pass behind the trunk and to avoid the stress on the back. *Procedure:* The therapist pushes the chin backward with the right hand. While maintaining the chin tuck in position the neck is flexed and is held at least for 6-10 seconds for significant stretching (Fig. 26.56).

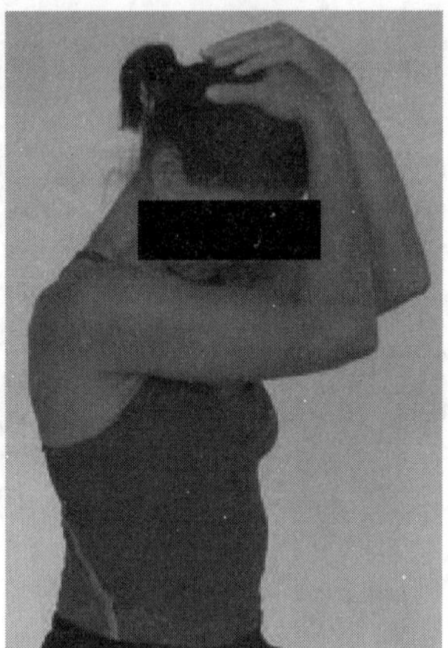

Fig. 26.56: Posterior neck muscle stretching in sitting

2. **Pectoralis Major:** In a standing or sitting position patient abducts the shoulders at 90° and then takes them back horizontally. Therapist can assist the patient and apply overpressure at the end range of motion. The exercise should be performed cautiously by patients with anterior instability. The patients may also perform the exercise by taking the shoulders backward at the 90 degree (Fig. 26.57).

3. **Levator Scapulae and Trapezius Upper Fibers:** *Position of Patient:* Sitting with comfortable back rest. The head is rotated to

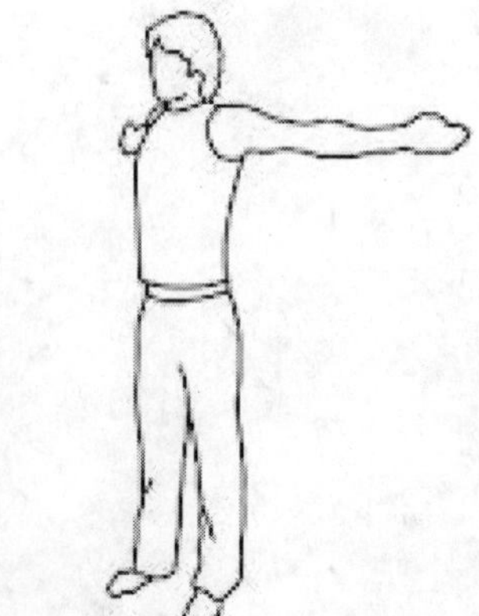

Fig. 26.57: Pectoralis major stretching

the opposite side. *Position of Therapist:* Therapist stands behind the patient. For an example, to stretch the right levator scapulae muscle the therapist stands behind the patient and places right hand on the patient's right shoulder and the left hand grasps the occiput (slightly to the right side). *Procedure:* While stabilizing the right shoulder with the right hand, the neck is flexed to the left shoulder with rotation (Figs. 26.58 and 26.59).

4. **Soft Tissue Manipulation:** The flexibility of the extensors can also be increased with soft tissue manipulation such as wringing, squeezing and kneading.

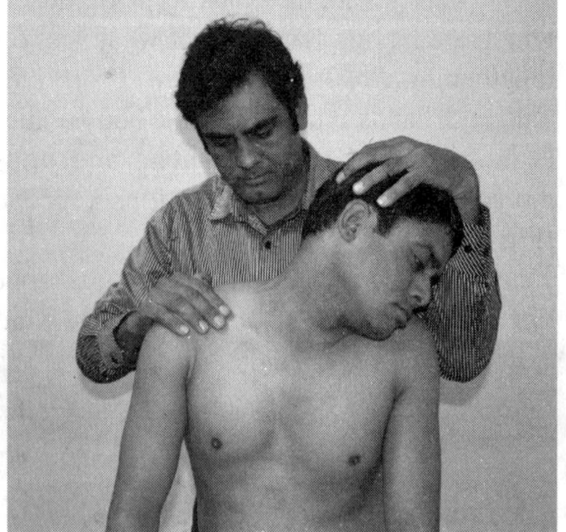

Fig. 26.58: Levator scapulae stretching in sitting

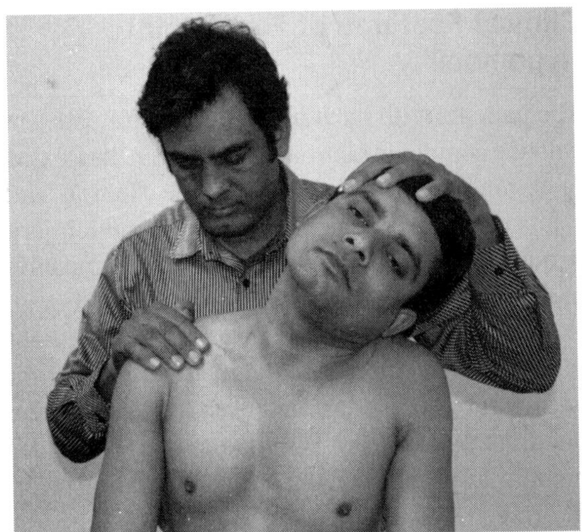

Fig. 26.59: Trapezius upper fibers stretching

Modalities

Moist Heat Therapy: This is one of the beneficial modalities helps in relieving pain and spasm and improving in flexibility of the muscles. The hot water bags easily available in the market may be used by the patient for at least 15-20 minutes twice daily. Patient should find the comfortable position such as sitting, prone or supine. **Short Wave Diathermy:** Short wave diathermy is one of the effective modalities to produce the heat to the deep structures such as ligaments, tendons and capsule. It helps in improving extensibility of the tissues. **Ultrasound Therapy:** Therapeutic ultrasound of 1 MHz, intensity between $1W/cm^2$ and $1.5W/cm^2$ with continuous mode shown good results in patients with cervicogenic headache. The continuous mode causes some heating effect which helps in improving the flexibility of the extensor muscles.

Mechanical Traction: *Position of Patient:* Supine with hip and knees flexion at $90°$. A towel roll is placed under the upper cervical spine. Upper cervical spine is flexed forward at least to $20°$, while maintaining this position a cervical halter is put on. An intermittent traction is more effective than the sustained traction as it produces stretching and relaxation of the static stabilizers of the spine. This may be recommended for at least 15 minutes of duration per treatment session. However, static traction is preferred over the intermittent to the patients with soft disc herniation as it helps in relieving sustained pressure on the nerve roots.

Surgical Management

The patients with soft disc herniation usually recovers with conservative treatment, but involvement of multiple level of disc herniation may cause severe motor and sensory nerve deficit. Such small percentages of patients require surgical intervention. The common surgical procedures for intervertebral disc herniation are: anterior decompression and fusion (ADCF), Laminectomy, Laminactomy-facetectomy and Laminoplasty.

Post Surgical Management

The post surgical treatment is divided into three phases:

Phase I: During the phase I the patient is advised to put on cervical collar, however, the collar may be removed during the exercises and modalities. The collar may be soft or hard that depends upon the surgical procedure. To decrease the pain and spasm, cryotherapy is advised initially for 15 minutes thrice daily. Soft tissue manipulation such as wringing and squeezing is performed on the trepezius upper fibers and posterior neck muscles. Gentle stretching of erector spinae trapezius and levator scapulae may be initiated in pain free range. Strengthening exercises of deep neck flexors, serratus anterior and rhomboids in the form of isometric should also be started. Exercises which aggravate the symptoms should be discontinued immediately.

Phase II: To progress to the phase II, the patient should have minimal pain and spasm; and improved neuromuscular control, range of motion or may be limited with pain in the end range. Grade

2 and 3 mobilization to improve the range of motion and intensive isometric may also be initiated at this stage to regain normal posture. Resistance may be applied manually.

Phase III: To progress to the phase III, the patient should restore full range of motion and neuromuscular control without pain and symptoms. The patient is withstand the demands of activity, work and practice. The exercises such as PNF techniques, dynamic strengthening, and conditioning programme in conjunction with activity, work, or practice are initiated during this phase.

FACET JOINT HYPOMOBILITY

The movements in the mobile segment greatly depends upon the orientation of the facet joints, hence, these are determined largely by the direction in which the articular joints face. The zygapophyseal joints (facet joints) face or slant upward and posteriorly at an angle of 45 degree, lying halfway between the horizontal and the frontal plane. Such a slant would seem to favour rotation and lateral flexion and to be unfavorable to flexion and hyperextension. However, flexion and hyperextension occur as freely as lateral flexion while rotation from the second cervical vertebra down occur only as moderate in terms of range of motion.

The facet joints in the cervical spine are diarthrodial synovial joints with fibrous capsules, surrounded by a capsule of connective tissue and produces synovial fluid to nourish and lubricate the articular cartilage.

Table 26.7: Facet joint movements in the cervical spine

Movement	Plane of movement
Flexion	The upper facet slides up and forward on the lower facet
Extension	The upper facet slides down and back on the lower facet
Side flexion	The upper facet slides down and back on the same side and up and forward on the opposite side
Rotation	The upper facet slides down and posterior on the same side and up and anterior on the opposite side

Clinical Features of Facet Joint Hypomobility

The patients with facet restriction usually present with the complaint pain and limitation in the flexion or extension combined with side flexion and rotation. They reveal the history of sudden jerk or quick movement followed by pain and limitation in the range of motion in a typical pattern. For an example, following sudden jerk or movement injury; the neck may stuck in the forward flexion with right rotation and right side flexion. The quadrant test (spurling) will be positive. Tender points may also be present on corresponding facet. The facet hypomobility produces two types of restrictions–opening and closing.

Opening and Closing Facet Joint Restriction

Following jerk, twist or sudden movement there is excessive slide of one of the facet joints. The excessive sliding of the facet stretches the facet capsule and stucks in a new position which may limit the range of motion either in flexion or in extension. The flexion opens the facet joint; hence; restriction in flexion is termed as opening facet restriction. On the other hand the extension closes the facet joint; hence, restriction in the extension is termed as closing facet restriction. These restrictions flexion or extensions are usually combined with rotation and side flexion.

In an opening restriction the superior facet joint does not glide up and forward on the inferior facet, thereby, limiting the flexion of that segment. In a close restriction, the superior facet stucks in flexion and unable to glide down and backward on the inferior facet, thereby, limiting the extension of that segment.

Management of Facet Joint Hypomobility

The treatment is aimed at smooth gliding of the facet joint in the treatment plane. Many techniques have been developed to bring the smooth gliding of the facet joint back to the normal. Before exploring the techniques the practitioners should be awared of the orientation of the facet joints plane and should also practice on the normal subjects before administering to the patients.

1. **Mobilization:** This has translatory and oscillatory glides performed on the patients in a most comfortable position.

   a. ***For Opening Restriction:*** The patient is positioned prone with the forehead resting on a towel with the cervical spine in pain free position. The therapist stands at the side of the facet which is being mobilized. As an example, for a patient who has a C_6 and C_7 level facet opening restriction on the right side, the therapist stands on the right side and places the thumb on the superior aspect of the C_6 and C_7 facet and applies pressure in the direction of the treatment plane. The oscillating glides are applied at end range which may last upto 30-60 seconds three to five times per treatment session (Fig. 26.60).

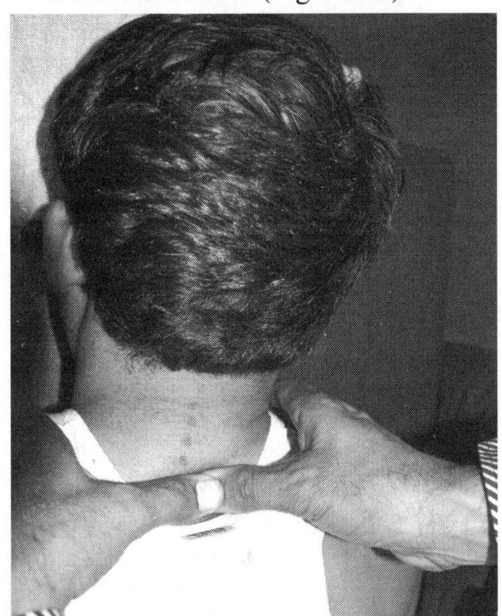

Fig. 26.60: Mobilization for opening restriction of C_6-C_7 facet joint

   b. ***For Closing Restriction:*** The position of patient remains same as for opening restriction. Therapist stands at the level of head, and places the thumb on the superior facet of the segment. As an example, for a patient who has closing restriction at right C_6 and C_7 segment, the therapist stands at the right side of the segment which is being mobilized and places the thumb on a superior facet of the C_6 and C_7 segment. The therapist applies a force down and backward in the treatment plane (Fig. 26.61).

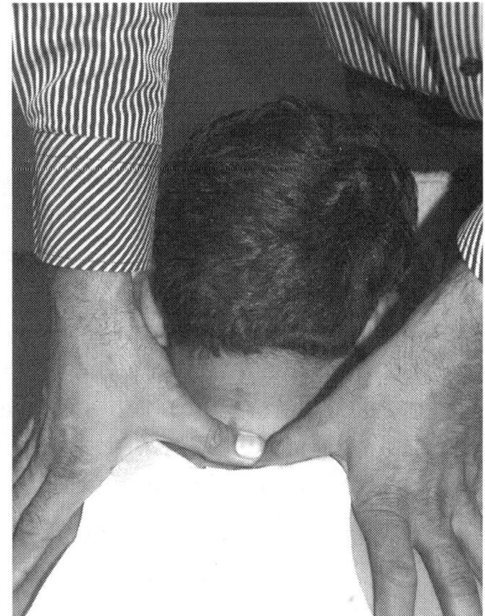

Fig. 26.61: Mobilization for closing restriction of C_6-C_7 facet joint

2. **Muscle Energy Techniques:** The muscle energy techniques involve isometric contraction of muscle or group of muscles which are responsible for loss of range of motion. For an example, if right side flexion and rotation is limited, the left side flexors and rotators are allowed to contract isometrically, as they are holding the neck to the left side flexion rotation. This strong isometric contraction causes same degree of relaxation that improves pain and range of motion.

a. ***For Opening Restriction:*** The patient has limitation in the range of flexion with rotation and side flexion. As an example, for a patient with right C_6 and C_7 opening restriction the patient may have restriction in the flexion, left side flexion and left rotation. ***Position of Patient:*** Supine; head out of the edge of the table. The therapist stands at the head. Head of the patient rests on the waist or thigh of the therapist. Therapist places right hand on the chick and left hand under the occiput, and then brings the neck in the extreme restricted positions (flexion, left side flexion and left rotation). ***Procedure:*** While maintaining the above position the therapist instructs the patient to move the head into extension, right side flexion and right rotation against the resistance for 3-6 seconds applied by the therapist. The patient is allowed to relax the muscles. In the next step, the neck is brought into the further improved positions (flexion, left side flexion and left rotation). Therapist maintains the position and again instructs the patient to bring the neck into extension, right side flexion and right rotation for 3-6 seconds against the resistance applied by the therapist. Several isometric contractions may be performed to reduce the muscle spam and increase in the range motion (Figs. 26.62 and 26.63).

b. ***For Closing Restriction:*** For a patient with right side C_6-C_7 closing facet restriction, the extension, right side flexion and right rotation may be limited. In this case the neck will be stiff in flexion, left side flexion and left rotation. To perform the technique the patient is positioned in supine with the head out of the edge of the table. Therapist stands at the head, and places right hand under the occiput and left hand on the

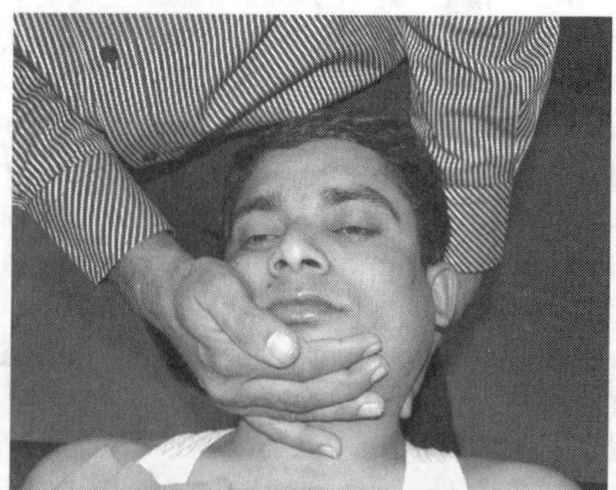

Fig. 26.62: Muscle energy technique for opening restriction at the level of right C_6-C_7

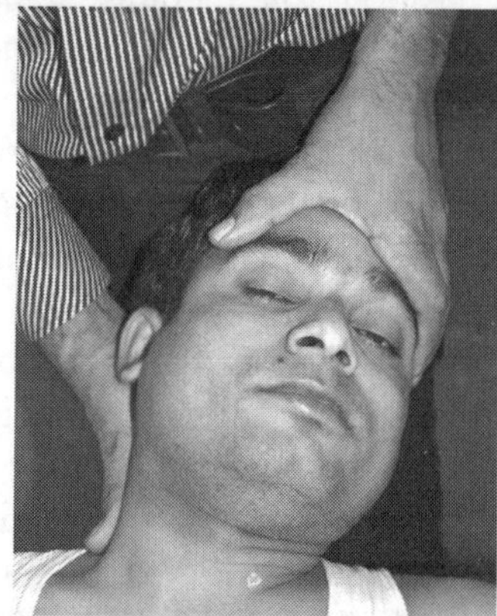

Fig. 26.63: Muscle energy technique for closing restriction at right side C_6-C_7

forehead (fingers on the forehead and hypothenar on the left side of head). The head of the patient rests on the therapist's thigh or waist. The therapist instructs the patient to bring the neck in the extreme limited positions (extension, right side flexion and right rotation). ***Procedure:*** While maintaining the above position the therapist instruct the patient to move the head into flexion, left side flexion and left rotation for 3-6 seconds against the resistance applied by the therapist. Patient is instructed to relax the muscles and neck is brought into the further improved positions (extension, right side flexion and right rotation). The therapist maintains the positions and instructs the patient to bring the neck into flexion, left side flexion and left rotation against the resistance applied by the therapist for 3-6 seconds. Several repetitions of isometric contractions may be performed to improve pain and range of motion.

Box 26.3
Muscle Energy Techniques: Strong isometric contraction of spasmodic group muscles is followed by same degree of relaxation of the same group of muscles.

3. **Side Glide Mobilization for Opening Restriction:** The patient lies supine with the head out of the edge of the table. Therapist stands at the top of the head of the patient and makes the *web space* of both the mobilizing and stabilizing hands. The stabilizing hand is placed on the distal and the mobilizing hand on the proximal part of the restricted mobile segment. As an example, for a C_6-C_7 opening restriction, the stabilizing hand is placed on the C_7 vertebra (distal mobile segment) and the mobilizing hand is placed on the C_6 vertebra (proximal part of the mobile segment). The patient's head rests on the therapist thigh or waist. *Procedure:* The therapist flexes the cervical spine with distraction to allow the mobile segment to open as much as possible. A gliding force is applied with the mobilizing hand towards the same side of the facet joint at the proximal mobile segment. This allows opening of the facet joint of the C_6-C_7 mobile segment opposite of the mobilizing hand, and closing of same side of the facet joint of the C_6-C_7 mobile segment (Fig. 26.64).

4. **Sustained Natural Apophyseal Glides (SNAGs):** The much talked about technique SNAG has been given by Brain Mulligan, a Neazeland based physical therapy practitioner. These techniques are performed

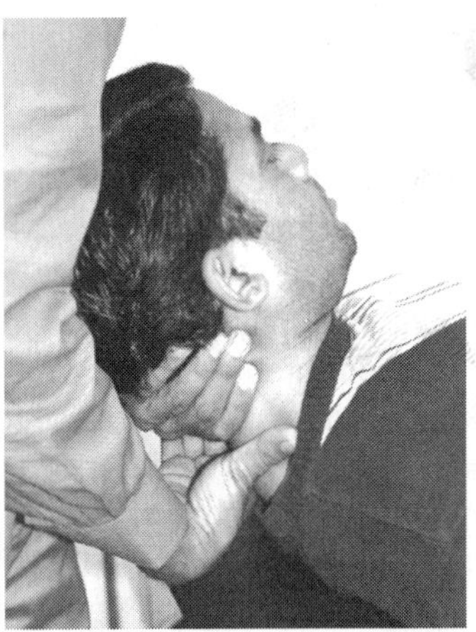

Fig. 26.64: Side glide mobilization for opening restriction

in weight bearing positions. These are very effective if the therapist can identify the exact site of facet dysfunction. The thumb is placed under the spinous process or direct on the facet and then it is glided in the treatment plane. Patient may have relief in sign and symptoms instantly. Unlike Maitland and other conventional techniques which are performed in most relaxed position (lying), the $SNAG_S$ are performed in the weight bearing position either in sitting or standing because when improvement in the sign and symptoms are achieved in a functional position they are likely to be retained. These mobilization techniques may also be performed with the movements (active or passive). At the end of active range of motion the therapist applies gentle overpressure. The important part of the technique is that the therapist should identify the location where from pain is originated, then the spinous process of the superior vertebra is palpated and thumb is placed under that. The therapist applies pressure through the thumb up in the direction with the movement along the treatment plane.

a. ***SNAGs to Improve Rotation and Decrease Pain Associated With It:*** For an example C_5 and C_6 is the intervertebral joint where from pain is originating and that is also limiting the rotation. The therapist places the medial border of one of the thumbs under the spinous process of C_5 and it is reinforced by other thumb. The spinous process of C_5 is pushed up in the direction of treatment plane through the reinforced thumb and then the patient is instructed to rotate the neck to the restricted painful direction. At the end of limitation a gentle overpressure is applied and is held atleast for 6-10 seconds. The head is returned to the neutral position with the gentle pressure. Improvement in the pain and range is assessed and several repetitions are performed. In case where pain aggravates, the therapist should stop and perform the technique on other level or discontinue (Fig. 26.65).

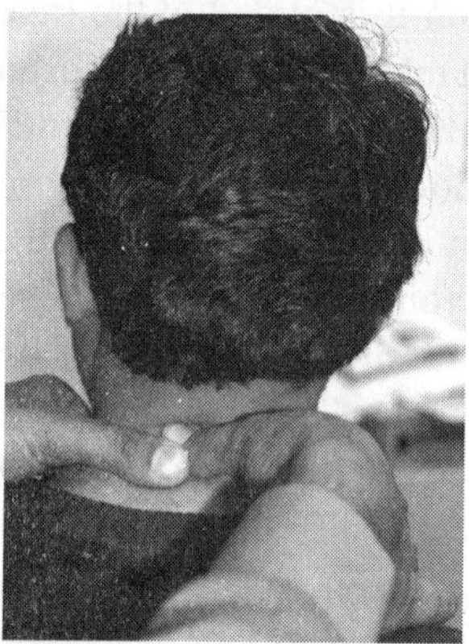

Fig. 26.65: SNAGs to improve rotation

b. SNAGs to Improve Flexion and Decrease the Pain Associated With It:
Position of Patient: Sitting on a stool.
Position of Therapist: Therapist stands behind the patient, faces the cervical spine. Similar to previous technique therapist identifies the site where from pain is originating, for an example C_6 and C_7 is the site. The medial border of the thumb is placed under the spinons process of C_6. The spinous process of C_6 is pushed up

along the treatment plane with the thumb and patient is asked to flex the neck forward. At the end of restriction overpressure is applied and is held for few seconds. The neck is then returned to the neutral position with the pressure (Fig. 26.66).

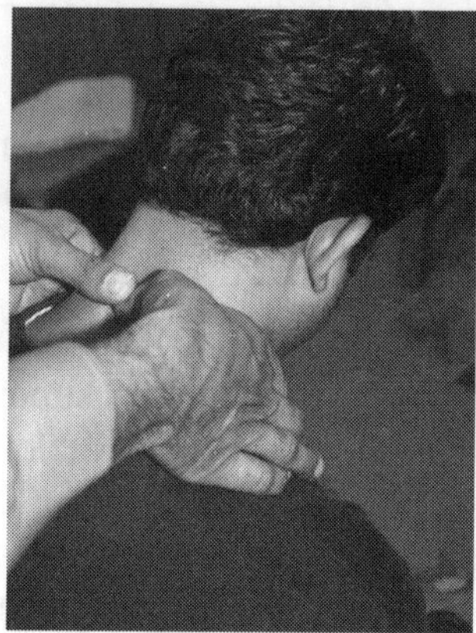

Fig. 26.66: SNAGs to improve flexion

c. SNAGs to Improve Extension and Decrease Pain Associated With It: Similar to the previous technique (flexion), the spinous process of the superior vertebra is pushed up along the treatment plane and patient is instructed to extend the cervical spine. At the end of motion where restriction starts, the therapist applies overpressure and sustains for few seconds. The cervical spine is then taken into the neutral position with the pressure (Fig. 26.67).

d. SNAGs to Improve Side Flexion and Reduce Pain and Symptoms Associated With It: The position of patient and therapist remains same as above. The therapist places thumb under the spinous process of the superior vertebra and pushes it up along the treatment plane. Patient is instructed to bend the neck to the restricted and painful side. At end of restriction the therapist applies

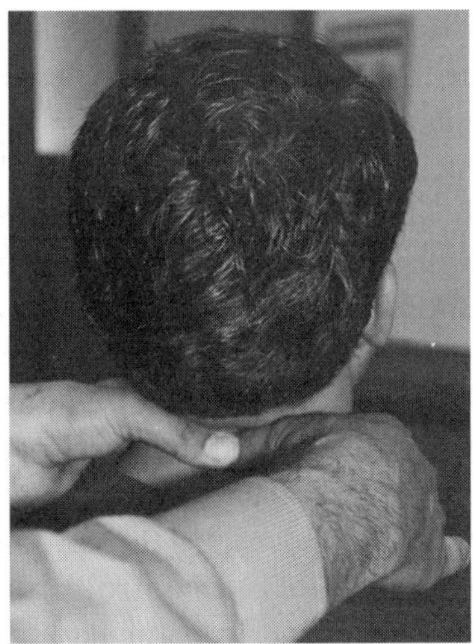

Fig. 26.67: SNAGs to improve extension

overpressure and sustains for few seconds. The neck is then returned to the neutral position with the pressure (Fig. 26.68).

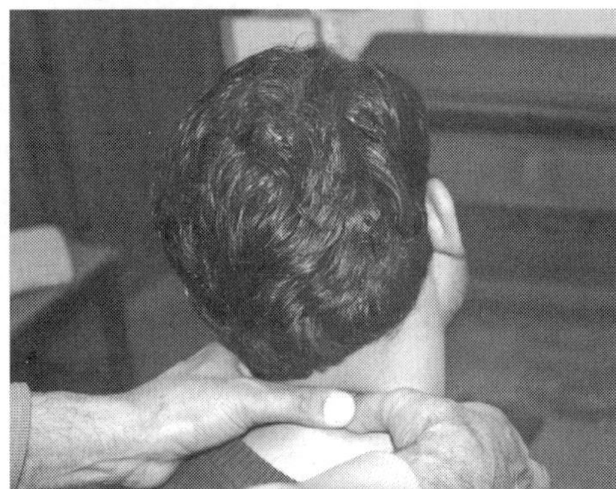

Fig. 26.68: SNAGs to improve side flexion

e. ***Spinal Mobilization with Arm Movement: Position of Patient:*** Sitting on a stool. ***Position of Therapist:*** Stands behind the patient. The facet which is producing the symptoms is identified. For example C_4 and C_5 is the site where from symptoms are produced to the right shoulder and aggravated with the arm movement. The therapist places the thumb on the left lateral side of the spinous process of C_4 vertebra. ***Procedure:*** The therapist applies pressure on the spinous

process to rotate it to the right and sustains it and allows the patient to adduct the shoulder joint horizontally with elbow flexion (Fig. 26.69).

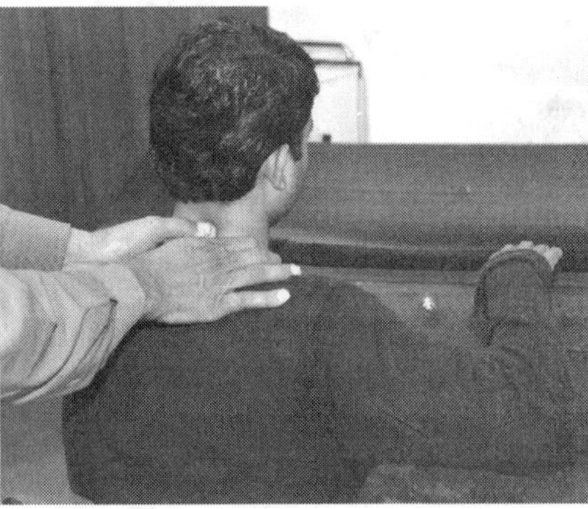

Fig. 26.69: Spinal mobilization with arm movement

f. ***Facet Down Slide:*** Patient lies supine with the head out of the edge of the table. The therapist places mobilizing hand under the neck with second metacarpophalangeal joint directly on the posterior pillar (apophyseal joints or transverse process) which is being mobilized. ***Procedure:*** While maintaining the above position; the neck is bent to the same side of the facet which is being mobilized. As soon as the movement reaches its limitation and patient starts complaining pain, the therapist glides the facet joint in the plane of facet through second MCP joint. The technique is effective in closing facet restriction and improving pain and range of motion. Therapist should be more cautious when it is used in acute inflammation and muscle guarding. It should be discontinued in case pain is aggravated (Fig. 26.70).

g. ***Facet Up Slide:*** The position of patient and therapist remains same as facet down slide. ***Procedure:*** The neck is flexed to the opposite side of the facet which is to be mobilized upto the pain and limitation starts. To glide the facet joint, the therapist

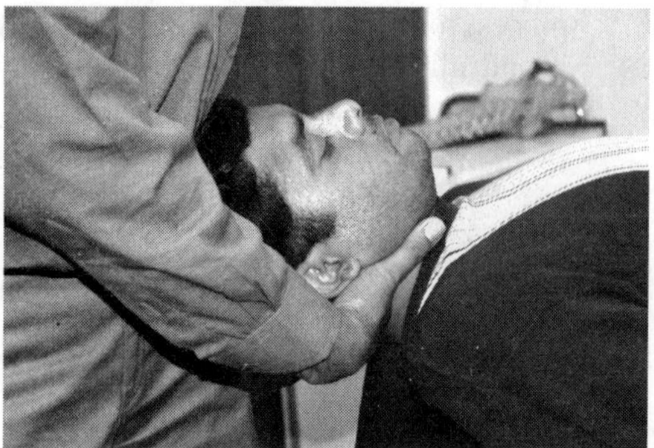

Fig. 26.70: Facet down slide mobilization

creates a force to the superior and anterior direction (towards the opposite eye) in its treatment plane. Facet up slide helps in opening facet restriction (Fig. 26.71).

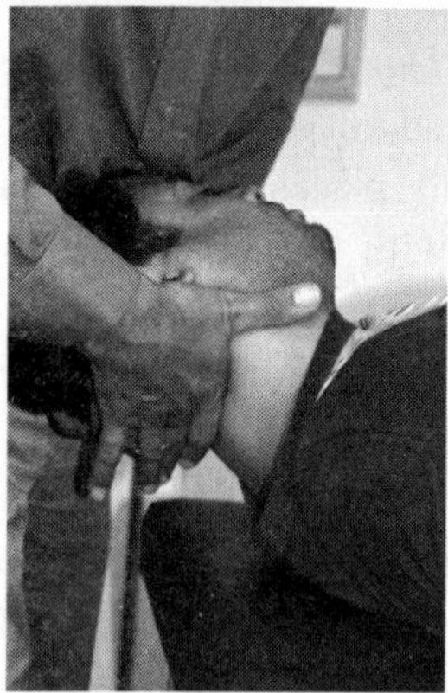

Fig. 26.71: Facet up slide mobilization

CERVICOGENIC HEADACHE (CH)

Introduction: Cervicogenic headache is described as a syndrome that is "a final common pathway" not an entity. Thus CH is a syndrome that can have many contributing factors. The World Cervicogenic Headache Society has defined CH as referred pain perceived in any part of the head and caused by a primary nociceptive sources in the musculoskeletal tissues that are innervated by the C_1, C_2 and C_3 spinal nerves. Pain associated with CH has been attributed to physical impairments of the joint, muscle and neural structures in the cervical region, and in particularly the upper cervical region.

The studies have demonstrated that the patients with CH had significantly less strength and endurance of the deep neck flexors compared to age-matched controls. They have also identified a decrease in strength of the deep neck flexors in patients with CH; when compared to able bodied individuals. In a recent clinical involving patients with CH, Jull *et al.* (JOSPT, 2005) compared the effect of specific active exercises directed at improving the strength and endurance of the deep neck flexors to manual therapy, or a combination of active exercise and manual therapy, displayed better outcomes than a control group who received no treatment. In particular, the group who received active exercise improved in both pain behavior and strength of deep neck flexors.

Pathogenesis: A forward head position with increased extension of the upper cervical region is commonly observed. This extended alignment is of particular importance because some investigators have described how cervical extension may contribute to increased stress on the cervical facet joints as a result of approximation of the facet joint surfaces. It has also observed that patients with CH frequently extend their neck when they perform unilateral or bilateral shoulder flexion (Jan, 2005, JOSPT) (Figs. 26.72a-b).

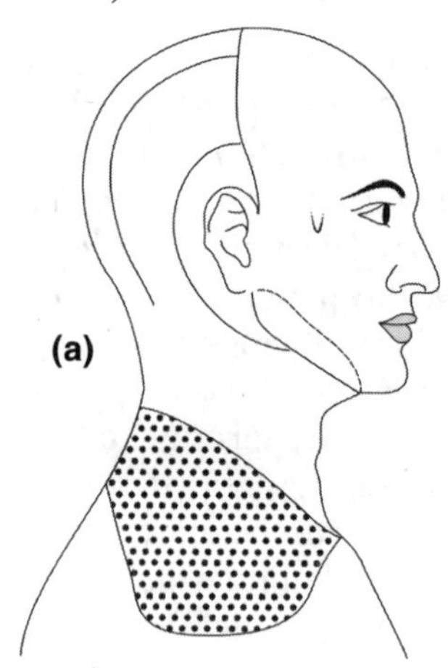

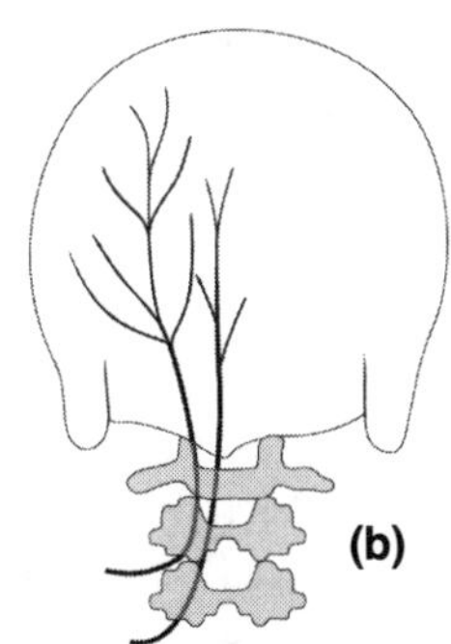

Fig. 26.72: C_2 and C_3 nerve supply

In the scapulothoracic region it has been noted that patients with CH often display an alignment of scapular abduction and depression indicating lengthened levator scapulae and trapezius muscles. This scapular alignment is often associated with concomitant weakness of some or all portions of the trapezius as well as the rhomboids and levator scapulae (Mary Kate Mc Donnell *et al.* 2005, Jan JOSPT). This suggests that impairments not only lies in the cervical region, but also in the scapulothoracic and lumbar region, may be important to consider when treating a patient with cervicogenic headache. The compensatory head position associated with a slumped, round upper back results in extension of the cervical spine (hyperextension of the upper cervical spine). The tight muscles (erector spinae) will produce hyperextension at the C_0-C_1, C_1-C_2 and C_2-C_3, which cause approximation of the posterior pillars (facet joints). This will irritate the pain sensitive structures, territories of the anterior and posterior rami of C_1, C_2 and C_3 which distribute the pain in the suboccipital, temporal and supraorbital region.

Common Characteristics of Cervical Headache

- The cervicogenic headaches are most often unilateral but as the disease progresses these can become bilateral.

- Tenderness can be palpated over the facet joint ipsilateral to the headache which may be present bilaterally with the time.
- The extensor muscles show tightness and limit the cervicocranial flexion and produce some sort of stretching feeling in the neck.
- Soft tissue manipulation and hot water fermentation improves the symptoms.
- Pain is perceived in the occipital, temporal or supraorbital regions.
- Pain does not change the location as it is common in migranous headache.
- Extension will aggravate the symptoms as it causes further approximation to the facet joints and irritation to pain sensitive structures.
- *Cervicogenic headache* is similar to migraine headache due to the ipsilateral pain and the typical migraine like symptoms such as nausea, vomiting and ocular. It differs from migraine in two ways:
  1. It never alternates sides.
  2. Initiates from neck.

Types of Cervicogenic Headache

A. Occipital – Headache: The greater occipital nerve which is both sensory and motor supplies the semispinalis and splenius capitis muscles. Pain is experienced in the occipital and can radiate to vertex. It corresponds to the territories of the posterior rami of C_2 and C_3 facet joints are the highest that can palpate. *It represents 20% of headaches.* ***Friction sign of scalp:*** It consists of pressing firmly with the pad of the fingers against the scalp and mobilizing it with small to and fro motions. Maneuver is painless in normal scalp, but it is very disagreeable and even painful in the cases of an occipital headache of cervical origin (Fig. 26.73).

Clinical Features
- Tenderness present on the ipsilateral to C_2-C_3 facet joint.

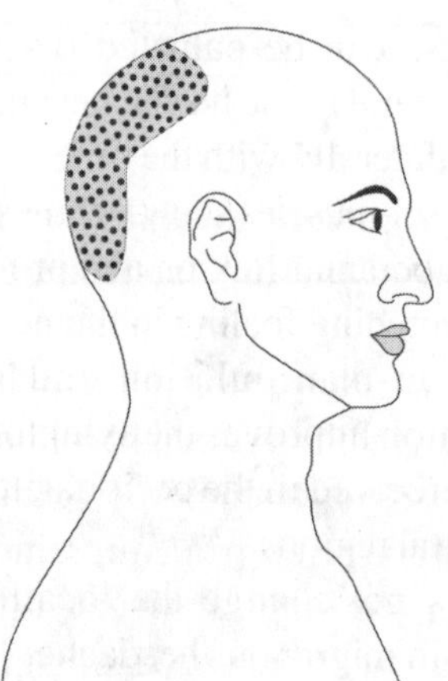

Fig. 26.73: Occipital cervicogenic headache

- The territory that is painful to friction can correspond to the posterior ramus of C_3 and C_2.
- C_3 – innervates – paramedian zone.
- C_2 – innervates – lateral part of the occiput, it can be more diffused but it does not go beyond the bi-auricular line. The periauricular region also receives innervations from anterior rami of C_2-C_3.
- The extension of the neck can reproduce the symptoms.
- Upper cervical goes into hyperextension and lower into flexion.
- Shoulder became rounded and protracted.
- The thoracic spine assumes in a kyphotic posture.

B. Occipito Temporomaxillary Headache (5%): It is felt on the retroauricular mastoid and parietal region and radiates towards the inferior maxilla. Tenderness and pain presents on ipsilateral to the C_2 and C_3. The painful scalp in the retroauricular territory is innervated by the superficial cervical plexus (anterior ramus of C_2, sometimes of C_3). The angle of jaw is innervated by the anterior ramus of C_2 and C_3, not by the trigeminal nerve. Friction sign on the scalp (retro-auricular) and pinch rolling at the angle of Jaw is positive (Fig. 26.74).

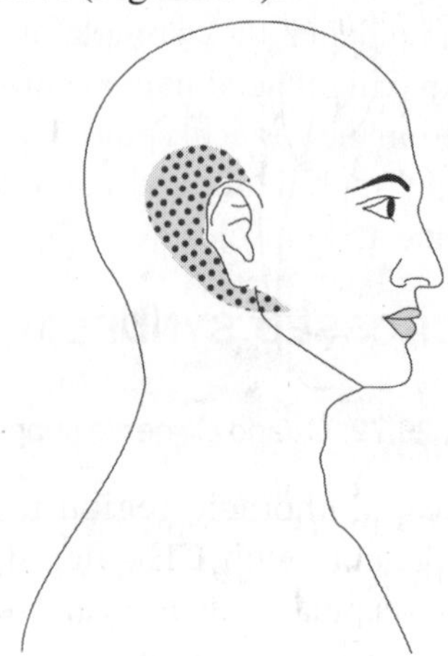

Fig. 26.74: Occipito temporomaxillary cervicogenic headache

C. Supraorbital Headache (67%): The topography of the pain is usually supraorbital, sometimes occipito-supraorbital, and in a few cases retro-orbital. *Eyebrow sign is present:* The eyebrow is pinched between the thumb and index finger and kneaded and rolled like a cigarette. It is explored from one end to the other, going over the forehead skin. In patients with *supraorbital headaches:* The roll is painful and thickened throughout all or part of the brow on the side of the usual headache, generally the side of C_2-C_3 articular pain (Fig. 26.75).

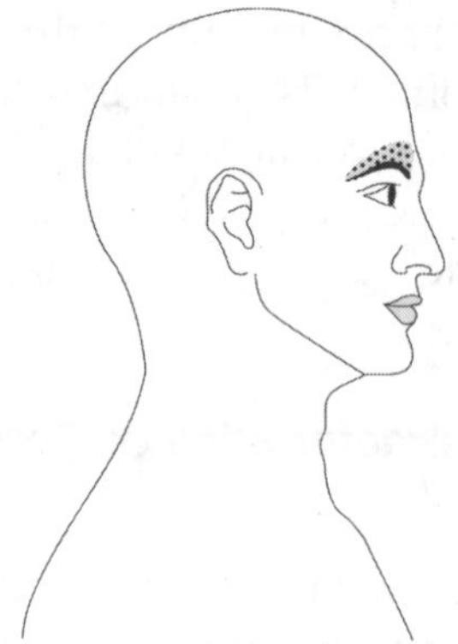

Fig. 26.75: Supraorbital cervicogenic headache

Chick Sign: Sometimes pain may also experienced in chick. When the skin of the neck is rolled and pinched they complaint tenderness below the maxilla. Facial pain syndrome is also has origin from the cervical spine. The syndrome is relieved by mobilizing and manipulating the cervical spine and muscles.

UPPER CROSSED SYNDROME

Introduction

Janda named this syndrome "Upper crossed" because when the weakened and shortened muscles are connected in the upper body, they form a cross. The upper crossed syndrome involves the tightness of the trapezius (upper fiber), upper cervical extensors, pectoralis major and levator scapulae and weakness of the rhomboids, serratus anterior, middle and lower trapezius and deep neck flexors (Fig. 26.76).

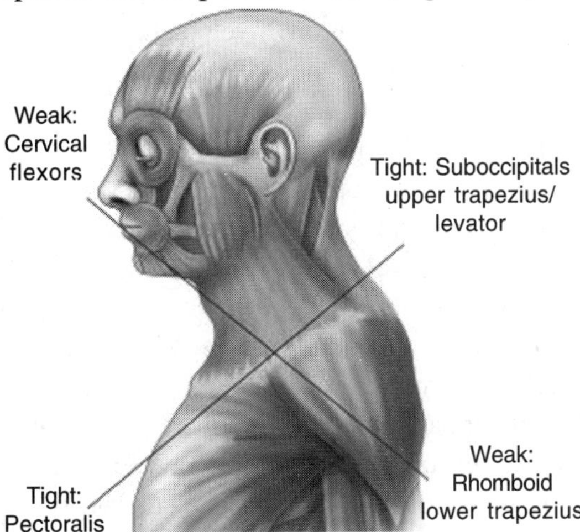

Fig. 26.76: Upper crossed syndrome

This muscular imbalance produces elevation and protraction of the shoulders, winging of the scapula and protraction of the head (forward head). Upper crossed syndrome places overstress on cervical cranial junction, the C_4-C_5 and T_4 segments and the shoulder due to altered motion of the glenohumeral joint.

Box 26.4

Migraine

A typical migraine headache is unilateral and pulsating lasting from 4 hours to 72 hours.

Symptoms: Nausea, vomiting, photophobia – increased sensitivity to light, phonophobia – increase sensitivity sound. Approximately 1/3rd of people who suffer from migraine headache perceive an auro-unusal visual, olfactory, or other experience that are the signs that the migraine will soon occur.

Pathophysiology: Cause is idiopathic. An accepted theory is that is a disorder of the serotonergic control system, a PET scan demonstrated the aura coincides with diffusion of cortical depression consequent to increased blood flow (upto 300% greater than baseline).

There are some migraine headache variants, soms originate from the brainstem (featuring inter celluler transport dysfunction of calcium and potassium), and some are genetically disposed.

Kim Christiansen (chiropracticener) states that "postural patterns are maintained by a complex arrangement of proprioceptive input modified by habits, somatotype and even psychogenic factors such as self esteem". Christiansen proposed that sustained malalignment results in muscular imbalance (shortening and lengthening of group of muscles). The end result of muscular imbalance is development of common postural patterns, such as forward head posture, elevation and protraction of the shoulders, protraction of head, increase thoracic kyphosis and cervical lordosis.

Ideally, when the posture is viewed from the side in standing, the plumb line should pass through the earlobe, midway through the shoulder joint, midway through the trunk, greater trochanter, slightly anterior to the mid point of the knee joint and slightly anterior to the ankle joint. In patient with upper crossed syndrome and cervicogenic headache the plumb line passes anterior to the shoulder joints and if the distance of the plumb line is high from the shoulder to the anterior, the condition may be graded as severe. If the distance of the plumb line from the shoulder to the anterior is very low the syndrome may be graded as mild and it may remain asymptomatic.

Management: The patients with UCS are managed by postural correction exercises. Strengthening of deep neck flexors, upper thoracic extensors, rhomboid and stretching of pectoralis major, upper cervical extensor, SCM, upper trapezius and levator scapulae muscle.

Table 26.8: Upper crossed syndrome

Weak muscles	Shortened muscles
- Serratus anterior	- Pectoralis major
- Lower and middle trapezius	- Upper trapezius and levator scapulae
- Deep neck flexors	- Sup occipitalis
	- Sternocleidomastoid

CERVICAL SPONDYLOLITIC MYELOPATHY

The gross osteoarthritic changes may project the osteophytes into the spinal canal and can contribute to narrowing of the canal. It is not at all uncommon for a patient with myelopathy to have associated radicular symptoms and produce the mixed type of symptoms such as lower motor neuron and upper motor neuron lesion symptoms. A pure myelopathic syndrome is rarely produced by the chronic disc degeneration with posterior osteophytes alone. A pure myelopathic syndrome within the cervical spinal cord is produced if the degenerated changes are combined with a congenital small bony spinal canal, degeneration in the cervical motion segment with annular bulging and osteophytes, facet joints hypertrophy, ligamentum flavum infolding, abnormal cervical

segment motion (i.e., forward or backward subluxation, and vascular impairment of the substance of the spinal cord.

The congenital small bony spinal canal, degeneration in the cervical motion segment with annular bulging and osteophytes and facet joint hypertrophy cause compression while vascular impairment causes ischaemia in patients with cervical spondylolitic myelopathy.

Clinical Features

The patients with cervical spondylolitic myelopathy present with mixed type of symptoms in the upper and lower extremities.

Upper Extremities: In upper extremity two types of radicular and myelopathic symptoms are produced. The lower motor neuron lesion (radicular) symptoms are experienced in the course of nerve root whose nerve root is compressed in process of osteophytes or spurs. The upper motor neuron (myelopathic) symptoms are produced below the lesion.

In the process of degeneration the osteophytes will project posteriorly first to the nerve roots and then to the spinal cord, therefore, below the lesion (at spinal cord) the symptoms will be myelopathic but at same level of lesion where nerve root is compressed there will be lower motor neuron (radicular) type of symptoms such as pain, paresthesia, weakness, and diminished reflexes. The myelopathic symptoms will be same as upper motor neuron such as exaggerated reflexes, increased muscle tone, spastic gait and spastic weakness in the hand often described as clumsiness (Figs. 26.77a-c).

As an example osteophytes at C_5-C_6 may compress the C_6 nerve root and can cause pain, weakness and diminished biceps reflexes, and paresthesia in the thumb and index finger. This is because of lower motor neuron lesion in C_6 nerve root. The lesion is below the anterior horn

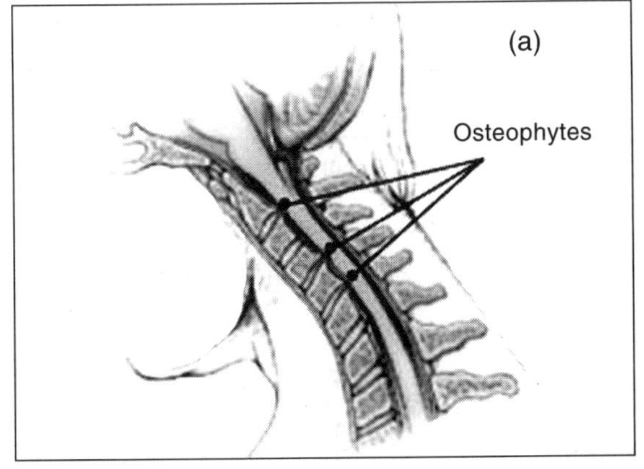

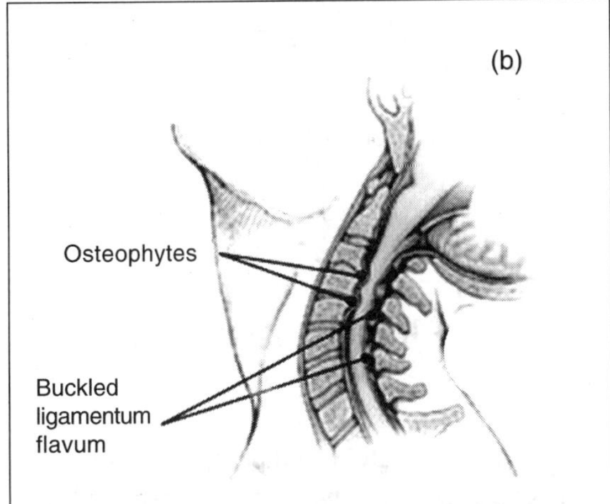

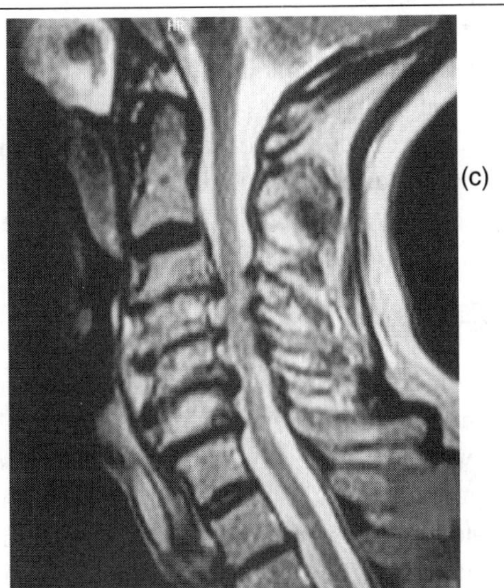

Figs. 26.77a-c: Cervical spondylolitic myelopathy

cell of the C_6 nerve root, therefore, the lower motor neuron lesion symptoms are produced, whereas, compression on spinal cord will produce upper motor neuron symptoms because, corresponding nerves are compressed above their anterior horn cells.

Lower Extremities: In the lower extremities symptoms will be upper motor lesion type. The patients find difficulty in walking, stair climbing and scuffing of shoes. As the disease progresses the gait becomes broad based and jerky. Patients often flex the cervical spine to open the intervertebral foramen in order to relieve the symptoms.

Conservative Management

The patients with CSM do not respond significantly to the conservative treatments. Symptoms such as pain and spasticity can be reduced temporarily by advising hot water fermentation and passive movements respectively. Core strengthening should be taught to maintain the posture. Gait may also be improved.

Cervical Traction: Manual and mechanical traction will not improve the myelopathic symptoms but it may help in stretching of the ligaments and other soft tissues and in maintaining the range of motion. Traction may help in relieving the pressure on the nerve roots and in improving the symptoms of radiculopathy. It rarely helps in improving the symptoms of myelopathy.

Strengthening Exercises: Strengthening of weak muscles such as deep neck flexors, rhomboids, trapezius and serratus anterior should be taught to prevent disuse atrophy of the muscles.

Surgical Management

Surgical intervention should only be advised when the symptoms are deteriorating and patients are having difficulty in performing activities of daily living. It is not there that surgical intervention will reverse the myelopathic deficit completely, but it is advised to improve the functions of patient and to stop further progression of the disease. The surgical procedures demand removal of the posterior vertebral bodies, removal of the lamina, removal of the ligamentum flavum and decompression of the nerve roots.

TORTICOLIS (WRY NECK)

Torticolis is a side flexion with rotation of the neck due to tightness or contracture of the sternocleidomastoid muscle. It is almost always a condition in children and is a symptom and/or sign not a disease. Torticolis may also occur as a result of intracranial lesion or intraspinal pathology. The torticolis may be of several types but the most common torticolis are congenital muscular, spasmodic and paralytic (Fig. 26.78).

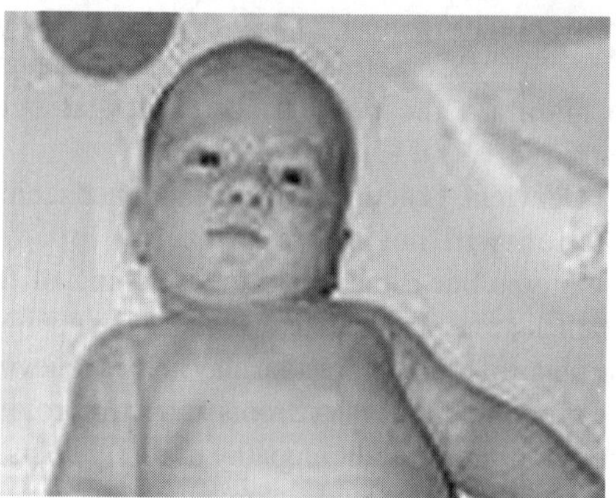

Fig. 26.78: Torticolis

Paralytic Torticolis

Unilateral cervical muscle movement in poliomyelitis is rather unusual. When it does occur the head is rotated towards the side of paralysis.

Spasmodic Torticolis

Severe spasm and pain in SCM, trapezius and splenius muscle may produce torticolis in adult patients. These patients often associated with severe psychiatric disturbances.

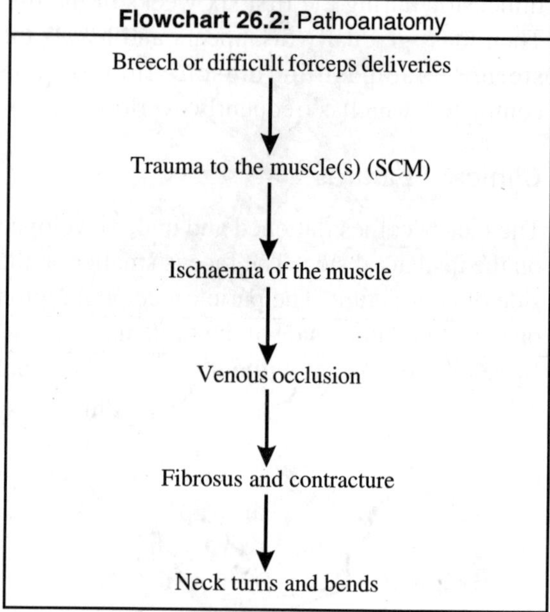

Congenital Muscular Torticolis

The shortening or tightness of the sterno-cleidomastoid muscle will flex the neck to the same side and rotate it to the opposite side. The exact cause is unknown but it is believed that following factors may contribute to the torticolis.

a. Intrauterine malposition.
b. Heredity.
c. Breech delivery or difficult forceps delivery.
d. Acquired muscular ischaemia/some mal-developmental deficits in the muscle.
e. Malposition in the uterus.

Examination

Children do not complain pain and other symptoms, however, mother or family members notice after two weeks of the birth that the head of the child is not on the neck it is flexed and rotated. A soft non-tender mass is frequently palpated within the substance of the involved sternocleidomastoid muscle. The overlying skin and subcutaneous tissue are freely movable and separated from the mass, which generally attains its greatest dimension during the first six weeks of the life. Then mass gradually disappears and leaves the sternocleidomastoid muscle injured and contracted, which is frequently overlooked.

Clinical Features

The face becomes flattened and underdeveloped on the ipsilateral side. The face is smaller on the side of contracture. The parieto-occipital region on the contralateral side of the skull also flattens. If the torticolis is left without treating, the facial and skull deformities increase due to inability of the soft tissues to keep pace with the bony growth of the skull and cervical spine. The corners of the eye and mouth are drawn down, eye itself appearing smaller than that on the sound side, and of a different shape. The nose deviates slightly towards the affected side. Shortening of bilateral sternocleidomastoid muscles is very rare but if present, the head is then bent forward, and kyphosis is a complication.

Management

Soft Tissue Manipulation: Stroking and finger kneading is performed on the sternocleidomastoid muscle where swelling is noticed.

Passive Stretching: It is one of the best treatments in terms of improvement in flexibility of the muscle. The child is placed supine on the plinth with the head out of the edge. The therapist holds the head well with both the hands. As an example, for a left torticolis child the head is rotated to the same side (left side) and then flexed to the opposite side (right side), as much as child allows or tolerates. The stretched position is held for at least six seconds to allow maximum effects of stretching. Several repetitions may be performed in a session. Sometimes child will cry or straggle with the maneuver, hence, the

stretching should be quick. The therapist can also teach the same to the patient care givers to perform the exercise at home. Precautions should be taken not to hurt the child.

Manual Traction: As the child grows older, traction may also be indicated. In a supine position with head out of the edge the therapist holds the chin and occiput of the child and distracts the cervical spine, which must be held for at least six seconds to allow the maximum effect of stretching.

Surgical Intervention

Torticolis in older children is very rare or if it is present it may be due to neglected congenital torticolis or may be an acquired. These children do not respond to the soft tissue manipulation and stretching, they must be treated by surgical intervention. The sternal and clavicular head of the sternocleidomastoid muscles are divided close to their origins, and any contracted bands of fascia are also severed. After releasing the contracted muscle and fascia the head is positioned in the overcorrected position with the help of splint, orthosis or plaster of paris until the stitches are removed (at least for 10-14 days).

Postoperative stretching exercises should be started after removal of the stitches or after consultation with the surgeon. Initially exercises should be mild in intensity. In sitting or supine position the head is bent to the opposite side with rotation to the same side of the operated muscle. The intensity of exercise may be increased as the healing improves.

MANUAL THERAPY FOR THE THORACIC SPINE

Similar to cervical and lumbar spine degenerative changes take place in the thoracic spine also. Symptoms such as pain and limitation in the range of motion particularly in rotation are the dominant clinical features of the degenerative changes of the thoracic spine. Following pain and symptoms the patients adapt a posture which relieves the symptoms. This is the first step of malalignment or faulty posture. As the disease progresses the patient develops "upper crossed syndrome". This involves hyperextension at the upper cervical, protraction at the shoulders and flexion at the lower cervical and upper thoracic spine kyphosis. These are two points where patients feel more stresses. Sometimes a hump can also be seen on the upper thoracic spine. T_2 and T_3 segment bears more unwanted stresses.

It is thought that manual therapy at thoracic spine can improve the mobility and pain at cervical, thoracic and sometimes at the shoulders. The improvement in the mobility of the thoracic spine, significantly takes stress off adjacent, hyper mobile cervical spine or shoulder joints.

SNAGs to Improve Rotation at Upper Thoracic Spine: Patient sits on a stool with the hands clasped behind the neck. As an example, for a patient with pain and limitation in the right rotation due to D_{10} and D_{11} mobile segment, the therapist stands behind the patient, wraps left arm around the chest. The ulnar border of the right hand is placed under the spinous process of D_{10} vertebra. The patient is instructed to rotate the neck to the right side as much as possible. During the movement (right rotation) the spinous process of D_{10} vertebra is pushed up and superiorly. The right hand around the chest encourages the movement and also helps in applying overpressure if indicated (Fig. 26.79).

SNAGs to Improve Flexion: Patient sits on the stool with the hands resting on the thighs. As an example, for a patient with pain and limitation in the flexion range, resulting from lesion in the D_{10} and D_{11} mobile segment, the therapist stands behind the patient (slightly to the right side) and wraps the left arm around the trunk at the level of D_{10} and D_{11} level. The ulnar border of

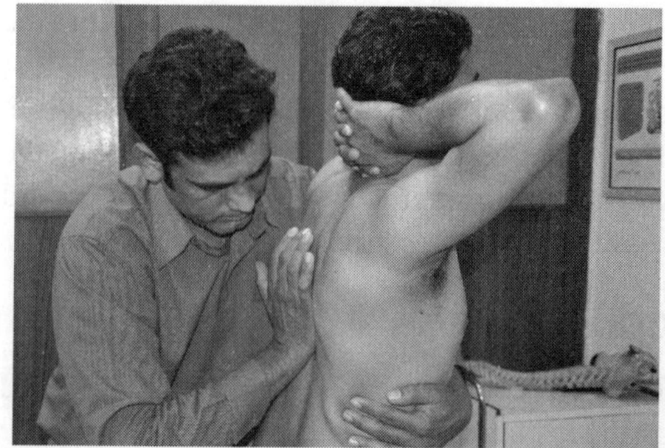

Fig. 26.79: SNAGs to improve rotation at upper thoracic spine

the right wrist is placed under the spinous process of D_{10}, which applies gliding force along the facet plane. The patient is asked to flex the thoracic spine as much as possible within the painfree range. The gliding force is applied through the wrist while the left arm acts as a fulcrum for flexion. The gliding force is maintained throughout the range of motion till the movement returns to the neutral (Fig. 26.80).

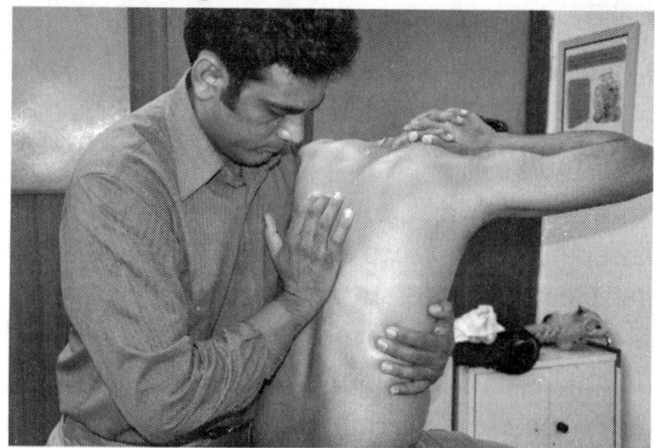

Fig. 26.80: SNAGs to improve flexion at upper thoracic spine

To improve an extension the position of the patient, therapist, and hands remain same as for flexion. The patient is asked to extend the spine as much as possible within the painfree range. The gliding force is applied through the ulnar border of the wrist throughout the movement till the movement returns to the neutral position (Fig. 26.81).

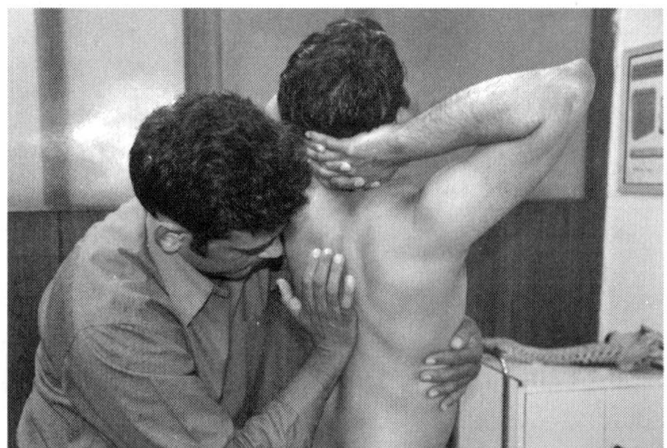

Fig. 26.81: SNAGs to improve extension at upper thoracic spine

Upper Thoracic Thrust Manipulation: The patient sits on a stool comfortably with the hands clasped behind the neck. The therapist stands behind the patient with slight flexion of the knees, and loops the hands through the patients arms and places over the patient's hands. A towel or sheet can be placed between the therapist chest and patient's back for cosmetic purposes. The therapist chest should rest on the patients back. A thrust is delivered to the upper thoracic spine by leaning backward and extending the knees. The technique is discarded if patient complains discomfort and pain in the shoulders. This technique not only improves pain and range at upper thoracic but also helps in relieving pain in the cervical spine.

Mid Thoracic Thrust Manipulation: The patient sits comfortably on a stool with both the hands grasping opposite scapula (posterior shoulder), so that the elbows are parallel and rests on the lower sternum. The therapist stands behind the patient and grasps the patients lower elbow. A small towel may be placed on the desired segment between patients back and therapists chest. The therapist takes up slack by adducting the arms, retracting the shoulders and pushing the chest to the desired segment (thoracic spine). A high velocity thrust is delivered by the therapist through the patients arms from anterior to posterior direction.

Thoracic Thrust Manipulation in Standing: The patient stands with both the hands clasped behind the shoulders on scapula. The therapist stands behind the patient places a small towel piece between his chest and the patient's thoracic spine, grasps the patient's lower elbow. Similar to the mid thoracic thrust manipulation, therapist takes up slack by adducting the arms, retracting the shoulder girdles and pushing the chest to the patients thoracic spine. While maintaining, position the therapist produces high velocity thrust by lifting the patient with extension of knees and leaning backward.

CHAPTER-27

Low Back Pain

INTRODUCTION

Back pain is a complex phenomenon and it is not always possible to determine its source reliably as it may originate from several structures of the mobile segment. However, it is possible to recognize basic patterns and presentations of pain and this certainly helps to facilitate provisional diagnosis. Pain experienced in the spine with radiation such as sciatica, may have one or more of four origins: Spinal, vascular, visceral and psychogenic.

The hectic life-style (daily busy schedules) long and indefinite working hours are eventually the predisposing factors to various health and stress related ailments among metropolitan youth. People do not find time to walk even for a mile, this life-style causes loss of flexibility of the muscle fibers.

The most common cause of back pain is a minor strain to muscle and/or ligament, but people suffering from this type of back pain usually do not seek medical treatment as most of these soft tissue injuries resolve naturally. Sometimes injury or strain to the muscle and ligament can cause further damage to the mobile segment that leads to dysfunction of the apophyseal joint and intervertebral joint the exact balance being uncertain.

Almost 80% of the population experience low back pain sometimes in their life, that each year 2% to 5% of adults seek treatment or lose time from work because of low back pain. Some of these individuals become disabled and need long term treatment, therefore, we can realize how significant an issue of low back pain is in our society. At least 70% patients recover completely within one month but some are prone to the recurrence of low back pain.

To manage the low back pain we have specialists: such as spine surgeons, physicians, physical therapists and occupational therapists. With all this high energy and intellect dedicated to the low back pain care, the society can expect improved results. The reasons of our failure to cope with the low back pain may be following:

(a) It is fact that we are dealing with the symptoms.
(b) Subjective low back pain is not always associated with objective physical findings.

It is, therefore, necessary to have a very clear concept of possible source of pain when presented with the problem of a patient seeking relief from the irksome burden of constant low back pain. In order to differentiate these lesions and to facilitate a provisional diagnosis, the clinician must diligently elicit an accurate and lucid history, and conduct a routine subjective and objective physical examinations.

Classification of Low Back Pain

Pain experienced in the low back region with or without peripheral radiation is a symptom not a disease, which may have origin within or outside of the spine. The causes of low back pain are many but it may broadly be classified into four major groups:

1. Spondylogenic.
2. Viscerogenic.

3. Vasculogenic.
4. Psychogenic.

The spondylogenic type of pain is originated from the spine itself due to trauma, pathology or degeneration. (Pain in the lumbar region due to the above other causes lies outside of the spine.)

Viscerogenic Low Back Pain: Viscerogenic back pain may originate from viscera such as kidneys, the pelvic viscera, lesions of the lesser sac, and retroperitoneal tumors. The pain perceived in the low back region is referred from the viscera, neither is aggravated by activities or movements of lumbar spine, nor is relieved by rest. Indeed, with severe pain, the patient whose symptoms are visceral in origin, will walk around to get relief, whereas the patient suffering from the tortures of a septic discitis will prefer to lie still.

Vascular Low Back Pain: Pathological changes in the vessels and arteries (vascular bundles) may produce similar symptoms as of sciatica or spinal pain. The symptoms may be boring type of deep-situated lumbar pain unrelated to activities (abdominal aortic aneurysms). Superior gluteal artery insufficiency may produce buttock pain of claudication nature. The important feature of abdominal aortic aneurysm and superior gluteal artery insufficiency is that symptoms may aggravate by walking and relieved by rest. (While walking the pain may radiate from the buttocks to the leg). However, the pain is not aggravated by the activities such as bending, stooping, lifting etc. In patients with intermittent claudication the pain is experienced in the calf, which is aggravated while walking and relieved by standing still. In case of spinal canal stenosis the pain is similar to peripheral claudication (Sciatic distribution) is frequently initiated and aggravated by the act of walking a short distance but not relieved by standing still.

Psychogenic Low Back Pain: Although pure psychogenic back pain is rarely seen in clinical practice but failure to consider it in the assessment of low back pain might lead to serious errors in diagnosis and management. The patients with psychogenic back pain are very anxious, tend to overexpose their problem. They are usually demonstrative, the hands being used to point out various painful areas almost without prompting. The pain distribution is often atypical and not specific to the particular dermatome. The reflexes are almost always hyperactive and hypersensitive to the touch. Diffuse tenderness even to slightest touch will be presented. In such patients, although the task may be difficult, the therapist must be prepared to accept the possibility of an underlying pathological process and investigate its probability thoroughly.

Mechanical Low Back Pain: *Spondylogenic referred pain:* It is a non-radicular pain which originates from any of the components of mobile segment including face joints, intervertebral joint, the intervertebral disc, muscles, ligaments, and the dura mater. Similar type of pain may also be referred from viscera to the low back region, proximal thigh and groin; therefore, it is important to distinguish the spondylogenic referred pain from visceral referred pain. The spondylogenic pain is deep dull aching which is relieved by rest and aggravated by the movements of the lumbar spine. The local tender points may not be elicited. *Radicular pain:* The radicular pain is a type of mechanical low back pain which has origin in the intervertebral foramen (nerve roots) and experienced in the course of the nerve root/s. It is characterized by pain, parasthesia, numbness (anaesthesia), loss of reflexes and muscle power. Sometimes the symptoms are more severe in the legs then in the spine.

Anatomical and Pathological Aspects

The spine is a flexible, multisegmental column bridging the interval between the base of the skull and the pelvis. It maintains not only the posture but also protects the neural structures. In addition to this it allows movements in the vertebral column.

The Mobile Segment: The mobile segment of the lumbar spine is of static stabilizers which are divided into two parts anterior and posterior segments. The anterior mobile segment contains anterior longitudinal ligaments, intervertebral joints, intervertebral discs, and intervertebral bodies. The posterior mobile segment contains posterior longitudinal ligaments, apophyseal joints, interspinous and supraspinous ligaments. The mobile segment works as a single functional unit during movements and rest. If any one structure of mobile segment is damaged due to trauma or in the degenerative process, it can decrease the stability of the lumbar spine and can contribute to the low back pain and symptoms (Figs. 27.1a-b).

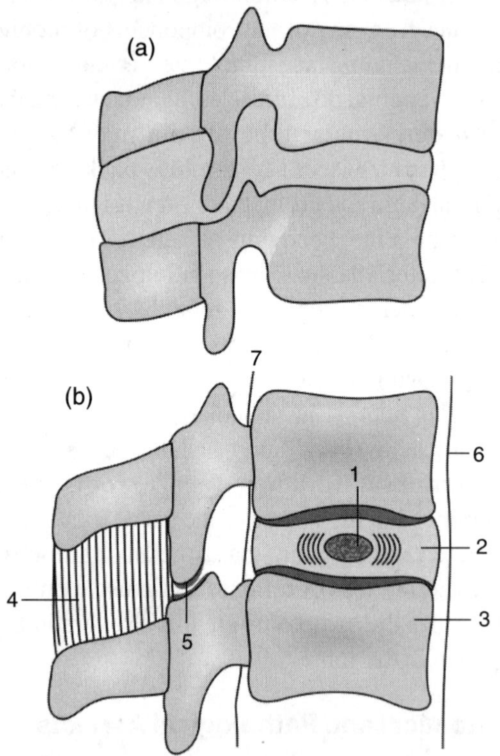

Figs. 27.1a-b: Mobile segment (1) Nucleus pulposus, (2) Annulus fibrosus, (3) Vertebral body, (4) Interspinous ligament, (5) Facet joint, (6) Anterior longitudinal ligament, (7) Posterior longitudinal ligament

Minor Intervertebral Derangement (MID) Theory of Maigne: Maigne pointed out that the functional ability of the mobile segment depends intimately upon integrity of the I.V.D. Thus if the disc is injured, other elements of the segment will also be affected. For an example, disc herniation reduces the intervertebral joint space, which in turn causes approximation of facet joints and laxity in the ligaments.

Vertebrae: The lumbar spine has got five vertebrae with posterior concavity joined with the sacrum vertebra. The vertebral bodies are connected to the intervertebral discs, and the neural arches are joined by the facet joints. The size of the vertebral bodies increases from first lumbar vertebra to the fifth lumbar vertebra as the load increases from L_1 to L_5. The lumbar vertebrae have massive bodies, suitable for supporting the entire superimposed weight of the head, trunk and arms. The total mass of five lumbar vertebrae is approximately twice that of the seven cervical vertebrae (Fig. 27.2).

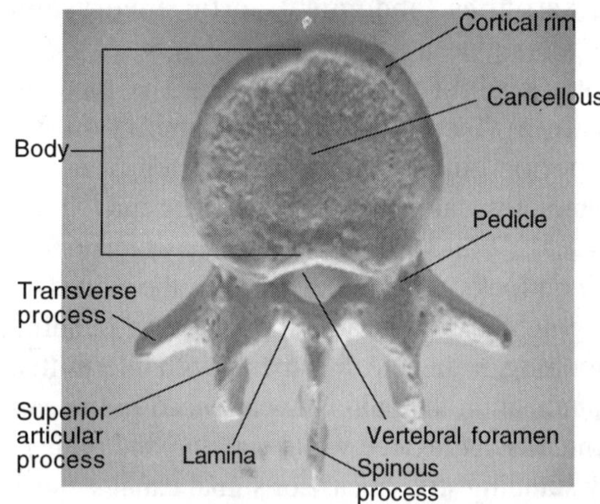

Fig. 27.2: Lumbar vertebra

Facet Joints: There are two facet joints at each mobile segment. The articular surface of the facets of the lumbar vertebrae is oriented nearly vertical. The superior facets are moderately concave, facing medial to posteromedial. The facet surfaces of the upper lumbar region tend to be oriented close to the sagittal plane. The superior facet surface in the mid to lower lumbar region tends to be oriented midway between the sagittal and frontal planes.

The inferior articular facets are slightly convex, facing generally lateral to anterolateral. These are reciprocally matched to the shape and orientation of the superior articular facets. The inferior facets of L_5 articulate with the superior facets of the sacrum and the joints are typically oriented much closer to the frontal plane than the other lumbar facet joints articulations. The anteroposterior lumbosacral stability to the lumbosacral junction is provided well by the $L_5 - S_1$ apophyseal joints.

The facet joints typically demonstrate changes with aging. The change may result from forces related to the development of bipedal gait in early childhood. Side-to-side joint asymmetry is common in adults and *lead articular troops, i.e.,* developmental alteration in the joints shape in a certain percentage of the population. Some investigators feel that tropism may alter the biomechanics and increase the forces in some portions of the intervertebral discs, thereby predisposing them to injury (Fig. 27.3).

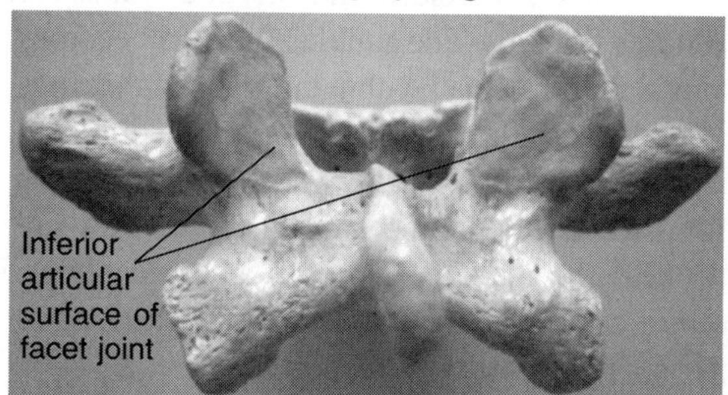

Fig. 27.3: Lumbar vertebra showing the facet surfaces

The facet joints are richly innervated from the medial branch of the posterior primary rami. The capsule of the facet joint receives a number of tiny branches from two segmental nerves. The malalignment of the facet joints causes stretching of the capsule, and produces dull to severe pain depending upon the severity of malalignment. The facet joints can produce the pain in the low back region and that may be referred to any part of the lower limb as far as the calf and ankle but most commonly pain is referred to the gluteus region, proximal thigh and groin. The entrapment of the medial branch of posterior ramus can occur and could refer pain to the structures that it innervates.

Apophyseal Glides During Spinal Movements: The facet joints glide to facilitate the lumbar movements. In case of facet joints malalignment these can block the movements of lumbar spine. *During Flexion:* The upper facet slides up and forward on the lower facet that opens the facet joint. *During Extension:* The upper facet slides down and back on the lower facet that closes the facet joint. *During Side Flexion:* The upper facet slides down and back on the same side to the movement "closing the joint" and up and forward on the side opposite of the movement (opening the joint). *During Rotation:* The upper facet moves up and anterior on the opposite of the movement (opening the facet) and moves down and posterior of the same side of the movement (closing the joint).

Intervertebral Disc: The intervertebral space of the lumbar spine involves portions of two vertebral bodies and an intervertebral disc. The intervertebral disc is the largest avascular structure of the body which is situated between two vertebral bodies. It comprises annulus fibrosus (AF), a nuclease pulposus (NP) and an end plate. The central part of the disc, a nucleus pulposus is comprised 70% to 90% water, depending on a person's age. It functions as a modified hydraulic shock absorber that dissipates and transfers loads between consecutive vertebra. The nucleus pulposus is thickened by relatively large branching proteoglycans. Each proteoglycan is an aggregate of many water binding glycosaminoglycans linked to core proteins. The nucleus also contains type II collagen fibers, elastic fibers and other non-collagenous protein. The annulus fibrosus consists of 10 to 20% concentric layers or rings of collagen fibers. The end plate is associated more strongly with the IVD then with the vertebral body. It is situated on the superior and inferior part of the intervertebral disc. It is the weakest part of the intervertebral disc in compression (Fig. 27.4).

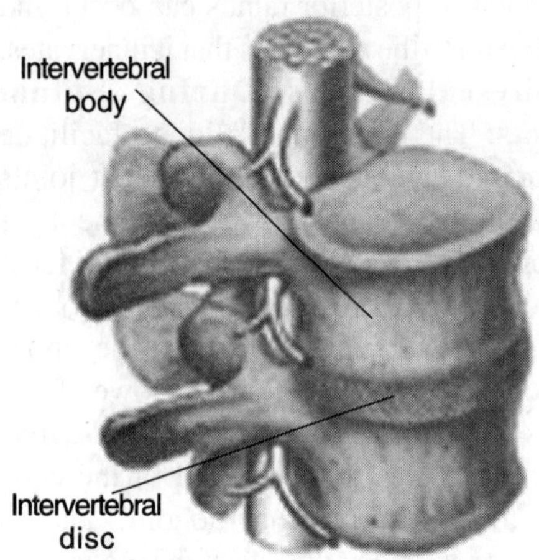

Fig. 27.4: Intervertebral disc

The intervertebral disc is the largest avascular structure of the body and its nutrition depends on diffusion. It receives its blood supply from the two *closest vessel sources,* which are those beneath the vertebral end plate and those at the periphery of the annulus fibrosus. Certain movements possible those in and out of the flexion, may facilitate nutrition of the disc (one of the benefits of exercise may be to facilitate the nutrition of the intervertebral disc). The intervertebral discs have a blood supply upto 8 years, but, thereafter, they are dependent on diffusion of tissue fluids. As the intervertebral disc is avascular and its nutrition depends on the diffusion and movements its healing transpires, but complete healing takes months to years.

The disc was generally believed to be non pain sensitive and consequently inert structure. Recently it has been found that the superficial layer of the annulus fibrosus in the lumbar region has significant innervations from the sinuvertebral nerves and stimulation of those nerve endings can result in pain.

As the load is transmitted to the nucleus through the hyline cartilage plate the load of axial compression is distributed not only in vertical direction but also radially throughout the nucleus as well. The intervertebral discs add considerable stability to the vertebral column as well as being shock absorber.

The stability to the vertebral column is primarily provided by the structural configuration of the collagen fibers within the annulus fibrosus. The annulus fibrosus is the part of intervertebral disc primarily composed of collagen fibers. The collagen fibers are organized in such a way that they inhibit radial expansion of the nucleus pulposus. They are arranged in multiple concentric layers, with fibers in every other layer running in identical directions. The orientation of each collagen fiber is about $30° + 90° = 120$ degrees from the vertical.

The compressive forces on the intervertebral disc are generated by the body weight and the contraction of the muscles, they push the end plate inward and toward the nucleus pulposus. The nucleus pulposus deforms radially and against the annulus fibrosus. The annulus fibrosus becomes tensed and stretched within the walls of the rings of collagen and elastic fibers. The internal resistance reinforces the walls of the annulus fibrosus. The entire mechanism creates pressure back to the nucleus pulposus and end plates, reinforces the entire disc and passes the load to the next vertebra.

Movements

Osteokinematics and Arthrokinematics: The range of motion of the lumbar spine differs at various levels as it depends on orientation of the facets of intervertebral joints. The movement does not occur independently at one motion segment

Flowchart 27.1: Mechanism of load transmission

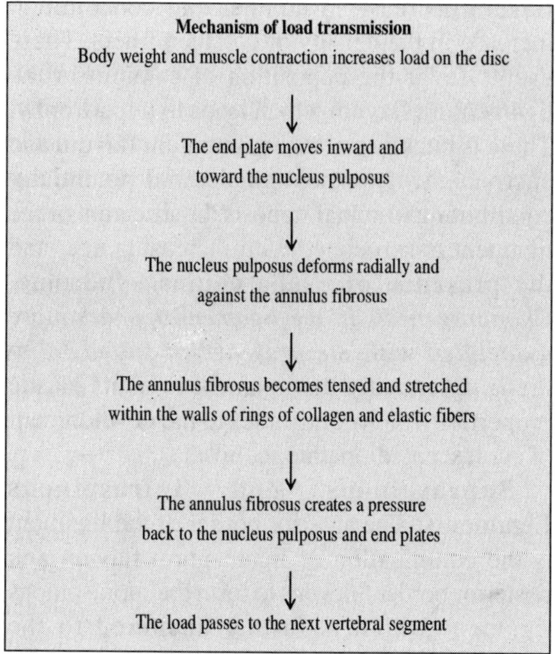

but it involves the combined action of several motion segments. *Spinal coupling:* Movement of the vertebral column in one plane is usually associated with an automatic and at times nearly interceptible movement in another plane as well. (During axial rotation and lateral flexion the spinal coupling takes place) (Figs. 27.5a-b and 27.6).

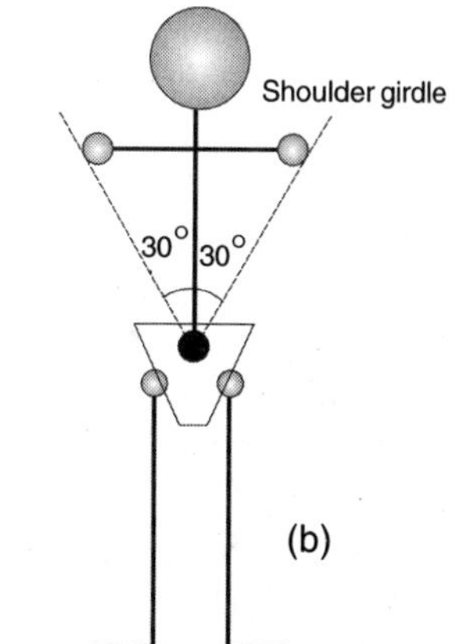

Figs. 27.5a-b: Lumbar spine range of motion (side flexion)

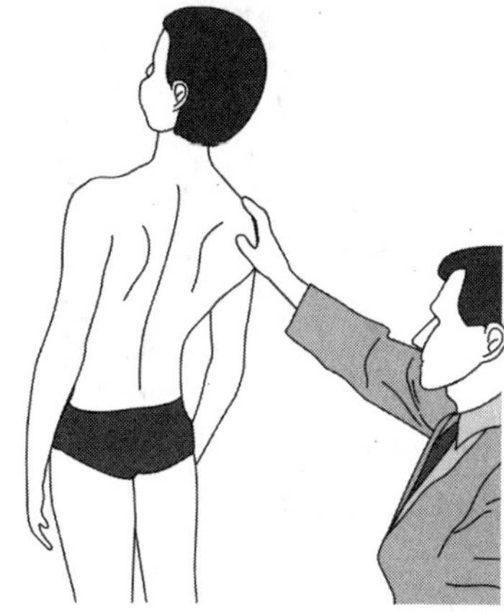

Fig. 27.6: Lumbar spine range of motion (side flexion)

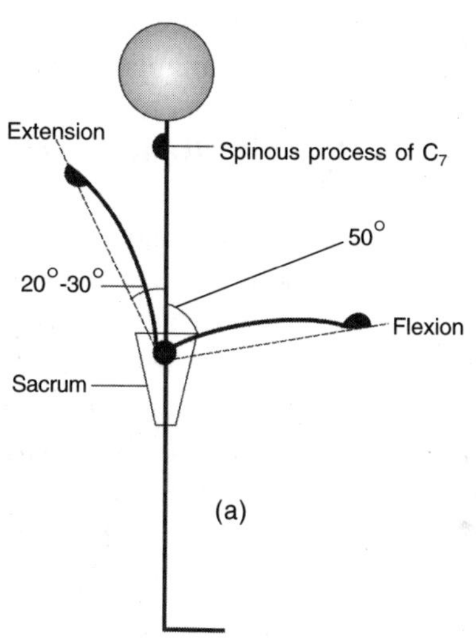

Table 27.1: Movements of the lumbar spine

Movement	In degrees	Plane
Flexion	50	Sagittal
Extension	20-30	Sagittal
Rotation	05	Horizontal
Lateral flexion	30 (Each)	Frontal plane

Ligaments

The various ligaments of the lumbar vertebral column form a continuous, dense, connective tissue stocking surrounding the vertebrae, and extending to the sacral area. In humans the ligament can best be described as a fan. It extends between borders of the spinous process of adjacent vertebrae. These are divided as under:

1. Neural arch ligaments
   - Ligamentum flavum.
   - Interspinous ligament.
   - Supraspinous ligament.
2. Articular capsular ligament.
3. Ligaments ventral to the facet joints
   - Anterior longitudinal ligament.
   - Posterior longitudinal ligament.
4. Inter-transverse ligament.
5. Ileolumbar ligament (Fig. 27.7).

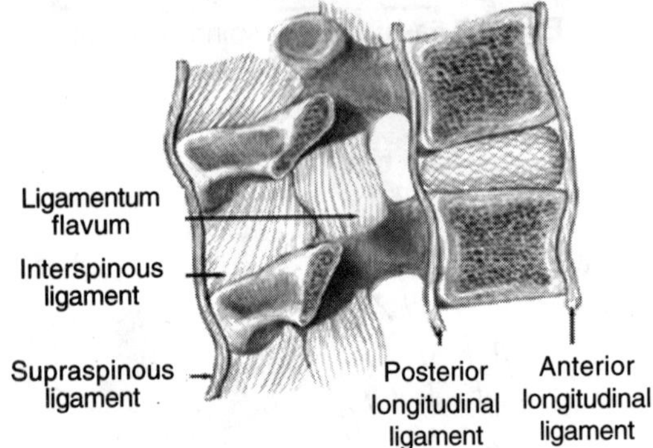

Fig. 27.7: Ligaments of the lumbar spine

Ligamentum Flavum

This ligament is composed of elastic fibers (80%) and collagenous fibers 20%. The elastic fibers imparting the ligament its yellow color and flexible nature forms a significant portion of roof of the spinal canal. The ligamentum flavum bridges the interlaminar interval attaching to the interspinous ligament medially and the facet capsule laterally. Superiorly it attaches to the anterior surface of the lamina above and inferiorly it establishes a cup-like grasp on the superior margin of the lamina below.

Normally, the ligament maintains a taut configuration, stretching for flexion and contracting its elastic fibers at neutral, therefore it provides a roof for the vertebral canal that does not buckle during extension-flexion movements of the vertebral column (in this way it covers but never infringes on the epidural space).

With aging the elastic fibers of the ligamentum flavum decrease in number and concomitant increase in the density of collagen fibers. These events favor the deposition of calcium in the ligamentum flavum which leads to hypertrophy. There is buckling of the ligamentum flavum and encroachment on the spinal canal potentially contributing to spinal stenosis. Ossification of the ligament is associated with increasing age, and the presence of cauda equina syndrome. *Chondrogenesis in the ligament appears more associated with the presence of spondylolisthesis.* Eventually the ligament loses its elastic properties which contributes to the development of adolescent idiopathic scoliosis.

Supraspinous and Infraspinous Ligaments: The anterior border of the ligament is the continuation of ligamentum flavum and posterior border thickens to form the supraspinous ligament which is further anchored to the thoracolumbar fascia. The fan shaped arrangement of the ligament not only allows the ligament to expand without rupture but also prevents the separation of vertebral column during flexion. The supraspinous ligament is tightly adhering to the posterior border of the lumbar spines and interspinous ligament.

Anterior Longitudinal Ligament: It runs the whole length of the anterior aspect of the spine and attaches to anterior annular fibers of each disc.

Posterior Longitudinal Ligament: It extends from the base of occiput (as the membrane tectorial) cervical to the sacrum caudally. The ligament is much thinner both in width and thickness than the anterior longitudinal ligament in the lower lumbar region, therefore, the main opposition to flexion of the lumbar spine comes from ligament flavum. This contributes to the lumbar disc problem at lower region.

Intertransverse Ligaments: Intertransverse ligaments are centrally membranes that extend between an adjacent transverse processes. These ligaments constitute a part of fascia system which separates the ventral compartment muscles from posterior muscles.

Iliolumbar Ligament: The iliolumbar ligament is a substantial ligament that binds the transverse process of the L_5 vertebra to the sacrum and resists forward sliding, lateral flexion and axial rotation of the L_5 vertebra on sacrum. Initially the ligament is muscular and represents the L_5 components of iliocostalis lumborum and as age progresses it undergoes fibrous metaphasis.

Muscles

The structural unit of the skeletal muscle is the muscle fiber, a cylindrical cell with hundreds of nuclei. Each muscle is composed of many hundreds of muscle fibers, which provide stability and mobility to the mobile segment. Weakness or tightness of the muscles can alter the stability and mobility of the mobile segment.

The Lumbar Multifidus: The lumbar multifidus is the largest and most medial muscle of the lumbar muscles and consists of repeating series (five separate bonds) of fascicles that stem from the laminae and spinous processes of the lumbar vertebrae and exhibit a constant pattern of attachments caudally.

The deepest fibers of the muscle in the lumbar arise from the posterior inferior aspect of the each vertebral lamina and articular capsule of the facet joint. The deep fibers insert into the maxillary process two levels below the deep fiber of the L_5 lamina inserts on an area on the sacrum just above the first dorsal sacral foramen as the L_5 lamina has no maxillary process (Figs. 27.8a-f).

Dick N and *et al.* department of rehabilitation sciences and P.T. Ghent University, Campus Hymens, state by using MRI study that the deep multifidus has a higher percentage of slow twitch fibers compared to the superficial multifidus. *No differential reenlistment has been found following trunk extension with and without pain induction.*

The superficial fibers have combined effect on the spine, they exert compression loading of the spine to enhance its stiffness and produce an effective moment arm for extension of the lumbar spine and control the lumbar lordosis. The laminar deep fibers can be considered to stabilize the two overlying functional segments. They control intervertebral shear and torsion via intervertebral compression. The attachment of the deep fibers of multifidus to the facet joints have an advantage in allowing multifidus in keeping the capsule from being impinged during movements caused by the multifidus.

Decrease in the size of the multifidus has been constantly documented in people with low back pain. Wallwork TL and *et al.* conducted study aimed at to compare both the size (cross-sectional area) and the ability to voluntary perform an isometric contraction of the multifidus muscle at four vertebral levels in 34 subjects with and without chronic low back pain by using the ultrasound imagings. The study shown a significantly smaller cross-sectional area of the multifidus muscle for the subjects in the chronic low back pain group compared with normal healthy subjects at the L_5 vertebral level and a significant smaller percent thickness contraction for subjects with the chronic low back pain group of the same vertebral level.

Hides J, Gilmore C, *et al.* have also conducted the similar type of study by recruiting 40 asymptomatic and 50 chronic low back pain subjects. Their results showed that the greatest asymmetry between sides was seen at the L_5 vertebral level in patients with unilateral pain presentation. The smaller multifidus cross-sectional area was ipsilateral to reported side of pain in all cases.

Recent advances in the understanding of the biomechanics of low back pain have highlighted the importance of muscular stabilization of the "neutral zone" range of motion in the low back

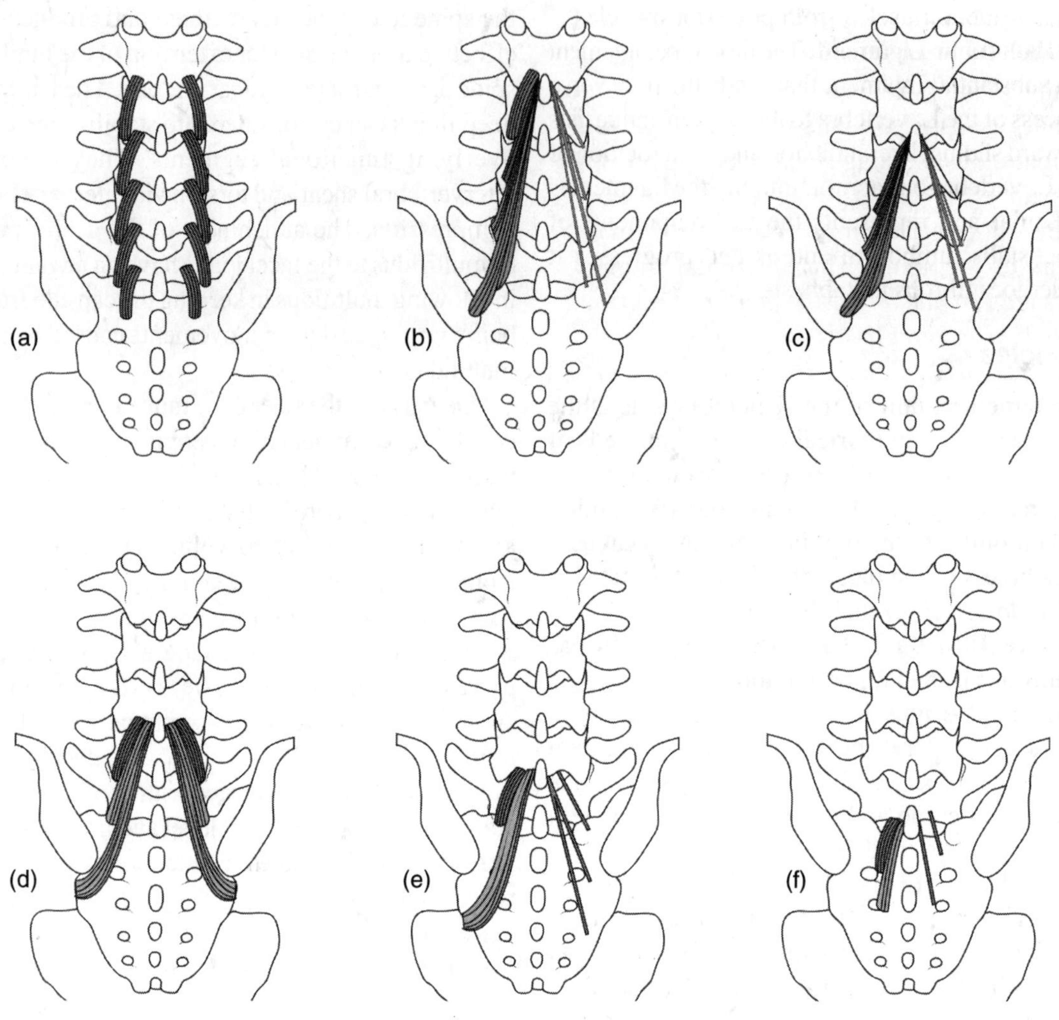

Figs. 27.8a-f: The component fasciculus of multifidus a. The laminar fibers of multifidus, b-f The fascicles from L$_1$ to L$_5$ spinous process, respectively

area. The lumbar multifidus muscles (LMN) are important stabilizers of this neutral zone and dysfunction in these muscles strongly associated with low back pain. The dysfunction is as a result of pain inhibition from the spine, and it tends to continue even after the pain has resolved, likely contributing to the high recurrence rate of low back pain.

The oblique abdominals are the primary rotators of the spine. The horizontal rotation occurs after *impaction* of the contralateral facet joint only if an appropriate shear force is applied to the intervertebral disc. The horizontal vector of the multifidus, however, is so small that it is unlikely that the multifidus would be capable of exerting such shear force on the disc by acting on the spinous process. Muscle training directed at teaching patients to activate their multifidus is an important feature of any clinical approach to the low back pain patients.

Transverse Abdominis: Studies have shown that strengthening of transverse abdominis helps in decreasing the pain and symptoms of low back pain as it is a key stabilizer of the lumbar spine. A coordinated contraction of the transverse abdominis, diaphragm, and pelvic floor muscles contributes to both unloading and stabilization of the lumbar spine. The transverse abdominis is optimally aligned for a posterior pull on the abdominal fascial complex. This posteriorly directed pull, especially around the slightly pressurized abdominal cylinder, compliments the more angled pulls of the external and internal abdominal oblique muscles. Thus the pull of the abdominal muscles cinches the abdomen with a corset-like effect and brings the abdominal contents posterior against the spine, which serves as another check to anterior shear of the lumbar vertebrae.

The fascicles of transverse abdominis originate from the inner surface of the lower six costal cartilages, the lumbar spine via the thoracolumbar fascia, the anterior two third of the inner lip of the iliac crest, and the lateral third of the inguinal ligament. The fascicles insert into the linea alba (Fig. 27.9).

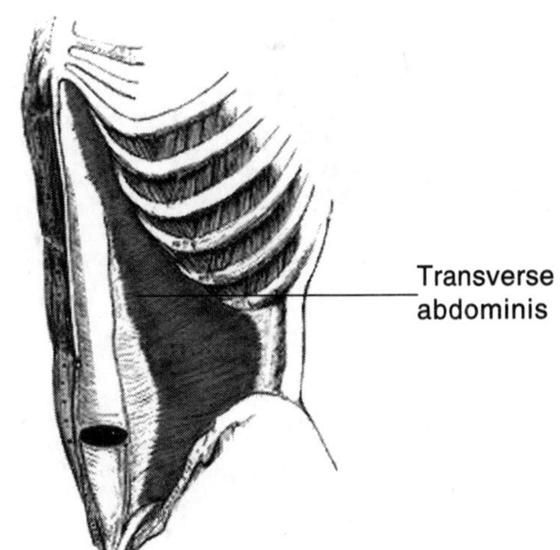

Fig. 27.9: Transverse abdominis

Thoracolumbar Fascia System

The muscles of the lumbar spine are enveloped by three layers of the fascia known as thoracolumbar fascia. The fascia consists of collagen fibers oriented in a variety of directions, with no particular orientation predominating. It is a dense network consisting of three layers of connective tissues–posterior, middle and anterior, which enclose the erector spinae, multifidus and quadratus lumborum muscles. Thoracolumbar fascia extends from the sacrum to the upper back and neck and is prominent in the low back region (Fig. 27.10).

Posterior Layer of the Thoracolumbar Fascia: The posterior layer of the thoracolumbar fascia is formed by the apponeurosis of the latissimus dorsi. It is thickest and strongest of the three layers which is attached to the spinous processes. It is a bilinear layer consisting of superficial and deep portions. The superficial portion is formed by the tendons of the ipsilateral latissimus dorsi, passing caudally and medially.

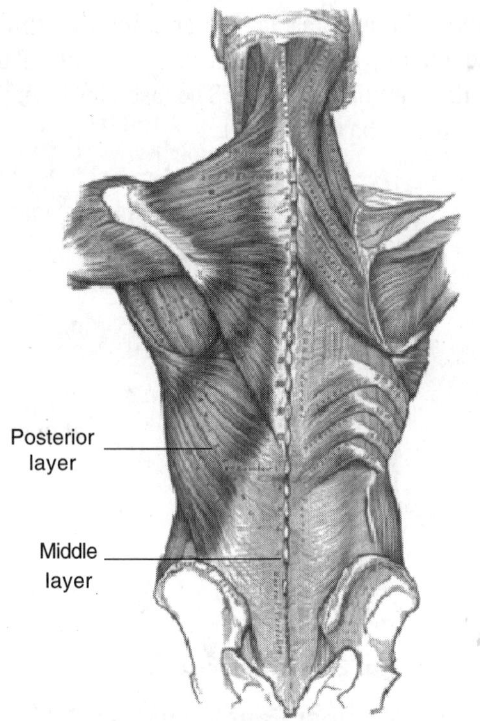

Fig. 27.10: Thoracolumbar fascia consisting three layers

The deep portion is formed by the tendons of the contralateral latissimus dorsi, passing downwards and laterally. The posterior layer extends into the thoracic region and lies posterior to the erector spine and multifidus muscles. The posterior layer of the thoracolumbar fascia is designed to transmit forces between the shoulder girdle, lumbar spine, pelvic girdle and lower extremity.

The Middle Layer of the Thoracolumbar Fascia: It is attached to the lumbar transverse processes and separates the deeper lumbar portion of the erector spinae muscle from quadratus lumborum muscles. It consists of tendinous fibers of the transverse abdominis. Between the transverse processes these tendons interlace to form the middle layer of thoracolumbar fascia.

The Anterior Layer of the Thoracolumbar Fascia: It is the thinnest layer of the thoracolumbar fascia which covers the anterior surface of the quadratus lumborum muscle and is formed by the deep fascia of this muscle.

The tension in fascia is created as a result of contraction of the muscles, which is within the fascial envelop. The increase in fascial tension results in stiffening of the spinal column which contributes to the stability of the spinal column. The coordinated contraction of the diaphragm, the transverse abdominis and pelvic floor muscle increases the stiffness (stability) of the spine by increasing intra-abdominal pressure.

There is a functional relationship between the shoulder girdle, abdominal musculature and the lateral raphe of the thoracolumbar fascia. There is continuation of the abdominal fascia with the thoracolumbar fascia. It is therefore, easy to visualize that abdominal or the oblique ventral muscle tendon sling has an impact on the function or tension of the thoracolumbar fascia and vice versa. The pectoral apponeurosis of the abdominal muscles often cross the midline to blend with the abdominal fascia on the opposite side and the superficial aspect of the rectus sheath.

ASSESSMENT

For an effective management of low back pain, assessment remains cornerstone of the clinical practice. It includes subjective and objective examination, provisional diagnosis and intervention.

General Information

The purpose of the medical practice is to relieve suffering. The first responsibility of the clinician is to understand the patient's problem irrespective of his or her religion. During the general information the clinician obtains the following information from the patient:

1. Age.
2. Sex.
3. Occupation.

4. Height : Weight ratio.

5. Reaction to stress and pain.

Consideration of Age: The prevalence of the certain conditions are at the certain ages. The disc degeneration starts at around age of 40 years, while onset of ankylosing spondylitis is before the age of 40 years. The patient over the age of 50 years presents with low back pain may be considered for the malignant disease, while, the patient below the age of 25-30 years with low back pain is considered for the mechanical or traumatic such as dysfunction at the intervertebral disc, apophyseal joints, ligaments, postural problems and malalignment and ruled out for the degenerative disease.

Sex: While obtaining general information, clinician must consider the sex of the patient. The prevalence of ankylosing spondylitis is higher in the males than females. If a female presents with a low back pain they may be considered for dysmenorrhoea, urinary and pelvic infection etc.

Occupation: People involved in the activities such as lifting and carrying objects may have dysfunction of the intervertebral disc, facet (apophyseal) joints etc., the prolong shortening of muscles and ligament to the concavity side and lengthening of the muscles and ligaments to the convexity side.

Subjective Examination

During subjective examination the examiner gathers information from the patient by asking questions such as: What is the problem? When it started? How it started? etc. The information collected during the subjective examinations depends on a greater extent by the quality of communication between the examiner and patient. Therefore, the examiner should establish a pleasant relationship with the patient to get an accurate information from the patient. Attempts are made to gather accurate information from the patient so that these may give clues in making the diagnosis and scheme of management. The examiner should ask the relevant questions. Every question need'nt be asked otherwise the patient will get irritated and may distort the information. The subjective examination involves following:

A.
 a. Chief complaint.
 b. Onset of complaint (Signs and symptoms).
 c. Mechanism of injury.
 d. Duration of symptoms (complaint).
 e. Area of symptoms.
 f. Nature and quality of pain and symptoms.
 g. Severity or intensity of the pain and symptoms.
 h. Depth of pain and symptoms.
 i. Irritability.
 j. Behavior of pain and symptoms.
 k. History
  – Previous history of treatment for pain and symptoms.
  – Past medical history including history of surgery, if any.

B. Observation of:
 i. Posture from all three planes.
 ii. Movement (active).
 iii. Swelling, redness, erythema and muscle atrophy.
 iv. Deformity.
 v. Gait.

Onset of Symptoms: The pain and other symptoms may start with gradual or sudden onset. Symptoms start with gradual onset indicates an active pathology such as infection or inflammation if they do not subside with the rest. The mechanical back pain such as disc degeneration and faulty posture has the gradual onset but they respond to the rest and heat modalities. The symptoms start with sudden onset speaks about traumatic lesion, and there is probability of the injury to the ligaments, intervertebral disc, apophyseal joints or muscle tear/rupture etc.

Mechanism of Injury: The patient explains how the injury took place. If patient is able to reveal the exact mechanism of injury, the clinician/examiner can reach to the exact site/structure level. Following mechanisms of injury are mentioned as under:

Forward bending and lifting the heavy weight: During forward flexion the line of gravity falls anterior to the midline which increases the extension moment arm, and requires more muscle work to stabilize the spine and lift the object. Initially the individual tries but fails to generate that much force in the midway, resulting tear of the muscles and posterior static stabilizers, that enables the intervertebral disc to prolapse posterior, and causes dysfunction at the facet joints.

Chief complaint or why has the patient referred for the treatment?

a. Pain.
b. Stiffness.
c. Giving way.
d. Instability.
e. Weakness.
f. Loss of function.
g. After:
   i. Trauma.
   ii. Surgery.
   iii. Manipulation under anesthesia (MUA).
h. Differential diagnosis.

Area of Symptoms: It is useful to record the area of the pain by using a body chart, because this helps in a quick visual reference. The patient may complain of more than one symptoms.

Severity or Intensity of Pain: The patient is asked to indicate according to the description as charted or number which best describes the intensity of their pain, from its least and at its worst.

- Mild.
- Moderate.
- Distressing.
- Horrible.
- Excruciating.

Depth of Pain: The depth of pain may give some indication as to the structure at fault but, like quality of pain, this can be misleading.

Irritability: This is the length of time for which the person has to perform the activity to increase the pain, and conversely how long it takes before the pain settles to its former intensity. It can be measured as high, moderate or low. ***High irritability:*** The aggravating factor causes the pain to increase very quickly or instantly and then the pain takes a long time to settle down. *Moderate irritability:* The aggravating factors take longer to increase the symptoms. *Low irritability:* The aggravating factor can be performed for a long time before exacerbating the patient's symptoms and then as the activity stops, the symptoms subside rapidly.

Behavior of Symptoms

Aggravating and Relieving: The movement or posture that produces or increases the symptoms.

Positional Factors: Most musculoskeletal pain is mechanical in origin and is therefore, made better or worse by adopting particular positions or postures that either stretch or compress the structure that causes pain.

Time Factors: Certain pathologies tend to be more painful at characteristic times of the day, for example, chronic changes are characteristically painful and stiff initially and arising from sleep.

Duration of the Symptoms

Constant: The symptoms persist all the time and there is no relief while rest and during activities. *Example:* In inflammatory/infection conditions the patient complaints pain in the day and night. Sometimes the symptoms are less severe in the day probably due to engagement in the activities.

Intermittent: Any relief in the symptoms even for a few minutes or low. *Example:* Mechanical pain. The patient complains less severe to no pain while resting in a particular position which releases the stress/load on the damaged structure.

History

Previous Treatments: Has the patient received any treatment for this condition in the past, if yes what treatment has been taken? Was it effective? or was the improvement partial or total? *Past Medical History:* Has the patient suffered any major illness? This might affect the tissues and be a contraindication to particular treatments. *Examples:*

i. Respiratory.

ii. Cardiac disease.

iii. Diabetes.

iv. Rheumatoid arthritis.

Is the patient receiving or *received oral* steroid medication? The patients having chronic respiratory diseases, inflammatory bowel diseases or RA, may receive oral steroid therapy. This treatment affects bone and produces tendency towards bruising. Medication used in the past or using for the present condition should also be noted.

Physical Observation: After taking the history next element of lower back pain assessment is careful physical observation of the patient posture. Here the examiner notes down the abnormalities of the posture and restriction in the active range of mention, if any, and the patterns of movements (such as compensatory movement and muscle substitutes to show the maximum results. The best way to find the abnormalities in the posture and movements is to have the normal picture of the posture and movements in the mind (practice to observe the posture and movements on normal subjects) or compare it with the normal. This is known as system review. For an instance the examiner finds the pulse rate of the patient 99 per minute and when it is compared with normal it is termed as tachycardia but if the examiner does not have the normal value in the

mind it cannot be said that it is high. The posture is reviewed (observed) from anterior, lateral and posterior view. During an observation the patient should be undressed. *Observation of the posture from anterior view:* The level of pelvis is viewed as one side of the pelvis is raised in case of scoliosis and leg length discrepancy (Fig. 27.11).

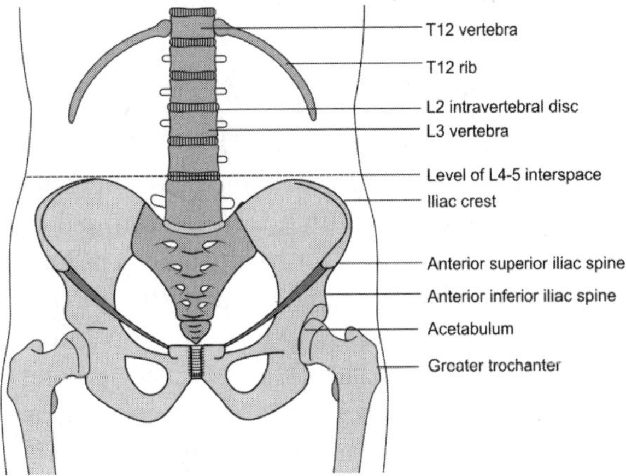

Fig. 27.11: Physical observation from anterior view

Outflare and Inflare from Lateral Side: The abdominals are viewed from this side, weak abdominals can produce hyperlordosis. The curve of the thoracic and cervical may also be viewed as it may change in order to compensate the lumbar spine curve.

Posterior View: Lateral tilling of *pelvis, unequal length of the legs, pelvic up slip and down slip, lumbar lordosis and side flexion (both sides) are observed from this view* (Fig. 27.12).

Observation of the Active Range of Motion: All active movements are observed from anterior, posterior and lateral view.

The lumbopelvic rhythm is the coordinated movement of the lumbar spine and hip during trunk flexion and extension. Ideal lumbopelvic rhythm is such that motion at the lumbar spine should be accompanied by motion of pelvis rotating over the hip. An appropriate rhythm is a lumbar flexion of 30° and anterior pelvic tilt (hip flexion) of 60°.

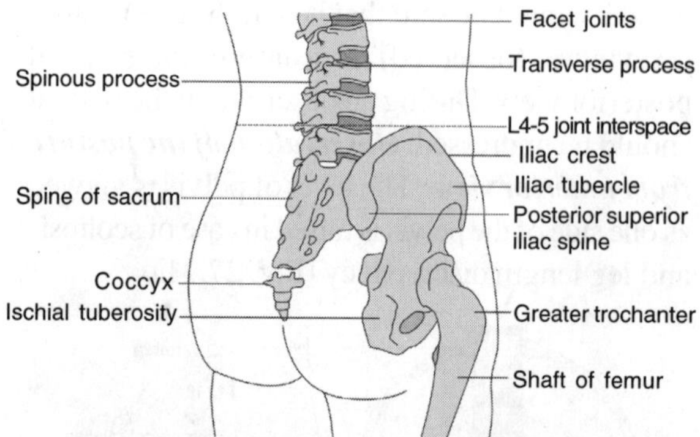

Fig. 27.12 : Observation from lateral view

In forward bending lumbar spine flexes first and when it reaches to its limit (30° flexion) pelvis starts rotating anteriorly on the hip joints. The total lumbopelvic rhythm is approximately 90° flexion of lumbar spine and pelvis on the hip joints (Fig. 27.13a). When the person returns to its erect standing from lumbopelvic flexion, the pelvis starts rotating posteriorly on the hip joints which is followed by extension of the lumbar spine to its neutral position (Fig. 27.13b).

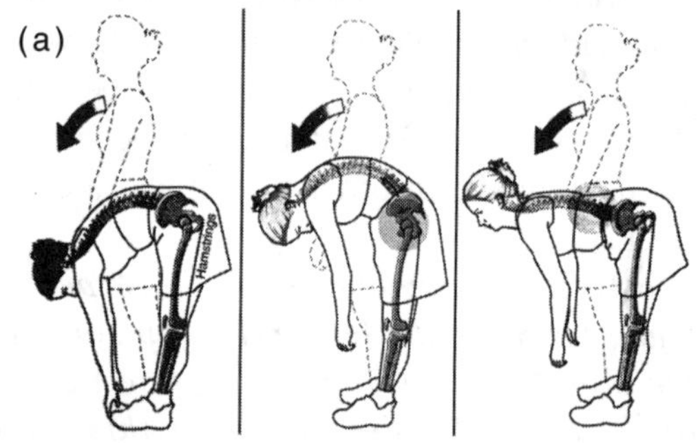

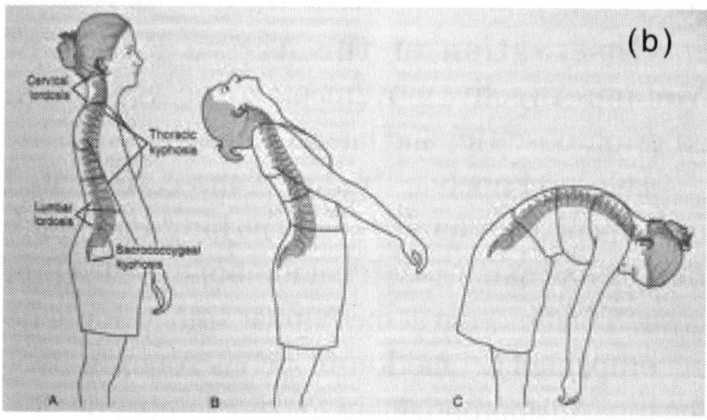

Figs. 27.13a-b: Lumbopelvic rhythm

Several factors such as tight hamstrings, erector spinae and excessive kyphosis can alter the lumbopelvic rhythm.

Observation of the Gait: The gait is observed from anterior, posterior and lateral views. The abnormality in the gait may be due to pain or weakness. The following conditions may alter the gait:

(i) *Prolapsed intervertebral disc with radiculopathy:* The patients will bend the trunk to the opposite side to relieve the pressure on nerve roots. He or she walks with slight hip and knee flexed position with more weight on the toes of the affected side this relieves the tension in the sciatic nerves.

(ii) *Facet block or malaligned:* The patient walks with flexed lumbar spine with slight bending to the opposite side. The spine will be fixed in one position, no significant movement is taken place beyond that position. Overall the patient walks with stiff back to the flexion.

(iii) *Chronic low back pain with lower crossed syndrome:* The hip joints remain slightly in flexed position with anterior tilling of the pelvis and exaggerated lumbar lordosis. Sometimes knees bucking inwards may also be noticed after a short walk.

Objective Examination

Palpation: The examiner should have the knowledge of anatomical structure and surface anatomy area which is being palpated. The lower back region is palpated to determine the level of the lesion and to detect the abnormalities in the bone structure (such as spina bifida and spondylolisthesis) and to establish the nature of the problems. There are two methods of palpation (i) Use of the tips of the thumbs and (ii) Use of the pisiform pad of hand. Which method and when it should be used depends on the area which is being examined. For small and delicate structures, tips of thumb or finger can be used but for larger areas such as glutei and lumbar both methods can be used. If the pressure is not sufficient with the thumb or pisiform pad than the other hand can be used as reinforcement.

The examiner should palpate the structures slowly and carefully starting with light pressure initially and working into high pressure to palpate deep structures. The palpation should start from distal part of the lesions and then progress to the central part so that the examiner has some idea of what to expect. Any difference or abnormality should be noted.

The examiner should be able to:

i.   Determine differences in tissue tension, e.g., effusion, spasm.
ii. Distinguish differences in tissue texture.
iii. Identify shapes, structures and tissue type and thus detects abnormalities.
iv. *Feel variations in temperatures and pulse.*
v.   *Feel tremors and fasciculation.*
vi. *Feel dryness or excessive moisture of the skin.*

The examiner must ensure that the area to be palpated is as develop a clear picture of what released as possible exactly (the structure) being palpated.

The lumbar spine is palpated to determine the:

(i) L_4 and L_5 Level: The patient must be releaxed in prone lying with an adequate exposure of the lumbosacral spine. Therapist stands behind the patient and places the fingers on the top of the iliac crests and thumbs at the same level of the midline of the back which crosses the level of fourth and fifth lumbar disc interspace. After palpating the top of the iliac crests an imaginary line is drawn from top of the left iliac crest to the top of the right iliac crest. The imaginary line where it crosses the lumbar spine is the intervertebral disc space between fourth and fifth vertebrae and the spinous process of fourth lumbar vertebra. After palpating the spinous process of fourth

lumbar vertebra the spinous process of L_3, L_2 and L_1 can be palpated by moving upward (Figs. 27.14 and 27.15).

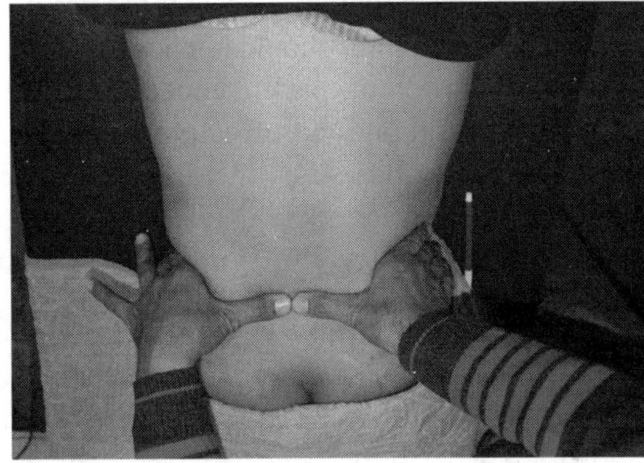

Fig. 27.14: Determination of the L_4/L_5 intervertebral space

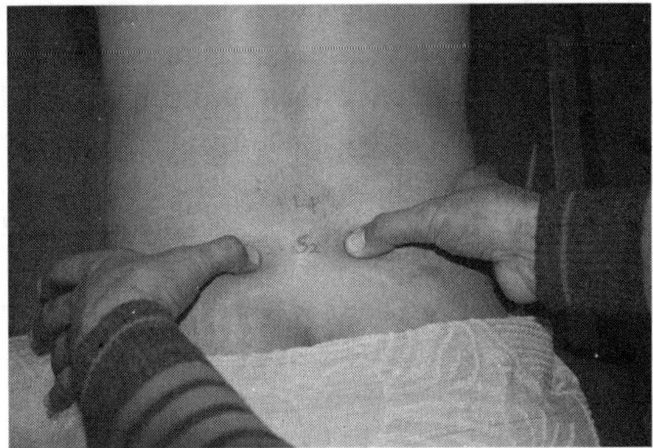

Fig. 27.15: Determining posterior superior iliac spine and S_2 level

(ii) Posterior Superior Iliac Spine and S_2 Level: Moving down from the top of the iliac crest, two depressions can be observed, these are the posterior superior iliac spines. When these are connected with an imaginary line, the line where it crosses the spine is considered as the second sacral verterbra. The other sacral vertebra can also be palpated by moving up and down of the second sacral vertebra.

Special Tests

The therapist must interpret the data collected during the history and subjective examination.

Based on the interpretation of the data it should be decided by the therapist which test and when it should be performed. The tests are performed to reproduce the symptoms. Tests those are not related to the symptoms should not be performed as it may discomfort the patient unnecessarily. A proper history taking and effective subjective assessment will allow the therapist to move forward to the exact special tests needed to perform to reproduce the symptoms and to confirm the diagnosis.

Quadrant Test: It is a useful compressive provocation test designed to determine if the origin of the pain is truly in the lumbar spine. The test should be performed when patient has no radicular symptoms but localized in the lumbar spine and active and passive movements fail to reproduce the symptoms. The quadrant test places greater stress on the articular pillars of the apophyseal joints, the posterior and lateral wall of the disc and posterior longitudinal ligament.

The patient stands comfortably and therapist behind the patient and places both hands on the shoulders of the patient. The therapist must ensure that the patient should not bend the knees throughout the procedure.

Procedure: The test is performed in three steps: (Figs. 27.16a-c)

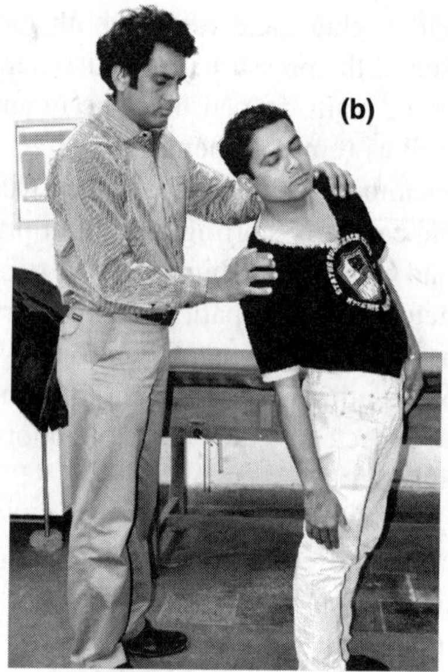

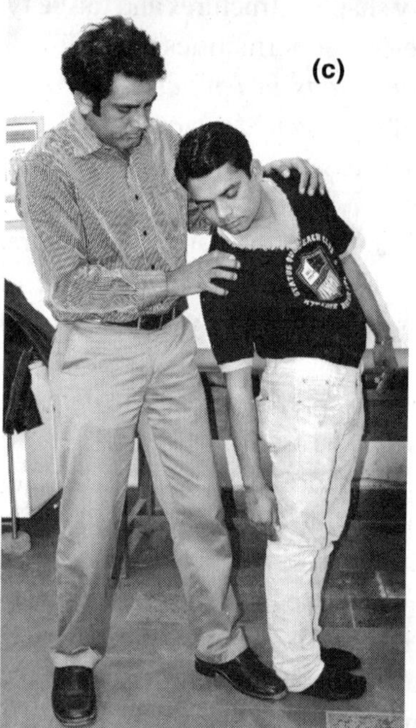

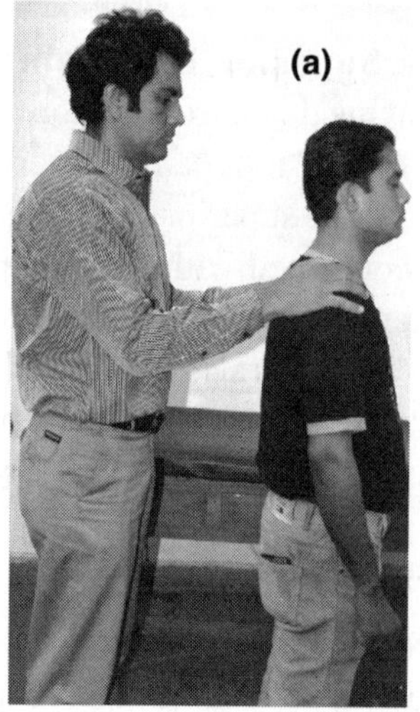

Figs. 27.16a-c: Quadrant test

1. While keeping the hands on the patient's shoulders, the therapist instructs the patient to extend the lumbar spine to its limit and applies over pressure by the hands.
2. The lumbar spine is bent (side flexed) to the affected side (painful side).

3. The last step is to rotate the lumbar spine to the painful side.

These three movements–extension, side flexion and rotation which place greater stress on the posterolateral part of the facet joint, intervertebral disc, and posterior longitudinal ligament are held at least for 20 seconds to allow for a delayed response. If patient complains pain then the test is considered to be positive and indicates involvement of the forementioned three structures.

Slump Test: It is a provocative test performed on the patient who has pain in the lumbar spine with or without leg pain, especially if leg pain includes posterior thigh pain. The test is designed to put the tension on sciatic nerve.

The patient is positioned in high sitting and therapist stands at the side of the patient which is being examined. The test is performed in five steps (Figs. 27.17a-e).

i. The patient slumps forward without excessively flexing the trunk. The test is negated by excessive flexion of the back from the lumbar area.

ii. The patient now places the chin on the sternum.

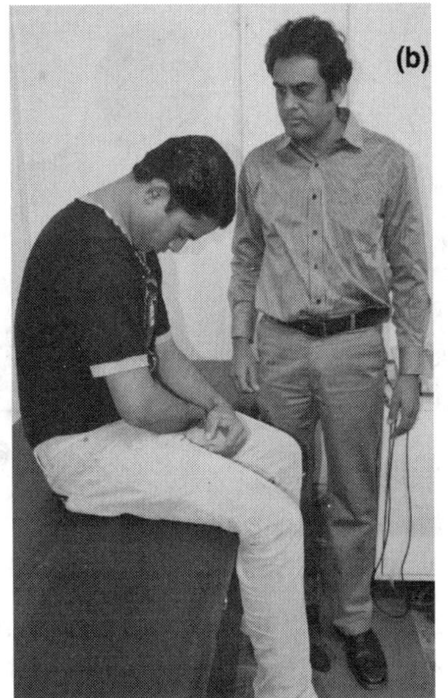

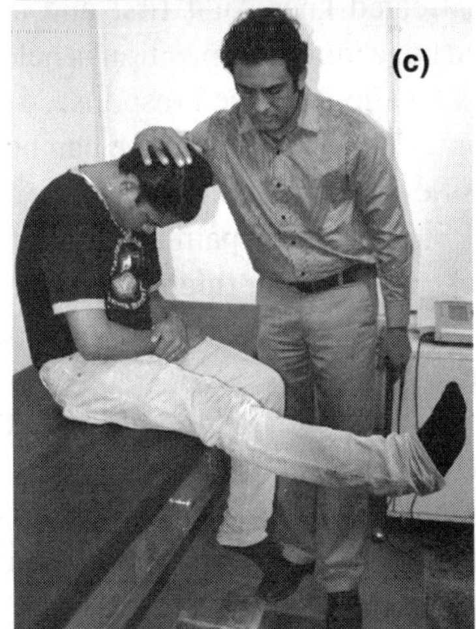

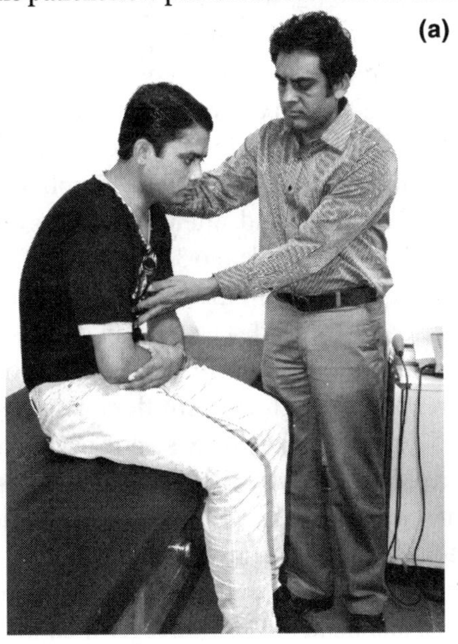

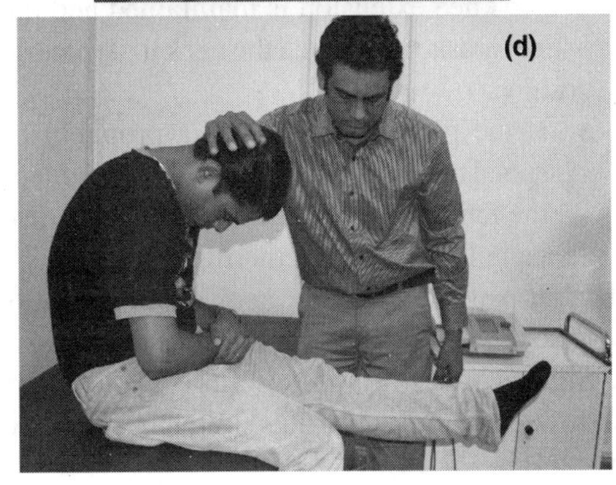

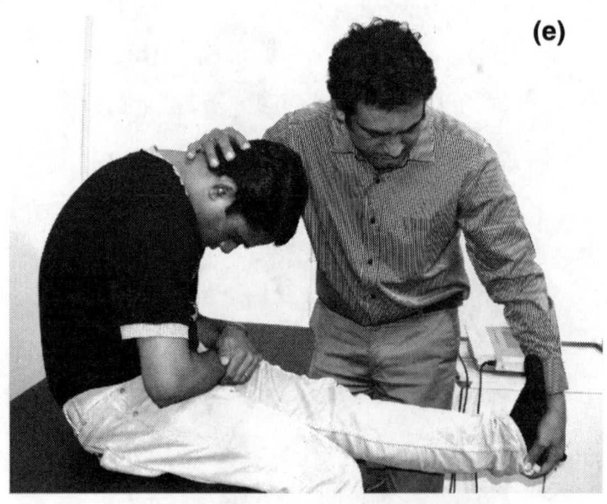

(e)

Fig. 27.17a-e: Slump test

iii. While maintaining the slump position and neck forward flexion, the patient is asked to extend the unaffected knee joint first and then the affected knee joint. The position is held for 20 seconds to allow delayed response.

iv. Further tension in sciatic nerve can be added by dorsiflexion of the ankle joint of the affected side, if it reproduces pain and symptoms in the back and posterior thigh, it may be due to sciatic nerve stretching or due to hamstrings tightness.

v. Passive dorsiflexion is also added to the last step. If it aggravates the symptoms in the posterior thigh and back, this further confirms, sciatic nerve root compression (sciatica).

To rule out the hamstrings pain from sciatic origin, knee extension is maintained and the patient is asked to extend the neck to its neutral position.

  a. If the pain disappears it is probably of spinal origin as the neck extension reduces the tension in the dura and indicates disc pathology or dura tethering (sciatica).

  b. If pain persist (after neck extension) it is due to hamstrings tightness.

Significance: It is the useful screening test for differentiating hamstrings stretch from sciatic stretch (Fig. 27.18).

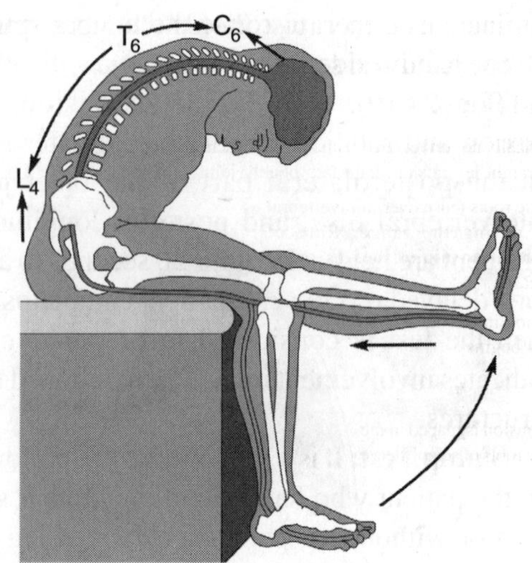

Fig. 27.18

The Straight Leg Raising (SLR) Test

The straight leg raising test is designed specially to put the tension in the sciatic nerve and dura to reproduce the symptoms. Initially it was performed only by raising the legs but now it is modified and dorsiflexion and neck flexion added to it (similar to slumps test).

SLR is a sciatic nerve stretching test performed by the therapist passively by raising the leg with knee extension. During the procedure the patient is asked to relax the quadriceps and not to raise the leg actively. As the test is designed to increase the tension in the sciatic nerve it is considered negative or normal if the patient complains pain before 30 degrees and after 75 degrees of hip flexion. This is because upto 30 degree hip flexion, no tension increases in the sciatic nerve and the nerve remains relaxed. The tension in the sciatic nerve starts increasing after 30 degree of hip flexion upto 75 degree of hip flexion and again after 75 degree tension in the sciatic nerve cannot be increased therefore SLR is considered positive only if the patient's symptoms are reproduced between 30 and 75 degrees.

Procedure: The patient lies in supine and therapist stands at side of the leg which is being examined. The therapist holds the leg at ankle with one hand and stabilizes the pelvic with other hand (Fig. 27.19).

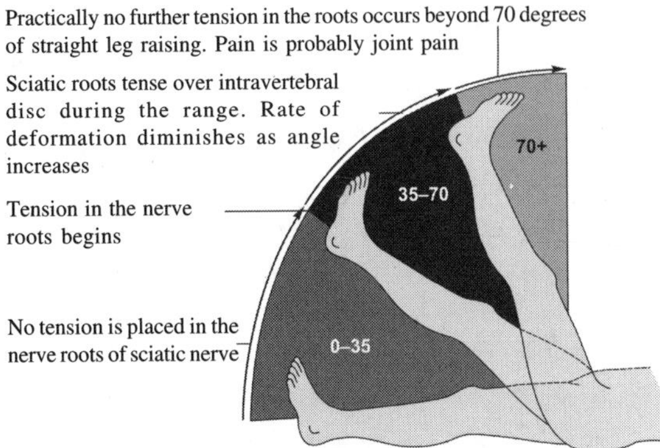

Fig. 27.19: The straight leg raising (SLR) test

The patient is instructed to relax the quadriceps and allow the therapist to raise the leg. The patellar movements can be checked by the stabilizing hand, if patella moves free then it is considered that the quadriceps muscles are relaxed. The therapist raises the leg gradually and notices the range where patient's symptoms aggravate. For example the pain and symptoms are aggravated at 60 degrees then the test is considered to be positive at 60 degrees.

For further confirmation the hip joint range is maintained at 60 degrees and sudden passive dorsiflexion is added to the SLR. If the dorsiflexion aggravates the symptoms, it further confirms the sciatic nerve pain. This is also known as Lasegue's test (adding dorsiflexion to SLR). If the passive dorsiflexion does not increase the posterior thigh pain symptoms then the pain is likely due to hamstrings tightness. Further tension in the sciatic nerve and dura can also be increased with neck flexion (Figs. 27.20a-d).

Significance: The test is an excellent sign of dural and irritation by lumbar disc protrusion. The test places a varying degree of tension on each of the lumbar spinal nerve roots in the dural sleaves from L_4 to S_2 but specially on S_1 nerve root.

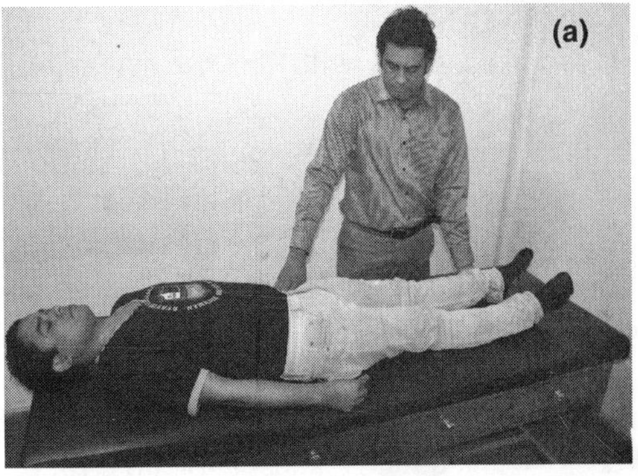
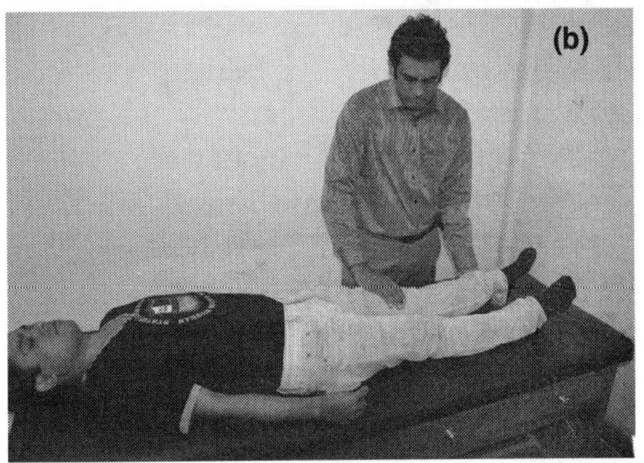
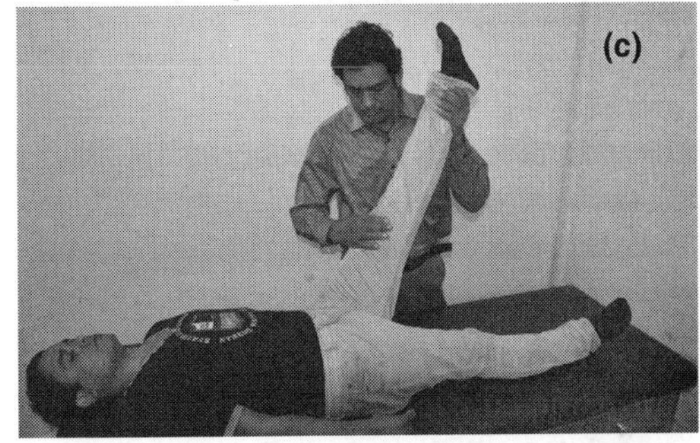
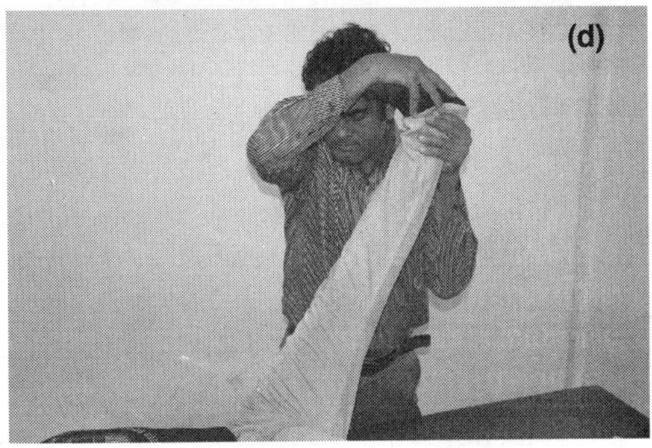

Figs. 27.20a-d: SLR, Lasegue's test

Crossover Sign or Cross SLR: The normal leg is raised passively with the knee extension. If the patient complains of radicular pain and symptoms on the contralateral leg it is known as crossover sign. This is present in patients with large soft disc protrusion. If the crossover sign is positive, it indicates surgical intervention as a choice of treatment.

Quick Tests: The tests are performed to examine the L_5 and S_1 nerve roots. The patient is asked to walk quickly and efficiently for 2-3 minutes.

a. *Walking on Heels:* The patient is asked to walk quickly and efficiently for 2-5 minutes on the heels. If patient cannot walk and drops the fore foot then the involvement of L_5 nerve root may be considered.

b. *Walking on Toes:* The patient is asked to walk on the toes as much quick as possible for 2-3 minutes. Inability of walking on toes indicates weakness of the gastrosoleus and compression on the S_1 nerve root.

Deep Tendon Reflexes

The deep tendon reflexes are performed to test the integrity of the nerve roots.

a. **Patellar Tendon Jerk:** The patellar tendon jerk is elicited to test the integrity of the L_3 nerve root. The L_3 and L_4 nerve roots supply the quadriceps muscles. The lower part including patellar tendon is supplied by L_3 nerve root. Compression on the L_3 nerve root can diminish the patellar tendon. The patellar tendon jerk/reflex will be absent if the motor nerve severely compressed. To test the patellar tendon reflexes the patient lies in high sitting position. The patient should look straight and not at the knee joint. The therapist stands at the side of the knee joint. The patellar tendon (between patella and tibial tuberosity) is felt. Therapist holds the percussion hummer with the right hand in loose grasp and strikes the

patellar tendon. The movement should take place in the wrist joint only. Both sides of the patellar jerks can be tested without changing the position (therapist). Some patients do not relax the quadriceps muscles and the results vary. These patients should be kept busy in talking or asked to clench their teeth or grasp the hands to divert the attention to allow the muscle to relax. The therapist should deceive the patient and strike the tendon to get exact results. This is known as Jendrasik maneuvre (Fig. 27.21).

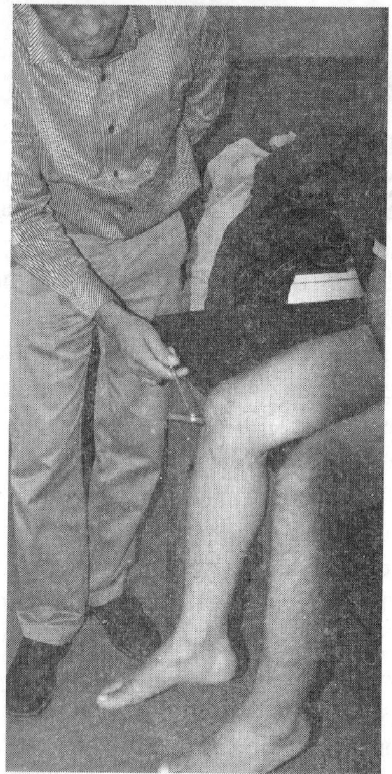

Fig. 27.21: Patellar tendon reflexes

b. **Ankle Jerk:** To test the integrity of the S_1 nerve root, the ankle jerk is tested.

Position of Patient: High sitting or prone with knee flexion upto 30°–40°.

Position of Therapist: Stands at the side of the patient, places left hand under the leg. Achilles tendon is palpated and then strike with the hammer with right hand. The therapist can test both side of Achilles tendons without changing the position and compare with the normal (Fig. 27.22).

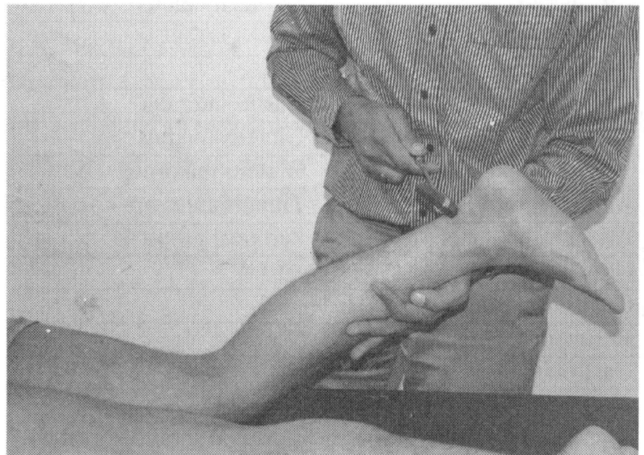

Fig. 27.22: Ankle jerk

POSTURAL PAIN

Pathology, poor workstation and injury can produce pain in the lower back region. The patient finds the compensatory movements or positions that reduce the pain. The compensation or adaptations lead to systemic and predictable patterns of muscular imbalance. The primary muscles responsible for specific joint movement may become weak or inhibited causing synergistic muscles to become hyperactive. The antagonistic group of muscles loses their flexibility and become tight.

The central nervous system regulates tonic and phasic muscle groups which oppose each other in action. The tonic muscle group functions as a facilitator while the phasic muscle groups work as inhibitor. The tonic muscles are also known as postural, have primary function to maintain upright (trunk) posture and the phasic muscles are responsible for rapid motions. Due to segmental dysfunction, pain and malalignment, the postural muscles become tight whereas, the phasic muscles have tendency to go into lengthened state, resulting in muscular imbalance, which eventually causes chronic pain and disability.

This situation alters the cooperative harmonious relationship between muscles and fascia leading to imbalance and articular compensation which further contributes to the change in movement patterns. The altered movement pattern is a movement pattern in which a change occurs in the coordination of the muscle firing sequences for a specific group of muscles facilitating a specific joint movement. *As a result of abnormal physiologic movements, motion patterns involving the fascial planes is altered, i.e., the paravertebral fascia of the cervical spine continues with the thoracolumbar fascia and is affected by its abnormal function. It means that cervical spine aberrant coupling patterns may be a function of abnormal thoracolumbar fascia loading.*

If the posture is not corrected in the initial stage the patient will continue to adapt the most suitable posture which will ease the symptoms and gradually develop a typical abnormal posture known as lower crossed syndrome.

LOWER CROSSED SYNDROME

Lower crossed syndrome is a postural distortion syndrome affecting the lower kinetic chain (lumbopelvic, hip complex, knee and ankle). The patient usually presents with anterior pelvic tilt, increased lumbar lordosis (sway back) and flexed hip joints. There is stress on the L_5-S_1 vertebral segment which produces pain and discomfort in the lumbar spine. This progresses to instability of the sacroiliac joints with increased lumbosacral angle, knee pain (anterior) and piriformis tightness (Figs. 27.23a-b).

Tonic Muscles: These types of muscles contain slow twitch type I fibers, a_2 motor neuron, high capillary density and high number of spindles. These fibers show slow fatigability and have tendency to become shorten due to dysfunction. These are involved in oxidative metabolism.

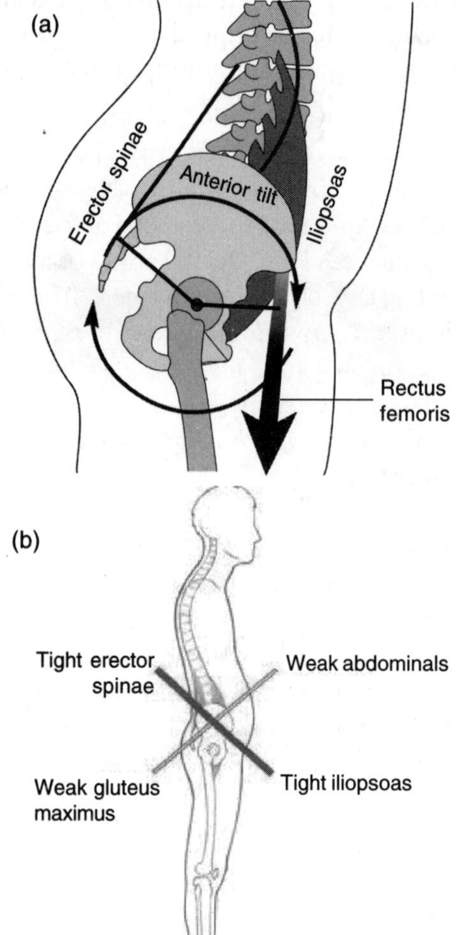

Figs. 27.23a-b: Lower crossed syndrome

Table 27.2: Lower crossed syndrome

Tight or facilitated muscles	Weak or inhibited muscles
Iliopsoas	Rectus abdominis oblique
Rectus femoris	Gluteus maximus
Tensor fascia lata	Gluteus medius
Adductor group	Hamstrings
Erector spinae	
Gastrocnemius	

Phasic Muscles: These are fast-twitch type II fibers, contain a_1 motor neuron, low capillary density and less number of spindles. These fibers show fast fatigability and have tendency to become weak due to dysfunction. These muscles involved in glycolytic metabolism.

Table 27.3: Tonic and phasic muscles

Tonic muscles	Phasic muscles
Lower extremity/pelvic area	Lower extremity/pelvic area
Biceps femoris	Vastus medialis
Semitendinosus	
Semimembranosus	
Iliopsoas	Vastus lateralis
Rectus femoris	Gluteus medius
Tensor fascia lata	Gluteus maximus
Adductor bravis	Tibialis anterior
Adductor magnus	Peroneal group
Gracilis	
Quadriceps femoris	
Adductor longus	
Gastrocnemius	
Soleus	
Trunk and shoulder girdle	Trunk and shoulder girdle
Cervical and lumbar erectors	Rhomboid muscles
Quadratus lumborum	Trapezius (ascending portion)
Scalene muscles	
Pectoralis major	Trapezius (horizontal portion)
Levator scapulae	
Trapezius (descending portion)	Pectoralis major (sternal portion)
Biceps brachii (short and long head)	Triceps brachii
	Thoracic erectors

SCIATICA

Sciatica is a symptom not a disease and is usually describes any painful condition along the course of the sciatic nerve. It may either be neuralgic or neuritis. **Neuralgic sciatica** is due to an external pressure on the nerve usually before it leaves the pelvis, as from a spinal cord tumor that exerts pressure within a canal, or metastatic tumors (that press the root, plexus or trunk), osteoarthritic spondylosis of the lumbar spine, prolapse intervertebral disc, and sacroiliac strain etc. **Neuritis Sciatica:** It is an inflammation of the sheath or connective tissue surrounding the axons themselves. Sciatic neuritis may be due to generalized toxaemia, from alcoholism or lead or arsenic poisoning, or it may be a result of systemic diseases, such as diabetes or syphilis. It is most commonly an interstitial neuritis, but in some cases the inflammation may spread to the axons, and set up a parenchymatous neuritis.

PROLAPSE INTERVERTEBRAL (SOFT) DISC (PIVD) SCIATICA

A prolapsed intervertebral disc or a disc protrusion is a herniation of the nucleus pulposus posteriorly or posterolaterally or centrally through the annulus fibrosus. This may occur at any level of the spine but most often it occurs at the lumbar spine L_4 and L_5 levels usually in young adult life.

Patho-mechanics: When an individual lifts a heavy object with forward flexion, excessive pressure is generated in intervertebral space. The center of gravity falls anteriorly, requires more muscle work from the extensors. If the load which is being lifted exceeds the force generated by the muscles, the muscles get strained which in turn transfers load to the posterior longitudinal ligament. The posterior vertebral segment opens excessively which allows nucleus pulposus to prolapse through the annulus fibrosus. The anterior part is compressed and the posterior part opens out. This tends to squeeze the nucleus pulposus posteriorly or posterolaterally. With or without undue stress the herniation may enlarge and impinge on a nerve root, thus producing symptoms and signs such as tingling sensation, numbness and weakness along the nerve root known as acute radiculopathy. The compressed nerve root becomes edematous, enlarged and often adherent to the protrusion. The extruded material from a ruptured disc appears to be more prone to irritate the tissue and set up an inflammatory reaction, with edema. There is increased redness on the dural sheath as well as on the epineurium.

Stages of Disc Protrusion

The disc may prolapse from mild to severe degree which is described in five stages:

1. **Protrusion:** Initial distention of the annulus occurs with posterior displacement of the nucleus, causing protrusion of the intervertebral disc (Figs. 27.24a-d).

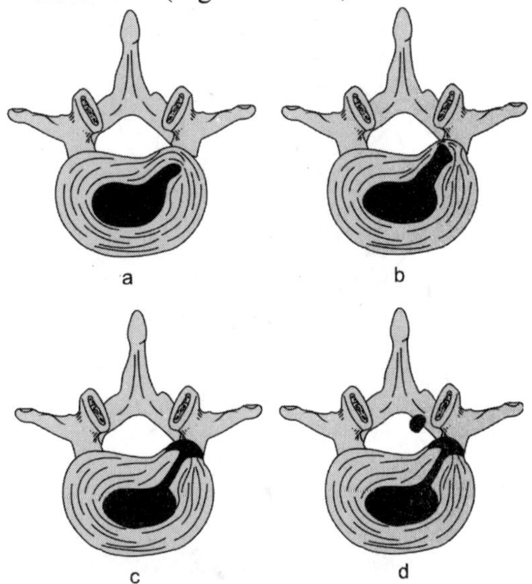

Figs. 27.24a-d: Stages of disc protrusion: a. protrusion, b. prolapse, c. extrusion, d. sequestrum

2. **Dehydration**, desiccation with early degeneration of the disc material.

3. **Herniation or Prolapse:** The radial tear of the annulus allows the nucleus to completely protrude posteriorly within the annulus and rest underneath the longitudinal ligament.

4. **Extrusion:** Subsequent protrusion through the annulus results in an extruded or uncontained disc herniation.

5. **Sequestration:** Eventually, a piece of the nucleus separates and migrates to form a sequestered herniation. The sequestrated disc material through both the annulus and posterior ligament, free to move within the spine .

Symptoms

The chief complaint of the patient is pain either sudden or gradual in onset. It is gnawing or burning and may be continuously present which occur in paroxysms. Pain is often extremely

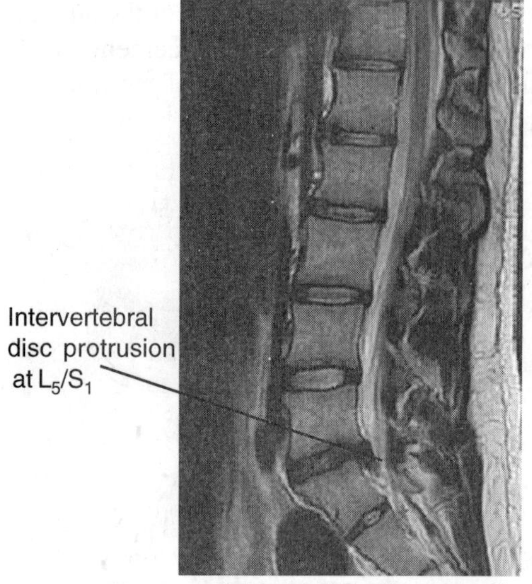

Intervertebral disc protrusion at L_5/S_1

(a) L_5 and S_1 disc protrusion

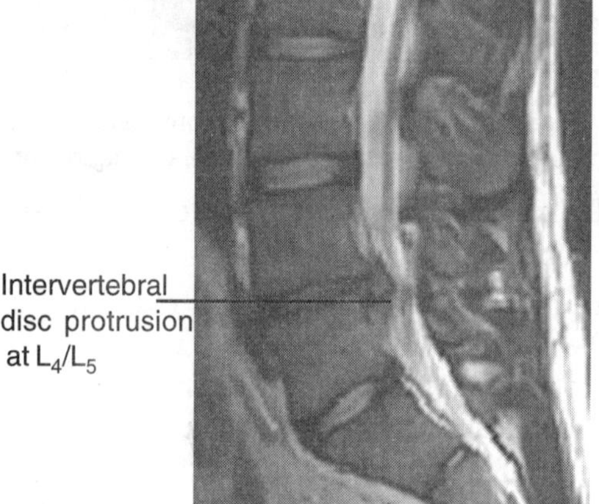

Intervertebral disc protrusion at L_4/L_5

(b) L_4 and L_5 disc prolapse

Figs. 27.25a-b: MRI showing disc prolapse and dural compression

severe especially in the leg and is worsened in any position that causes pressure on the nerve root such as sitting. Pain commences in the lumbar spine and radiates down the buttock, and posterior thigh which may never reach below the knee joint; but it may involve any or all branches of the nerve in its course. Special points of tenderness known as valley's points are found on the nerve and its branches: between the ischial tuberosity and the

greater trochanter, at the center of the posterior aspect of the thigh, just lateral to the middle popliteal space, the middle of the calf and last just behind the medial malleolus. Straight leg raising and Lasegue's sign may be positive in all cases. In severe cases patient walks on the affected side toes with the knee flexion and list is often produced. Muscle atrophy, parasthesia, hyperesthesia, loss of ankle jerk may also be seen.

Clinical Features

Pain: Pain is the most dominant feature which is more in intensity in the thigh and buttock rather than in the lumbar region. It is aggravated in any position which causes pressure on nerve roots such as sitting or which stretches the nerve such as standing on heels with knees straight. Diffuse tenderness may be present.

Gait: With severe symptoms the patients walk on toes with hip and knee flexion to avoid stretching on nerve. This produces a limp, but relieves pain while walking. The pelvis is lifted upon the affected side and a compensatory scoliosis list may develop.

Parasthesia: Parasthesia, most often described as 'pins and needles' is present in one or another in majority of cases, which may be localized by the patients.

Sensation: Some patients have complaints of diminished feeling of sensation partial or complete (rare) and numbness. Loss of other sensations–cold and warmth–although often demonstrable.

Muscle Wasting: Muscles which are innervated by the compressed nerve roots may show some degree of weakness and muscle wasting. For example compression of fifth lumbar nerve root may cause weakness in the extensor hallucis longus (EHL).

Deep Tendon Reflexes (DTRs): Loss of tendon reflex depends upon the severity of nerve root compression. Occasionally, the ankle jerk may totally be absent but even a slight reduction in the response to the threshold stimulus may be of significance.

Posture: The most common change in the lumbar spine is flattening of the lumbar curve, quite frequently noticeable even in relatively mild cases. Very rarely there may be an increase in lumbar lordosis.

Circumduction Test: Forward flexion of spine or circumduction away from the affected side may produce pain. This suggests lateral displacement of the nerve root. Flexion towards affected side does not stretch the root and is a movement of relative ease. A root stretched over the summit of the protrusion would give pain of flexion straight forwards, the more reliably the test indicates sideways displacement of the root. Straight leg raise test (SLR), Lasegue's test, Quadrant test may also be performed.

Sciatica (Disc Herniation) Management

There is a gradual resorption of the herniated disc without surgical intervention. The larger disc herniations were found to have more resorption. This favorable natural history shows why upto 75% of patients with confirmed, painful herniated discs recover without surgery within 6 months. These patients have found to have less recurrence rate than the patients who have managed with surgical intervention.

> **"Cause of the cause":** Unfortunately the sciatic nerve pierces the piriformis muscle in 10 percent population. Spasm and pain in the piriformis muscle is the most commonly associated with lumbar spine, sacroiliac and hip joint pathology. The piriformis muscle stabilizes the pelvis with increased motion in the sacroiliac joints or other forms of pelvic instability. Due to inflammation in the muscle, edema develops in the belly of muscle and passive external rotation will produce pain particularly at the end range as it stretches the tight muscle.

Relief of Pain: Sometimes in cases of insidious-onset, the gluteus medius muscle becomes weak; this may contribute to Trendelenburg gait and exacerbates the problem. After proper muscle testing, if the muscle is found weak it should be strengthened with resisted and closed kinetic chain exercises.

Cryotherapy for duration of at least 20 minutes may allow greater penetration and helps in healing of inflammation particularly in acute symptoms. Moist heat packs, shortwave diathermy, and interferential therapy may be advised to relieve pain and symptoms.

Bed Rest: Rest used to be the choice of the treatment in the past, but recent studies have shown that rest for more than three days has no healing effect but it encourages the muscle wasting. The compressive forces in the intervertebral disc decreases in lying and with the time, the nucleus potentially can absorb more water to equalize pressure. Lying with hip and knee flexion increases the intervertebral space posteriorly which allows accumulation of imbibed fluid in posterior increased space. The accumulated imbibed fluid in the posterior space increases the intradiscal pressure and produces pain and symptoms specially when patient rises from prolong bed rest. This is the reason that absolute bed rest is not recommended.

The Royal College's General Practice Guidelines state that prolong bed rest may lead to debilitation, chronic disability and increasing disability in rehabilitation. Advice to continue ordinary activity can give equivalent or faster symptomatic recovery from the acute attack and lead to less chronic disability and less time work than 'traditional' medical treatment with analgesics as required, advice to rest, and let pain be your guide for return to normal activity. Hence, bed rest should not be recommended for simple back pain.

Seventy-five percent patients with prolapse intervertebral disc resolve spontaneously within

Lateral shift: Lateral shift is the lateral displacement of the trunk and shoulders in relation to the pelvis. Displacement of the trunk and shoulders to the right side is termed as right lateral shift. The lateral shift is most commonly associated with the disc herniation with acute radiculopathy. The patient shifts or bends the trunk and shoulder to the opposite of the radiculopathy. For example the patient with left acute radiculopathy will shift the trunk to the right side to avoid pressure and irritation on the nerve root. Sometimes the muscles may also produce lateral shift.

McKenzie has described a technique to correct the lateral shift. The extension exercise alone cannot correct the lateral shift, therefore, he has described the technique which is followed by spinal extension exercise. The patient stands with the elbow flexion, and therapist stands at the side opposite to the disc herniation. In case of left lateral shift the therapist stands to the right side of the patient. Therapist places his right shoulder under the elbow and wraps the both hands around the top of the opposite pelvis. A force couple is created by pulling the pelvis with both the hands and by pushing the trunk to the midline simultaneously. The purpose of the technique is to centralize the symptoms. In case patient reports improvement in the sign and symptoms the technique should be continued followed by spinal extension exercise.

Self correction of the lateral shift: In standing, in case of right lateral shift the patient places his right hand on the right rib cage and left hand on the top of left illium. Both hands pushes the trunk and pelvis simultaneously to the midline. **In side lying:** The patient lies on the affected side, and a small pillow or towel is placed under the thorax. Patient should remain in this position till the pain centralizes. **In prone lying:** The patient lies on the prone position and therapist creates a force couple in opposite direction and glides the pelvis and thorax towards the midline.

six months. Only 5-10 percent patients with persistent radiculopathy (sciatica) require surgery. These patients have 10 times higher risk of developing subsequent disc herniation compared to the general public.

Ergonomics: The initial prevention of proplapsed intervertebral disc to further progression is the major part of the treatment. The patients with prolapse intervertebral disc are taught all the positions which aggravate and relieve the intradiscal pressure. Patient should be encouraged to use the position which produces least pressure on the intervertebral disc. The below mentioned positions are described in ascending order (lowest disc pressure to highest pressure):

a. *Supine with Knees Flexion and Supported on Pillows (Figs. 27.26a-b):* This position allows the iliopsoas muscles to relax and flattens the lumbar lordosis which decreases pressure on the intervertebral disc. In acute prolapsed intervertebral disc cases this is the choice of position which should be recommended during the bed rest. In supine the load produced by the body weight is eliminated.

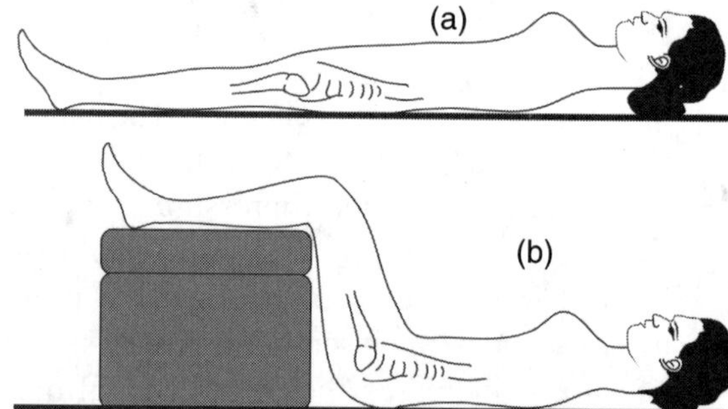

Figs. 27.26a-b: a. Supine with hip and knee at neutral b. Supine with hip and knee flexion supported on stool

b. *Sitting with Back Rest to 90°:* Initially when patient is moved from bed rest to sitting, it should be recommended only if the back rest support of the chair is inclined appropriately. Further placing a pillow under lumbar region reduces the intradiscal pressure. This is the ideal position for the patients with prolapse intervertebral disc who wants to attend office (Fig. 27.27).

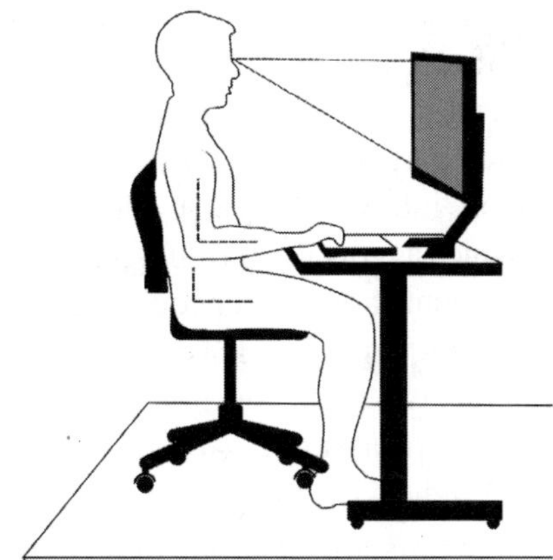

Fig. 27.27: "Ideal sitting" position

c. Standing: Patients with prolapse intervertebral disc can be allowed to stand without any hesitation as this position produces 100% load on the intervertebral disc.

d. Walking: Moderate walking is safe and perhaps ideal therapeutic exercise for those with these patients. If the speed of walking is increased from 90 steps/minute it further can increase the intradiscal pressure, therefore, walking should be advised but the speed should be limited to the normal cadence. The patient should be taught not to bend the trunk forward as it increases intradiscal pressure.

e. Sitting: The patients with prolapse intervertebral disc complain more pain, irritation and burning sensation in erect sitting because it increases the intervertebral disc pressure by 150%. The erect sitting should not be recommended as it may cause further disc prolapse.

f. Forward bending with weight lifting (Fig. 27.28).

Relative change in the pressure/load in the third lumbar disc in different positions in percentage (Figs. 27.29a-b).

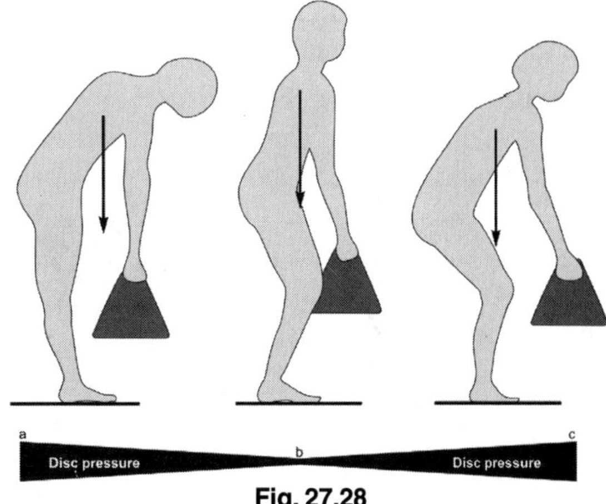

Fig. 27.28

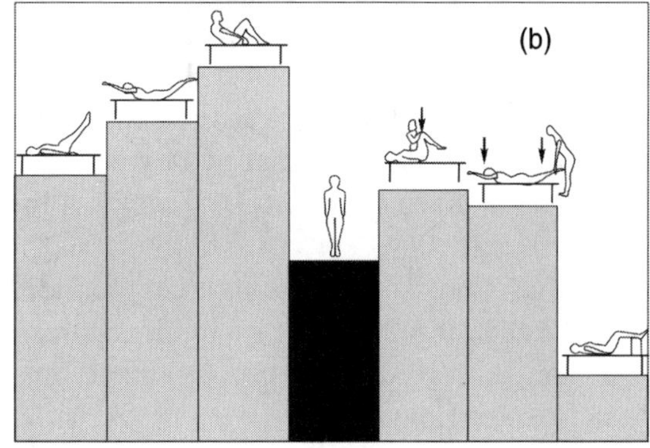

Figs. 27.29a-b

Therapeutic Exercises

As soon as patient finds improvement in the sign and symptoms exercises are started. Initially exercises which produce least pressure on the intervertebral disc should be started. These are progressed according to the improvement in pain and other symptoms of the patient.

Spinal Extension Exercises: In spinal extension the posterior part of the intervertebral space is compressed and the anterior part opens out. This tends to squeeze the nucleus pulposus anteriorly and reduces the protrusion/prolapse in the intervertebral disc posteriorly; for this reason spinal extension exercises are beneficial and safe for the patients with prolapse intervertebral disc. McKenzie has described spinal extension exercises as under:

McKenzie Method: McKenzie approach is not merely extension exercises. In its true sense, it is a comprehensive approach to the spine based on the principles and fundamentals that when understood and followed accordingly are very successful. In fact most remarkable, but least appreciated, is the McKenzie assessment process. Identification for the underlying disorders through objective findings and movements for each individual and then separating them with apparently similar presentations into definable mechanical syndromes is the key of the McKenzie approach. McKenzie has named three mechanical syndromes: Postural, dysfunction and derangement.

- **Postural:** It is the postural problem where patient remains asymptomatic unless and until a stress is given on the extreme range of the movement.

- **Dysfunction:** The symptoms are reproduced at the end range by placing a minimal stress, as the shortened structures ligaments and muscle get elongated.

- **Derangement Syndrome:** It is the anatomical disruption or displacement of the structure within the motion segment. The classical example is prolapse intervertebral disc. McKenzie approach uses the movements of the body to establish a diagnosis and the treatment. In derangement syndrome the

movements are identified which aggravate the symptoms from proximal to distal. According to the approach once these movements are identified they should not be used as treatment tool and avoided very well. On the other hand we identify the movement which can reduce the symptoms from distal to proximal. Such type of movements become the treatment tool and performed repeatedly. Increase in symptoms from proximal to distal is known as peripheralization, whereas, decrease in symptoms from distal to proximal is known as centralization. Movements which centralizes the symptoms are performed repeatedly.

McKenzie approach is based on sound principles and fundamental, for example forward flexion compresses the anterior part of the disc and opens out the posterior part of the disc which allows further prolapse of the disc posteriorly which may increase further pressure on the nerve root, hence, the symptoms aggravate from proximal to distal part and logically this movement should be avoided as it may damage further. On the other hand, extension compresses posterior part of the disc and opens up the anterior part, which plays important role in relieving symptoms from distal to proximal.

(a) ***Prone on Elbows:*** The intradiscal pressure in a prone position with upper body supported on the elbows can be decreased to 50% of the body weight. The exercise may be advised even in acute stage when the patient is on bed rest (Figs. 27.30a-b).

(b) ***Bridging:*** The extension of the lumbar spine in supine position with hip and knee flexed to 60°; has great benefit as it does not produce pressure on the intervertebral disc, instead of it helps in recovering from prolapse.

(c) ***Spinal Extension with Pillows under Abdomen:*** The placement of pillows under the abdomen in prone position can decrease the arch of the back and allows the disc to

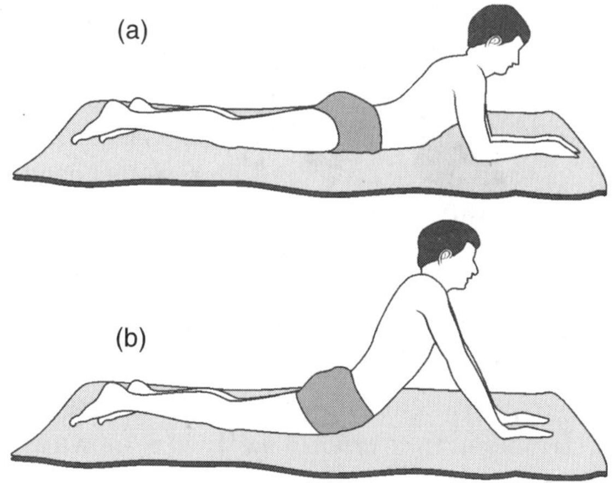

Figs. 27.30a-b

better resist stresses because the vertebrae are aligned with each other. Arching the back in prone position can greatly activate the erector spinae muscles but also produce such high stresses on the lumbar discs, which are loaded in an extreme position. Isometric contraction of erector spinae with pillows under the abdomen is the preferable position (Figs. 27.31a-b).

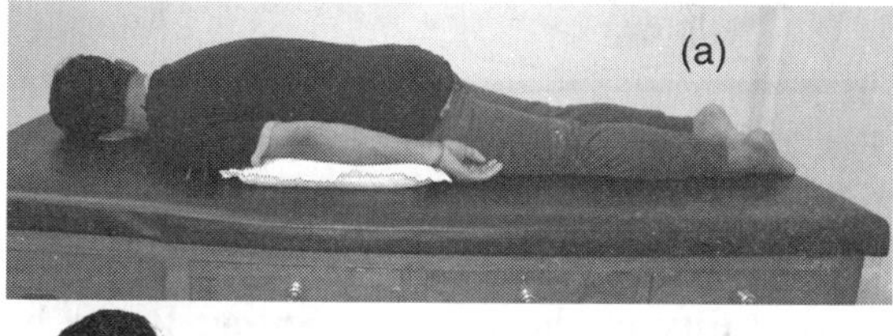

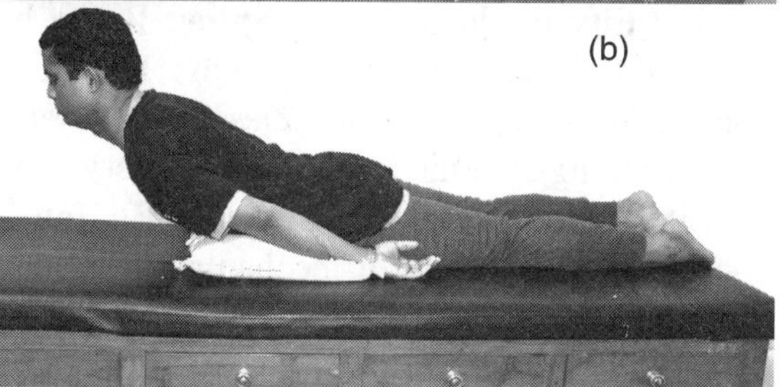

Figs. 27.31a-b: Spinal extension pillow under abdomen (a. starting, b. extension)

(d) Slump to Erect Sitting: Sitting with slight forward flexion with relaxed shoulder girdle is the slump position. When coming back to the erect sitting from slump allows

strengthening of the erector spinae muscles especially upper back extensors.

Spinal Flexion Exercises: The extension exercises are progressed to flexion exercises when patient as soon as patient achieves full range of motion in sagittal plane with minimal pain. These exercises should be progressed from the exercises which produces least intradiscal pressure to the highest intradiscal pressure. Flexion exercises are often advised to provide core stability following spinal extension exercises (Figs. 27.32 and 27.33).

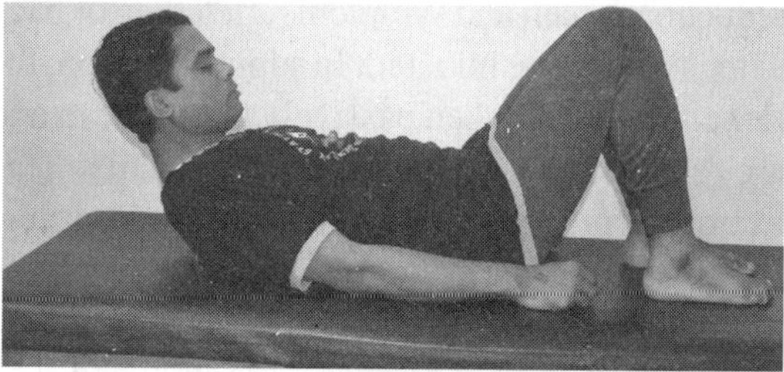

Fig. 27.32: Curl up

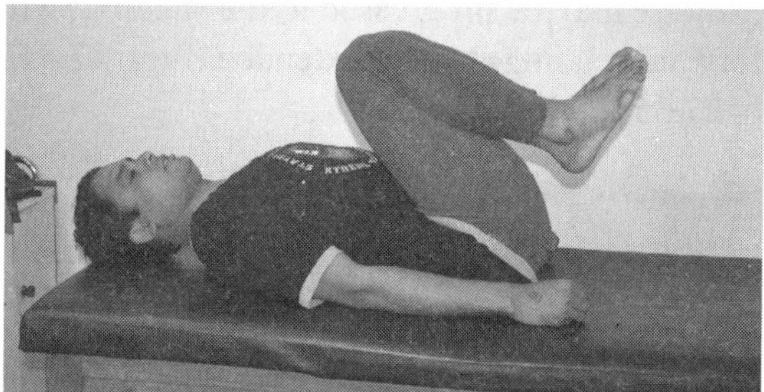

Fig. 27.33: Reverse curl up

(a) Curl up: This exercise is advised to strengthen the upper portion of rectus abdominis and external oblique muscles. In supine position with knees flexed to 90°, the head and shoulders are lifted off the plinth. The load on the lumbar spine remains minimal as the patient is allowed to clear the shoulder blades only minimizing the lumbar motion. A greater movement is produced by raising the arms or placing hands behind the head, as the center of gravity of the upper body shifts farther away.

(b) Twisting Curl up: The patient lies in supine position with one leg flexed to 90° and other

leg (ankle) is placed on top of the flexed knee joint. Patient is asked to lift the head and shoulder off the plinth. Patient places both hands on the occiput and then turns to the opposite side of flexed knee joint.

(c) Reverse Curl up: A reverse curl isometrically performed, provides efficient training/strengthening of the lower abdominals, and produces moderate stresses on the lumbar discs.

Stretching Exercises: After significant reduction in pain and symptoms stretching of back extensors may be initiated. In supine position, the flexed knees are taken passively to the chest, and are repeated at least 25 times, thrice daily. This exercise is progressed to stretching in long sitting. In long sitting the patient is asked to touch the toes with the knees straight. In this position both hamstrings and back extensors are stretched. The exercise may be progressed to the standing with forward bending at knees extended (Figs. 27.34a-b, 27.35 and Fig. 27.36).

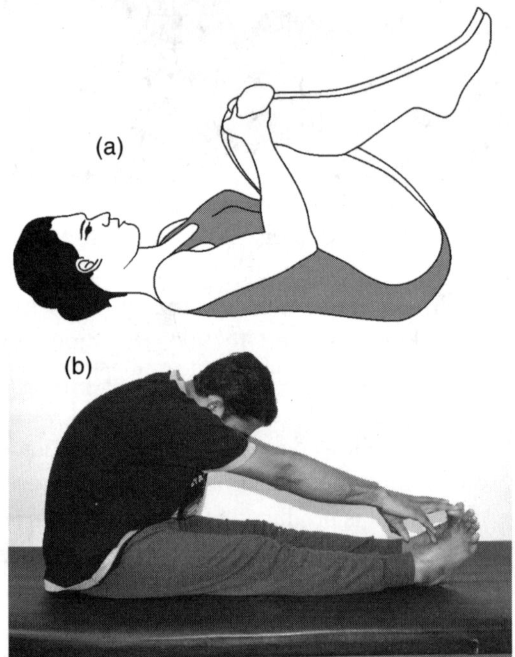

Figs. 27.34a-b: Back extensor stretchings

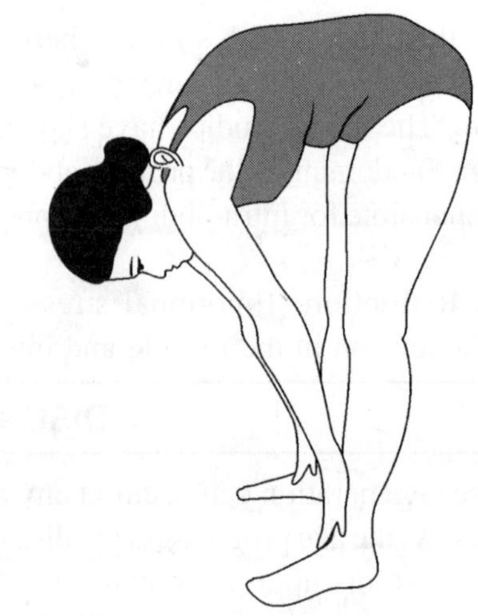

Fig. 27.35: Long sitting with toe touch

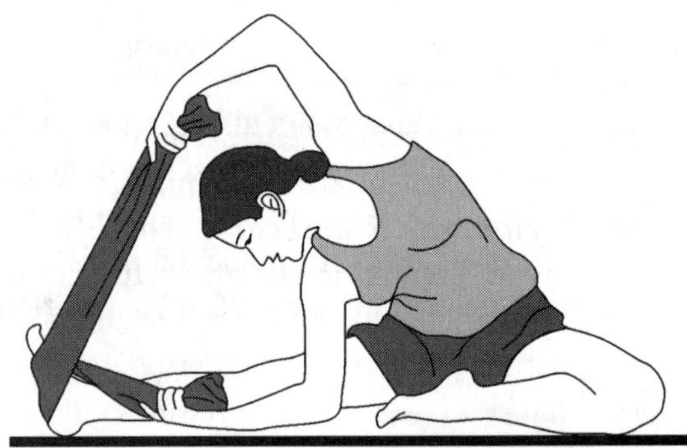

Fig. 27.36: Degenerated disc prolapsed (a) Annulus tear, (b) Circumferential tear, (c) Peripheral tear, (d) Radical tear, (e) Disc prolapsed

Stability of the Lumbar Spine: It can be achieved through several means: IAP, co-contraction of the trunk muscles core muscles strengthening external support and surgery.

Intra-Abdominal Pressure (IAP): Intra-abdominal pressure is a mechanism that may contribute to both unloading and stabilization of the lumbar spine. IAP is the pressure created within the abdominal cavity by a coordinated contraction of the diaphragm, the abdominals and pelvic floor muscles. This creates an extension moment that lies the compression forces on the lumbar spine. The intra-abdominal pressure reduces the load on the intervertebral discs.

Therefore, the patients with soft disc herniation should be encouraged to improve an IAP mechanism. The recent studies have shown that the transverse abdominis is the primary abdominal muscle responsible for intra-abdominal pressure generation.

Stress Reduction: Emotional stresses can increase the tension in the muscle and interfere with or delay the recovery process. Try to eliminate stress as much as possible by placing non-urgent jobs on hold. Obtaining counselling for major life stresses and seeking support from family, friend or health providers.

Adverse Effects of Bed Rest: In lying, intradiscal pressure decreases with time, the nucleus potentially can absorb more water

---

DISC DEGENERATION

Age: Disc degeneration can occur at any age, but it is more common in older discs, usually after forty years. As the age progressess the disc looses its water binding capacity and physical properties. There is a gross disruption of collagenous network (fibers). The disc becomes less resistant to the repeated stresses. In the process of degeneration, there are formation of tears and fissures in the annulus fibrosus and nucleus pulposus respectively.

A. *Annulus Tears:* There are three types of tears often occur in the degenerated annulus of the disc.

   (a) Circumferential Tears: These may represent the effect of interlaminar shear stresses, possibly arising from compressive stress concentration in older discs.

   (b) Peripheral Rim Tears: These are also known as 'rim lesions' consist of focal circumferential avulsions of the peripheral annulus. They are twice as common in the anterior annulus compared to the posterior, and typically affect the upper anterolateral margin of the disc. The peripheral tears may occur due to trauma.

   (c) Radial Fissures: These fissures commences from the nucleus and extends to the posterior or posterolateral. The radial fissures are associated with nucleus degeneration and with disc radial bulging but is not clear which comes first.

B. *Disc Prolapse:* In the process of degeneration there are formation of radial fissures of the annulus which may be associated with degeneration in the nucleus. The gross radial fissures allow the nucleus to migrate posteriorly or posterolaterally to the extent that the disc periphery is affected, then the disc is said to be prolapsed or herniated, which contains primarily the nucleus pulposus displaced down a radial fissure. The disc prolapse may be protrusion, extrusion or sequestration depending on the extent of migration of nucleus.

The degenerative process of disc has been divided into three stages with relatively destine findings:

Stage I: The first stage is dysfunction which is seen before the age of 45 and is characterized by circumferential and radial tears in the disc annulus and localized synovitis of the facet joints.

Stage II: It is the stage of instability which is common in patient between 35 and 70 years age. This stage is characterized by internal disruption of the disc, progressive disc resorption, degeneration of the facet joint with capsular laxity, subluxation and joint erosion.

Stage III: It is the stage of stabilization. The progressive development of hypertrophic bone around the disc and facet joints leads to segmental stiffening.

contents to equalize pressure (imbibition). On the other hand, lying with flexed spine allows the imbibed fluid to accumulate posteriorly in the intervertebral disc where there is greater space. when patient stands, pain and symptoms from a disc protrusion are accentuated, as the accumulated fluid in the disc spaces will increase the intradiscal pressure. Therefore, to avoid exacerbating symptoms absolute bed rest during acute phase should not be advised. Bed rest for 1-2 days may be advised, but it should be interspersed with short intervals of standing.

Extension Exercise Bias: Patients with lumbar disc protrusion are often comfortable and may have partial or full relief with extension of the spine. The patients with extension bias often assume a flexed posture with or without side flexion. The impairment may be due to a contained intervertebral disc lesion, fluid stasis, a flexed injury or a muscle imbalance from a faulty flexed posture.

Therapeutic Modalities: SWD, MWD and moist heat therapy may also be beneficial in reduction of muscle spasm. Moist heat therapy is the most convenient and feasible which may be used at home also. These help in relieving pain and increasing flexibility and range of motion of the lumbar spine. Interferential Therapy at 80-100 Hz (analgesic effect) may also be advised for relieving pain and m uscle spasm.

CORE STABILITY

Core stability is the combination of global and local stability system. The global stability system involves the larger and superficial muscles such as rectus abdominis, paraspinals and obliques. The local stability refers to the deep intrinsic muscles such as the transverse abdominis and multifidus. The global stability system provides mobility whereas local stability system provides segmental stability to the lumbopelvic region. Weakness of the muscles of these systems can grossly cause the loss of stability and mobility of not only the proximal (lumbopelvic) region but also the distal region (extremities). A strengthening of core muscles will *not only prevents injuries* but also improves the performance of the athletes who participate in sports activities.

Core muscles provide stability and mobility mainly to the lumbopelvic joints which involves the intervertebral sacroiliac and hip joints and it also *encompasses the scapulothoracic* junction. The mobility and stability of the lower extremities depend upon the core stability. For example weakness of the abdominals allows the pelvis to rotate anteriorly which causes lightness of the quadriceps and produces anterior knee pain. Anterior knees pain can cause adverse effects on the stability of the knee joint (lower extremity).

Evaluation of the Core Stability

Evaluation of muscles of lumbopelvic region before *commencing strengthening*, should be the prime objective, because it helps in determining the area where the therapist and patient needs to work more. The functional movement screen (FMS) test which *involves stepping, lunging, squatting, striding, reaching, anterior posterior core stability and core stability*, are used in evaluating the core stability.

a. **Biering–Sorenson Extensor Endurance Test:** (Fig. 27.37)

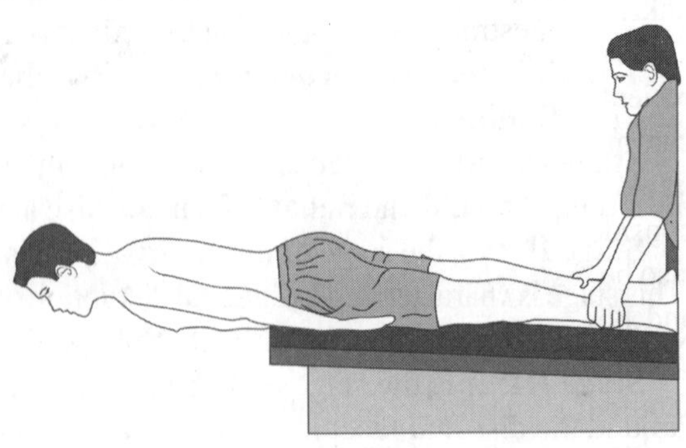

Fig. 27.37: Extensor endurance test

Position of Patient: Prone with trunk off the table.

Position of Therapist: Standing at the side of the feet of the patient, places both the hands on calves.

Procedure: The patient is asked to maintain the upper torso paralleled to the plinth (floor) time is recorded till the patient maintains the position. Once the patient falls below the level of plinth the test is completed and time is recorded.

b. Flexor Endurance Test: (Figs. 27.38a-b)

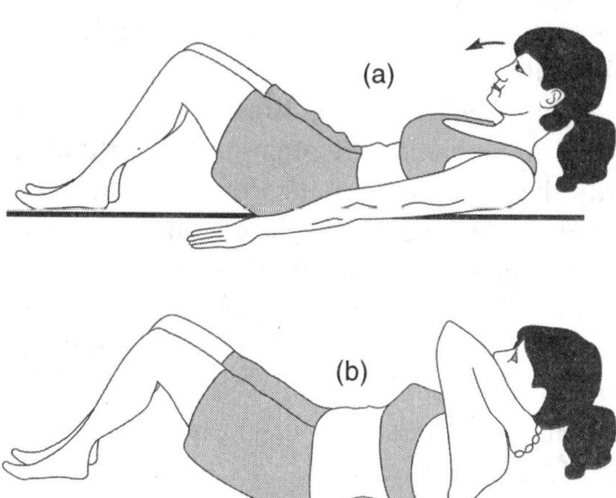

Figs. 27.38a-b

Position of Patient: Sitting inclined with 55° angle. Hands placed on the opposite shoulders. Hips at 30° and knees flexed to 90°.

Position of Therapist: Standing, stabilizes the ankle and legs.

Procedure: The back rest removed and patient is asked to maintain the position. If patient can maintain the position without touching the back to the table (the flexors strength is considered as good). Abdominal endurance can also be tested in supine position with both the hip and knees flexion to 90 degrees. Endurance is considered fair if the subject can lift the head and shoulders ten times with both the hands at side. Endurance may be considered good if the subject

clears the shoulder blades off of the ground ten times with both hands behind the neck.

c. Lateral Endurance Test: (Fig. 27.39)

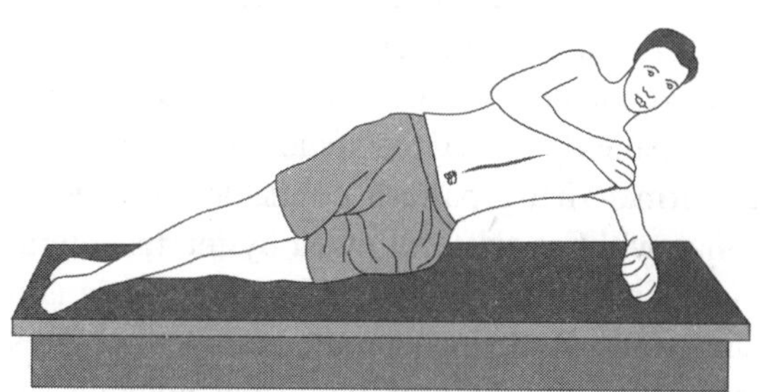

Fig. 27.39: Lateral endurance test

Position of Patient: Side lying. Top foot is placed in front of the bottom foot. The body rests on the elbow. Top hand may be placed on the opposite shoulder.

Procedure: The patient takes the hips off the plinth, so that the body comes in a straight line. The lateral stability is considered poor if the patient finds difficulty in lifting the hips.

d. Normal Firing Pattern of the Pelvis (Fig. 27.40).

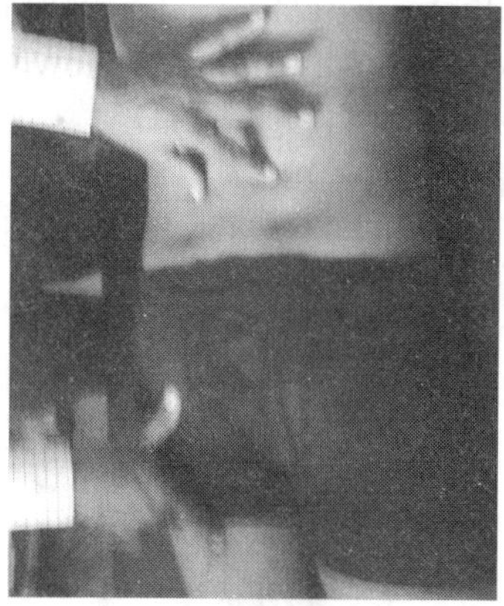

Fig. 27.40

Patient Position: Prone lying with adequate exposure of gluteus maximus and erector spinae muscles.

Therapist Position: Stands at the side, facing the lumbosacral spine. To test the left gluteus maximus therapist stands at the left side, places thumb and index finger of left hand on erector spinae of each side. The right hand thumb is placed on the gluteus maximus and little finger on the hamstrings of the same side.

Procedure: While maintaining the position of hands patient is asked to extend the left hip joint. In normal firing pattern contralateral erector spinae will fire first, followed by the ipsilateral gluteus maximus, ipsilateral erector spinae and hamstrings. If the ipsilateral erector spinae fires before the gluteus maximus this indicates an inhibited gluteus maximus.

[*Normal Firing Pattern:* Contralateral erector spinae, ipsilateral gluteus maximus, ipsilateral erector spinae and hamstrings.]

Inhibited Gluteus Maximus: Contralateral and ipsilateral erector spinae, gluteus maximus and hamstrings.

e. **Overhead Squat Test (Global Assessment Test):** It is the full body functional analysis test which tests the total kinetic chain, neuromuscular efficiency, integrated–functional strength, dynamic flexibility and involves a degree of muscular fatigue, that is why the test is known as global assessment test (Fig. 27.41).

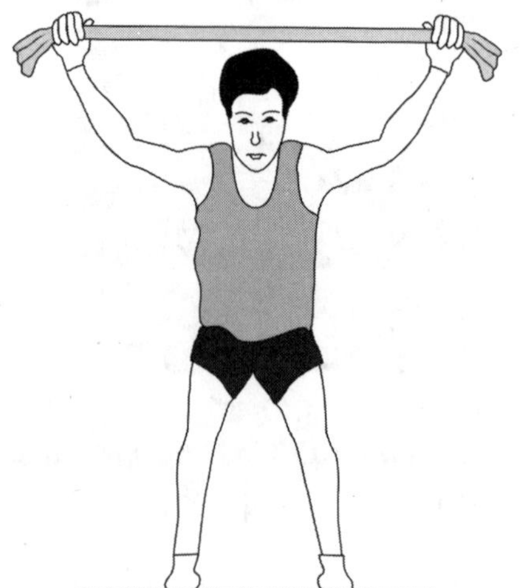

Fig. 27.41: Overhead squat test

Patient Position: Standing with feet and shoulders (shoulders abduction 120) apart.

Therapist Position: Standing behind the patient, walks around during the test. Checks the feet, knees, lumbar curve, arm movement, chin elevation and stomach protrusion.

Procedure: The patient is asked to slowly squat down to a comfortable position for 6-15 repetitions.

Deviations: In case of lower crossed syndrome feet flattened, toes flaring out, knees buckling inward, and low back arching are the common deviations. These may be unilateral or bilateral.

Non-Weight Bearing Bias: The patient with soft disc herniation are often more comfortable with the traction and lying down. Because this relieves the load on the facet joints and also reduces pressure on the nerve roots by reducing the intradiscal pressure. For such patients traction and rest may be the choice of treatment until the patient feels comfortable in weight bearing. The patient is progressed to weight bearing as pain and healing improves.

CORE STRENGTHENING

The core stabilizers are strengthened in different positions. The exercises are progressed from minimal load to maximum load as the symptoms improves. Exercise which exacerbates the symptoms should not be performed.

Crunch or Curl up: Crunch exercises are designed to strengthen the abdominals as strong abdominals can unload the lumbar spine stress. The exercises are started with one knee flexed and other leg remains extended. The head and shoulder blades are lifted off the plinth and the hand position is changed as the crunch exercises progress. Every position is held up to 6 seconds to allow optimal contraction of the abdominals. 10 repetitions of three sets may be performed at a session (Figs.27.42a-e).

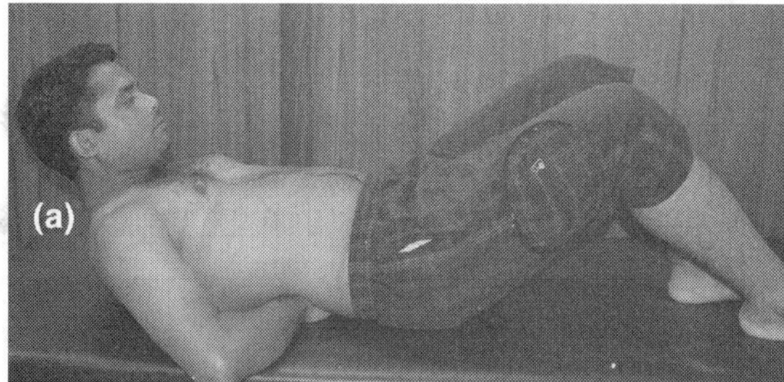

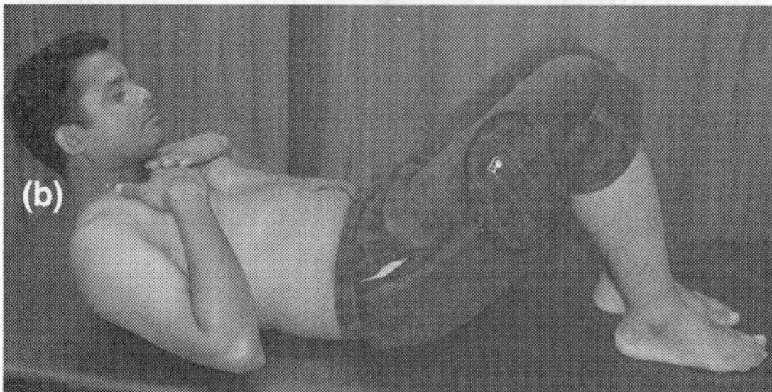

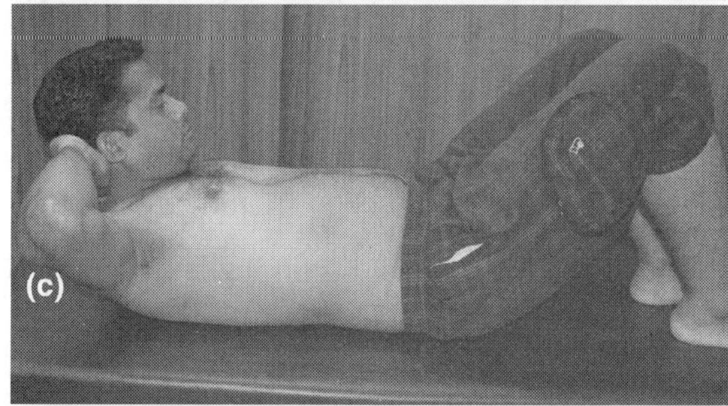

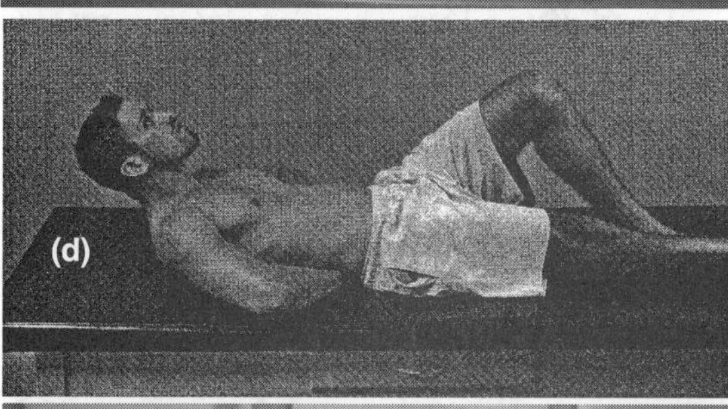

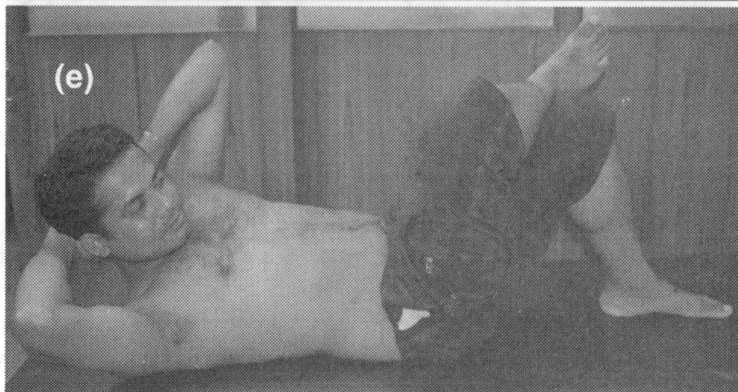

Figs. 27.42a-e: Cural up

a. A supine with one or both legs flexed to 90°. Hands under the lower back region with elbows on the plinth. The head and shoulder blades lifted off the plinth for 6 seconds (Fig. 27.42a).

b. Supine with both legs flexed and hands on the chest. The head and shoulder blades lifted off the plinth for 6 seconds (Fig. 27.42b).

c. Supine with both legs flexed, head and shoulder blades lifted off the plinth, the hands are placed on the occipital region. The position is held for 6 seconds (Fig. 27.42c).

d. Supine with both legs flexed, hands placed under the lower back region with elbow lifted off the plinth. The head and shoulder blades lifted off the plinth for 6 seconds (Fig. 27.42d).

e. Supine with one leg flexed and other is raised and placed on the top of it. Both hands are placed on the head. The patient lifts head and one shoulder to opposite of the raised leg (Fig. 27.42e).

Planks: Plank exercises are designed to improve endurance and strength of the abdominal wall and the extensors including multifidus. The patient is positioned prone on elbows and then trunk, legs and arms are alternatively lifted off the ground as the planks progress (Figs. 27.43a-e).

a. Prone on elbows (90° flexed) with hips off the plinth weight is taken on the elbows, knees and toes (Fig. 27.43a).

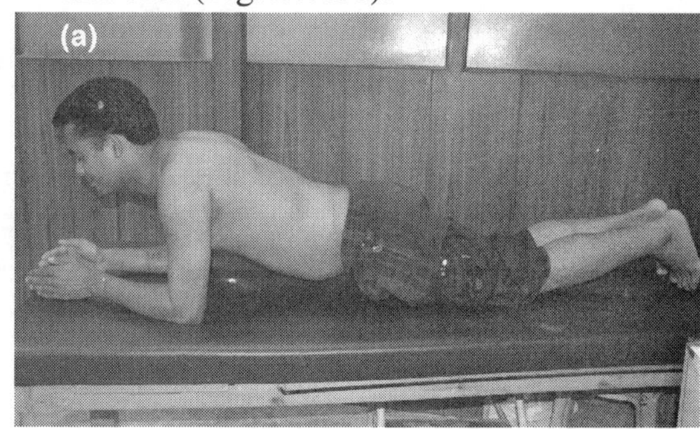

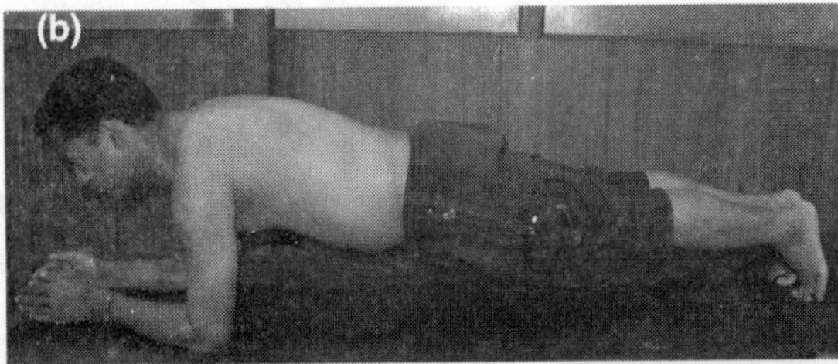

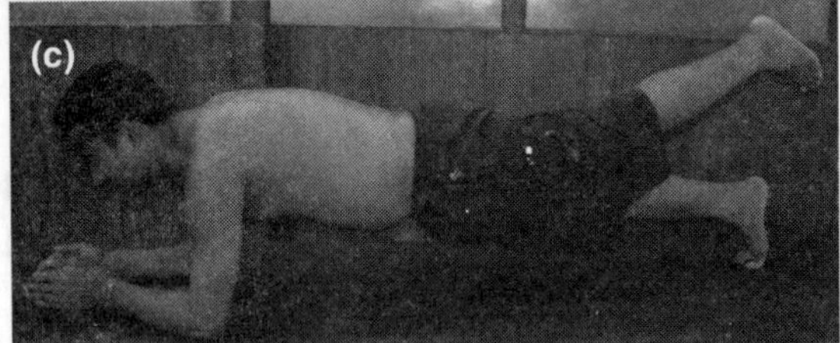

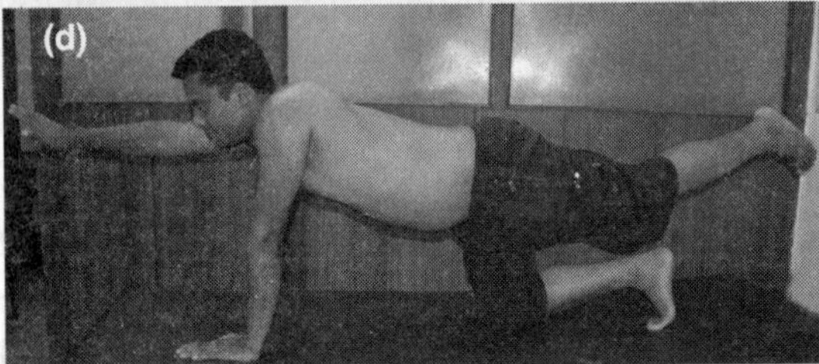

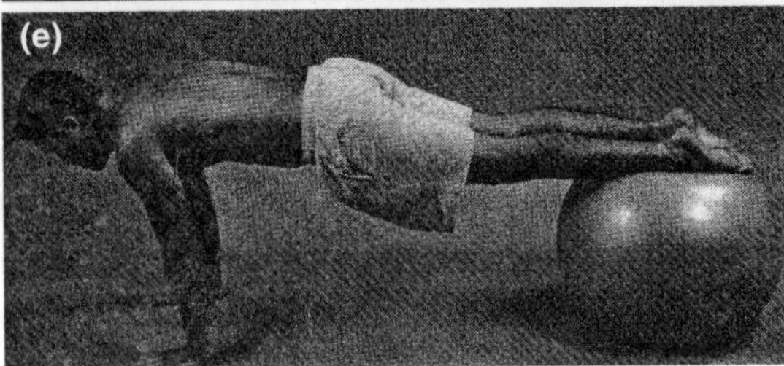

Figs. 27.43a-e: Planks

b. Prone on elbows (90° flexion) with hip and knees off the plinth, weight is taken on the elbows and toes (Fig. 27.43b).

c. Prone on elbows, weight is on the elbows and toes. One leg is raised to the level of hip joint (Fig. 27.43c).

d. Prone on elbows, weight is on the elbows and toes. One arm is raised to the level of shoulders (Fig. 27.43d).

e. Both the legs placed on the medicinal ball and the weight of upper body is taken on the hands (Fig. 27.43e).

Birddog (Four-Point Kneeling) Exercises: The four-point kneeling exercise is designed to strengthen the large number of the core muscles such as transverse abdominis multifidus, internal and external obliques, gluteus maximus, erector spinae and quadratus lumborum. All exercises commence from quadruped position and progressed to the raising of arm and leg alternatively (Figs. 27.44a-e).

a. Quadruped position with forward flexion of the spine-camel position (Fig. 27.44a).

b. Quadruped position with extension of the trunk-cat position (Fig. 27.44b).

c. Quadruped position with trunk at neutral, one arm is raised to the level of shoulder joint for 6 seconds (Fig. 27.44c).

d. Quadruped position with trunk in neutral position, one leg is raised to the level of hip joint for 6 seconds (Fig. 27.44d).

e. Quadruped position with trunk in neutral position, left arm and right leg is raised upto the level of trunk. This is followed by right arm and left leg raising (Fig. 27.44e).

Dead Bug: Dead bug exercises are also designed to recruit the muscle fiber of rectus abdominis, external oblique, internal oblique upper and lower extremities. The exercises are performed on mat in supine (hook) lying. The legs and arms are moved alternatively to allow the

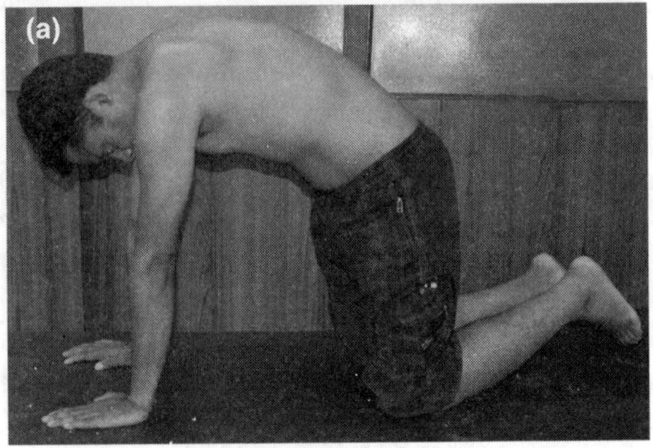

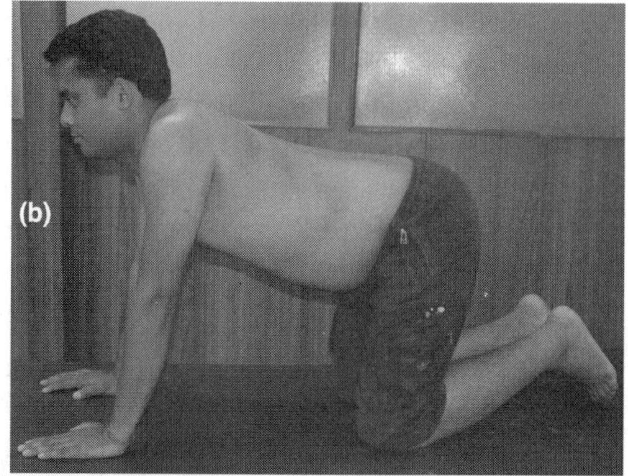

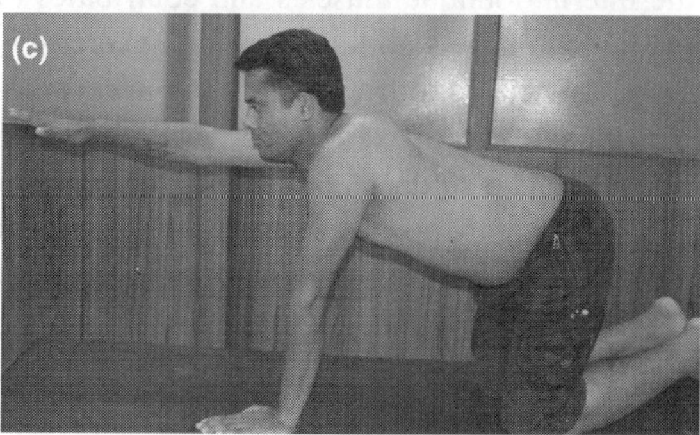

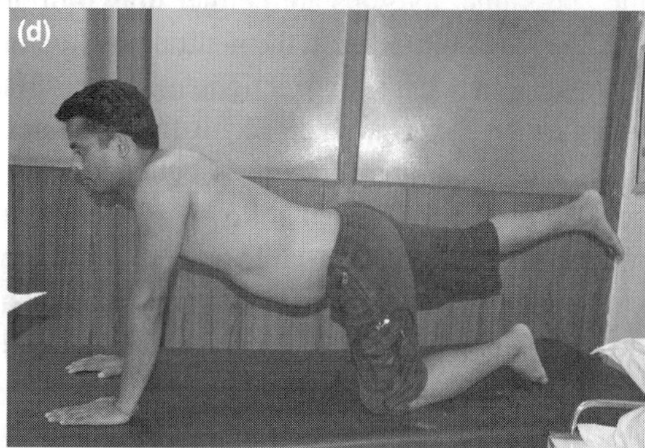

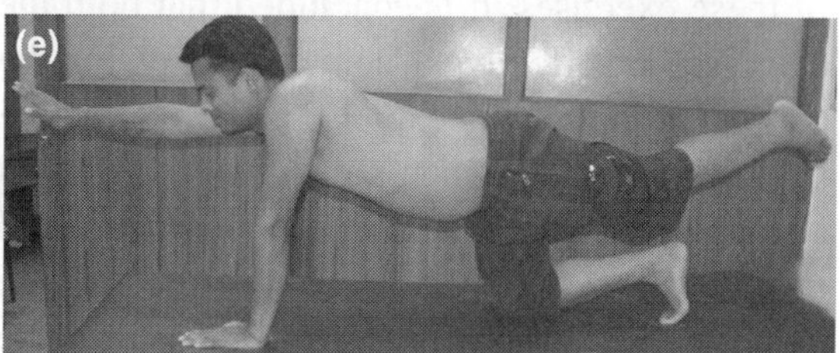

Figs. 27.44a-e: Birddog exercises

contraction of the muscles. The weight cuffs can also be added (to the patient) to increase the activity of the muscles (Figs. 27.45a-b).

a. Hook lying with alternate movement of the arms and legs (Fig. 27.45a).

b. Hook lying with cuff tied on the ankle joint and hands. Alternate movement of legs and arms (Fig. 27.45b).

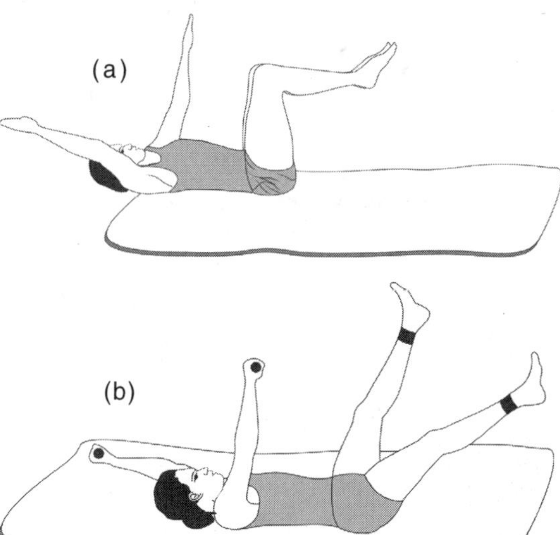

Figs. 27.45a-b: Dead bug exercises

Overhead Squat: The exercise is recommended to the athletes as it challenges and integrates all aspects of the core such as hip, trunk and shoulders. The exercise should not be recommended to the older patient with patellofemoral osteoarthritis as it increases the patellofemoral ground reaction forces on the knee complex (Figs. 27.46a-d).

a. In standing both the hands are placed on the occiput and the patient squats. The exercise should start with mini squat and progressed to half squatting. In case of pain and other symptoms the exercise should be discontinued.

b. In standing both the hands are raised over the head and the same procedure is repeated.

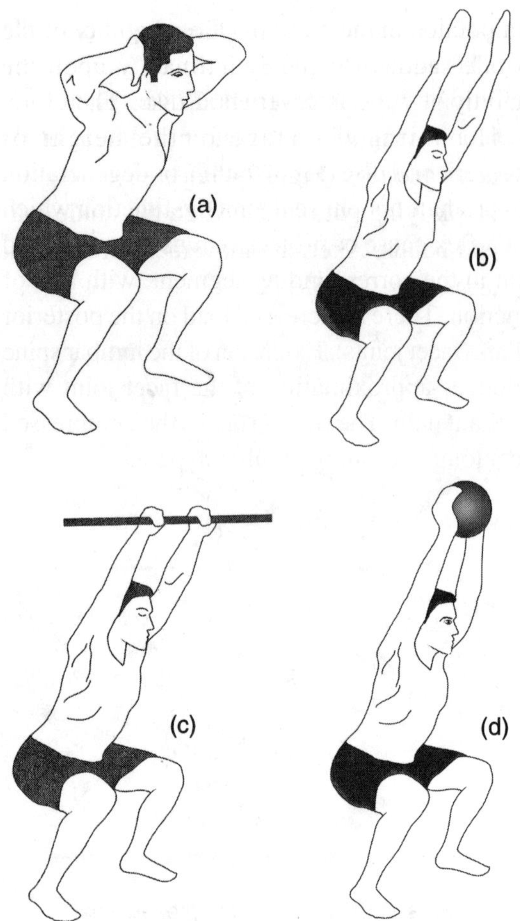

Figs. 27.46a-d: Overhead squat

c. In standing, a rod is held with both the hands over the head and the same procedure is repeated.
d. In standing, a football sized ball is held with both the hands over the head and the same procedure as above is repeated.

Transverse Abdominis Strengthening: The patient lies supine with the knees flexed. The therapist instructs the patient to pull the umbilicus in towards the spine. The exercise is repeated atleast 20-30 times thrice daily. The exercise is progressed in sitting position after significant improvement in the strength. Finally the exercise is progressed to the prone position. A tennis ball is placed under the umbilicus. Therapist instructs the patient to draw the umbilicus up and in towards the spine, attempting to lift the stomach off the tennis ball, without moving the pelvis.

Abdominal Hollowing versus Abdominal Bracing

Abdominal hollowing is the exercise in which tummy is taken in or the umbilicus is drawn up in at the neutral position of the lumbar spine. This exercise coactivates the transverse abdominis and the internal oblique muscles and contributes to the lumbar spine stability, therefore, exercise is also known as core stabilizing exercise. Unfortunately this exercise activates only two muscles and also does not activate the muscles to high enough levels to cause a training effect in healthy individuals.

On the other hand abdominal bracing is the contraction of all the abdominal muscles that contribute to the abdominal wall. In this exercise the abdominal muscles are neither drawn in or out, they are contracted at the neutral position in a similar situation like a boxer tightens his muscles when other boxer is about to hit the abdomen wall. The abdominal bracing is believed to be superior to the abdominal hollowing in terms of recruiting more muscles while performing more challenging dynamic stability exercises. It also provides more stability to the spine during rapid perturbations.

There was much debate over effectiveness of these exercises. It is concluded that both the exercises are effective in spinal stability, but the abdominal hollowing exercise is more effective in the acute stage when pain is the concerned because it increases the abdominal pressure and in turn decreases intra-discal pressure. As the pain improves the abdominal hollowing exercise should be progressed to the abdominal bracing.

LUMBAR FACET SYNDROME

Facet syndrome is one of the major cause of low back pain which contributes 15% to 40% to the chronic back pain. Approximately 80% of patients with facet syndrome have association with prior disc disease. Pain comes suddenly with the history of trauma such as lifting weight with a sound of click in posterior pillars; which may radiate upto the buttocks but not below the knees. The pain aggravates in extension and rotation of the lumbar spine and may be by lumbar flexion.

Clinical Features

The patients may experience pain or tenderness in the lower back region that increases with twisting or arching. The patient may also feel stiffness and difficulty with certain movements, such as standing up straight or getting up from a chair.

Mechanism

The superior facet articular surface moves up and forward on the inferior facet articular surface during lumbar flexion. Lifting of heavy objects causes excessive opening of the superior facet articular surface. When the person returns to the neutral position from the lumbar flexion with the object, the superior facet articular surface fails to slide backward and downward on the inferior facet articular surface, and stucks in a particular position. The facet joint is said to be malaligned. The muscles guard the facet joint by preventing the movements of that motion segment.

The lumbar facet syndrome occurs often with the intervertebral disc protrusion. There is a gradual resorption of the herniated disc with the time, but the facet malalignment remains untreated. Patient recovers with the sign symptoms of radiculopathy, but left with facet syndrome symptoms.

Minor Intervertebral Derangement (MID) Theory: Maigne has given this theory and pointed out that the functional ability of the mobile segment depends intimately upon the condition of the intervertebral disc. Therefore, even a minimal change in the height of intervertebral disc due to trauma or degeneration can produce apophyseal joint dysfunction which is a reflex cause of protective muscle spasm and pain in the corresponding segment, with loss of function. There is increased load on the posterior pillars (facet joints). Extension of the lumbar spine produces approximation of the facet joint with resultant pain. The flexion opens the compressed facet joints, resulting to relief in pain.

Types of Facet Restrictions

The facet restrictions are named according to the position in which the facet joint is stuck. There are two types of restrictions. It may be stuck/restricted either in flexion or extension position, combined with side flexion and rotation. In case, the facet joint is stuck in the flexed position, which limits extension of the lumbar spine, in other words it limits the closing of the facet joint, hence it is termed as closing restriction. If the facet joint is stuck in extension with side flexion and rotation it means the flexion will be limited, hence it is termed as 'opening restriction' (Fig. 27.47).

1. **Opening Restriction:** The facet joint is stuck in extension, rotation and side flexion, so the segment has limited mobility in flexion, rotation and side bending.
2. **Closing Restriction:** If the facet joint is stuck in flexion combined with side flexion and rotation of the same side.

Management

Flexion Bias: This exercise is most commonly used in patients with facet syndrome. As per McKenzie approach the position or movement patterns that relieves the symptoms should be repeated. In these patients flexion exercise may

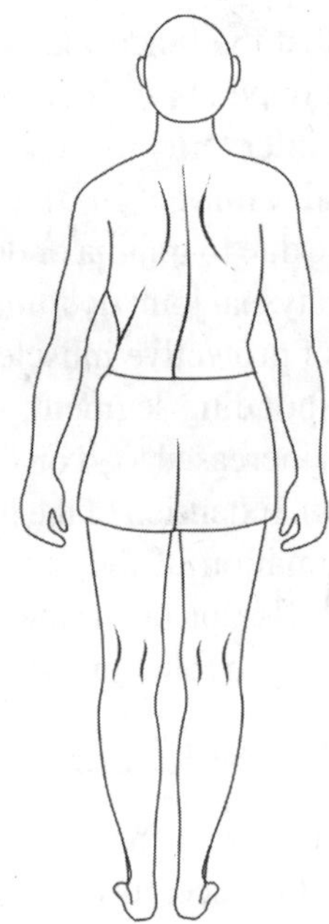

Fig. 27.47: Patient with facet joint restriction

act to reduce facet joint compression and provide stretch to lumbar musculature, ligaments and myofacial structures. The repeated flexion of lumbar spine in pain free range may centralize the symptoms in patients with facet syndrome. The cyclic range of motion exercises usually passive are the cornerstone of the McKenzie program.

Techniques for Opening Restriction

A. Left Side (L_4-L_5) Opening Restriction

Position of Patient: Left side lying.

Position of Therapist: Facing the patient.

Procedure: The therapist palpates the intervertebral space of L_4-L_5 with the right hand and flexes the hip and trunk with left hand. As soon as therapist feels the opening of L_4 and L_5 intervertebral space, he usually around 90° stops flexing the hip and spine further. The knees of the patient rest on the therapist thighs and the therapist holds the ankles of the patient with left hand. At the last step the therapist pulls the

patient's feet and legs toward the patient's head, creating a side bending movement in the spine which opens the left facet joint of L_4 and L_5 and closes the right facet joint at L_4 and L_5 and improves the range of motion (Figs. 27.48a-b).

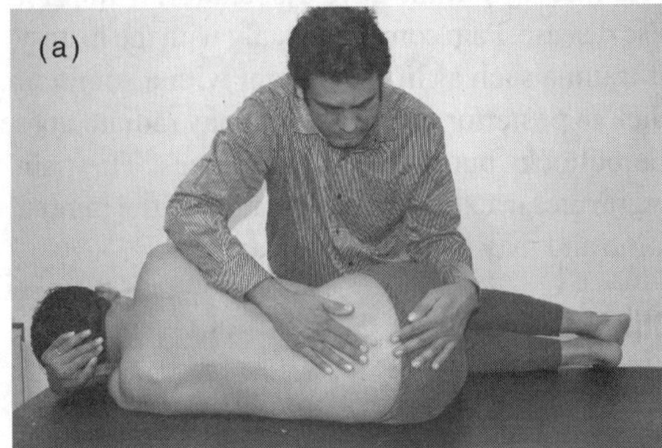

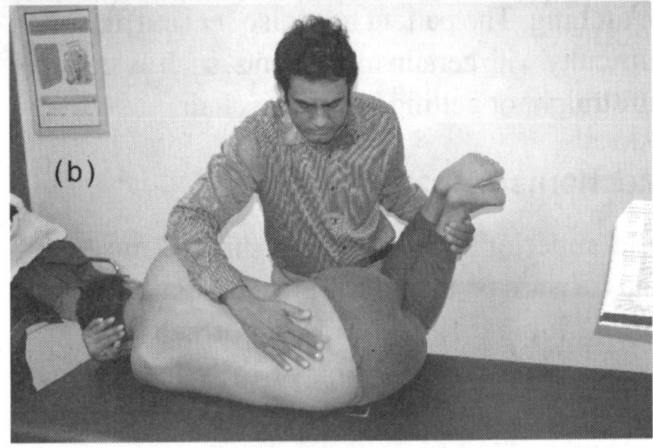

Figs. 27.48a-b: a. Left side lying with hip and knees flexion to 90°, therapist feels the opening of L_4/L_5 facet joint. b. The spine is bent to the right by bringing the legs to the head to open the left L_4/L_5 facet joint

B. Both Sides (Left and Right Open Restrictions)

Position of Patient: Supine a towel roll is placed under the spine at the level of L_3. Hip and knees flexed 90° to 100°.

Position of Therapist: Kneel standing on the plinth at the side of the patient (Fig. 27.49).

Procedure: The therapist places both the hands on the top of knees of the patient and applies downward force through the femur, creating motion at the lumbar spine. This opens both the facet joint at the level of L_3 and L_4 and increases the range of motion (Fig. 27.49).

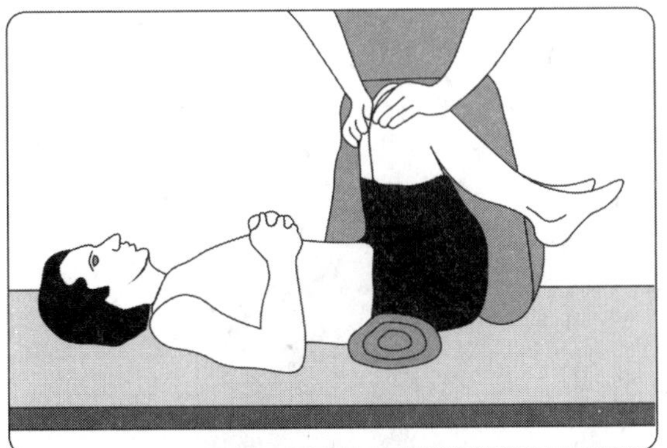

Fig. 27.49: Technique for opening restriction at left and right L_3/L_4 level

Techniques for Closing Restrictions

Common Complaints: Patient has complaint of pain and stiffness with extension limitation.

A. Left L_4-L_5 Level Closing Restriction

The side flexion and rotation of the same side will be limited when patient attempts to extend the lumbar spine. Pain deviates to the opposite side of the restriction as the facet joint is stuck on that side and does not close as well as the other side.

Position of Patient: Prone with extension of the lumbar spine till the restriction starts. To maintain this position a wedge is placed under the chest of the patient. Arm rests on the wedge.

Position of Therapist: Therapist stands at the side of the patient.

Procedure: The therapist places pisiform aspect of the right hand on the spinous process of the restricted vertebra. Keeping the arms straight gentle rhythmic oscillations are applied through the arms to the vertebra (Fig. 27.50).

Note: The same procedure can be done by changing the position of wedge from chest to thighs. Rest of procedure remains same (Fig. 27.51).

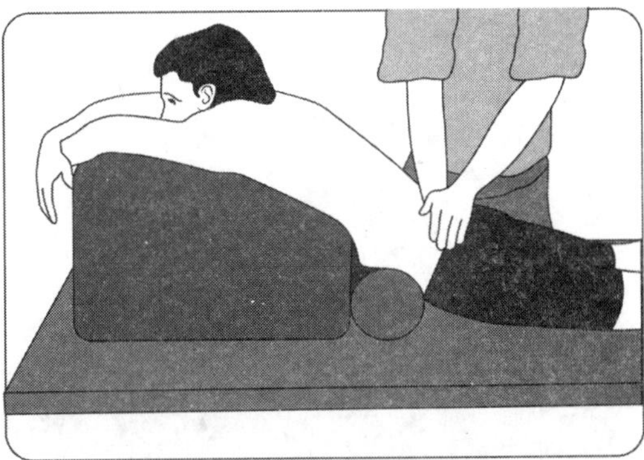

Fig. 27.50

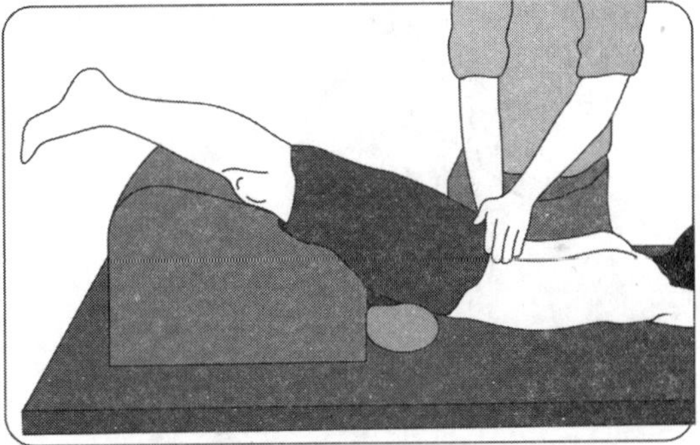

Fig. 27.51: Technique for closing restriction at L_4-L_5

B. Physiological Mobilizations for Opening and Closing Restrictions at L_3-L_4 level

Position of Patient: Side lying with upper most hip and knee flexed to 90-100.

Position of Therapist: Standing facing the patient, places right arm under the axilla and right hand on the L_3-L_4 level. The therapist places left arm on the gluteal region and the fingers of left hand on the space between L_3-L_4.

Procedure: A force couple is applied through the hand creating rotation at the lumbar segment. Right hand pushes the chest backwards and left hand pulls the pelvis anteriorly. This creates a rotation on the desired segment (Figs. 27.52a-b).

Muscle Energy Techniques for Opening and Closing Restrictions: The use of voluntary contraction of the muscles in a controlled direction against the counter force applied by the therapist can decrease the muscle spasm, and increase flexibility and range of motion.

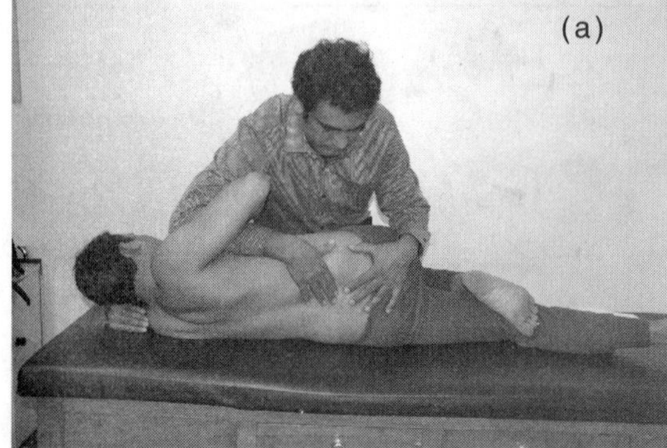

(a)

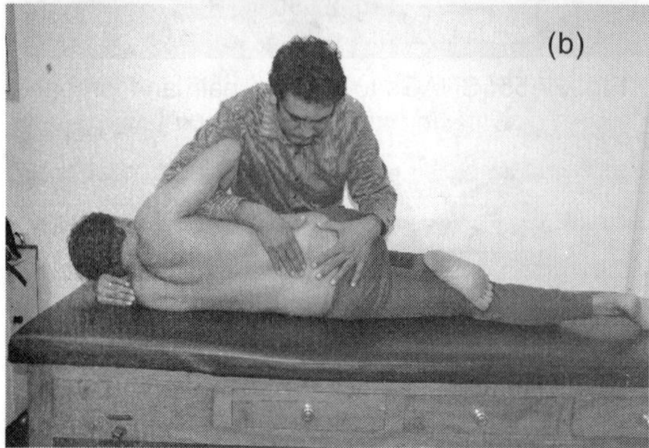

(b)

Figs. 27.52a-b: Technique for opening and closing restriction at left L_4-L_5 level

A. Muscle Energy Technique for Flexion Restriction (Open Restriction): At the level of L_4-L_5 right rotation, right bending.

Position of Patient: High sitting, grasps both the hands and holds the edge of the plinth to the right side, creating forward flexion, right side flexion and right rotation.

Position of Therapist: Standing, facing the patient, places right hand on the left scapula and left hand on the right scapula.

Procedure: The patient is asked to flex, side bend and rotate the spine to the limited side as much as possible.

Therapist maintains the position at the extreme limitation range with both the hands and asks the patient to extend, rotate and bend to the left side isometrically against the resistance applied by the therapist. The whole procedure involves the sub-

maximal isometric contract for 3-5 seconds followed by a relaxation. The isometric contraction and a relaxation consists of onset. After completing onset the patient should be placed further into flexion, right side bending and right rotation upto the pain free range 3-5 repetitions should be performed (Fig. 27.53).

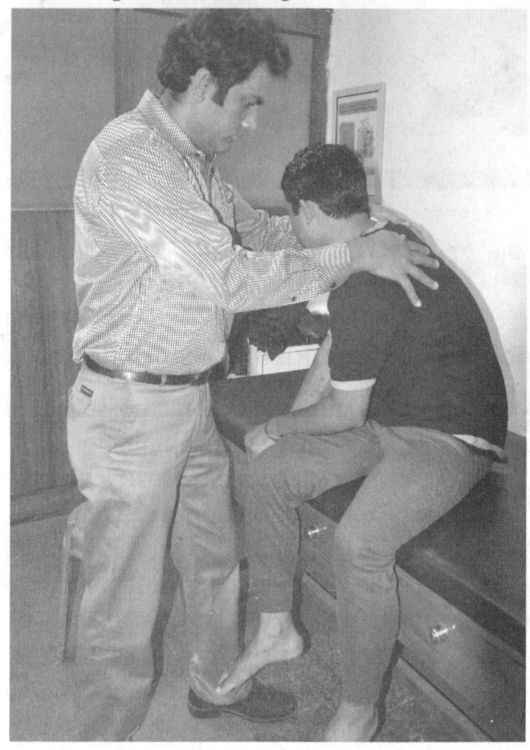

Fig. 27.53: Muscle energy technique for flexion restriction (open restriction)

B. Muscle Energy Technique for Extension Restriction of the L_4-L_5 Level Extension, Right Rotation (Right Side Flexion) (Fig. 27.54)

Position of Patient: High sitting with right hand on the left thigh.

Position of Therapist: Standing behind the patient, place right forearm on the chest and hand on the left shoulder of the patient. The therapist place left hand on the L_4-L_5 level. Spine is extended with right side flexion and rotation until the restriction is felt or symptoms start aggravating.

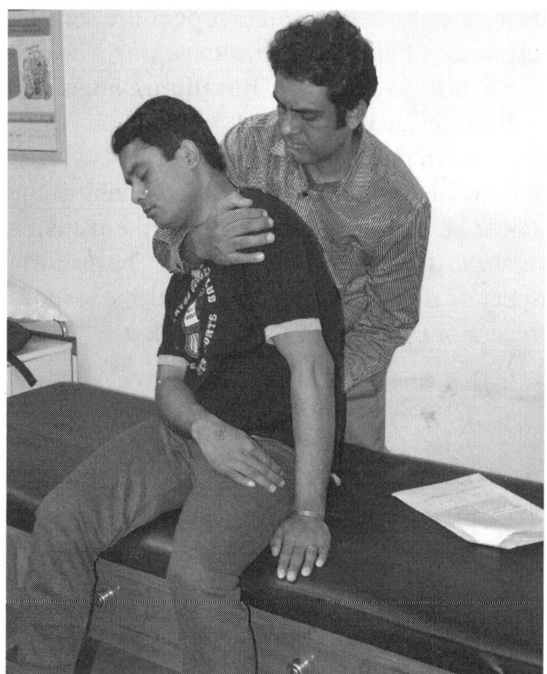

Fig. 27.54: MET for extension restriction at L$_4$-L$_5$ level

Procedure: The patient is asked to flex the spine with left side flexion and rotation against the resistance applied by the therapist. A submaximal isometric contraction is held for at least 3-5 seconds, followed by relaxation. The procedure is repeated 3-5 times.

Sustained Natural Apophyseal Glides (SNAGs)

A. SNAGs to Improve Pain and Lumbar Flexion at L$_3$-L$_4$ Segment

Position of Patient: Sitting, hands rest on the anterior thighs.

Position of Therapist: Standing behind the patient, facing the dorsal aspect of L$_3$-L$_4$ level. A belt is wrapped around the patient's waist just below the anterior superior iliac spine and over the sacrum of the therapist. The spinous process of the L$_3$ vertebra is palpated, and the pisiform aspect of the wrist is placed under it (Fig. 27.55).

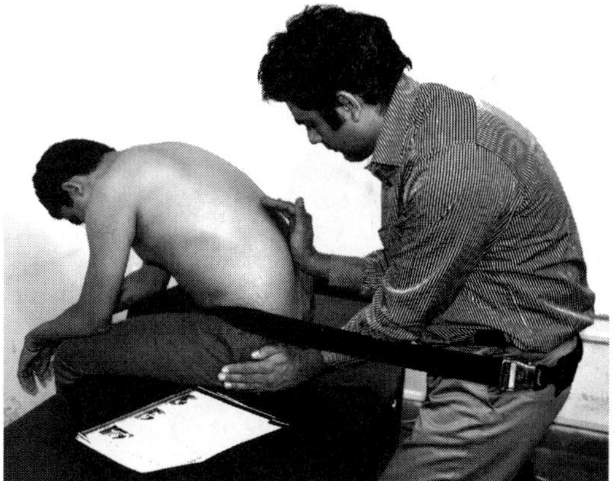

Fig. 27.55: SNAGs to improve pain and lumbar flexion at L$_3$-L$_4$ segment

Procedure: Therapist applies an accessory gliding force up along the treatment plane while the patient flexes the spine forward until the pain is felt, at this point the movement is sustained for few seconds and then returns to the starting position. An accessory gliding force up along the treatment plane is maintained throughout the range of motion until the patient returns to starting position. It is unadvisable to relieve the force in the mid range, it can produce pain. As per this approach three repetitions are enough in the first visit which can significantly reduce the pain and improve the flexion range. The same can be performed on other lumbar spine segments, but for the L$_4$-L$_5$ and LS segments instead of pisiform aspect of wrist, thumb can be used and it is reinforced with other thumb. The same procedure may be performed in standing with slight knees extension.

B. SNAGs to Improve Extension Range and Pain at L$_3$-L$_4$ Segment

Position of Patient: Standing.

Position of Therapist: Standing, behind the patient slightly to the left side of the patient to allow the patient to extend the spine, facing the L$_3$-L$_4$ segment. The pisiform aspect of wrist is placed under the spinous process of the L$_3$ vertebra (superior spinous process of the segment). A belt is wrapped around the patient's and therapist's waist similar to previous technique (Fig. 27.56).

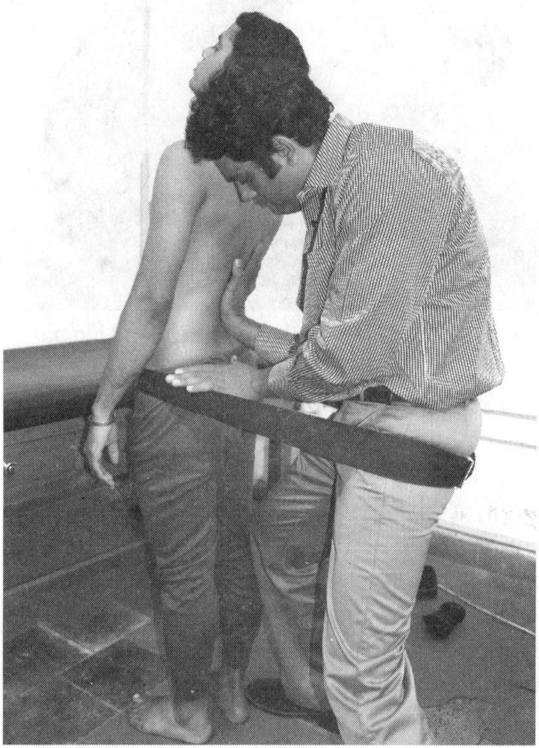

Fig. 27.56: SNAGs to improve pain and lumbar flexion at L_3-L_4 segment

Procedure: Patient extends the lumbar spine gradually and at the same time with the extension therapist pushes the L_3 spinous process up along the treatment plane; until the patient feels pain, at this point the movement is sustained for few seconds then returns to the starting position. The accessory gliding force up along the treatment is maintained throughout the range until patient returns to starting position. If the pressure/force is released in the mid range before reaching to the starting position it may produce unwanted pain and symptoms. The same procedure can be performed in sitting position.

As per this approach three repetitions are enough in the first visit and patient should be called after one day. The same procedure can be performed on the other segments.

C. SNAGs to Improve Rotation Range and Pain at L_3-L_4 Segment

Position of Patient: Standing.

Position of Therapist: Stands behind the patient. A belt is wrapped around the patient's waist and therapist's gluteal region. The pisiform aspect of right wrist is placed over the spinous process of L_3 vertebra (Fig. 27.57).

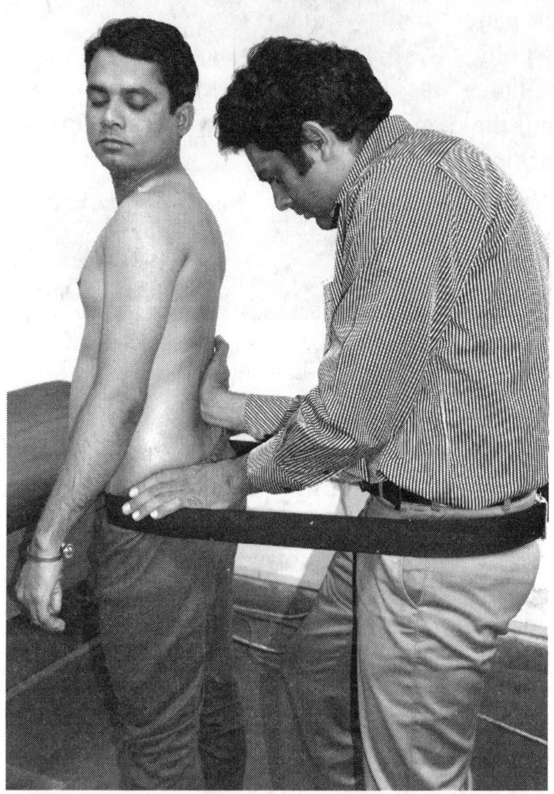

Fig. 27.57: SNAGs to improve pain and lumbar flexion at L_3-L_4 segment

Procedure: For restriction in rotation to the left side the patient rotates the trunks to the left side. The right arm of the therapist encourages the movement. The therapist applies an accessory glide in the treatment plane on L_3 until the patient complains pain and symptoms. At the end range of rotation the therapist may add overpressure.

An accessory gliding force in the treatment plane must be maintained throughout the range until the patient returns to the starting position. Three repetitions in the first visit are sufficient for significant improvement.

D. Self SNAGs to Improve Lumbar Flexion at L_3/L_4 Level

In standing the patient holds the belt and wraps it around the L_3-L_4 level and stabilizes both the hands in front of the chest with the elbows flexed. The patient applies a gliding force up at the L_3-L_4 by pulling the belt with both hands. The patient maintains the gliding force and bends forwards until the pain is felt, then returns to the starting position (Fig. 27.58).

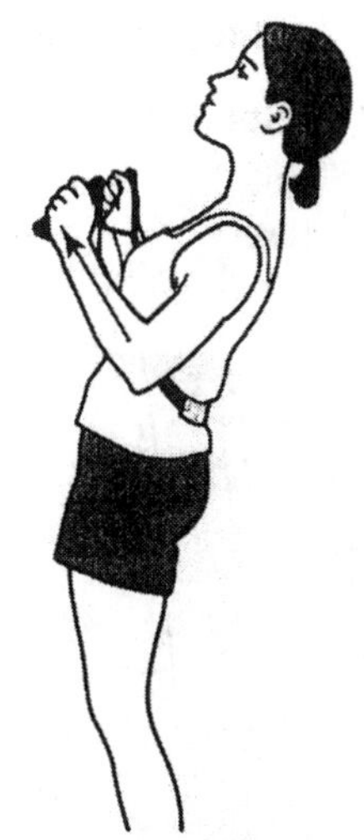

Fig. 27.59: Self SNAGs to improve extension and pain L_3-L_4 level

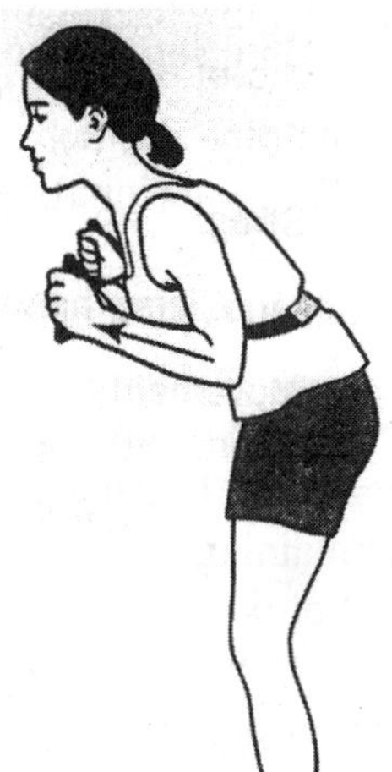

Fig. 27.58: Self SNAGs to improve flexion and pain of L_3-L_4 segment

E. Self SNAGs to Improve Lumbar Extension at L_3/L_4 Level

In standing position similar to previous technique, while maintaining the gliding force, the patient bends backwards until the pain is felt, then the patient returns to the starting position (Fig. 27.59).

PIRIFORMIS SYNDROME

The sciatic nerve passes underneath piriformis muscle at the level of greater trochantor. Spasm and tightness in the muscle can cause pressure on sciatic nerve. Bulky wallet in the hip pocket can also cause pressure on the piriformis muscle and in turn irritates the sciatic nerve. The presentation is identical to prolapse intervertebral disc radiculopathy but pain is localized on the buttock which may radiate down the course of sciatic nerve. Some patients present with the tight trousers with bulky wallet in their hip pocket may also have the symptoms of radiculopathy. Symptoms aggravate in the sitting position as the wallet puts more pressure. Typical symptoms are tingling and numbness along the sciatic nerve course. Shortwave diathermy, on the gluteal region and continuous ultrasound with 1 MHZ at high intensity may help in relieving inflammation. If the root cause is tight trousers with bulky wallet the patient should be advised to wear loose trousers. Stretching of the piriformis muscle is the cornerstone of the treatment. In supine position the hip joint is internally rotated and taken to the opposite shoulder with knee flexion. If the diagnosis is correct, the patient will respond to the treatment even in one sitting of stretching (Fig. 27.60).

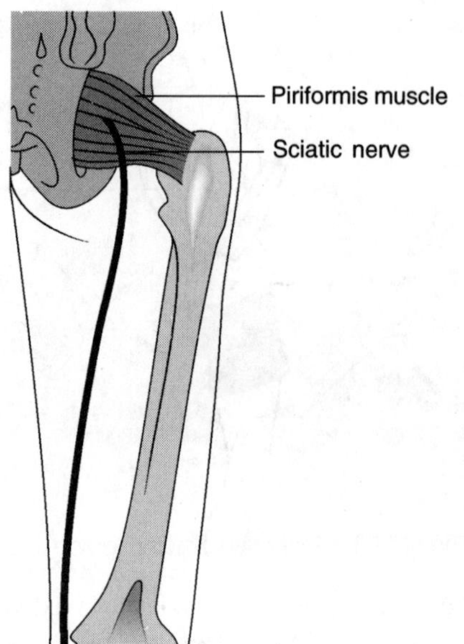

Fig. 27.60: Piriformis syndrome, piriformis muscle and sciatic nerve

SPONDYLOLYSIS

Spondylolysis is a stress fracture of the pars interarticularis. The classic theory of causation for spondylolysis has been that an individual is born with a weakness in the pars-interarticularis, and at approximately 6 years of age, a fatigue injury occurs that breaks the pars in children involved in the repetitive flexion extension activities such as back-walkovers in gymnasts causing excessive load on the pars-interarticularis (eventually fractures the pars). Later in high school with the history of weight lifting football play or the extension stresses of gymnastics or wrestling, the lateral fracture becomes irritated and symptomatic. 5% of the general population remain asymptomatic (Fig. 27.61).

Clinical Features

1. Age: Usually children below *the age of eighteen years.*
2. Gradual onset, sometimes acute.
3. Hereditary predisposition.

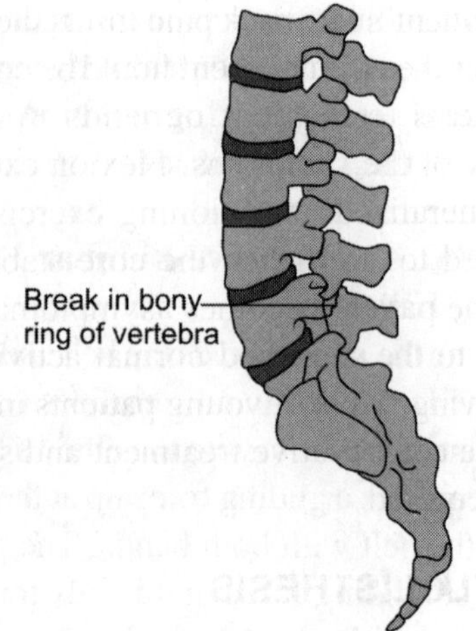

Fig. 27.61 : Spondylolysis

4. Symptoms usually low back pain dominant to one side, but more often is in line with the lumbosacral junction.
   a. Occasionally posterior thigh pain with hamstrings tightness.
   b. No neurological signs and symptoms.
5. Stork test:
   (a) The patient stands on one leg with the other leg on the weight bearing knee.
   (b) While maintaining the above position the patient hyperextends the lower lumbar spine.
   (c) Reproduction of the symptoms suggest spondylolysis.
6. Single-photon emission computed tomography (SPECT) scan can show involved area.
7. Oblique radiographs may help in determining the defect.
8. The next element of investigation is C.T. scan which requires only if aforesaid techniques fail to detect the site of lesion.

Management

1. If the patient has no symptoms of low back pain (despite the results of radiographs, bone scan and C.T. scan), do not limit the activities of the patient let him play the sport.

2. If the patient's low back pain limits the sports activities then the children should be on brace.

3. In general, treatment depends upon the severity of the symptoms. Flexion exercises and generalized conditioning exercises are instituted to strengthen the core stabilizers. Once the patient becomes asymptomatic, he returns to the sport and normal activities of daily living. Most of young patients improve with the conservative treatment and surgery is not required.

SPONDYLOLISTHESIS

It is defined as slip of one vertebra on another. The forward slip of vertebra is resisted by the posterior facet joints, intact neural arch and pedicle, normal bone plasticity preventing stretch of the pedicle and the intervertebral discs. The breakdown of this normal locking mechanism causes forward slip of the vertebra which is known as spondylolisthesis (Fig. 27.62).

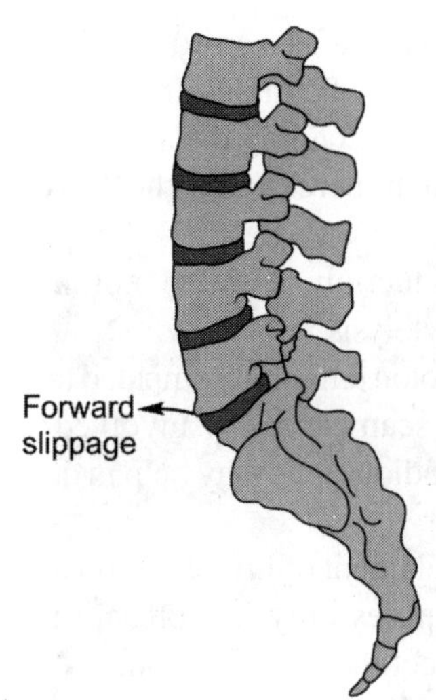

Fig.27.62: Spondylolisthesis forward slip of L_4 vertebra or the L_5 vertebra

The amount of slip of one vertebra on another is graded in percentage as mentioned below: (Meyerding grading) (Fig. 27.63).

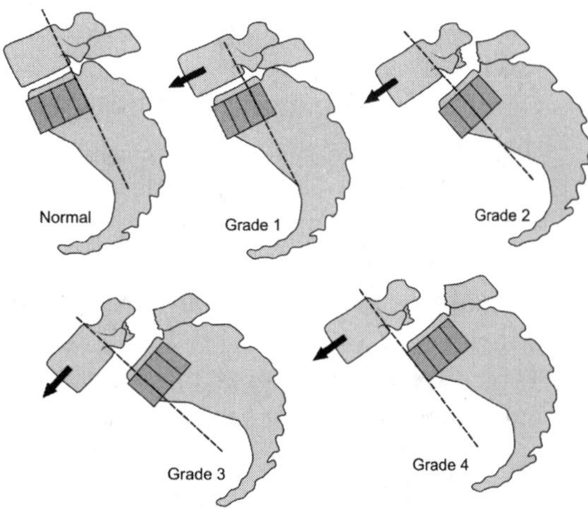

Fig. 27.63: Meyerding grading, grade 1, 2, 3 and 4

Grade I – 25%.
Grade II – 25% - 50%.
Grade III – 50% - 75%.
Grade IV – 75% - 100%.

The complete slip or dislocation of vertebra is called as spondyloptosis.

Assessment of displacement or slip of vertebra on another is represented in percentage (%).

A/B × 100 = Slip of vertebra in percentage.

Wiltse Classification

Table 27.4: Commonly accepted clinical classification of spodylolisthesis

Type	Classification	Descriptions
I	Dysplastic	Congenital abnormalities of upper sacrum or arch at L_5
II		Lesion in pars interarticularis
III		Facet joint degeneration
IV		Fracture in areas of arch other than pars
V	Pathologic	Secondary to generalized or localized bone

Adopted from Macnab's Backache

Clinical Features

- The patients experience a sudden onset of backache with restriction in the motion of the lumbar spine, commonly associated with functional scoliosis.

- On observation buttocks look like "Heart shaped".
- Slip visualized on standing "spot" lateral.
- Often patient complains of spasm in the hamstring muscles.
- Coughing and sneezing can intensify the symptoms.
- Typical physical changes that occur in an individual with lumbar spondylolisthesis is a general stiffness of the back and tightness in the hamstrings with change in both posture and gait.
- In most advanced cases, the gait of the patient may change to give the appearance of more of a "waddle" then a walk where the individual rotates the pelvis more due to decreased flexibility of the hamstrings.

Isthmic Spondylolisthesis

Approximately 5 to 7% of population has either a fracture of the pars interarticularis or a spondylolisthesis. 80% of these patients remain asymptomatic. Isthmic spondylolisthesis occurs most commonly at L_5-L_1.

The etiology of this lesion is unknown. The congenital defects in the pars interarticularis of the neural arch occurs mostly between the 5 and 7 years, and forward slipping of the vertebral body occurs between 10 and 15 years. Once this has occurred it rarely continues to many of the patients experience occasional back pain but so does the vast majority of people without isthmus spondylolisthesis.

A more contemporary theory of pain generation is excessive tension on the annulus of the inferior disc and foramenial stenosis at the level of the slip. However this theory does not explain why some patients have symptoms while others do not, since the inferior discs of all the patients are subjected to similar forces.

Degenerative Spondylolisthesis

It affects the elderly people. As the age progresses usually after fourth decade of life, degenerative changes start at the intervertebral disc and articular cartilage of the facet joints become incompetent and allows vertebral body to slip forward on the other. Not all slips remain asymptomatic but if they are associated with spinal canal stenosis they can produce symptoms such as neurogenic claudication. But the neural arch remains intact. The degeneration causes gross segmental instability (Figs. 27.64a-b).

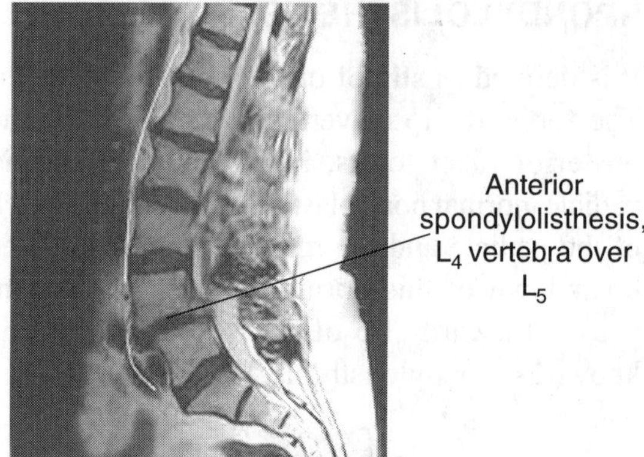

Fig. 27.64a: MRI–spondylolisthesis L_4 vertebra over L_5 vertebra

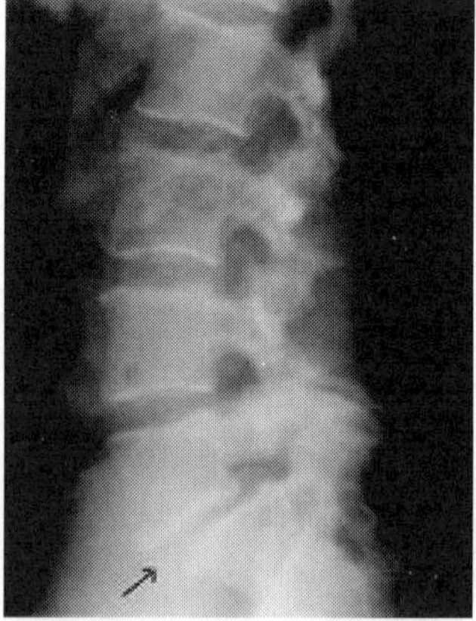

Fig. 27.64b: X-ray–spondylolisthesis L_4 vertebra over L_5 vertebra

Traumatic Spondylolisthesis

Forward slipping of a vertebral body may occur as a result of trauma to the spine. Trauma can cause dislocation of the posterior joints or a fracture of spinous process extending into the lamina of the pars interarticularis which may produce slipping of one vertebra over other. A true traumatic spondylolisthesis is very rare (fracture through pars interarticularis with forward slip of the vertebra).

Congenital or Dysplastic Spondylolisthesis

It is a true congenital spondylolislithesis that occurs because of malformation of lumbosacral junction with small, incompetent facet joints. It is associated with multiple congenital anomalies. In a true congenital or dysplastic spondylolisthesis the lesion may be either dysplasia of the upper sacrum specifically may be either of the upper sacrum, specifically in the facet joints, or an attenuation of pars interarticularis that gets pulled out and thinned as taught it were made of a malleable plastic. Due to lack of stability there is forward slip of the L_5 on the sacrum. As the forward slip progresses, the pars interarticularis becomes increasingly stretched, it may eventually break the pars interarticularis and produces spondylolisthesis. This break/fracture is secondary to the slip and is not the cause of spondylolisthesis.

The aforesaid concept represents a slight deviation from the Wiltse-Newman-Macnab classification. According to this theory due to lack of stability development of first sacrum of the first sacral arch, with absence or dysplasia of the superior aritcular facet of the sacrum the only lumbosacral disc prevents the forward slip of the L_5 vertebra. When the lumbosacral disc breaks there is forward slip of the L_5 vertebra with the inferior facets gliding over the rudimentary superior articular facets. In the next process slipping involves attenuation and elongation of the pars interarticularis.

Management–Conservative

Flexion Exercises: William Flexion exercises generally help in reducing the slip of the vertebra. The exercises can be performed in many positions (Figs. 27.65 a-c).

(a)

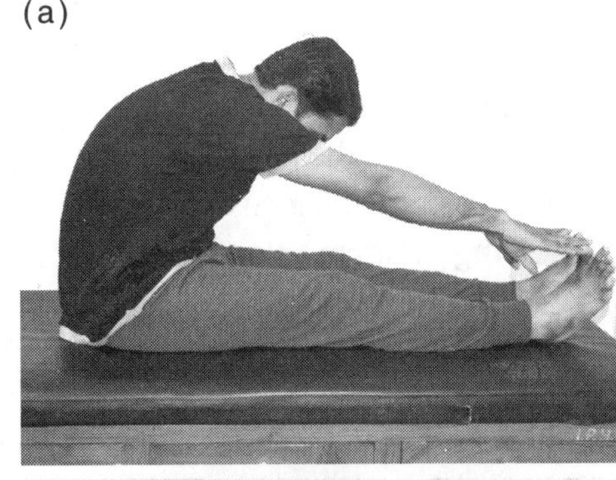

(b)

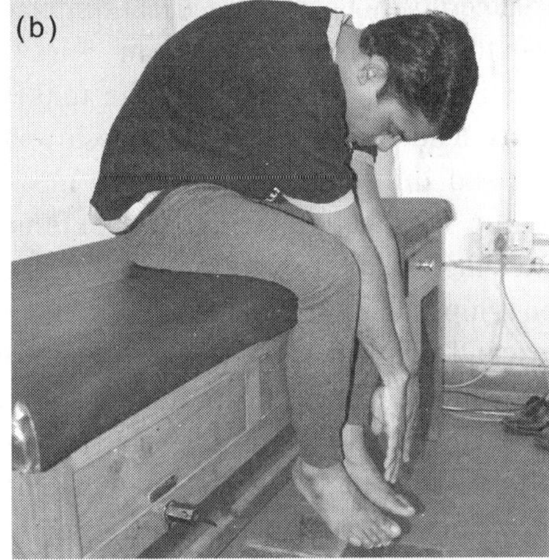

(c)

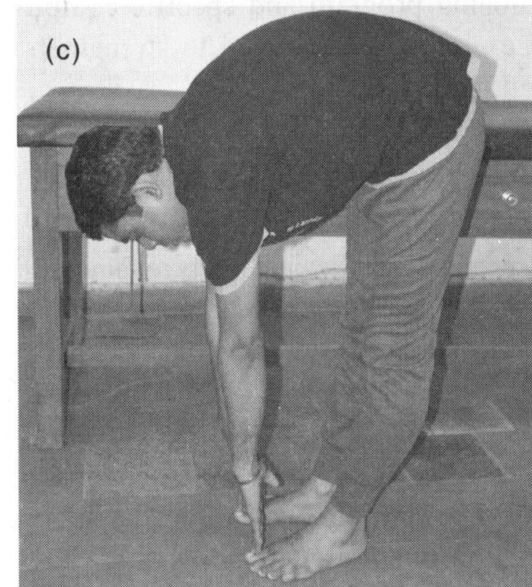

Figs. 27.65a-c: Flexion exercises, a long sitting with toe touch, high sitting with toe touch, standing with toe touch

1. Supine lying:
  i. The patient is asked to bend the knees and touch to the chest by holding both the knees.
  ii. With the flexion of both hip and knee joints the patient lifts the head and shoulders.
  iii. Bilateral straight leg raising.

2. Long sitting: Patient attempts to touch the toes with the fingers.

3. Standing: Patient attempts to touch the toes with the fingers.

Modalities: The modalities such as short wave diathermy, hot packs, electrical stimulation can ease the pain and muscle spasm.

Soft tissue manipulation of the muscles, ligaments, tendon can reduce the muscle spasm tension and improves the range of motion. Stretching of the hamstring and extensors increases the flexibility and improves range of motion at hip and lumbar spine.

Brace: During the stage when symptoms such as pain and instability are there the patient should obtain from the aggravating activity which in itself may be the most important treatment.

Once symptoms start to improve a generalized conditioning program and specific equipment based exercises are initiated to strengthen the core muscles.

Surgical Management

The young patients improve with the flexion exercises and modalities and rarely require surgical intervention.

Surgical treatment is only considered after at least 6 weeks to one year of non-operation treatment fails to improve the symptoms. However in cases of a bilateral radiculopathy in a dermatome distribution as well as radiological evidence of slip progression.

Posterior Lateral Fusion: Fusion with decompression.

SACRALIZATION

Sacralization is a *developmental anomaly* in which one or both transverse processes of the fifth lumbar vertebra generally become disproportionally large and strong. Sometimes they become so large that they extend into the base of the sacrum or ileum and form a connection with them. This union forms a foramen between the lower margin of the transverse process and the upper free edge of the sacrum instead of the normal broad and irregular cleft (Fig. 27.66).

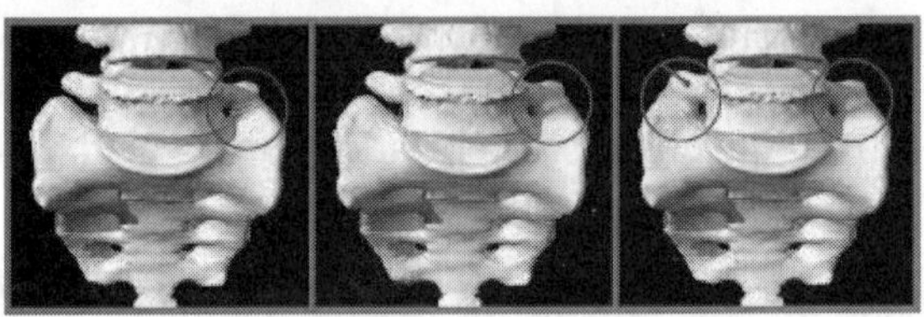

Fig. 27.66: Sacralization

INTERMITTENT CLAUDICATION

Claudication is a pain and/or cramping of the lower leg due to inadequate blood flow to the muscles. The word claudication comes from the Latin "claudicate" meaning to limp. The pain in the muscles is felt during exercises or walking, and subsides at by rest. Hence it is called as intermittent claudication as the pain comes and goes. However in severe cases the pain persists during the exercises or walk as well as at rest. Intermittent claudication is of two types—vascular and neurogenic.

Vascular Claudication

Vascular claudication is a condition involving insufficient blood circulation due to narrowing of the arteries in the legs.

Clinical Features: Commonly, the calf muscles are the most affected, and patients describe a cramping discomfort as characteristic of pain. In the initial stage of the disease, the patient may walk with the pain, but as the disease progresses further, this is not possible and claudicating pain causes limping which is relieved by rest. Symptoms can worsen when walking barefooted or wearing *flat slippers,* climbing stairs or up hills. In short symptoms aggravate whenever muscles are required to work more. Patient frequently rests in between the walk/work to relieve the symptoms. In cases where blockage is severe the pain is not relieved by rest and persists all the time.

Causes

The most common cause of vascular intermittent claudication is the atherosclerosis. There is deposition of cholesterol in the innermost layer of the artery, that decreases the diameter of the artery. Over the years the cholesterol and calcium builds up in the arteries. The narrowing or blockage of the artery will reduce the blood supply to the muscles. The muscles demand more oxygen when patient walks; the demand of oxygen is completed by the blood. In the patients with narrowing of arteries there is an inadequate blood supply to the muscles and that is why the patient starts complaining of pain during continued walk.

In some patients the blood flow is so restricted that the symptoms are not relieved even during rest. These patients also complain of night pain which disturbs the sleep. The symptoms are eased when the leg is hanged down over the edge of the bed. This is the critical stage where ischemia has developed and the leg is at risk of avascular necrosis.

Pathophysiology

The normal artery consists of three layers. The inner layer known as intima is the surface in contact with flowing. A single layer of *cells (endothelial cells) lines the whole* of the arterial (and venous) system. The initial trigger for the development of atherosclerosis is probably damage to the endothelial *cell layer lining the artery.* The damage is usually by smoking, viruses, chemicals and drugs. In the initial stage, yellow *fatty streaks* develop in the blood vessels caused by the deposition of fats in the wall. They are yellow due to deposited cholesterol. At this stage there is complaint of pain, these can progress to the development of atherosclerosis plaques. There is thickening of the innermost wall of the artery that limits the blood flow to the muscles/tissues. The plaques are caused by the accumulation of low density lipoprotein (LDL, a type of cholesterol).The increased LDL in the blood stream will lead to transport into the artery wall where it is retained. Moreover, other cells such as monocytes are attracted towards this *attired* LDL which further accelerates the accumulation. A fibrous plaque develops as smooth muscle cells and monocyte accumulate.

Furthermore, the monocytes also transform into another cell type called macrophases which absorb the cholesterol and fats deposited in the arterial wall. The plaques can become so thick that they protrude into the artery and can interfere with normal blood flow. In more advance cases calcium is also deposited and the plaques become very hard. **Embolisation:** Sometimes the plaque surface becomes ulcerated, that leads to fragmentation of the plaques. These are carried downstream to block a smaller blood vessel–this is the complication of atherosclerosis. **Collateral Arterial Supply:** When the plaques become large they can block the artery completely and in that situation the blood is diverted into smaller arteries, known as collateral arteries. These small arteries, although not the major blood vessels to the leg, usually carry enough blood to prevent severe disability.

Prognosis: Overall about one third of patients with intermittent vascular claudication will improve, one third will remain stable and rest of patients will deteriorate. In majority of cases

(> 65%) the symptoms will remain stable or improve.

Amputation: In the advance stage or severe cases the symptoms become constant (not relieved by rest, pain at rest and at night), and there are ischemic ulcerations (critical limb ischemia). These changes indicates means that the patient has developed problems that are putting the leg at risk of amputation.

Physical Examination: The patient should be examined for high blood pressure, heart abnormalities, blockage in the arteries of neck, and abdominal aneurysms. In addition to above patient should also be examined for ulcer and colour changes of the skin.

A. **Ankle Brachial Index:** The systolic blood pressure of the arm is measured. Then the systolic blood pressure of the leg is also measured at four different sites and passes a Doppler probe over arteries in the foot. The signal emitted from the strongest artery is recorded as the cuffs are inflated and deflated. This is considered as the ankle's systolic pressure. The systolic blood pressure of the arms divided by the systolic blood pressure of the leg. The result is called the ankle-arm pressure index (API) or ankle-brachial index (ABI).

Results: If the result is 90 or above, this result often rules out peripheral artery disease (*PAD*). If the result is below 90, this is usually sufficient information to diagnose the PAD. ABI between 50 and 40–highly associated with impaired leg functions. ABI below 40–highly risk of gangrene.

Patients with ABI above 90 may further undergo *freomil test. The systolic B.P. of arm and leg* is measured following treadmil. If the ABI falls or drops, the case may be diagnosed as PAD. The lower the ABI, the greater the risk for heart attack, strike or other serious circulatory diseases.

B. **Invasive Angiography:** It is a conventional angiography in which angiogram *uses dye, that is injected* through a catheter in the groin.

C. **Magnetic Resonance Angiography:** It is the non-invasive method which gives as accurate results as invasive angiography. Gadolinium is given through an intravenous to provide more clear images. The magnetic field and radiofrequency waves are used in this method that provides images of the arteries. MRI is the test which is used frequently in the clinical practice.

D. **Computed Tomography:** In this method X-rays are used to test the flow of blood. This is more advanced method but is used only on the patients those are contraindicated to MRA, as it causes radiation exposure.

Management

Medical: The effect of medicines on the clot is negligible, that cannot unblock the arteries. Aspirin 25 mg, clopidogrel and cilastazol are some of the drugs advised to dilute the blood or make the blood less sticky.

Exercises: Regular exercises can improve the walking distance. The patients with intermittent claudication are advised to walk as much as till the pain is perceived after that tries little. Once the pain becomes severe stop walking and take rest till the pain subsides. Again repeat the same. Measure the distance at the same pace for one week. On the next week the distance can be increased. On the third week increase the distance slightly further. This exercise program will improve the distance covered in walking. Regular exercises can help to lower the blood cholesterol levels as well as improve walk and general well-being.

Buerger Exercises: There is good evidence that patients with intermittent claudication who take regular exercise can increase their walking distance (the distance that they can walk before they have to stop because of pain in the muscles. Buerger exercises are the postural exercises specifically recommended for patients with arterial insufficiency to enhance circulation in the lower extremity. These exercises are also known as Buerger-Allen exercises as described by them. The exercise is started in the supine position with the legs raised to 45 degrees. Patient maintains the raised legs for three and performs ankle pump exercises for at least one minute or until blanching occurs. Once blanching occurs the leg is lowered on the treatment table at the level of the heart and again patient performs ankle pump exercises for at least one minute, and then once the feet become warm (redness appears) the leg is hanged with the knee flexion for three minutes with one minute of anklc pump exercises. If the exercise is performed for both the legs the patient has to sit and hang the legs for three minutes and do the ankle pump exercises for one minute. The patient then returns to the supine position with the lower extremities "flat" for another 3 minutes and performs an active muscle contraction for 1 minute in this position.

Cholesterol: The increased level of cholesterol low density lipoprotein (LDL) should be the patient's first priority to reduce it. The patient should cut down the fat in diet. The drugs which reduces cholesterol level in the blood should be advised.

Smoking: There are lot of evidence that tobacco is the basic cause of the trouble, moreover smoking clamps down the small collateral blood vessels and reduces the blood supply and oxygen to the tissues. The patient must make efforts to give up smoking.

Surgery

Angioplasty: Sometimes short blockages can be stretched open with a balloon in the radiology department under local anaesthesia.

Bypass Graft: In advanced stages where patients develop critical limb ischemia, the bypass graft is the choice of surgery to restore blood flow to the leg and of course to avoid amputation. The larger blockages are bypassed using a vein from the leg under general anaesthesia.

Neurogenic Claudication

It is the neurological entity which is caused by spinal stenosis or inflammation of the nerves. As with intermittent vascular claudication, the neurogenic claudication is also intermittent but in severe nerve root cases, the neurogenic claudication is not intermittent but painfully persistent.

Clinical Features

Pain is felt in the unilateral or bilateral calf muscles, buttock and thigh. The pain may be associated with weakness of the thigh and calf muscles. The pain is aggravated or precipitated by walking and prolonged standing and is not relieved by resting. After few yards of walk pain starts in the back and lower extremity. To relieve the pain patient bends forward and then walks another few yards. The forward flexion opens the intervertebral foramena and reduces the pressure on the nerve roots. This is the reason that the patients with neurogenic claudication have less disability in climbing steps, pushing carts and cycling.

Spinal Stenosis

Spinal canal stenosis is the narrowing of the spinal canal with subsequent neural compression and is frequently associated with symptoms of neurogenic claudication, such as pain paraesthesia, numbness in the leg and thighs.

Pathology: Lumbar spinal stenosis usually occurs in middle aged and elderly people. It generally takes long time for the stenosis to develop and the symptoms of neurogenic claudication to appear. The symptoms of neurogenic claudication are unusual before the sixth decade of life.

The first factor which contributes to the spinal stenosis is narrowed spinal (vertebral) canal. However, alone (small spinal canal) rarely produces the symptoms of neurogenic claudication. The degenerative changes form osteophytes, which causes thickening of the ligamentum flavum. As the age progresses, usually after sixth decade of life, the thickened (hypertrophied) ligamentum flavum may bulge into the spinal canal, degenerated osteophytes also extend into the spinal canal and contribute to the significant narrowing of canal which eventually produces pressure on the spinal cord or cauda equina; resulting manifestations of neurogenic claudication.

Vertebral displacement with an intact neural arch will critically narrow an already small canal. Spondylolisthesis due to degeneration effectively reduces the canal size at the level of displacement. It is more common in women. Whereas, bilateral neurogenic claudication is more common in men, and approximately 50% bilateral neurogenic claudication in men is caused by degenerative spondylolisthesis.

Patients with neurogenic claudication do not have symptoms of claudication at rest as oxygen supply remains adequate, but symptoms aggravate during exercises or walking due to an inadequate oxygenation or accumulation of metabolites in the cauda eqiuna.

Many patients may have radiological evidence of spinal canal stenosis but remain asymptomatic or do not have neurogenic claudication symptoms, hence, it is not necessary for the spinal stenosis to have symptoms of neurogenic claudication, such as a large central disc protrusion can block the canal without claudication, and single level stenosis from degenerative changes at L_3-L_4, L_4-L_5 may occlude the dural sac and yet produce only back pain.

Assessment of Neurogenic Claudication and Spinal Stenosis: Not all patients with lumbar spinal stenosis have symptoms of neurogenic claudication, but usually after six decades of life, presence of leg pain in walking, classically relieves by flexion of the spine and not simply relieved by rest, are the common clinical finding of the spinal stenosis with neurogenic claudication. The studies have shown that no firm conclusion on the diagnostic performance of clinical or radiological tests can be drawn; hence expensive imaging may therefore, be unnecessary except where surgical intervention is advised. There are some physical tests useful in making the diagnosis of neurogenic claudication following lumbar spinal canal stenosis. There are the simple clinical tests of exercise tolerance either using a static bicycle or a walking test.

A. Static Bicycle Test: The patient is asked to lumbar extension (erect sitting, no forward flexion). After 2-3 minutes if he finds difficulty in further cycling, he or she is asked to flex the lumbar spine and do cycling. If the symptoms or leg pain relieves in forward flexion the test may be considered positive for neurogenic claudication with stenosis.

B. Walk Test: The patient is asked to walk with lumbar extension as much as possible. He or she is asked to flex the lumbar spine, if there is any leg pain or difficulty in erect walking. The test may be positive for intermittent claudication if the patient complains of leg pain in erect walking but feels comfortable in forward flexed walking. In the next step the patient is asked to walk on the ramp (hill) up and then down. Complaint of leg pain on walking down on the hill or ramp is the indication of intermittent claudication.

Management of Neurogenic Claudication

It is universally recommended that conservative treatments are used as the first line of treatment for patients with neurogenic claudication. A fair trial of conservative treatment relieves the pain symptomatically and increases range of motion and strength of muscles. The patient is educated about the progression of the diseases and measures to control the progression. The physiotherapist should emphasize on flexion based exercises, core stability strengthening exercises and general fitness exercises. To relieve pain superficial heat therapy, deep heating modalities such as short wave diathermy and interferential therapy are usually recommended. Surgical intervention may not always be the choice of treatment, except in cases presenting with severe and persistent pain and disability or where there are sign of progressive neurological deficit or cauda equina compression.

CHAPTER-28

Sacroiliac Joint Pain

A sacroiliac synovial joint comprised sacrum and ilium is a plain joint which absorbs the weight of the trunk and transfers it to the ilium and lower extremities. The joint is surrounded by number of muscles and ligaments which contribute to the stability and play an important role in shock absorption. The joint has physiologically normal ridges and depressions, which can be seen easily on X-rays. Tension in the ligaments can be increased by strong contraction of the muscles as there are fibrous connections between the ligament and muscles. For an example; there is a fibrous connection at ischial tuberosity between sacrotuberous ligament and biceps femoris muscles. Tension in the sacrotuberous ligament can be increased by contraction in biceps femoris or vice versa. The sacrotuberous ligament also has attachments to the multifidus muscle. The tension in the sacrotuberous ligament is also increased as a result of contraction (tension) in multifidus muscles. This potentially increases the ligamentous stabilizing mechanism of the sacroiliac joint.

Mobility: Many authors have different opinions on the mobility of the SI joint whether motion can occur at SI joint or not. The studies have proven that a small amount of motion range from 2 degrees to 4 degrees is possible in three planes, sagittal, frontal and transverse. The normal sacroiliac joint cartilage has intra-articular ridges and depressions; which show friction coefficient (particularly by the complimentary ridges and depressions) motion takes place within the ridges and depressions.

Under abnormal stresses the sacroiliac joint is forced into a new position, ridges and depressions are no longer complimentary. This new position can block the motion at sacroiliac joint. This blocking results to asymmetrical opposition of the SI joint surfaces and can cause unilateral SI joint hypermobility or hypomobility.

Nutation: It is also known as sacral flexion. The base of sacrum moves anteriorly and inferiorly while the apex of sacrum moves posteriorly and superiorly. The attachment of the superficial erector spinae to the sacrum provides a potential force for sacral nutation. The superficial erector spinae plays a major role in force closure of the sacroiliac joint. The rectus abdominis and biceps femoris muscles rotate the innominate or ilium posteriorly on the sacrum and produces nutation at the sacroiliac joint. The nutation provides stability to the sacroiliac joint.

Counter Nutation: Counter nutation is also known as sacral extension. The base of the sacrum moves posteriorly and inferiorly while apex moves anteriorly and superiorly. Pubococcygeus and levator ani originating from the pubic rami and inserting into the coccyx rotate the sacral base posteriorly (counter nutation). Iliacus, rectus femoris and tensor fascia lata/iliotibial band complex rotate the ilia forward or anteriorly relative to the base of the sacrum (counter nutation). The counter nutation decreases the stability of the sacroiliac joint (Figs. 28.1 and 28.2).

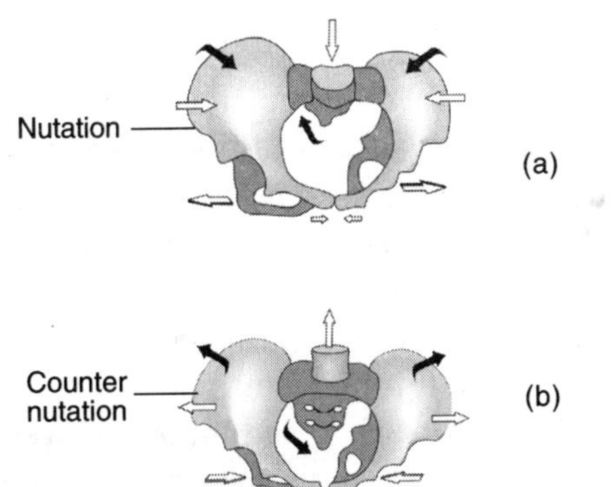

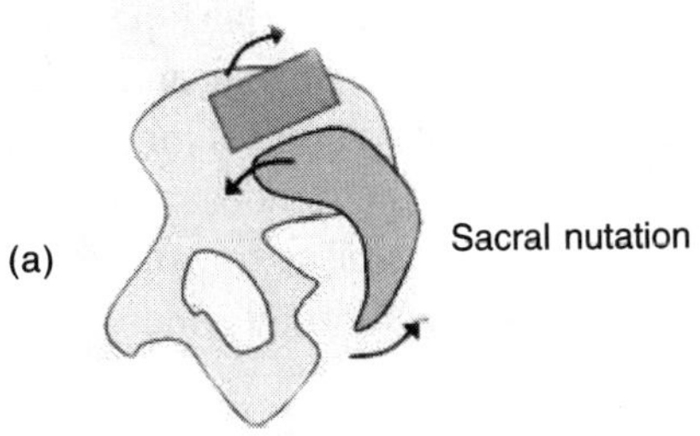

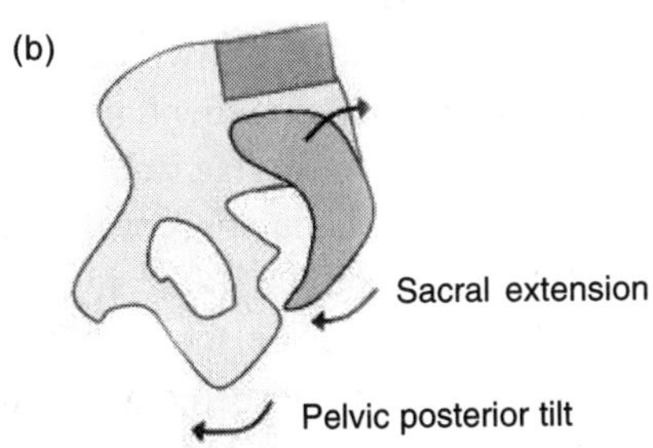

Figs. 28.1a-b: Nutation and counter nutation at sacroiliac joint, anterior view

Figs. 28.2a-b: Nutation and counter nutation at sacroiliac joint, lateral view

In standing, forward flexion of lumbosacral spine causes forward rotation of the ilia and base of the sacrum (nutation). After 50-60 degrees, the ilia continues to rotate anteriorly while the base of sacrum rotates posteriorly and the apex of sacrum rotates anteriorly (counter nutation). In sitting forward flexion of the lumbar spine rotates the pelvis or ilia anteriorly with respect to the base of sacrum (counter nutation). Further,

trunk flexion causes tension in the long dorsal sacroiliac ligament resulting in posterior rotation of the ilia with respect to sacrum (nutation). Hence, in sitting trunk flexion causes counter nutation initially, but it is replaced with the nutation due to tension in the ligaments.

In standing, initially, trunk extension rotates the ilia posteriorly with respect to the base of sacrum. This increases lumbar lordosis and the lumbosacral angle. In sitting, trunk extension does not rotate the ilia initially but further extension will result in anterior rotation of the ilia as tension in the sacrospinous and sacrotuberous increases.

Stability: The sacroiliac joint is stabilized by the static and dynamic structures, termed as form closure and force closure respectively. These structures help in preventing friction in the sacroiliac joint by increasing the joint friction coefficient and joint compression.

Form Closure: The shape, structure or form of the joint provides the stability.

(i) The specific anatomical structures such as interlocking ridges, grooves and roughening of the joint surfaces helps in increasing the friction.

(ii) The triangular shape of the sacrum fits between the ilia, helps in increasing compression and minimizing shear on the SI joint as its lateral arches are firmly connected to ilia, sacrotuberous and sacrospinalis ligaments, the coccygeus and piriformis muscles.

Force Closure: The force closure is a mechanism in which the stability of the sacroiliac joint is provided mainly by the dynamic stabilizers by the force generated within and outside the SI joint. The muscles such as multifidi, sacrospinalis (extensor spinae) produce anterior rotation of the base of sacrum (nutation), and the contraction of rectus abdominis and hamstrings produce posterior rotation of the pelvis (nutation) with respect to the base of sacrum. The contraction of the aforesaid muscles produce nutation which contribute to the force closure mechanism, thereby increasing the compression on the sacroiliac joint surfaces, which in turn increases the stability of the joint for load transfer. The inner unit consists of multifidi, thoracic diaphragm, transverse abdominis, and pelvic floor muscles. These specific muscles are coupled with pelvic floor muscles. The simultaneous contraction of these two groups of muscles (force couple) affects the stability of the sacroiliac joint and lumbosacral junction, and may also move the sacrum into stable or unstable position. For an example, the contraction of multifidus muscle causes nutation, whereas, contraction of iliacs and ischiococcygeus causes counter nutation.

The oblique muscles have connections with hip joint muscles via their corresponding fascia, which helps in stabilizing the SI joint. The posterior oblique muscle, latissimus dorsi connects the contralateral gluteus maximus through thoracolumbar fascia. The contraction of these two muscles produces compression on the sacroiliac joint through the thoracolumbar fascia. The internal abdominal and external abdominal oblique also known as anterior oblique, connects the contralateral adductors of the hip joint through anterior abdominal fascia. The contraction of these muscles help in the stabilizing the SI joint.

The gluteus medius and minimus and the contralateral adductors play important role in stabilizing the pelvis on the femur while standing and walking. Weakness of these muscle contribute to the instability of the pelvis and sacroiliac joints.

The erector spinae muscles is connected to the sacrotuberous ligament and biceps femoris through the deep lamina of the thoracodorsal fascia. Contraction of these muscles increases tension in the sacrotuberous ligament, which in turn compresses the sacroiliac joint and increases its stability.

PELVIC MALALIGNMENT

The stability of sacroiliac joint and positions of pelvis is greatly affected by the spine and extremities alignments. The pelvis may show rotational malalignment along with upslip. The rotational malalignment and upslip may also occur in isolation 80% and 10% respectively. The rotational malalignment may also occur in association with outflare and inflare, however, outflare and inflare may also occur in isolation.

Rotational Malalignment

The pelvis rotates anteriorly and posteriorly in sagittal plane during normal walk and activities of daily living. Excessive rotation of innominate may affect the kinetics of the lumbosacral spine. The most common presentation of rotational malalignment is that of right anterior and left posterior innominate rotation with locking of the right sacroiliac joint. The opposite sacroiliac joint (left) may show compensatory hypermobility. The studies have shown that there are two major causes of the pelvic rotation malalignment, the repeated or direct trauma and muscular imbalance. As discussed earlier, there is nutation of the sacrum during forward bending upto 50-60° in standing. Beyond 50-60° forward flexion, the base of sacrum rotates posteriorly and inferiorly (counter nutation of the sacrum), this contributes to the instability of the sacroiliac joints as relaxing of the posterior pelvic ligaments. The caudal glide of the SI joint is impaired and the joint becomes vulnerable to dysfunction. If forward bending is combined with the side bending and axial rotation, anterior rotation of the SI joint of the contralateral side is restricted due to increased tension in the sacrotuberous ligament because of strong contraction of the biceps femoris and piriformis (attached to the sacrotuberous ligament). Whereas, the anterior rotation of the SI joint, on the ipsilateral side is increased; which leads to asymmetrical loading of the spine and pelvis. There is acute pain often felt on trying to get back to the standing. This dysfunction can be prevented to some extent if the spine bends forward prior to the pelvic anterior rotation and innominate rotates posteriorly before the spine extension. This is also known as lumbopelvic rhythm (Fig. 28.3).

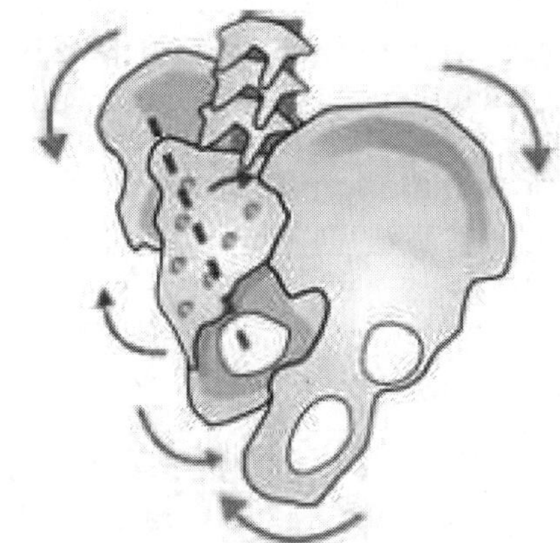

Fig. 28.3: Rotational malalignment a. Anterior, b. Posterior

The rotational malalignment either anterior or posterior also depends upon position of the innominate at the time of trauma. For example a posterior directed force at the anterior or superior aspect of the pubic bone and an anterior directed force of the level of posterior iliac crest can cause anterior malalignment of the pelvis. Similarly a posterior directed force at the anterior iliac crest and anterior directed force at the ischial tuberosity can cause posterior malalignment of the pelvis.

The forces transmitted by the extremities through the hip joints to the sacroiliac joint may also cause significant rotational malalignment of the pelvis. In this regard the position of the leg is very important at the time of trauma is to understand the exact mechanism. For an example, if the hip joint is flexed and force is transmitted from the leg to the pelvis through the hip joint, it may place significant anterior rotation of the pelvis on sacrum. These forces from the leg usually come when an athlete or individual falls on knee joint, casual jump on one leg, misses a step when going downstairs etc.

In addition to the position of extremities, the lumbar spine also contribute to the malalignment of pelvis. For example, rotation of the L_5 vertebra either left or right will put the tension on the ligaments and cause posterior rotation of the pelvis. For an instance, right rotation of the L_5 vertebra on sacrum, will rotate the right transverse process posteriorly and left transverse process anteriorly. The rotation of transverse processes put the tension on iliolumbar ligaments. Therefore the right tensed iliolumbar ligament will pull the right pelvis posteriorly, and left iliolumbar ligament pulls the left pelvis anteriorly.

Muscular Imbalance: The muscles such as gluteus maximus, medius, abdominals, psoas major and hamstrings play important role in nutation by rotating the pelvis posteriorly with respect to the sacrum. It also helps in achieving the closed packed position of sacroiliac joint. In closed packed position a joint has maximal resistance to distraction and translation or shear and demonstrates greater load bearing stability. Weakness of these muscles allows the pelvis to rotate anteriorly with respect to the sacrum and produces counter nutation. It has already been mentioned that counter nutation decreases the stability of the sacroiliac joint. This is because in counter nutation the joint goes into the loose packed position. This is a position (loose packed) of minimal congruency between the articular surfaces with greatest potential for separation of joint surfaces. The loose packed position of the sacroiliac joint is provided by the contraction of iliocostalis, tensor fascia lata and rectus femoris muscles.

Upslip and Downslip: In normal gait, the sacroiliac joint may permit pelvis to translate upward and downward approximately two degrees. Upslip and downslip are the abnormal positions of innominate in which one side of the innominate will exert excessive translation (more than two degrees) and stuck either in upward or downward direction respectively in relation to the sacrum. Upslip is more commoner than the downslip which may be 10-20% in isolation, and 5-10% in association with rotational malalignment. The upslip most commonly occurs when the traumatic force is transmitted from the extended leg through the neutral hip joint to sacroiliac joint. This mechanism produces upslip instead of rotational malalignment as the hip and knee joints remain neutral. Situation may be like falling on the foot with hip and knee neutral. Sometimes if patient falls or lands directly on the ischial tuberosity on one side, that may also cause upslip. In compare to upslip, downslip occurs rarely. The pelvis may translate excessively downward and stuck, if there is a traction force on the leg. The typical mechanism may be like one foot has sunk into a hole and the individual tries hard to extract it. This may cause excessive downward translation (downslip) of the innominate in relation to the sacrum.

Outflare and Inflare: The pelvic outflare and inflare occurs in the transverse plane around a vertical axis. The outflare and inflare of the innominate refers to the outward and inward movements respectively. Normally these movements occur in combined with rotation of the pelvis. The outward or outflare occurs with the anterior and posterior rotations of the pelvis. Inward movement or inflare also occurs with anterior and posterior rotations. For an instance, during anterior rotation of the innominate, the innominate flares out as it is allowed by the anterior widening of the sacrum. Interestingly, even in posterior rotation of the pelvis, there may be outflare of the innominate because the posterior narrowing of the sacrum glides innominate medially.

In patients with sacroiliac joint dysfunction, outflare and inflare may exist in isolation or in combination with anterior and posterior rotations. If there is an excessive outward movement of the pelvis in a transverse plane, it may stuck in an outflare position. In combined with rotation malalignment, outflare occurs with anterior rotation of the innominate and the compensatory inflare occurs with the opposite posterior rotation of the pelvis.

Sacral Torsion: It is the normal movement of the sacrum as the part of daily activities. It occurs with the movements of trunk, pelvic bones, lower extremities and by the contraction of piriformis and iliacus muscles. Excessive sacral torsion can also cause sacroiliac joint dysfunction or malalignment.

Sacral Torsion Combined with Lumbar Vertebra: The right side of the L_5 vertebra on the sacrum will rotate the right transverse process of the L_5 vertebra posteriorly and left transverse process of the L_5 anteriorly. This rotation of the transverse processes of L_5 vertebra will increase the tension on the iliolumbar ligament by virtue of their attachments to the transverse processes and ilium, which in turn bring the surfaces of L_5-S_1 facet joints increasingly closer together. If there is further rotation of the L_5 over the sacrum the L_5-S_1 facet joints compressed maximally and starts acting as a fulcrum, so that any further rotation of L_5 will now cause torsion of the sacrum around the right oblique axis. The piriformis muscle which has its diagonal orientation, inserts on the anterior aspect of the base of sacrum. This muscle rotates the sacral base posteriorly with relation to the innominate. The strong contraction or shortening of the piriformis muscle can cause torsion of the sacrum and loss of mobility between the ilium and sacrum.

Subjective Examination of Lumbosacral Spine: The important part of the assessment is the understanding of complaint of the patient as much as possible. The patient will reveal the mechanism of injury, whether the pain and symptoms started with trauma or accident. In case of trauma, was the force transmitted through extremities to trunk? If force transmitted through extremities, then what was the position of extremity? Flexed or extended? This will help in establishing the diagnosis of malalignment of sacroiliac joint.

The second part of the assessment is the careful observation of the pelvis and lumbosacral spine. This includes observation of the height of iliac crests, pubic bones, Anterior Superior Iliac Crests (ASIS), Posterior Superior Iliac Crests (PSIS), dimples of venus on the buttocks (about 1 cm above the PSIS), ischial tuberosities, inferior lateral angle of the sacrum and sacral sulci (Fig. 28.4).

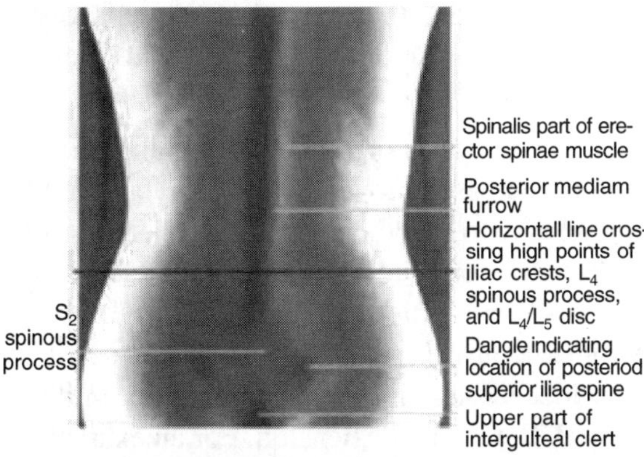

Fig. 28.4: Bony landmarks observed in sitting and lying

Pelvic Obliquity: The level of the iliac crests is observed in standing, sitting and lying. In case of leg length discrepancy, the lengthened (leg) side iliac crest will be raised in standing, but both the iliac crests will be leveled in the sitting. On the other hand, in case of malalignment the iliac crest will be raised in both standing and sitting. In more evident malalignment cases, the opposite iliac crest to that noted in standing, is raised in sitting position.

Range of Motion: The active range of motion of the lumbosacral spine is observed carefully from anterior, posterior and lateral views. In normal lumbopelvic rhythm, initially motion occurs in the end then at the pelvis. In case of tightness of extensors of spine, the innominates rotate prior to the flexion of the spine, this can produce dysfunction of the sacroiliac joint.

Observation of Outflare and Inflare: In supine position, the distance of both the anterior superior iliac spines is measured from the umbilicus. In case of presence of outflare the one side of the ASIS will have more distance from the umbilicus than the opposite ASIS (Inflare). Outflare and inflare can also be observed in prone lying. In case of outflare the corresponding posterior superior iliac spine will move inwards with respect to the midline or gluteal cleft, and for inflare the PSIS moves outward from the gluteal cleft.

The examiner should develop a hypothesis regarding the contribution of faulty lumbopelvic posture to pathomechanical cause of symptoms and the relationship of other body regions in perpetuating the faulty lumbopelvic posture. For an example a lordotic posture with anterior pelvic tilting elongates external oblique.

Objective Examination

The sacroiliac joint and innominates are palpated for tenderness, any kind of crepitus and temperature. For tenderness, the examiner can place the thumb or pisiform aspect of the wrist on the corresponding area. To deliver more force the thumb and pisiform can be reinforced with other hand thumb and pisiform respectively.

The passive movements of lumbosacral and sacroiliac joints are performed to reproduce the symptoms. In order to localize the symptoms, the examiner should test the sacroiliac joints, hip joints, lumbar spine and also supporting soft tissue structures, however, emphasis is given on sacroiliac joints and its supporting soft tissues. The tests which can compress the sacroiliac joints, are more likely to reproduce the symptoms from sacroiliac joint, and tests which distract the sacroiliac joint are more likely to reproduce the symptoms from ligaments and capsule.

Flexion and Extension Tests: The tests are designed to evaluate the movement of pelvic girdle and lumbosacral junction in standing and sitting. The therapist stands behind the patient and places tip of both thumbs on each dimples of venus (inferior aspect of the posterior superior iliac spine). In normal cases the thumbs move up in lumbosacral flexion and down in extension by an equal amount. In standing, when the lumbosacral spine is flexed, the one side of PSIS will be raised than the other. In case of upslip, the right and left PSIS still will move in unison and to an equal extent (Figs. 28.5a-b).

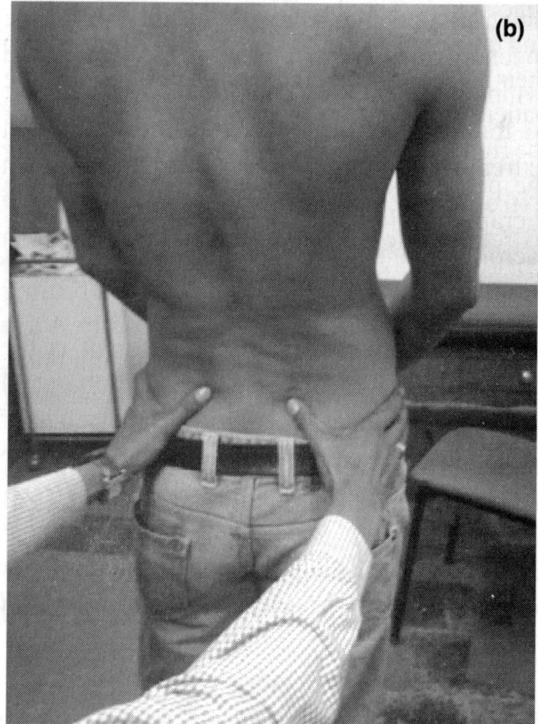

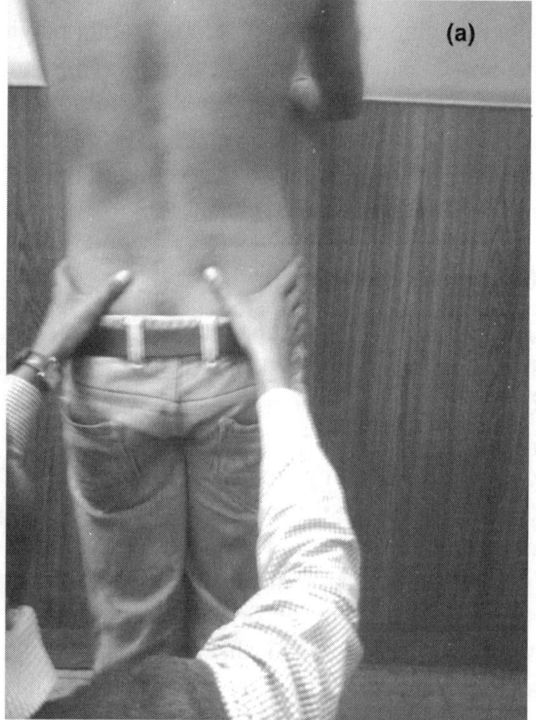

Figs. 28.5a-b: Flexion and extension test

In the presence of rotational malalignment, there is decreased movement possibly at one SI joint relative to the other or even complete loss of movement referred to as locking of the sacroiliac joint. No movement takes place at locked sacroiliac joint, instead of that ilium and the sacrum of the locked sacroiliac joint moves as one unit as on trunk flexion and extension. For an example, if right sacroiliac joint is locked, the right sacrum and ilium will move as a one unit, higher than the left on trunk flexion and lower on trunk extension. It may be concluded that the PSIS of locked or hypomobile sacroiliac joint will show more movement than the normal sacroiliac joint.

Walk Test: This test evaluates the mobility of the sacroiliac joint in non weight bearing position. The patient stands with both hands on a wall or chair to balance himself or herself. The therapist crouch down so that the eyes are at level with the sacrum and the posterior superior iliac spines. The therapist tucks each thumb up and under the PSIS on either side to firmly locate their position. To test the right sacroiliac joint, the patient is asked to stand on the left leg and flex the right hip joint upto 90 degrees, without tilting the pelvis, as if taking a marching step. The therapist notices the movements on both the sacroiliac joints. If normal, the physiotherapist would expect an PSIS on the non weight bearing right leg to rotate posteriorly and inferiorly. A test may be positive if the right posterior superior iliac spine fails to rotate posteriorly relative to the sacral base. If the hip joint (right side) is flexed further (above 90 degrees), the right PSIS moves upwards rather than downwards, this is because the locked right sacrum and right innominate (right sacroiliac joint) rotate as one unit counter clockwise in the frontal plane. If the joint is not locked completely some movements (downward rotation) can be expected, but is less on the right compared with what occurs when the test is performed on the normal left leg (Figs. 28.6 and 28.7).

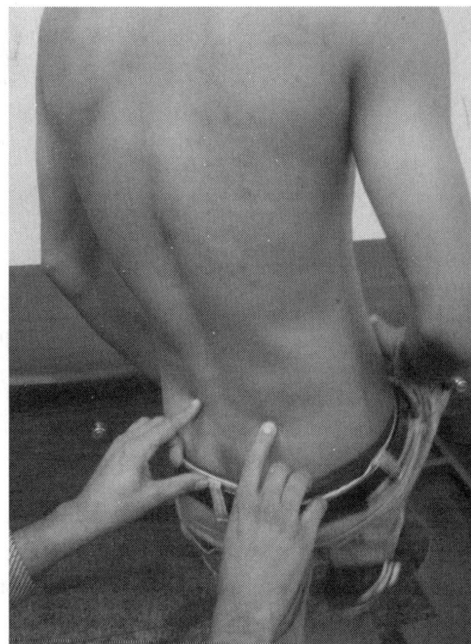

Fig. 28.7: Walk test with right hip and knee flexion, right PSIS with the finger tip moves posterior and inferior. Test is considered normal. If right PSIS moves superior and anterior instead of posterior and inferior, test is considered positive for right SI joint hypomobile

Patrick or Faber Test: This is one of the provocative tests, useful in making a diagnosis of sacroiliac joint pathology. It places greater stress on the sacroiliac as well as hip joint; hence, it should not be performed on geriatric patients where osteoporotic changes are evident. The patient lies supine on the treatment couch, and affected side foot is placed on the opposite knee joint so that the hip joint (affected side) can be brought into flexion, abduction and external rotation. The therapist stands at the affected side and places one hand on the flexed knee joint and other hand on the opposite ASIS. While maintaining the position, the therapist gently presses the knee and opposite ASIS downwards simultaneously. If low back pain or buttock pain is reproduced the cause is likely to be a disorder of sacroiliac joint (Fig. 28.8).

Winged Compression Test: The patient lies supine on the treatment couch. The therapist

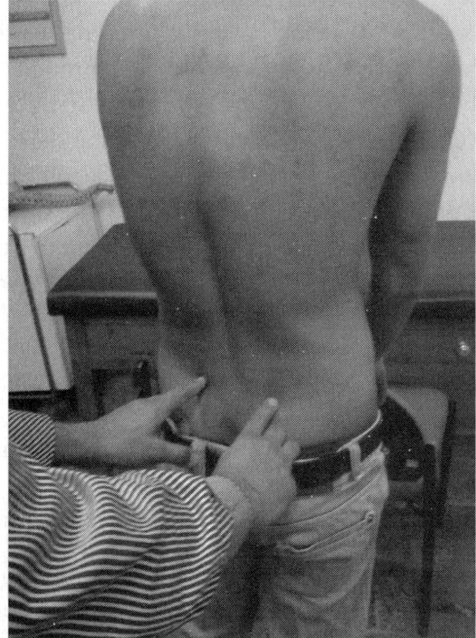

Fig. 28.6: Walk test starting, finger tips on the leveled PSIS

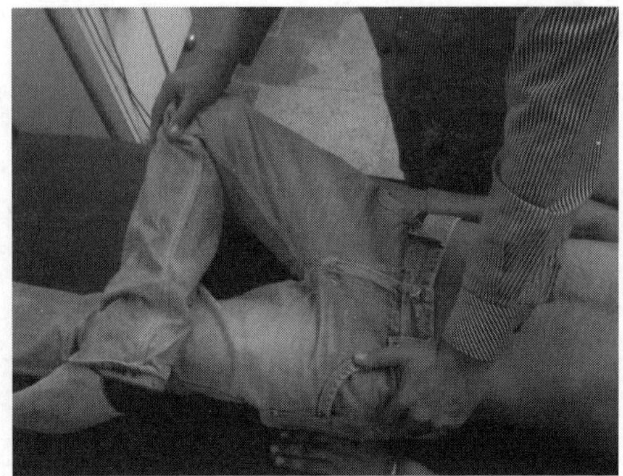

Fig. 28.8: Patrick or faber test

stands at the side and places hands on both the anterior superior iliac spine with crossed arms. The therapist separates the iliac crests with a downwards and outwards pressure. The test places compressive forces on the sacroiliac joint and provokes pain in case of sacroiliac joint pathology (Fig. 28.9).

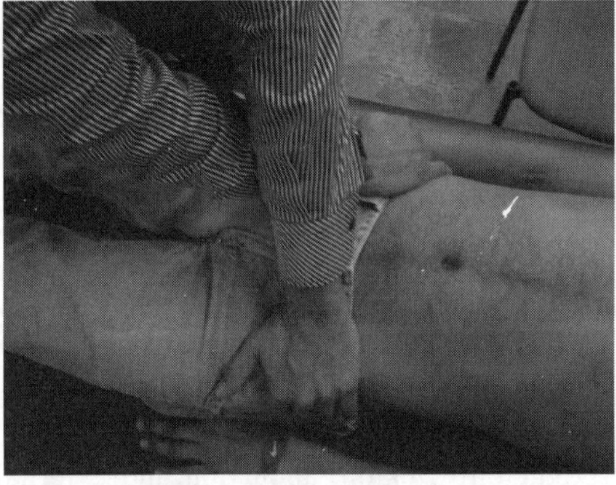

Fig. 28.9: Winged compression test

Compression and Distraction Test: The patient lies supine on the treatment couch. Therapist stands at the side and places hands on both the anterior superior iliac spine. In the first step of the test both the iliac crests are separated by pushing them downwards and outwards. In the second step of the test the iliac crests are brought towards each other by pulling them in order to relieve pressure on the sacroiliac joint.

In case of sacroiliac pathology, the compression test should provoke the symptoms while distraction test relieve the symptoms.

MANAGEMENT OF SACROILIAC JOINT

Many approaches such as mobilization, manipulation and muscle energy techniques are administered to correct the alignment of the joint. The core stability strengthening programme should also be incorporated to mobilization as muscle weakness is very common following pain and malalignment of the sacroiliac joint.

Direct Oscillation (Mobilization): The patient lies supine on the treatment couch. Therapist stands at the side of the sacroiliac joint which is being mobilized; and places the heel of the right hand on the sacrum with reinforcement by the left hand. Direct oscillation is helpful in achieving nutation and counter nutation movements of sacrum with reference to the innominate. To produce nutation, the therapist places the heel (pisiform aspect) on the base of the sacrum (over the posterior proximal part of sacrum) and exerts anterior pressure through the body momentum, there should not be any movement at the wrist, elbow and shoulders. To improve counter nutation, therapist places the heel over the apex (posterior distal part) of the sacrum and exerts anterior pressure through the body.

Direct Central Pressure with Hyperextension (Mobilization): This technique is effective in correcting the posterior rotational malalignment of the innominate. The technique combines the use of anterior directed central pressure and extension of the lumbar spine through hyperextension of the hip joint with the leg. The therapist stands at the opposite side of the sacroiliac joint which is being mobilized and places heel of one hand on the posterior superior iliac spine and holds the leg with other hand at the lower thigh. The therapist hyper extends the hip joint with the one hand by using the leg as a lever and applies downward pressure with the heel of other hand. The hyperextension of the hip joint should be upto the pain free range (Fig. 28.10).

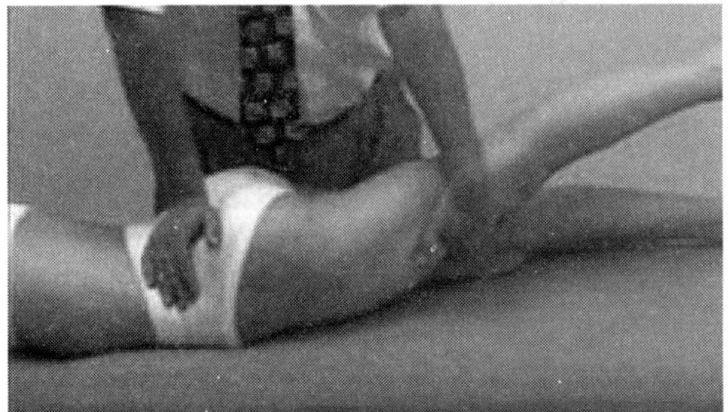

Fig. 28.10 : Direct central pressure with hyperextension

Muscle Energy Techniques: The muscle energy techniques are also effective in correcting rotational malalignment of the sacroiliac joint by using the strong isometric contraction of the muscle or group of muscles.

Correction of Right Anterior Pelvic Malrotation (MET): The right anterior rotation of the innominate can be corrected by strong contraction of the right gluteus maximus muscle. The patient lies on the left side with affected side uppermost; and flexes the right hip joint in diagonal manner as much as possible. The lower leg (left) is pulled backwards to the point where sacrum just begin to move. The therapist stands at the front side of the patient and places right hand on the lumbar spine and left hand on the distal thigh to resist the hip extension. The patient is asked to grasp the table with right hand. The therapist maintains the position of the patient's trunk with the right hand and forearm and asks the patient to move the hip joint into extension. The left hand resists the movement of hip joint (Figs. 28.11 to 28.13).

When thigh is free, the strong contraction of the gluteus maximus will extend the hip joint; but by resisting hip extension, the action can be

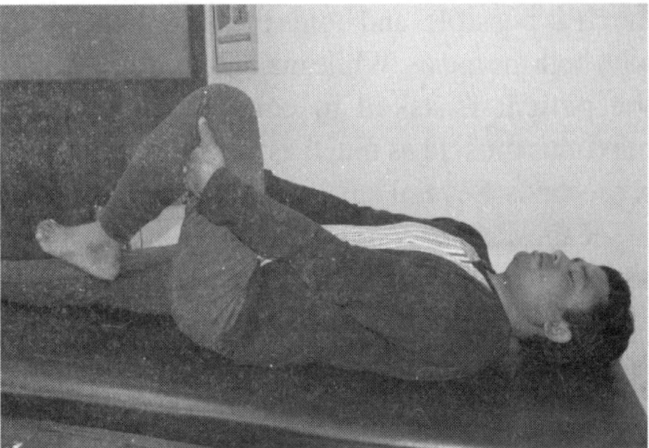

Fig. 28.11: Self-correction of left anterior malrotation by using gluteus maximus MET. The patient places the hands on the distal posterior thigh

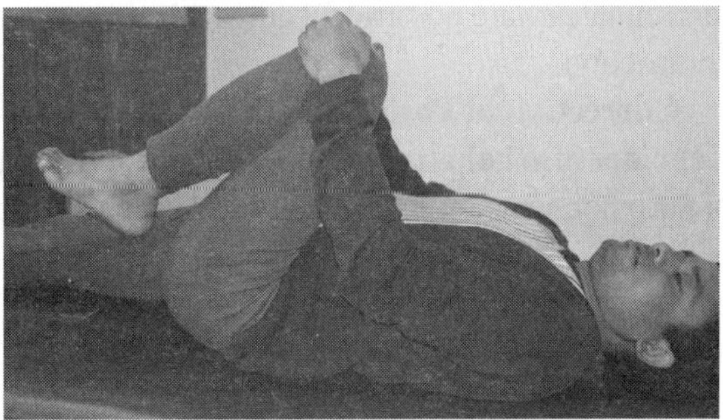

Fig. 28.12: Correction of left anterior pelvic malrotation by muscle energy technique

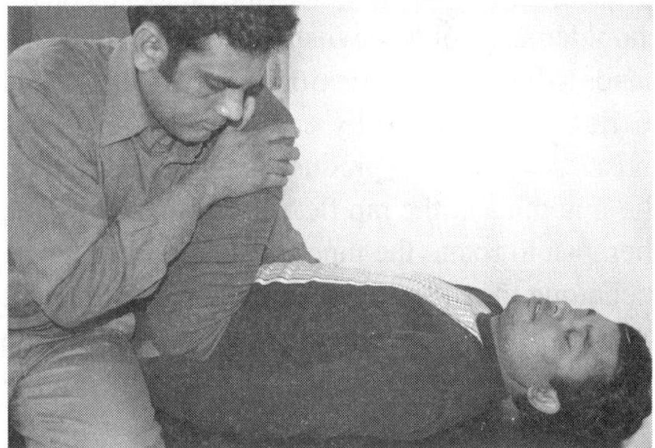

Fig. 28.13: Correction of left anterior malrolation in supine lying by gluteus maximus muscle energy technique

reversed to the origin. Now gluteus maximus will exert a posterior rotational movement on the right innominate, as it is free to move.

The technique may also be performed in supine lying. The patient flexes the hip and knee joint as much as possible, and holds the flexed knee joint with both the hands. While maintaining the position the patient is asked to contract the gluteus maximus muscle as much as possible for at least six seconds. Several repetitions may be performed to see the desired results; and hip is taken further to the chest and opposite shoulder after every repetition. In order to produce posterior rotation on the desired innominate the distal attachment (insertion) of the gluteus maximus needs to be fixed (by holding the knees with the hands) and the proximal attachment (origin) of the gluteus maximus muscle remains free to allow the innominate rotate posteriorly during the isometric contraction.

Correction of Posterior Tilt: Muscle energy technique also helps in correcting the posterior tilt of the innominate by using the isometric contraction of the iliacus and rectus femoris muscles. For iliacus contraction patient lies supine comfortably on the treatment couch. The therapist also sits on the edge of the plinth at the affected side, approximately at the knee joint. The affected side knee and hip is flexed to 90°. Therapist places the flexed leg on his shoulder and holds the distal thigh with both the hands to block the hip flexion. The patient is asked to flex the hip joint by contracting the iliacus muscles. In order to produce anterior rotation on the innominate, the hip flexion is blocked by the therapist to rotate the innominate anteriorly. The technique may also be performed by the patient himself or herself without the assistance of the therapist by pushing the knee joint with both the hands (Figs. 28.14a-d).

The rectus femoris muscle originates from the anterior inferior iliac spine (AIIS) and anterior rim of the acetabulum. The muscle inserts on the superior pole of the patella and then to the tibial tubercle through patellar tendon. Rectus femoris is a principle extensor of the knee joint. It also has a secondary action on the hip joint, i.e., flexion. To correct the posterior

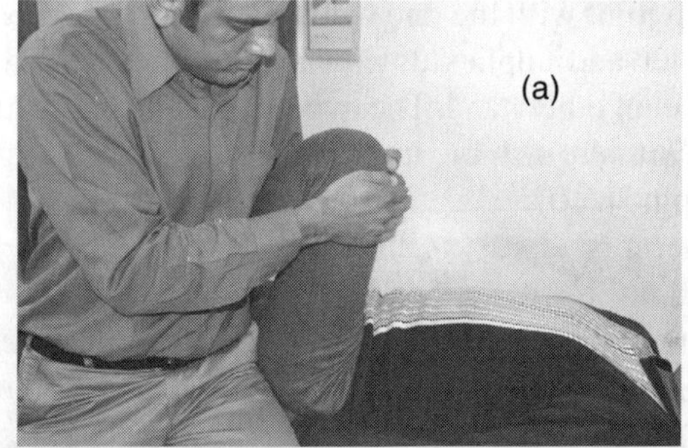

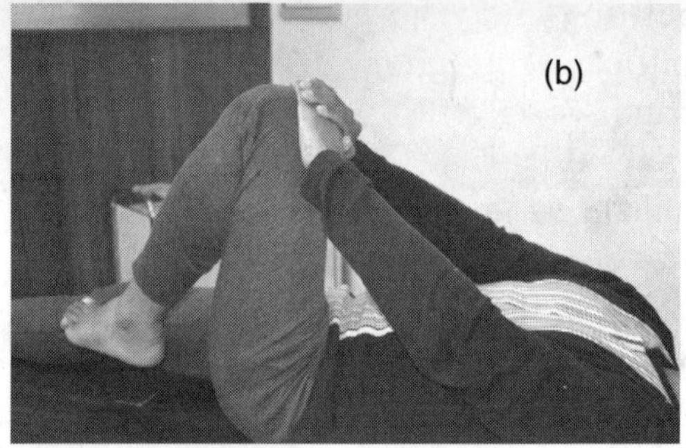

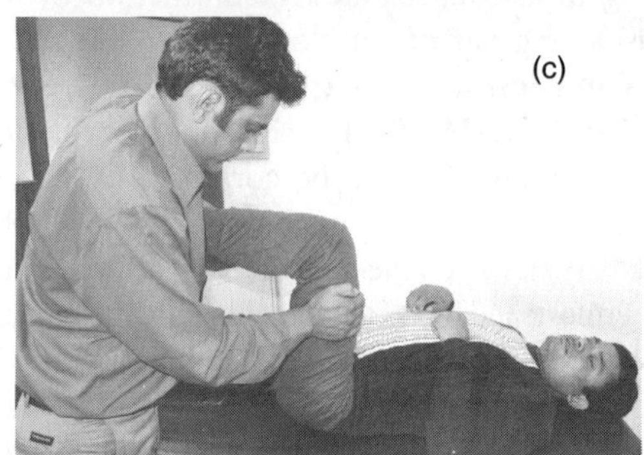

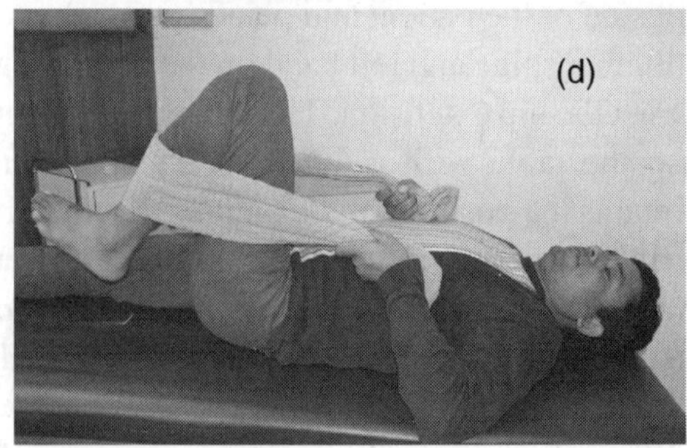

Fig. 28.14a-d: Correction of posterior malalignment by using a. iliopsoas MET, b. self-iliopsoas MET, c. rectus femoris MET, d. self rectus femoris MET

malrotation of the innominate the distal attachments of the rectus femoris is fixed and proximal attachment is left free to produce the movement on the innominate. The patient lies supine with hip $90°$ flexion and knee full flexion. Therapist stands at the opposite side of the leg and holds the flexed knee and ankle joint. The patient contracts the rectus femoris as much as possible, and the therapist resists the movement and maintains the hip and knee flexion. Several repetitions may be performed to produce significant correction of the innominate on sacrum.

Sacral Thrust (Manipulation): It is the manipulative technique with a low amplitude and high velocity thrust to the base of sacrum to correct the rotational malalignment. The patient sits comfortably on the treatment couch. For left sacroiliac joint hypomobility the patient sits comfortably on the treatment couch with the left hand on the right shoulder and trunk rotation and bending to the right side. The therapist stands behind and to the right side of the patient, and places left hand on the left base of the sacrum. The therapist grasps the patient's left arm and locks the spine into side bending and right rotation including the sacrum with the right hand. This will cause the left sacral base to move forwards which can be felt with the left hand. While maintaining the position the therapist applies a low amplitude high velocity thrust with the left hand in an anterior direction. The small arc of movement must be applied at a full stretch (Fig. 28.15).

Simultaneous Correction of Right Anterior and Left Posterior Rotation

(i) The patient lies supine with both legs out of edge of the treatment table. Patient flexes the right hip and knee as much as possible and holds at the knee joint with both the hands in order to bring it to the chest. The left leg hangs

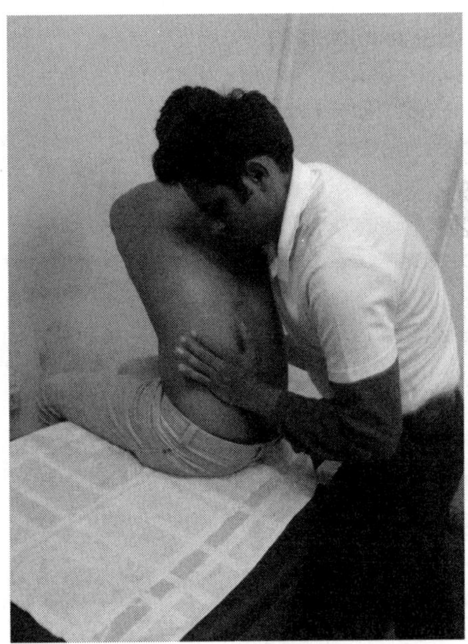

Fig. 28.15: Sacral thrust

freely into the hip extension. The right hip flexion corrects the right anterior rotation as it rotates the right innominate posteriorly on the sacrum. The left leg which hangs, freely extends the left hip and rotates the left innominate anteriorly on the sacrum, corrects the posterior rotation of the left innominate (Figs. 28.16a-b).

(ii) The patient stands and places right foot up on the stool with flexion of hip and knee joint. The left foot remains on the floor with full extension of the left hip and knee joint. The patient holds the chair with the right hand. The right hip and knee flexion with slight trunk flexion rotates the right innominate posteriorly on the sacrum and helps in correcting the right anterior malrotation. The left extended hip corrects the posterior rotation of the left innominate by rotating the left innominate anteriorly on the sacrum.

Correction of Upslip: The patient lies supine with the ankle joint slightly out of the table. He or she holds the table with both the hands. Therapist stands at the foot of the patient and grasps the

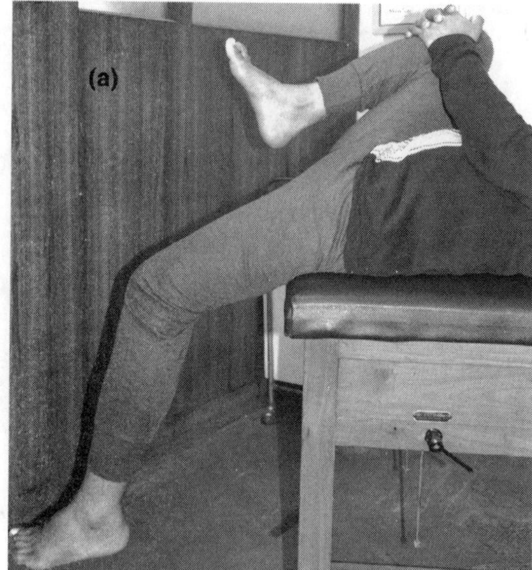

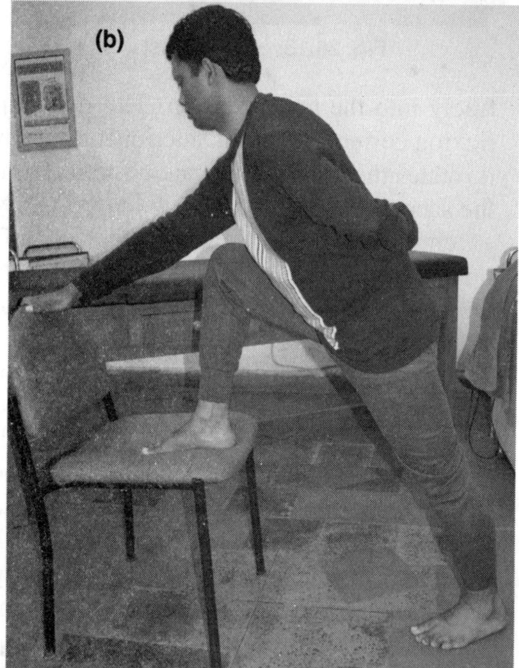

Figs. 28.16a-b: Simultaneous correction of right anterior and left posterior rotation

affected side ankle firmly with both the hands, and lifts the leg slightly off the table. The therapist keeps the patient busy with conversation and then a sharp high velocity tug is applied to the leg, in the plane of the sacroiliac joint.

Note: The therapist should ensure complete relaxation of the girdle muscles. To achieve complete relaxation the therapist can flex hip and knee three to four times before the traction.

- It should not be used in case of pain in the ankle, knee or hip joint.
- The patient should be warned that there may be increased discomfort for a few days (Fig. 28.17).

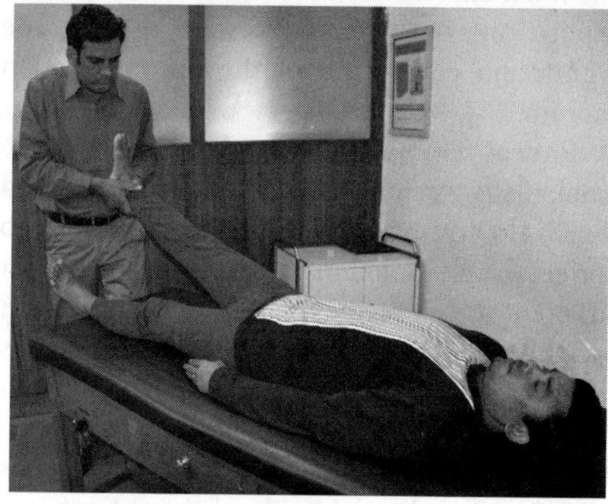

Figs. 28.17: Correction of upslip (right)

Correction of Outflare: The most common clinical presentation is existence of outflare on one side (usually with the posterior rotational malalignment) and inflare on other side (with the anterior rotational malalignment), however, outflare or inflare may exist in isolation. To correct the right outflare, the patient lies supine with both the knees and hips flexion. The right ankle is placed on the anterior aspect of the left knee joint. Now the right leg is in the position of figure of four; with abduction, external rotation and flexion of the hip joint. The therapist sits on the table at the same side, and places left hand on the lateral aspect of the right knee joint and right hand on the left knee joint. The patient pushes the therapist's left hand outwards by contracting the external rotators, abductors and extensors against the resistance applied by the therapist's left hand. Several repetitions may be performed. Each repetition should have 5-6 seconds contraction. After each contraction the therapist should flex the left leg to bring the right hip joint into more flexion, abduction and external rotation so that tension in the external rotators may be maintained (Fig. 28.18).

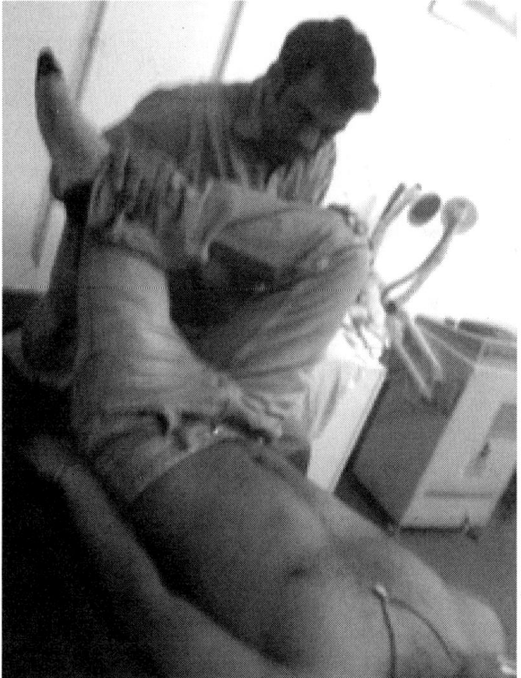

Fig. 28.18: Correction of sacroiliac outflare

Correction of Inflare: The patient lies supine with both the hips and knees flexion. To correct right inflare, the right ankle joint is placed on the anterior aspect of the left knee joint. Now the right leg will be in figure of four position with hip flexion, abduction and external rotation. The therapist stands opposite of the right side, and places right hand on the medial aspect of the right knee joint and left hand on the ankle joint. The patient contracts the flexors, and internal rotators against the resistance applied by the therapist with the right hand. The contraction is followed by further progression of hip flexion and external rotation. Several repetitions may be performed (Figs. 28.19 and 28.20).

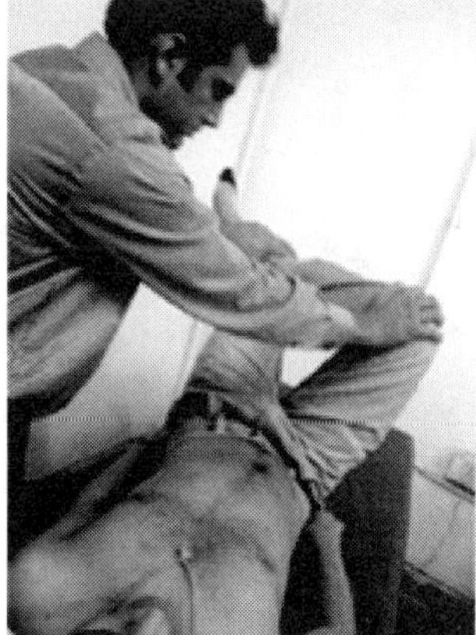

Fig. 28.19: Correction of sacroiliac inflare

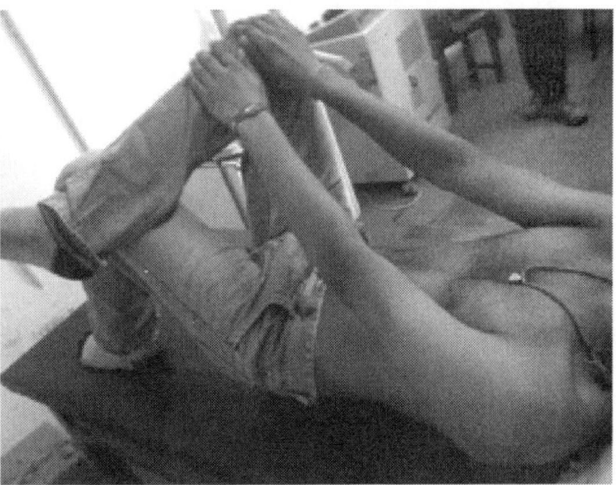

Fig. 28.20: Self-correction of sacroiliac inflare

Index

A

A beta fibres 107
A delta fibres 106
Abdominal
  bracing 500
  hollowing 500
Abnormal postures 49-51
  excessive lordosis 49, 54
    flat back 51
    flat neck 51
    forward head 51
    kyphotic lordosis 50
    scoliosis 51
    sway back 50
Accessory insertion 97
ACL 313
Acromian
  process 392
  anomaly 393
Active
  assistive
    movements 16, 19, 20
    resisting 16, 20
  free movements 16, 16-26
    classification 16
    lower extremity 24, 25
    movements 299
    resistance test 94
    resistive movements 16, 20-22
    stretching 181
  upper extremity 25, 26
Acute
  radiculopathy 434, 488
  strain 304
Adhesion-cohesion 367
Adhesive capsulitis 405, 406
ADL
  evaluation 250
  goal of training 250
  instrumental 249
  sequence of ADL training 251
  basic 249
    principle of training 251

Adson's test 436
Adventitious bursa 321
Age 293
Aggravating
  and relieving 296
  factors 299
Agonists 8, 181, 199
Alar 412
Alimentary 296
American physical therapy
  association 298
Amputation 514
Angioplasty 515
Angular motion 11
Ankle
  brachial index 514
  jerk 482
  pump exercise 335
Annulus
  fibrosus 413, 415, 464, 465
  tears 493
Antagonists 8, 199
Antalgic gait 75
Anterior
  crcuciate ligament sprain 313
  drawer test 309, 316, 372
  instability 369, 407
  laxity 369
  pelvic malrotation 527
  scalene muscle strain 306
  stabilizers 370
  superior iliac spine 53
  talofibular ligament (ATFL)
    sprain 308
  trunk bending gait 71
Anzina pectoralis 437
Apana 290
Apical 412
Apley's scratch test 408
Apophyseal glides 465
Apprehension test (crank test) 371
Area of symptoms 295, 299
Arthroplasty 361

Arthroscopic reconstruction of the
  anterior cruciate ligament 318
Arthroscopy 313, 339
Arthrotomies 313
Articular cartilage 328
Asanas 285
Ashtanga
  vinayasa yoga 288
  yoga 283, 284
Assessment 293, 472
Ataxic gait 75
ATFL 310
Atlas 412
Auto
  stretching 181
  genic training 177
Available range of motion 93
Axial fixation 157
Axis 412

B

Baker's cyst 348
Balance
  constraint in maintenance of 221
  definition 221
  dysfunction
  anatomical lesions leading to 221
  diagnostic condition
    manifested by 221
  evaluation for 222
  exercises
    dynamic 228
    for movement strategies 226
    for weakness 226
    static 226
  vestibular dysfunction 232
Ballistic stretching 183
Bankart
  arthroscopic 386

lesion 384
Base width 68
Basic fundamental positions 38-46
    knealing 41
    lying 38, 39
    sitting 40, 41
    standing 43-45
Beating 150, 151
Behavior of symptoms 295, 299
Berg balance scale 223
Bhakti yoga 284
Biceps
    femoris 518
    jerk 424
    load test for SLAP 407
    tendinitis 407
Biering–Sorenson extensor
    endurance test 494
Bija mantras 286
Biomechanics 11
Biphasic material 328
Birddog exercises 498
Bobath approach
    concepts 264
    introduction 264
    principles 266
    theories 265
Body wraps 167
Boutonniere
    or button-hole deformity 353
    splint 360
Bow legs 53
Bracing 319
Break test 93
Breathing exercises 131-134
    classification 131
    definition 131
    goals 131
    indications 131
Bridging 490
Bristow procedure 386
Brunstrom's approach
    goals 261
    guidelines for treatment 263
    introduction 259
    principles 259
    techniques 262

Buerger exercises 514
Buoyancy 164, 165, 170

C

C fibres 106
Cadence 67
Calcaneofibular 308
    ligament (CFL) 308
Cane exercises 90-92
Canes 77
    adjustable cane 78
    definition 77
    gait pattern 79
    measurement 79
    offset cane 78
    quadruped cane 78
    standard cane 77
Capsular
    fibrosis 328
    pattern 418
Capsuloligamentous restraints 367
Cardiac disease 296
Cardiopulmonary 19
Cardiovascular 136
    and respiratory 296
Carpal tunnel syndrome 355
    destruction 329
    permeability 329
Cartilage stiffness 329
Cemented 340
Cementless 340
Centre of gravity 12, 72, 157
    lateral displacement 66
    stability 12
    vertical displacement 65, 67
Cerebellar ataxia 75
Cerebrovascular accident
    (CVA) 70
Cervical
    rib syndrome 435
    spondylolitic myelopathy 456
    traction 457
Cervicogenic headache (CH) 452
CFL 310

Chick sign 455
Chief complaint 294, 299
Chin tuck 429, 442
Chronic strain 304
Circular friction massage 155
    technique, indications 155
Circumduction test 389, 487
Circumductory gait 70
Clapping 150
Clark sign 343
Cleat 159
Clinical decision making 299
Closed
    kinetic chain exercise 317, 319
    packed 308
Closing
    facet
        joint restriction 446
        restriction 446, 447, 448,
          501, 503
Cocontraction 8
Collagen fibers 106, 328, 431
Compression 308, 311
    and distraction test 526
Computed tomography 514
Condroitin sulphate 328
Congenital 511
Congruence angle 343
Constant intermittent or
    fluctuating 295
Contract relax 173, 411
Contracture 74, 180
Contrast
    bath 168
    method 176
Contusion 320
Coordination
    exercise 240
    introduction 234
    tests 238
Coracohumeral space 392
Core
    stability 494
    strengthening 496
Coronal plane 11

Costal breathing 131-133
   apical 131
   lower costal 131, 133
   posterior basal 133
   upper costal 131-133
Costo-clavicular syndrome 435
Counter nutation 518-520
Crepitus 297, 299
Critical zone 395
Cross SLR 482
Crossover sign 482
Crunch or curl up 496
Crutches 79
   axillary crutch 80
   exercises 90
   forearm crutches 80
   gait patterns 82
   measurement 81
   preparatory exercises 91, 92
Curl up 491
Curvilinear 11
Cyriax 153
Cyst formation 330

D

Dandasana 289
Dead
   bug 498
Deep
   breathing 288
   effleurage 142
Deformities of hand and fingers 352
Degenerated articular cartilage 332
Degenerative
   changes 431
   disease 328
   spondylolisthesis 510
Degenetration 401
Depth of pain 295
Derangement syndrome 430, 490
Dermatomes 423
Dharana 285
Dhyana 285
Diabetes 296

Diagnosis 293, 298
Diagnostic criteria for rheumatoid arthritis 350
Diaphragmatic breathing 133
Differential diagnosis 294
Disability
   concepts of 245
   definition 245
   models of 245
Disc
   degeneration 431, 493
   herniation 464, 487
   prolapse 494
   protrusion 485
Diseases 297
Dislocation 369, 387
   of shoulder 381
Disorder 297
Doppler arteriography 436
Double support 67
Drop arm test 398
Dural compression 486
Duration of symptoms 296, 299
Dynamic
   stabilizers 366
   stretching 182
Dysfunction 490
   syndrome 430
Dysplastic spondylolisthesis 511

E

Eccentric strengthening exercises 319
Ecchymosis 309
Eden-hybinede procedure 386
Effleurage 141-144
   deep effleurage 142
   definition, classification, superficial, longitudinal strokes, reverse longitudinal 141
   difference 144
   effects, uses, cautions, contraindications 144
Elastic range 304
Elevation 308, 311

Elongation 304
Embolisation 513
Emergency muscles 8
Empty cane 398
   test 398
End feel 101, 297, 299
   firm 102
   hard 102
   pathological 102
   soft 102
End plate 415, 465
Epilepsy 296
Erector spinae muscles 520
Ergonomics 488
Evaluation 293, 298
Examination 293
Excessive lordosis posture 49, 54
Excision arthroplasty 361
Exercise 514
   active assisted exercises 16, 19, 20
   assisted resisted exercises 16, 20
   exercises 16
   free exercises 16
   resisted exercises 16, 20-22
   balance exercises 226
   closed and open kinetic chain 272
   crutch and cane exercises 90
   definition 5
   for vestibular occular reflex 233
   Frenkel's exercises 240
   gait training exercises 86-90, 171
   group exercises 219
   heavy resistance 272
   isokinetic resistance exercise 23
   isometric resistance exercise 23
   isotonic resistance exercises 22
   mat and bed exercises for crutches 91
   multiple angle isometric exercise 23

muscle setting exercise 23
parallel bar exercises 92
plyometric exercises 272
progressive resisted exercise
    (PRE) 23, 271
stabilization exercise 23
vestibular ocular reflex
    exercise 233
wheel chair exercises 92
Williams flexion exercise 275
to improve extension lag 338
to improve flexion 339
Exercise therapy
definition 5
goals .6
Exhalation 288
Exhaling 288
Extension
bias 428
exercise 490
lag 341
External
auditory meatus 49
force 11
rotation stress test 312
Extra
articular 351
fusal fibres 172

F

Facet
down slide 451, 452
joint 464
    hypomobility 446
restrictions 501
up slide 451, 452
Facilitation techniques 256
proprioceptive 257
tactile 256
Fast breathing 288
Fatigue 305
state 376
wear 330
Femoral and tibial tunnel 318
Festination 75
Finger pad kneading 145, 146
First
class lever 14, 15
degree sprains 309

Fissuring of the annulus 431
Fixators 9
Flat
acromian 393
back posture 51
neck posture 51
Flexed knee gait 74
Flexion
and extension tests 524
bias 501
exercises 511
Flexor endurance test 495
Foot
baths 167
drop gait 73
flat 62, 64
Foraminal compression and
distraction 418
Force
closure 519
couple 393
Forced passive movements
27, 28
Form closure 519
Forward head posture 51
Freezing phase 406
Frenkel's exercise 238
Friction 152
classification 153
resistance 157
Frontal plane 11
Frozen phase 406
Function 249
Functional
reach test 224
rehabilitation in orthopaedics
    281
tests 299

G

Gait 62-76, 299
abnormal 69-76
assessment 76
canes 79
characteristics 65-69

crutches 82-84
four point gait 82
partial weight bearing
    gait 83
swing to and swing
    through 83, 84
three point gait 83
two point gait 82
cycle 62
definition 62
energetic consideration 76
length 68
muscular activity 63-65
phases 62, 63
training 86, 170, 171
with cane 87
with crutches 88-90
Gate control theory 107
General
information 293, 299
relaxation 176
well-being 296
Genitourinary 296
Giving way 294
Glenohumeral
force couple 394
suction cup 367
Glossopharyngeal breathing 134
Gluteus
maximus set 334
medius muscle strain 306
Glycosaminoglycans 106, 403
Goniometers 99
electro goniometers 100
fluid (bubble) goniometer 101
gravity dependent
    goniometers 100
inclinometer 100
pendulum goniometer 101
universal goniometer 99, 100
Goniometery 99
contraindications 102
introduction 99
precautions 102
Grading system 94-96

Ground substance 106
Group exercise 219
   disadvantage 219
   rationale 219
Group
   formation 219
   muscle action 8
Guthrie Smith 157

H

Hacking 151
Hallux valgus 355
Hammer and claw toes 355
Hamstrings
   graft 318
   strain 305
Hand to knee gait 72
Hatha yoga 283, 284
Heel
   off 63
   strike 62, 64
   to toe pattern 73
Hemiplegia 70, 170
Herniated discs 487
Herniation 416
High
   impact wear 330
   sitting/sitting on table 335
Hill sachs lesion 382
Hip hiking 70
Hold relax 173, 182, 411
Horizontal
   cleavage 332
   pelvic dip 66
   plane 11
Howkins Kennedy 397
   test 398
Hubbart tank 168
Human locomotion 62-76
Hyaluronic acid injections 339
Hybrid prosthesis 340
Hydrodynamic pressure 165
Hydrostatic pressure 164, 165

Hydrotherapy
   introduction, history, rationale
      164
   physiological effects 165, 166
   pool 168
   unit 168
   uses, risks, cautions,
      contraindications,
      techniques 166
Hyperextended knee gait 72
Hypermobility 518
Hystack arrangement 106

I

Ice 308
Ideal posture 49
Iliacus 518
Iliopsoas
   bursitis 323
   or iliopectineal bursitis 322
Iliotibial band friction syndrome
   347
Ilium 518
Impaired blood supply 402
Impingement
   sign 397
   syndrome 392, 407
   test 397
Incoordination
   occurs due to 234
   signs of 235
Inferior capsular
   shift 391
   stretching 400
Inferior instability 390
Inflammatory bowel diseases 296
Inflare 522, 531
Information 293
Infrapatellar bursitis 324
Infraspinatus muscles 374
Inhaling 288
   exhaling 288
Innominate 520, 528
Instability 294, 369
Intensity of symptoms 299

Interfacial wear 330
Intermittent claudication 512
Internal
   force 12
   torsion of tibia 333
International classification of
   functioning (ICF) 247
Interosseous membrane 312
Interposition arthroplasty 362
Intervention 293, 299
Intervertebral disc 413, 415, 465
Intra-abdominal pressure 492
Intrafusal fibres 172
Invasive angiography 514
Irritability 295, 299
Ischial tuberosity 518
Ischiogluteal bursitis 323
Isometric
   stretching 182
   tests 299
Isthmic spondylolisthesis 510

J

J sign 343
Jendrasik maneuvre 482
Jerk test 389
Joint
   contour 299
   flexibility 6, 17
   mobility 6, 17
   play tests 299
   stiffness 107

K

Karma yoga 284
Keratin sulphate 328
Kinematics 11
Kinetics 11
Klippel Feil syndrome 416
Kneading 145-147
   classification 145
Kneeling 41
   half kneeling 42
   kneel sitting 41

538 Exercise Therapy

prone kneeling 42
  side sitting 41
Knuckle kneading 145, 146
Kumbhaka 288
Kyphotic lordosis posture 50

L

Lachman test 316
Lasegue's test 481, 487
Lateral
  endurance test 495
  pelvic shift 66
  shift 488
  thinking 299
  trunk bending gait 69
Laxity 369
Laya yoga 284
Levator ani 518
Levers 13, 15
  classification 13
  effort arm 13-15
  elements, fulcrum 13-15
  first class 14, 15
  mechanical advantage 15
  resistance arm 13-15
  second class 14
  third class 14, 15
Lift off 410
Ligamentous sprain 307
Ligaments 467
Ligamentum flavum 468
Linear motion 11
Load and shift test 373
Local relaxation 173-175
Locomotors 296
Longitudinal
  plane 11
  tear 332
Loose
  bodies 331
  packed 308
Lordotic gait 74
Loss of
  function 294
  joint space 331
Lower crossed syndrome 483

Lumbar
  facet syndrome 501
  spine 54
Lumbo-pelvic musculature strain 306
Lying 39
  across-prone lying 39
  crook half lying 39
  half lying 39
  leg lift lying 39
  prone lying 39, 138
  side lying 39, 139
  stride crook lying 39
  stride lying 39
  supine lying 39
  with pelvis raised 39
Lymphatic system 136

M

Magnetic resonance angiography 514
Magnitude 11
Maitland 438
Make test 93
Mallet finger 354
Management 293
Manipulation 106
  definition 106
Mantra yoga 284
Manual muscle strength
  testing 93
  contraindication 93
  general rules 96
  introduction 93
  precautions 93
  resistance application 97
  uses 93
Manual therapy 431, 437
  for the thoracic spine 459
Massage 135
Mat activities
  bridging 214, 216
  half kneeling 214, 218
  hook lying 214, 215
  kneeling 214, 217
  prone on

elbows 214, 215
  hands 214, 215
  quadruped 214, 216
  rolling 214
  sitting-long, -short 214, 217
Matsen's preferred method 384
McKenzie 277, 428, 488, 490, 501
Mechanical
  low back pain 463
  response 136
Mechanism of injury 294, 299
Medial arch 48, 53
Median nerve dominant test 420
Medical history 296
Medication 297
Medicinal ball 22
Meditation 177, 283
Mental attitudes 291
Mid
  stance 62, 64
  thoracic thrust manipulation 461
Middle and lower trapezius strain 306
Migraine 455
Milch's technique 384
Mild sprain 307, 308
Mobile segment 462, 464
Mobilization 105-131, 526
  contraindications 108
  definitions 105, 106
  effects 106
  grades 108, 109
  indications 106, 107
  introduction 105
  methods 108
  oscillatory 108
  principles 109
  sustained translatory 108, 109
  techniques 111
    acromioclavicular joint 111, 112
    ankle joint 128-129
    carpometacarpal joints 119
    elbow joint 116, 117
    hip joint 120-122
    intercarpal joints 119
    intermetatarsal 130

interphalangeal joints 130
intertarsal joint 129
knee joint 122-135
metacarpophalangeal joints 120
patellofemoral 125
scapula 112, 113
shoulder girdle complex 113-116
sternoclavicular joint 111
tibiofibular 123
    inferior 127
    superior 126
    wrist joint 118
Mobilizations 503
Moderate sprain 307
Modified impingement test 397
Moist heat 168
Mortise 308
Motor
    development, sequence 253
    introduction 267
    limitation of 270
    recovery, stages 261
    strategies 221
    theoretical basis 267
    therapeutic intervention 269
Movement strategies 221
Movers 8
    principal, assistant 8
Mulligan 278
Multidirectional instability 391
Multifidi 519
Multifidus 469, 518
Muscle
    atrophy 299
    cramp 320
    endurance 6, 17, 23
    energy techniques (METs) 447, 503, 504, 527
    effects 274
    principles 274
    uses 274
full range 9
inner range 9, 10
middle range 9, 10
outer range 9, 10
spasm 170
strain 304
strength 6, 17, 23
tension 6, 172
wasting 417
wasting 433
work 9, 10
Muscular
    contraction 5-7
    imbalance 521
    isometric 6
    isotonic 5
    static, concentric, eccentric 7
    system 137
Music therapy 177
Myofascial release (MFR) 280
Myositis ossification 320

N

Nature and quality of symptoms 299
Naviaser 405
Neck retraction 429
Neer 392, 393
Negative muscle work 7
Nervous system 48, 136, 298
Neural movement tests 299
Neuralgic sciatica 484
Neuritis sciatica 484
Neurogenic claudication 515, 516
Neutralizer 9
    mutual 9
New bone (osteophyte) 328
Newton's law
    first law 12
    econd law 12
    third law 12
Niyama 287
Nodding 442
Non-inflammatory 328
Nuclease pulposus 413
Nucleus pulposus 464, 465
Nutation 518, 519, 520

O

Objective 293
    assessment 297
    examination 293, 297, 523
    physical examination 462
Oblique muscles 520
Observation 297, 299
Occipital–headache 453
Occipito temporomaxillary headache 454
Occupation 294
Odontoid process (dens) 412
Olecranon bursitis 328
Onset of symptoms 294, 299
Open
    kinetic chain exercises 317
    restrictions 502
Opening 446
    and closing restrictions 503
    facet restriction 446
    restriction 447, 448, 501, 502
Orthosis 360
Osteoarthritis 328
Osteoarthrosis 328
Osteophytes 329, 331, 432
Osteotomy 339, 363
Outflare 522, 530
    and inflare 475
Overhead
    activities 402
    squat 499, 500
    test 496
Overuse 305
    syndromes of the knee (OSKs) 347
Oxford scale 169

P

Padmasana 289
Painful arc syndrome 408
Palmer kneading 145, 146
Palpation 297, 299
Panarticular arthritis 332
Pannus 349
Paralytic torticolis 458

Parascapular muscles 392
Parasthesia 486
Parkinson gait 75
Passive
   accessory 27, 28
   manipulation 27, 28
   movements 27, 37, 173
      classification, uses, goals,
         indications 27
   stretching 181
Patanjali 284, 288
Patellar
   mal tracking 342
      tests 343
   tendon
      bone autograft 318
      jerk 482
Patellofemoral
   angle 343
   joint osteoarthritis 341
Patrick or Faber test 347, 525
PCL 313
Pelvic malalignment 520
Pelvic obliquity 523
Pelvis 54
   horizontal dip 66
   lateral shift 66
   list 66
Pendular suspension 158
Pes planus 342
Pet therapy 177
Petrissage 145
   contraindication 150
   definition, classification 145
   effects, uses 149
Physical
   activity 5
   fitness 5
Picking up 147, 148
Piriformis
   muscles 519
   syndrome 507

Pivot shift test 316
Planks 497
Plastic range 304
Plus and minus grades 98
PNF 198
   basic procedures 199
   principles, patterns, diagonals
      198
   stretching 182
Poses 286
Positional factors 296
Positive muscular work 7
Posterior apprehension 389
   capsule stretching 337
   capsule stretching 400
   instability 387
   talofibular 308
   tilt 528
   trunk bending gait 71
Postural
   pain 483
   syndrome 429
Posture 47-61, 140, 299
   anterior view 52
   assessment 52-61
      adult 52-54
      infant 55-61
   centre of gravity 48
   control 48
   definition 47
   development 47, 55-61
   dynamic 48
   ideal posture 49
   lateral view 54
   posterior view 53
   primary curve 47
   secondary curve 47
   stability 48, 49
   standard posture 49
   static 48
   types 48
Potter's knee 355

Pounding 152
Prana 288
Pranava mudra 289
Pranayama 286, 288
   body gesture 289
Pranic activities 288
Pratyahara 285
Prepatellar bursitis 324
Prevention 313
PRICE 307, 320
Primary osteoarthrosis 331
Prognosis 293, 298
Progressive resistive exercise
   (PRE) 23, 269
Prolapse intervertebral (soft) disc
   413, 485
Proprioception 198, 199
Proprioceptive training 311
Proprioceptors 48
Proteoglycans 328, 431, 465
Protrusion 485
Provisional diagnosis 293, 462
Psychogenic 463
   low back pain 463
Pubococcygeus 518
Pulleys 12, 13
   anatomical 12
   movable 12, 13
   single 12, 13
Puraka 288
Pursed-lip breathing 134
Push
   off 62, 64
   ups 379
Putti platt procedure 386

Q

Quadrant test 478, 487
Quadriceps
   ('Q') angle 53
   sets 334
   strengthening 337

Quick tests 482
Quiet breathing 288

R

R.A. 297
Radial
   fissures 493
   nerve root dominant test 421
Radicular 415
   pain 463
Radiological examination 299
Raja yoga 284
Rebound phenomenon 97
Rechaka 288
Reciprocal inhibition 177
Rectus femoris 518
Recurrence rate 385
Recurrent dislocations 384
Redness, muscle atrophy, posture,
   active movements and gait 297
Reflexes 423
Reflexive response 136
Reinforced kneading 145, 147
Relaxation 17, 170, 172-177
   indications, physiological
   manifestations, techniques
   173
Relaxed passive movements
   27-37
Release test 372
Relocation test 372
Repetition maximum (RM) 271
   closed and open kinetic
      chain 273
Resistive movements 20
   isokinetic resistance
      exercise 23
   isometric resistance
      exercise 23
   isotonic resistance exercise 22
   resistance apparatus 21
   types 22

Respiratory diseases 296
Resting splints 359
Reverse curl up 492
Rheumatoid arthritis 296, 349
Ridges and depressions 518
Rolling 149
Rood's approach
   introduction 254
   levels of motor control 254
   method of treatment 254
   principle 254
   sensory input 254
Roos test 436
Ropes 159
Rotational malalignment 520, 521
Rotator cuff 374
   injuries 401
   muscles 393
   tears 401
   tendinitis 407
   shoulders 417

S

Sacral extension 518
   flexion 518
   nutation 518
   thrust 529
   torsion 522
Sacralization 512
Sacrospinalis ligaments 519
Sacrotuberous 519
   ligament 518, 520
Sacrum 518
Sagittal plane 11
Samadhi 285, 288
Samana 288
Scalenus anticus syndrome 435
Scapula
   force couple 393
   stabilizers 376
   winging 416
Scapulohumeral rhythm 368

Scoliosis 51
Screw home mechanism 333
Second
   class lever 14
   degree sprain 309
Secondary osteoarthritis 331
Self SNAGs 507
Sensation 297, 299
Sequestration 485
Serial plaster 360
Serratus anterior 393
   muscle 377
   strengthening 378
Severe sprain 307, 309
Severity or intensity of pain 295
Sex 294
Shaking 156
   indications, contraindications 156
Short step gait (Parkinson) 75
Side
   glide mobilization 449
   leg raising 335
Single support 67
Sitting 40, 41
   forward lean sitting 41
   half sitting 40
   long sitting 40
   stride sitting 41
   with legs unsupported 40
Sitz baths 167
Skin 136
Slings 159
Slump test 479
Social modality 177
Somatosensory loss
   management 234
Spasmodic torticolis 458
Spastic diplegia gait 74
Spasticity 70, 170, 173, 180
   extensor 71
Special tests 293, 299
Speed test 407
Spinal stabilization 274

concepts 275

stenosis 515

Splints 359

Spondylogenic 462

referred pain 463

Spondylolisthesis 509

Spondylolysis 508

Sprengel's scapula 371

Spurling test 418

Squatting 336

Squeeze test 312

Stability of the 519

ankle 308

shoulder 366

Stabilizers 9

Stance phase 62

foot flat 62, 64

heel strike 62, 64

mid stance 62, 64

push off 62, 64

Standard posture 49

Standing 43-45

head rest standing 45

lax stoop standing 44

lumbar rest standing 45

neck rest standing 45

one leg standing 44

reach standing 45

standing with feet apart 43

step standing 44

stoop standing 44

toe and heel standing 44

walk forward standing 44

wing standing 45

yard standing 45

Static

bicycle test 516

cycling 336

stabilizers of shoulder 366

Step length 68

Steroid medications 296

Stiffeners 294

Stimson's technique 384

Straight leg

raise test 487

raising (SLR) test 480, 481

raising 335

Strain 462

Strengthening exercises 374, 399, 442

Stretch

reflex 200

stimulus 200

Stretching 178, 427

biceps 196

common extensors 196

contraindication 180

digitorum longus and brevis 189

exercises 443, 492

extensor hallusis longus, extensor 189

flexor hallucis longus, flexor digitorum 189

gluteus maximus 184

hamstrings 186

hip adductors 184

iliacus and psoas major 184

indications 179

infraspinatus, latissimus dorsi 194

interossei 197

longus and brevis 189

lumbricals 197

neurological changes 179

parameters 180

pectoralis major 193

physiological changes 179

pirifornis 190

plantar fascia 190

purpose 178

rectus femoris 186

soleus 188

supraspinatus 193

techniques 181, 183

tendoachillis 188

TFL 187

tibialis anterior, peroneus longus 189

tibialis posterior peroneus tertius 189

trapezius, rhomboids 192

triceps 196

trunk 191

wrist and finger flexors 197

wrist flexors, extensors 196

Stride length 69

Subacromial

bursitis or sub deltoid bursitis 327

space 392

Subchondral cyst 331

Subcutaneous nodules 350

Subgluteal bursitis 322

Subluxation 369

Subscapularis

bursitis 326

tendinitis 409

Substantia geletinosa 107

Subtle strain 305

Sulcus angle 343

Sun salutation or surya namaskar 285

Superficial effleurage 141

Superior stability 367

Supinator jerk 424

Supplements 339

Suprahumeral space 394

Supraorbital headache 454

Suprapatellar bursitis 323

Supraspinatus 374

Surgical reconstruction of the ATFL 313

Surya 286

Suspension therapy 157

devices 158

lower limb 159
upper limb 162
uses, types 157
Sustained natural apophyseal
glides (SNAGs) 449, 505
splint 359
Swan-Neck deformity 353
Swastikasana 289
Sway back posture 50
Swelling 297, 299
Swing phase 63, 66
acceleration 63, 66
deceleration 63, 66
mid swing 63, 66
Syndesmosis sprains 312
Synergists 8, 9
true, helping 9
Synergy 259
lower extremity 260
upper extremity 260
Synovectomy 361
Synovitis 353
Synovium 349
System review 296, 297

T

T cells 106, 107
Tactile stimulation 201
Talar tilt test 310
Talofibular ligament 308
Tapotement 150
definition, classification 150
effects, contraindications 152
Temperature 297, 299
Tenderness 297, 299
Tendon
action 97
reflexes 486
Tensor fascia lata 518
Thawing phase 407
Theraband 22

Therapeutic
classification, clinicians
preparation 137
drapings 138-140
effects 6
effleurage 140-145
exercise 6, 489
friction 152-155
introduction, history,
development, definitions 135
massage 135-156, 173
petrissage 145-150
physiological effects 136
shaking 156
tapotement, percussion 150-152
vibration 155
Third
class lever 14, 15
degree sprain 309
Thoracic
outlet syndrome 435, 437
thrust manipulation 461
Thoracolumbar
fascia 520
fascia system 471
Thumb pad kneading 145, 146
Tibial torsion 53
Tibiofemoral joint osteoarthrosis
331
Tibiofibular ligaments 312
Tibiotalar shuck test 312
Tightness 180
Time factors 296
Toe off 63
Torticolis (wry neck) 458
Total
hip replacement 362
knee replacement (TKR) 339
Traction 426
Translation motion 11
Transverse
abdominis 471

friction massage 153
ligaments 412
plane 11
procedure 154, 155
strengthening 500
technique 153, 154
uses 155
Traumatic
bursitis 327
spondylolisthesis 510
Treatment plinth 137
Trendelenburg
gait 69
sign 69
Triceps jerk 424
Trick movements classification
97
Triphasic medium 329
Trochanteric bursitis 322
Turbulence 165
Twisting curl up 491

U

Udana 288
Ulnar drift 352
Universal goniometer 99, 100
Upper
crossed syndrome 455, 456
limb tension tests 420
thoracic thrust manipulation
461
Upslip 522, 529
and downslip 521

V

Vajrasana 291
Vascular
claudication 512
low back pain 463
Vasculitis 350
Vasculogenic 463

Vasoconstriction 310

Vasodilatation 165, 166, 310

Vastus medialis obliques
    (VMO) 345

Vaulting gait 73

Vertebrae 464

Vertebro basillary insufficiency 421

Vertical
    fixation 157
    pelvic tilt 65
    thinking 299

Vibration 155
    indications, contraindications
      156

Vicarious motions 97

Viscerogenic 462
    low back pain 463

Visual analogue scale (VAS) 295

Vyan 288

W

Waddling gait 70

Walk test 516, 524, 525

Walkers 84-86

Walking aids 77-92
    classification 77
    indications 77
    introduction 77
    mechanism of action 77

Walking on
    heels 482
    toes 482

Warm up 284

Water 431

Weakness 294

Weight bearing 319

Wide base gait 75

Wiltse classification 509

Winged compression test 525

Winging 148
    of the scapula 370

Y

Yama 284

Yargason test 407

Yoga 177, 283
    postures 285
    sutra 285

Yogasana 284, 286

Yogasutras 288